Vaccinology

Vaccinology

An Essential Guide

EDITED BY

Gregg N. Milligan, PhD

James and Vicki McCoy Professorship in Vaccinology
Professor, Departments of Pediatrics and Microbiology & Immunology
Associate Director, Sealy Center for Vaccine Development
University of Texas Medical Branch
Galveston, TX, USA

Alan D.T. Barrett, PhD

John S. Stobo Distinguished Chair
Professor, Departments of Pathology and Microbiology & Immunology
Director, Sealy Center for Vaccine Development
University of Texas Medical Branch
Galveston, TX, USA

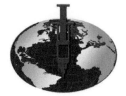

WILEY Blackwell

This edition first published 2015 © 2015 by John Wiley & Sons, Ltd.

Registered office: John Wiley & Sons, Ltd, The Atrium, Southern Gate, Chichester, West Sussex, PO19 8SQ, UK

Editorial offices: 9600 Garsington Road, Oxford, OX4 2DQ, UK
The Atrium, Southern Gate, Chichester, West Sussex, PO19 8SQ, UK
111 River Street, Hoboken, NJ 07030-5774, USA

For details of our global editorial offices, for customer services and for information about how to apply for permission to reuse the copyright material in this book please see our website at www.wiley.com/wiley-blackwell.

Library of Congress Cataloging-in-Publication Data
Vaccinology : an essential guide / edited by Gregg N. Milligan, Alan D.T. Barrett.
        p. ; cm.
   Includes bibliographical references and index.
   ISBN 978-0-470-65616-7 (pbk.)
   I. Milligan, Gregg N., editor.   II. Barrett, A. D. T. (Alan D. T.), editor.
   [DNLM: 1. Vaccines–pharmacology.   2. Vaccines–therapeutic use.   3. Drug
Discovery.   4. Vaccination.   QW 805]
   RM281
   615.3′72–dc23

                                         2014011447

A catalogue record for this book is available from the British Library.

Wiley also publishes its books in a variety of electronic formats. Some content that appears in print may not be available in electronic books.

Cover images: Vial image: courtesy of Diane F. Barrett. Syringe image: Stock Photo File #5255912. © JurgaR.
Cover design by Andy Meaden

Set in 8.75/12 pt MeridienLTStd-Roman by Toppan Best-set Premedia Limited

Printed in the UK

Contents

Contributors

A. Paige Adams, DVM, PhD
Research Assistant Professor
Kansas State University
22201 West Innovation Drive
Olathe, KA 66061, USA

Christine M. Arcari, PhD, MPH
Associate Professor
Department of Preventive Medicine & Community Health
Robert E. Shope MD Professorship in Infectious Disease Epidemiology
Director, Public Health Program
University of Texas Medical Branch
Galveston, TX, USA

Alan D.T. Barrett, PhD
John S. Stobo Distinguished Chair
Professor, Departments of Pathology and Microbiology & Immunology
Director, Sealy Center for Vaccine Development
University of Texas Medical Branch
Galveston, TX, USA

David W.C. Beasley, PhD
Associate Professor, Department of Microbiology & Immunology
Sealy Center for Vaccine Development
Galveston National Laboratory Regulatory Compliance Core
University of Texas Medical Branch
Galveston, TX, USA

Nigel Bourne, PhD
Professor, Departments of Pediatrics and Microbiology and Immunology
Senior Scientist, Sealy Center for Vaccine Development
University of Texas Medical Branch
Galveston, TX, USA

Gavin C. Bowick, PhD
Assistant Professor
Department of Microbiology and Immunology
University of Texas Medical Branch
Galveston, TX, USA

Bridget E. Hawkins, PhD
Assistant Director
Sealy Center for Vaccine Development
University of Texas Medical Branch
Galveston, TX, USA

Robert M. Jacobson, MD
Medical Director, Employee and Community Health Immunization Program
Director of Clinical Studies, Vaccine Research Group
Associate Medical Director, Population Health Science Program
Professor of Pediatrics, College of Medicine
Consultant, Community Pediatric and Adolescent Medicine
Mayo Clinic
Rochester, MN, USA

Edgar K. Marcuse, MD, MPH
Emeritus Professor, Pediatrics
Department of Pediatrics
University of Washington
Seattle Children's Hospital
Seattle, WA, USA

Jere W. McBride, MS, PhD
Professor
Department of Pathology
Sealy Center for Vaccine Development
University of Texas Medical Branch
Galveston, TX, USA

Gregg N. Milligan, PhD
James and Vicki McCoy Professorship in Vaccinology
Professor, Departments of Pediatrics and Microbiology & Immunology
Associate Director, Sealy Center for Vaccine Development
University of Texas Medical Branch
Galveston, TX, USA

Martin G. Myers, MD
Professor
Department of Pediatrics
Sealy Center for Vaccine Development
University of Texas Medical Branch
Galveston, TX, USA

Contributors

Douglas J. Opel, MD, MPH
Assistant Professor of Pediatrics
University of Washington School of Medicine
Treuman Katz Center for Pediatric Bioethics
Seattle Children's Research Institute
Seattle, WA, USA

Caroline M. Poland, NCC, LCAC, LMHC
Licensed Clinical Additions Counselor, Licensed Clinical Medical
Health Counselor
Counseling Center
Taylor University
Upland, IN, USA

Gregory A. Poland, MD
Director, Mayo Vaccine Research Group
Mary Lowell Leary Professor of Medicine, Infectious Diseases, and
Molecular Pharmacology and Experimental Therapeutics
Distinguished Investigator of the Mayo Clinic
Mayo Clinic
Rochester, MN, USA

Jai S. Rudra, PhD
Assistant Professor
Department of Pharmacology
Sealy Center for Vaccine Development
University of Texas Medical Branch
Galveston, TX, USA

Richard E. Rupp, MD
Professor
Department of Pediatrics
Director, Clinical Trials Group
Sealy Center for Vaccine Development
University of Texas Medical Branch
Galveston, TX, USA

Dirk E. Teuwen, MD
Vice-President Corporate Societal Responsibility and Senior Safety
Advisor
UCB Pharma S.A.
Brussels, Belgium;
Research Associate Scientist
Department of Microbiology and Immunology
Katholieke Universiteit Leuven
Leuven, Belgium;
Invited Professor, Department of Health Sciences
University of Aveiro
Aveiro, Portugal

Alfredo G. Torres, PhD
Professor
Department of Microbiology & Immunology
Sealy Center for Vaccine Development
University of Texas Medical Branch
Galveston, TX, USA

Dennis W. Trent, PhD
Director, Regulatory and Scientific Affairs
Office of Nonclinical Regulated Studies
University of Texas Medical Branch
Galveston, TX, USA

David H. Walker, MD
The Carmage and Martha Walls Distinguished University Chair in
Tropical Diseases
Professor and Chairman, Department of Pathology
Executive Director, Center for Biodefense and Emerging Infectious
Disease
Sealy Center for Vaccine Development
University of Texas Medical Branch
Galveston, TX, USA

Preface

I remember my grandmother pointing out a large cedar tree near an abandoned homestead that served as a marker for the graves of two young girls that had died of diphtheria sometime in the early 1900s. I've often thought of her story and how different the world was for her when childhood mortality from infectious diseases was so common. Thankfully, the development and utilization of safe and effective vaccines against a number of important pathogens has made a tremendous impact on public health. However, much remains to be done, and vaccines are unavailable against a number of important pathogens that directly or indirectly impact the health and welfare of humanity.

The purpose of this textbook is to serve as a framework for educating the next generation of vaccinologists and is primarily aimed at advanced undergraduate, graduate, veterinary, and medical students. However, anyone with an interest in or desire to become involved in the vaccine development pathway would find this book beneficial. This book comprises 20 chapters that cover all aspects of vaccinology. The book content includes a complete introduction to the history and practice of vaccinology, including basic science issues dealing with the host immune response to pathogens, vaccine delivery strategies, novel vaccine platforms, antigen selection, as well as the important facets of clinical testing and vaccine manufacture. Importantly, determinants of vaccine development including safety, regulatory, ethical, and economic issues that drive or preclude development of a candidate vaccine are also discussed. The book also describes vaccine regulation and clinical testing from a global perspective and examines vaccine development against both human and veterinary pathogens.

Each chapter contains a section of abbreviations used in the text as well as definitions of important terms. Where possible, we have included relevant figures and tables to enhance the chapter text. We have also included textboxes that provide examples or further explanation of important concepts, and a list of "key points" can be found at the end of the chapter as a summary of the important issues covered. Each chapter ends with a "Further Reading" section in which the reader is directed to related published material to provide further details. The index facilitates quick location of topics of interest.

We'd like to thank the many contributors who made this book possible. The book is based on lectures given in a vaccine development pathway course at the University of Texas Medical Branch, and many of the UTMB faculty who participate in the course graciously consented to render their lectures into text. We'd like to especially thank Dr. Martin Myers, Professor Emeritus in the Sealy Center for Vaccine Development, for providing a historical perspective on infectious diseases; Dr. Dirk Teuwen for taking time from his incredibly busy schedule to contribute to the manufacturing and safety monitoring content; and Drs. Caroline Poland, Robert M. Jacobson, Douglas J. Opel, Edgar K. Marcuse, and Gregory A. Poland for their discussion of the political, ethical, social, and psychological considerations involved in vaccine development. We are also deeply indebted to Ms. Sandra Rivas for help with figure preparation, and we express our deepest thanks to Diane Barrett for her artwork on the front cover.

While we have tried to be as inclusive as possible of the most important aspects of vaccine development, we realize that it would take a book many times this size to provide all the pertinent information necessary for this task. We hope to refine as well as update vaccine development information in future editions of this book for the next generation of vaccinologists.

G.N.M.
A.D.T.B.

1 The history of vaccine development and the diseases vaccines prevent

Martin G. Myers

Sealy Center for Vaccine Development, University of Texas Medical Branch, Galveston, TX, USA

Abbreviations

CDC	US Centers for Disease Control and Prevention	MMRV	Measles, mumps, rubella, and varicella
CMI	Cell mediated immunity	MVA	Modified Vaccinia Ankara
CRS	Congenital rubella syndrome	PCV7	Heptavalent pneumococcal conjugate vaccine
HAV	Hepatitis A virus	PHN	Postherpetic neuralgia
HBIG	Hepatitis B immunoglobulin	PPS23	23-valent pneumococcal polysaccharide vaccine
HBsAg	Hepatitis B surface antigen		
HBV	Hepatitis B virus	PRP	Polyribosylribitol phosphate
Hib	*Haemophilus influenzae*, Type b	SSPE	Subacute sclerosing panencephalitis
HPV	Human papillomaviruses	TIV	Trivalent inactivated influenza vaccine
IPD	Invasive pneumococcal disease	VAPP	Vaccine-associated paralytic poliomyelitis
LAIV	Live attenuated influenza vaccine	VZIG	Human anti-varicella immunoglobulin
MMR	Measles, mumps, and rubella	VZV	Varicella zoster virus

The 18th century: vaccines for smallpox

> "In 1736 I lost one of my sons, a fine boy of 4-years-old, by the smallpox...I long regretted bitterly and I still regret that I had not given it to him by inoculation; this I mention for the sake of parents, who omit that operation on the supposition that they should never forgive themselves if a child died under it; my example showing that the regret may be the same either way, and that therefore the safer should be chosen."
>
> Benjamin Franklin, *Autobiography*, 1791

Attempts to prevent infectious diseases date to antiquity. The first successful prevention strategy was "variolation," the deliberate inoculation of people in the 16th century in India and China with the pus from smallpox sufferers. This was observed by Lady Mary Wortley Montague in 1716–1718 in Turkey, who had her children inoculated and introduced the method to England.

In 1721, Cotton Mather, an evangelical minister, persuaded a young physician named Zabdiel Boylston (the great-uncle of US President John Adams) to variolate 240 people in Boston, all but six of whom survived the procedure. In contrast, more than 30% died of naturally acquired smallpox. Although the two men were driven out of town and threatened with violence, ultimately variolation was widely used in Boston in the 18th century.

Vaccinology: An Essential Guide, First Edition. Edited by Gregg N. Milligan and Alan D.T. Barrett.
© 2015 John Wiley & Sons, Ltd. Published 2015 by John Wiley & Sons, Ltd.

Diseases caused by bacteria and viruses where the name of the organism and the disease is not the same
Chickenpox (varicella): Varicella zoster virus
Diphtheria: *Corynebacterium diphtheriae*
Intestinal tuberculosis: *Mycobacterium bovis*
Pertussis ("whooping cough"): *Bordetella pertussis*
Q fever: *Coxiella burnetii*
Shingles: Varicella zoster virus
Syphilis: *Treponema pallidum*
Tetanus ("lockjaw"): *Clostridium tetani*
Typhoid fever: *Salmonella typhi*

The vaccine era, however, really began in 1774 with the observation by a farmer named Benjamin Jesty that milkmaids who had had cowpox seemed to be immune to smallpox. He inoculated his wife and two sons about 22 years before Edward Jenner's first inoculation and publication in 1798. At some point in the 19th century, vaccinia virus (a mouse poxvirus) replaced cowpox in the vaccine.

Many lessons were learned from the smallpox vaccine: Initially, the vaccine was pus spread from a person who had been recently immunized to an unimmunized person, but syphilis also was passed this way. It was also recognized that loss of vaccine potency occurred after serial human passage (i.e., the virus changed when it was passed from human to human so that it was no longer immunogenic) so the vaccine began to be prepared in other animals; ultimately cattle were predominantly utilized. An imported batch of vaccine from Japan in the early 1900s caused an epizootic of Q fever (caused by *Coxiella burnetii*) among US cattle, which resulted in new quarantine laws and the creation of the US Department of Agriculture. In the 1920s, the need for standardization of vaccine production led to the designation of "strains" of vaccine viruses, such as the New York Board of Health strain in the USA and the Lister strain in Europe; both so-called strains, however, were a mix of viruses with different phenotypes, including many plaque variants with differing virulence. In 1903, the mandatory immunization of Massachusetts school children with smallpox vaccine in an attempt to protect the public

health was found to be constitutional by the US Supreme Court. The successful demonstration of "ring immunization" (the identification, immunization, and quarantine of all contacts of cases and the contacts of contacts) as a tool permitted the elimination and ultimately the eradication of smallpox, which was officially declared by the World Health Organization in 1980, 4 years after the last case. In 2001, because of concerns of bioterrorism, the US government embarked on the development of smallpox vaccines employing modern techniques: the development of a new plaque purified seed virus, cultivated in tissue cultures and then the development and testing of a safer human replication deficient strain of virus in 2010, termed "modified vaccinia Ankara," or MVA.

The 19th century: new understanding of infectious diseases and immunity

The concept of attenuation (weakening the virulence of the bacterium or virus) preceded Louis Pasteur's observations with hog cholera, anthrax, and rabies attenuation and vaccination, but those observations began the quest by many scientists to identify and prevent infectious diseases in animals and humans by using killed or inactivated vaccines (normally by chemicals such as formalin) and live attenuated vaccines for hog cholera, cholera, typhoid fever, and plague. At about the same time, late in the 19th century and early in the 20th century, great strides were also made in recognizing serum and cellular immunity, which led to the development of the concepts of passive and active immunity.

Diphtheria and tetanus toxins were recognized as the causes of those diseases and that antiserum made in horses against the toxins ("antitoxin") could neutralize the toxin effects; antitoxin was first used to prevent diphtheria in a child in 1891 and early vaccines against diphtheria and tetanus were developed at the beginning of the 20th century, which combined toxin with antitoxin.

The 20th century: the control of diseases using vaccines

During the 20th century, many infectious diseases came under control in many countries because of clean water, improved sanitation, and pasteurization of milk, which reduced exposure to *Brucella* sp. (the cause of brucellosis, a disease of animals transmissible in milk to humans), *Mycobacterium bovis* (the cause of most cases of intestinal tuberculosis), and *Salmonella typhi* (the cause of typhoid fever). Unfortunately, paralytic poliomyelitis also arose during this same period because of these same reasons—improved sanitation had the indirect effect of children acquiring the viruses that cause polio at later ages, causing about 1% to develop paralytic disease.

But the greatest change to the occurrence of infectious diseases occurred when vaccines were developed and became widely used. In the second half of the 20th century, vaccines substantially increased the life expectancy of children and prolonged life throughout society. For example, in the USA alone, before vaccines, there were half-a-million cases of measles with about 500 deaths each year. In 1964–1965, about 4 years before the rubella vaccine became available, there were more than 12.5 million people infected, causing 20,000 babies with congenital rubella infection to be born; of the children born with congenital rubella, 11,600 were born blind, and 1,800 were mentally retarded. In 1952, there were more than 21,000 individuals paralyzed by poliomyelitis in the USA. An overview of the reduction of vaccine-preventable illnesses in the 20th century is shown in Table 1.1.

Table 1.1 Vaccine-Preventable Illnesses Before and Since Routine Childhood Vaccination in the USA

Disease	Number of Cases Before Vaccine	Year Vaccine Recommended for Routine Use in Children	Number of Cases in 2009[a]
Smallpox	48,164	Early 1900s	0
Diphtheria	175,885	Mid-1940s	0
Pertussis[b]	142,271	Mid-1940s	16,858
Tetanus	1,314	Mid-1940s	18
Paralytic polio	16,316	1955	1[c]
Measles	503,282	1963	71[d]
Mumps	152,209	1967	1,981
Rubella	47,745	1969	3
Congenital rubella	823		2
Invasive *H. influenzae*, type b[e]	20,000	1985	38
Invasive *S. pneumoniae*[e]	17,240	2000	583
Hepatitis A (acute illness)	26,796	2009[f]	1,987
Hepatitis B (acute illness)	26,107	1991[g]	3405
Varicella	4,000,000	1995	20,480
Deaths	105		2

Adapted from Myers MG and Pineda D (2008). Do Vaccines Cause That?!. I4PH Press, Galveston (with permission).
[a]Centers for Disease Control and Prevention (2011). Summary of Notifiable Diseases—United States, 2009. MMWR: 58(53).
[b]Numbers of cases of pertussis were at a historic low of 1,010 in 1976. The rise in cases since then probably involves reduced immunity over time, plus an increased awareness of whooping cough in adolescents and adults for whom there is now a booster dose of vaccine.
[c]Vaccine-associated in an immunodeficient person.
[d]Measles has been largely eliminated from the USA. However, there were 21 importations of measles into the USA in 2009 (14 of whom were US residents traveling abroad), which spread to others in the community.
[e]Children younger than 5 years of age.
[f]Introduced incrementally after licensure in 1995.
[g]Introduced incrementally after licensure in1986.

In 2005, the total savings from direct costs saved (such as hospitalizations, clinic visits, lost ability from illness or death to fully function in society) from the routinely recommended childhood vaccines in the USA were estimated to be $9.9 billion per year. If the indirect health costs were also included (such as parents' time off from work or the need for caregivers), those vaccines saved $43.3 billion.

Vaccines

The term *vaccine* is derived from the Latin word, *vacca* (meaning cow), because cowpox was used to prevent smallpox. Vaccination is the deliberate attempt to prevent disease by "teaching" the immune system to employ acquired immune mechanisms. In the 21st century, vaccines are also being used to enhance existing immune mechanisms with the development of vaccines as treatments, so-called therapeutic vaccination. The properties of a vaccine are shown in Table 1.2.

Vaccines developed by trial and error
The smallpox vaccines were developed because of direct observation, first with the use of variolation, which, although sometimes a fatal procedure, was of lower risk than when smallpox was acquired in an epidemic, and then by the recognition that cowpox could provide immunity to smallpox. The vaccines for tetanus, diphtheria, and pertussis were prepared by trial and error in the early 1900s, but many other vaccines were also tested in this manner; however, many of these either failed to prevent disease or had severe adverse consequences.

Diphtheria
Diphtheria is a serious disease that can cause death through airway obstruction, heart failure, paralysis of the muscles used for swallowing and pneumonia. It is caused by the bacterium *Corynebacterium diphtheriae*, which produces toxins that cause cell death both at the site of infection and elsewhere in the body.

Diphtheria usually begins with a sore throat, slight fever, and swollen neck. Most commonly, bacteria multiply in the throat, where a grayish membrane forms. This membrane can choke the person—the source of its common name in the late 19th century as the "strangling angel."

Sometimes, the membrane forms in the nose, on the skin, or other parts of the body. The bacteria also release a toxin that spreads through the bloodstream that may cause muscle paralysis, heart and kidney failure, and death.

Approximately 5% of people who develop diphtheria (500 out of every 10,000) die from the disease and many more suffer permanent damage.

"Baby" Ruth Cleveland, first child of President and Mrs. Grover Cleveland died of diphtheria in 1904, at the age of 12 (see Figure 1.1). In the 1920s, before the diphtheria vaccine, there were 100,000 to 200,000 reported cases in the USA each year. For example, in

Table 1.2 Properties of Infectious Disease Preventive Vaccines

The following are properties of preventive infectious disease vaccines:
- An antigenic stimulus that elicits a specific adaptive immune response that can be recalled upon exposure to a specific agent
- Intentionally delivered
- Usually given to healthy individuals

This classic definition of a vaccine now needs to be enlarged to include therapeutic vaccines, such as:
- Herpes zoster vaccine, which restimulates immunity to varicella zoster virus in order to prevent reactivation of latent virus as shingles
- Cancer vaccines
- Vaccines for addiction

Diphtheria: The "Strangling Angel"

Brown County, MN, early 1880s:
"Louis Hanson lived southeast of town about five miles. He and his wife had five children. The scourge came and took all five. It was a sad sight to see Hanson driving up the road every day or two on his way to the cemetery, alone with his dead. All their children died between August 26 and September 5."

Davis, Leroy G (1934). A diphtheria epidemic in the early eighties. *MN History* 15:434–8.
With permission: Minnesota Historical Society.

1921 there were 206,000 cases of diphtheria and 15,520 diphtheria-caused deaths, mostly among children.

Early in the 20th century, diphtheria antitoxin became a powerful new tool for the prevention of diphtheria. Unfortunately, there was no oversight as to how it was produced and used, which led to the great tragedy of the St. Louis, Missouri, diphtheria epidemic in 1901. Equine diphtheria antiserum—

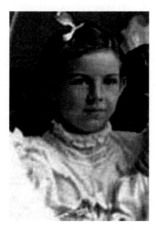

Figure 1.1 "Baby" Ruth Cleveland, first child of President and Mrs. Grover Cleveland, who died of diphtheria in 1904, aged 12 years. The former president and the remainder of the family were treated with diphtheria antitoxin and remained symptom free.

made from a horse that had died from tetanus—was given to children, causing fatal tetanus. Also, that year there were cases of tetanus among recipients of contaminated smallpox vaccine in Camden, New Jersey. These outbreaks led Congress to enact the Biologics Control Act of 1902, the predecessor to the Centers for Biologics Evaluation and Research of the US Food and Drug Administration, the beginning of vaccine regulatory control.

Active immunization employing diphtheria toxin and antiserum (so-called TaT) was effective but also associated with many adverse events, such as "serum sickness." However, in the early 1920s it was shown that toxin treated with heat and formalin lost its toxicity but was immunogenic. The production of diphtheria toxoid has evolved since then, but the process remains highly effective in providing protection against disease. However, the fully immunized person who is exposed to the bacterium can, in rare circumstances, still be infected as a "carrier" who usually only develops a mild case, or may not get sick at all. But if they are not fully vaccinated, the risk of getting severely ill after exposure is 30 times higher.

Because of the high level of immunizations now in the USA, only one case of diphtheria (or fewer) occurs each year. However, in areas where the immunization rate has fallen (such as Eastern Europe and the Russian Federation in the 1990s, as shown in Figure 1.2), tens of thousands of people suffered from diphtheria. Even

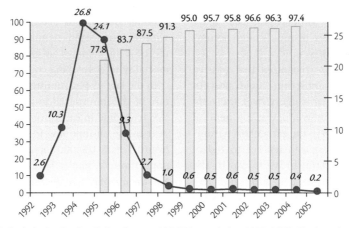

Figure 1.2 Cases of diphtheria in the Russian Federation per 100,000 population 1992–2006. The bars demonstrate the immunization coverage rate for children as measured by the Department of Sanitation, Russian Federation. Data provided by Dr. Olga Shamshava, 2007.

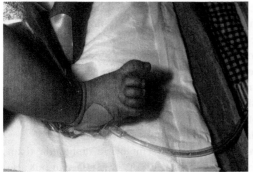 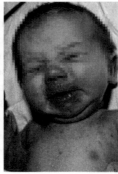

Figure 1.3 A 7-day-old infant with neonatal tetanus. Intense spasmodic muscle contractions shown as clenching of the feet (left) and of the facial muscles causing risus sardonicus, literally a "sardonic grin" (right). The child's mother had not previously been immunized. © Martin G. Myers

though we do not see many cases, the potential for diphtheria to reemerge is real.

Tetanus

Unlike the other vaccine preventable diseases, tetanus is not communicable person to person. Tetanus ("lockjaw") is caused by a potent neurotoxin produced by the anaerobic bacterium *Clostridium tetani*. The bacterium is a ubiquitous organism found in soil and the intestines of animals and humans. The organism multiplies in wounds—particularly dirty wounds with devitalized tissues—elaborating a plasmid-encoded exotoxin that binds to skeletal muscle and to neuronal membranes without causing an inflammatory response.

Generalized tetanus, the most common form of disease, usually begins with spasms of the face and chewing muscles causing trismus—or as it is popularly called "lockjaw"—causing a characteristic facial expression, the risus sardonicus or sardonic grin (see Figure 1.3). As the illness progresses, trismus is often accompanied by intense muscle spasms.

In the late 1890s it was recognized that passive prophylaxis with equine antiserum could prevent tetanus. This, plus aggressive surgery, was the only means to combat tetanus in World War I. Chemical inactivation of tetanus toxin in the early 1920s permitted the active immunization with tetanus toxoid to prevent tetanus by the US Army in World War II. The prophylactic use of vaccine plus post-injury management (a booster dose of tetanus toxoid, aggressive surgery, and passive prophylaxis with antiserum) dramatically reduced the occurrence—and therefore the mortality—of tetanus among the US Army in World War II compared to WWI (see Table 1.3).

Table 1.3 The Impact of Tetanus Toxoid Among US Soldiers

	Admission for Wounds	Cases of Tetanus	Cases per 100,000 Wounds
World War I	523,158	70	13.4
World War II	2,734,819	12[a]	0.4

Adapted from Long AP, Sartwell PE (1947). Tetanus in the U.S. Army in World War II. Bull U.S. Army Med Dept 7:371–385.
[a]Six of whom were unimmunized.

Neonatal tetanus (Figure 1.3)—generalized tetanus in newborn infants—occurs in infants whose mothers are not immune because they have not received vaccine. Because of nearly universal immunization with tetanus toxoid, neonatal tetanus is now rare in the USA but remains an important cause of neonatal mortality in developing countries.

In the late 1940s, routine tetanus toxoid immunization of children started in the USA. There has been a steady decline in cases from about 500 to 600 cases a year to the all-time low in 2009 of 18 cases—that is, from 0.4 cases/100,000 population to 0.01 cases/100,000 population. Mortality because of better wound care and the use of human tetanus immunoglobulin (which has now replaced horse antiserum) has decreased from 30% to 10%. Persons who recover from tetanus still need to be immunized against tetanus, however, as immunity is not acquired after tetanus. That is, so-called natural immunity to tetanus does not occur.

Almost all cases of human tetanus that occur in the USA now occur in adults who have either not been immunized or have not had a booster dose within 10 years.

Pertussis

Pertussis ("whooping cough") is a bacterial infection caused by *Bordetella pertussis*. It is spread in respiratory secretions when infected people cough or sneeze.

Children with pertussis have decreased ability to cough up respiratory secretions, and they develop thick, glue-like mucus in their airways. This causes severe coughing spells that make it difficult for them to eat, drink, or breathe. The child may suffer from coughing spells for 2 to 3 weeks or longer. Sometimes the child coughs several times before breathing; when the child finally does inhale, there may be a loud gasp or "whooping" sound. The disease is most severe when it occurs early in life when it often requires hospitalization; most of the deaths due to pertussis occur in very young infants.

Unlike many other vaccine preventable diseases, the bacterium that causes pertussis, *B. pertussis*, continues to circulate in the population even though most people have been immunized. Because pertussis is one of the most contagious human diseases, it is a great risk to those who are not vaccinated. Pertussis will develop in 90% of unvaccinated children living with someone with pertussis, and in 50% to 80% of unvaccinated children who attend school or daycare with someone with pertussis.

In the pre-vaccine era, pertussis was a universal disease, almost always seen in children. Between 1940 and 1945, before widespread vaccination, as many as 147,000 cases of pertussis were reported in the USA each year, with approximately 8,000 deaths caused by the disease. It is estimated that at the beginning of the 20th century as many as 5 of every 1000 children born in the USA died from pertussis.

In 1976, there were 1,010 case of pertussis in the USA, the lowest number of cases ever reported. Over the past few years the number of reported cases of pertussis has increased, reaching 25,827 in 2004; worldwide, there are an estimated 300,000 annual deaths due to pertussis. In 2009, there were 16,858 cases of pertussis in the USA with the greatest rate occurring in infants younger than 6 months of age but with about half of the cases occurring in adolescents and adults.

• The majority of pertussis-related deaths are in young infants. Approximately 50 out of every 10,000 children younger than 1 year of age who develop pertussis die from the disease.
• In 1997, adolescents and adults accounted for 46% of reported cases of pertussis, and they are often the ones who spread this disease to infants and children. Indeed, family members are often the source of pertussis exposure in young infants.
• In 2004, adolescents 11–18 years of age and adults 19–64 years of age accounted for 34% and 27% of the cases of pertussis in the USA, respectively. The true numbers are probably much higher in these age ranges because pertussis is often not recognized in adults. These cases are very important because teenagers and adults with pertussis can transmit the infection to other people, including infants who are at greatest risk for complications and death.

The initial pertussis vaccines were suspensions of formalin-killed whole organisms, first developed in 1914, which was shown to be effective in controlling epidemic pertussis in the early 1930s. It was combined with diphtheria and tetanus toxoids and recommended for routine administration to children in 1948. Despite the clear benefits of these vaccines at reducing pertussis, widespread parental concerns about vaccine safety arose, resulting in reduced immunization coverage. For example, in England and Wales the immunization levels dropped precipitously from 80% to 30% leading to a widespread epidemic involving more than 102,000 cases (see Figure 1.4). Although still used for control of pertussis in some countries, the whole cell pertussis vaccine is no longer used in many countries having been replaced by the acellular pertussis vaccine.

In 1991, the Food and Drug Administration licensed the acellular pertussis vaccines (diphtheria toxoid, tetanus toxoid, and acellular pertussis vaccine for use in young children [abbreviated DTaP]). These acellular pertussis vaccines consist of various components of the *B. pertussis* bacteria and cause much fewer side effects than the previous whole cell pertussis vaccines. Some of the newer DTaP vaccines have also included other vaccines, which allowed for a reduction in the number

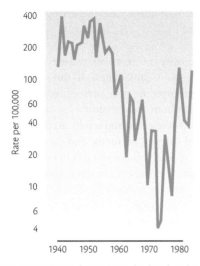

Figure 1.4 Pertussis attack rate in England and Wales (1940–1982). Reprinted from Cherry JD. (1984). The epidemiology of pertussis and pertussis immunization in the United Kingdom and the United States: a comparative study. Current Probl Pediatr 14(2), 80.

of injections. In 2005, new acellular pertussis vaccines were licensed for use in adolescents and adults (abbreviated Tdap because they contain less diphtheria toxoid and the pertussis components than the DTaP) in an attempt to reduce the number of pertussis infections in very young infants.

Testing the new acellular vaccines in the 1990s presented an ethical dilemma: As the USA had a licensed vaccine—the inactivated whole cell vaccine—that was known to be relatively safe and effective, how could the new vaccine be best tested for safety and effectiveness? This was solved by testing in countries that had stopped immunizing against pertussis because of parental concerns and that were then experiencing a resurgence of cases of pertussis.

Half of those vaccinated with DTaP will experience no side effects at all. About half of those vaccinated will experience mild reactions such as soreness where the shot was given, fever, fussiness, reduced appetite, tiredness, or vomiting. Some children may experience a temporary swelling of the entire arm or leg where DTaP was given; this reaction is more common after the fourth or fifth dose of DTaP but does not indicate that it will happen again after the next dose. Unfortunately, vaccines, particularly pertussis-containing

vaccines, have been incorrectly blamed for many things in the past. For example, the evidence does not support DTaP vaccines as a cause of asthma, autism, type 1 diabetes, brain damage, or sudden infant death syndrome. In addition, severe encephalopathy within 7 days after DTaP vaccination is usually explainable by another cause.

In 2004, one of the two manufacturers of tetanus toxoid-containing vaccines in the USA unexpectedly left the market because the cost of manufacturing limited the financial incentive to continue its manufacture. This caused a serious shortage of all tetanus toxoid-containing vaccines because about 9 months is needed to manufacture the vaccine.

Vaccines prepared by trial and error attenuation

Yellow fever

"From the second part of our study of yellow fever, we draw the following conclusion: The mosquito serves as the intermediate host for the parasite of yellow fever, and it is highly probable that the disease is only propagated through the bite of this insect."
Walter Reed, James Carroll, and Jesse Lazear. 1900. *The Etiology of Yellow Fever. A preliminary note.* Med Rec vi, 796. Quoted by RH Major. Classic Description of Disease, 3rd edition, 5th printing, 1959. Charles C. Thomas, Springfield, Ill.

Until the 20th century, epidemics of yellow fever repeatedly devastated seaports in North America and Europe. For example, 10% of Philadelphia, the new US capital city, succumbed in 1793 as graphically described by Longfellow in his poem about the travels of Evangeline in search of Gabriel, from whom she had been separated on their wedding day by the British forces who evicted Acadian men from Nova Scotia.

Until the hypothesis by Carlos Findlay and the experiments in 1900 by the Yellow Fever Commission in Cuba led by Walter Reed, the prevailing belief was that yellow fever was spread by filth, sewage, and decaying organic matter. In their experiments, Reed and his team showed that yellow fever was not a bacterial infection but was transmitted by the bite of the *Aedes aegypti* mosquito.

Yellow fever infection causes a wide spectrum of disease. Most cases of yellow fever are mild and similar to influenza, and consist of fever, headache, nausea, muscle pain, and prominent backache. After 3 to 4 days, most patients improve, and their symptoms disappear. However, in about 15% of patients, fever reappears after 24 hours with the onset of hepatitis and hemorrhagic fever. The "yellow" in the name is explained by the jaundice that occurs with hepatitis. Bleeding can occur from the mouth, nose, eyes, and/or stomach. Once this happens, blood appears in the vomit and feces. Kidney function also deteriorates. Up to half of those who develop the severe illness die within 10–14 days. The remainder recovers without significant organ damage.

In 1930, the regulatory function for biologics products (such as vaccines) was renamed the National Institute of Health (the forerunner of the National Institute of Allergy and Infectious Diseases). In 1934, because of a proliferation of potential new products, regulatory rules required that new biologics licensure would require the proof of both effectiveness and safety.

Only humans and monkeys can be naturally infected with yellow fever virus. Initial strains of yellow fever virus were established in 1927 in monkeys at the Rockefeller Institute in New York and the Institut Pasteur in Paris. Attempts at developing a vaccine were unsuccessful until Theiler and Smith at the Rockefeller Institute were able to attenuate the virus by subculture in mice—selecting for less virulent strains—followed by serial cultivation of the virus in chick embryo cell cultures. They used the lack of viscerotropism or encephalopathic effect in monkeys as "proof of principle" in 1936. Testing in humans quickly was begun in New York and then large field trials in Brazil in 1937.

Several important lessons were learned from yellow fever vaccine development in addition to the ability to attenuate its pathogenicity. Additional subculture of the vaccine virus in tissue cultures was found to lead to loss of vaccine immunogenicity, which led in turn to the recognition of the importance of using seed and vaccine pools in order to standardize passage level (discussed in detail in Chapter 11). Testing in monkeys became a regulatory requirement for new batches

of vaccine. In addition, the vaccine virus proved to be unstable unless serum was added to the vaccine. However, the use of human serum caused more than 10,000 cases of hepatitis B in the military in 1943.

Although the vaccine has been available for more than 70 years, the number of people infected over the past 2 decades has increased, and yellow fever is now once again a serious public health issue in a number of countries. Although epidemic yellow fever used to occur in the USA, the disease now occurs only in sub-Saharan Africa and tropical South America, occurring with increased risk during the rainy seasons (July to October in West Africa and January to May in South America). In those regions, it is endemic and becomes intermittently epidemic. It is estimated globally that there are 200,000 cases of yellow fever (with 30,000 deaths) per year. However, due to underreporting, probably only a small percentage of cases are identified. Small numbers of imported cases also occur in countries free of yellow fever; in the USA and Europe, these are usually in unimmunized travelers returning from endemic areas.

The risk to life from yellow fever is far greater than the risk from the vaccine, so people who may be exposed to yellow fever should be protected by immunization. However, if there is no risk of exposure—for example, if a person will not be visiting an endemic area—there is no need to receive the vaccine. The vaccine should only be given to pregnant and breast-feeding women during vaccination campaigns in the midst of an epidemic. Yellow fever vaccine should not be given to infants under 6 months of age due to an increased risk of viral encephalitis developing in the child and, in most cases, children 6–8 months of age should have travel and immunization deferred until the child is 9 months of age or older.

Yellow fever vaccine generally has few side effects; 10–30% of vaccinees develop mild headache, muscle pain, or other minor symptoms 5 to 10 days after vaccination. However, approximately 1% of vaccinees find it necessary to curtail their regular activities. Immediate hypersensitivity reactions, characterized by rash, urticaria, or asthma or a combination of these, are uncommon (incidence 1.8 cases per 100,000 vaccinees) and occur principally in persons with histories of egg allergy.

Rarely, yellow fever vaccine can cause serious adverse side effects. Encephalitis is estimated to occur in 0.8 per 100,000 vaccinees in the USA. Multiple organ system failure—which is a similar illness to yellow fever—following immunization (termed *yellow fever associated viscerotopic disease* [YEL-AVD] has been reported from around the world since 2001, particularly among people with certain immune deficiencies; in the USA the rate has been estimated to be 0.4 per 100,000 individuals. Both of these risks from yellow fever vaccine appear to occur more commonly in those who are over 60 years of age, and all cases have been seen in those being immunized for the first time; i.e., the risk of serious adverse events following yellow fever immunization is seen only in primary vaccinees and not in individuals who receive booster immunizations.

Poliomyelitis

Poliomyelitis was observed in antiquity, but the modern history of polio is the history of the rise of evidence-based medicine in the 19th and 20th centuries. Early in the 19th century, during the period when it was recognized that a physician could deduce a patient's pathologic findings from the physical examination, patients with "infantile paralysis" were recognized to have lesions in the anterior horn cells of the spinal cord detected on postmortem examination. In 1840, a German orthopedist, Jacob von Heine, provided a meticulous description of the clinical features of infantile paralysis, and in 1887, Karl Oscar Medin, a pediatrician in Stockholm, observed 44 cases and is credited for assembling the first comprehensive description of the disease (giving Sweden an unenviable reputation at that time as being a disreputable place). Figure 1.5 shows a clinical case of poliomyelitis. However, it would only be a few years until other countries had similar epidemics. Indeed, in 1893, two Boston area physicians published a letter titled "Is acute poliomyelitis unusually prevalent this season?" noting that most of the cases came from the suburban communities but not from the city of Boston.

In 1905, Sweden experienced 1,031 cases of polio that were closely studied by Medin's student Ivar Wickman. Wickman made the extraordinary observations that there were many asymptomatic and milder nonparalytic infections and that the disease was—in contrast to other infectious illnesses—not increased by crowding as a risk factor. This was confirmed by Wade

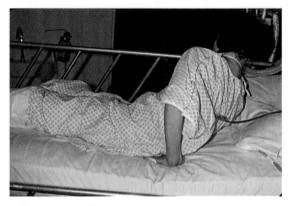

Figure 1.5 One of the last wild-type poliomyelitis cases in the USA, a 12-year-old girl in 1979, shown here with paralysis of her right leg and arm, the "tripod sign" when trying to sit up, and the epidemiologic link, her Amish cap. Poliovirus, type 1, was recovered from her. © Martin G. Myers

Hampton Frost in the 1920s in the USA; Frost is credited as being the first US epidemiologist.

In 1912, the identification of a filterable virus, the establishment of the monkey as an animal model, and that the spinal cords showed the identical pathologic findings as humans by American scientist Karl Landsteiner opened up new vistas for research. Landsteiner ultimately received the Nobel award for his description of blood groups in 1930. In the 1940s, anatomist David Bodian at Johns Hopkins, using serologic methods and many poliovirus isolates, demonstrated that there were three polioviruses.

Treatment of poliomyelitis was a therapeutic attitude of "do nothing to aggravate the disease" until the 1920s, when Phillip Drinker at Harvard invented the iron lung respirator followed by Sister Kenny—who is considered the originator of physical therapy—popularized her ideas about "orthopedic methods" after the acute illness had subsided.

But the rise of modern virology was ushered in by John Enders with two trainees in his laboratory at Children's Hospital in Boston in 1948 when they were able to cultivate each of the three polioviruses in monkey kidney tissue cultures, describing the histological changes they saw in culture as "cytopathogenic effects." Enders and his trainees, Tom Weller and Frederick Robbins, received the Nobel award in 1954.

By the early 1950s, the natural history of poliovirus infection had been shown to involve replication in the gastrointestinal tract, occasionally followed by viremia, which on occasion infected the spinal cord anterior horn cells. The formalin-inactivated polio vaccine developed by Jonas Salk was licensed in 1954 after large field trials (400,000 immunized) demonstrated effectiveness and safety of the vaccine.

Unfortunately, little was known about the complexities of scale-up or the kinetics of poliovirus inactivation by formalin. When the first inactivated vaccines were licensed, all the manufacturers experienced production and quality control problems, culminating in the "Cutter Incident" of cases of paralytic poliomyelitis in 1955, which were caused by residual infectious virus in some of the new vaccine lots, particularly those produced by Cutter Laboratories. This led to the temporary suspension of the polio vaccine programs in the USA and elsewhere. Inactivated vaccine was subsequently rereleased after additional safety tests demonstrated consistency in production and viral inactivation. As a consequence of the problems with the Salk vaccine, the regulatory functions at the US National Institute of Allergy and Infectious Diseases (part of the National Institutes of Health) were moved to a separate institute, the Division of Biologics Standards, ultimately becoming the modern Center for Biologics Evaluation and Research of the Food and Drug Administration.

In the 1950s, Albert Sabin in Cincinnati and investigators at a number of other laboratories took the three strains of polioviruses (one each for the three serotypes of poliovirus) and passaged them repeatedly in monkey tissue cultures, testing them for attenuation by inoculating monkeys. The least neurovirulent of these, the Sabin vaccine candidate, was ultimately selected. Sabin field tested his oral vaccine in 75 million people in the former Soviet Union.

Immunologically, the inactivated vaccine differs substantially from the attenuated vaccine in that inactivated vaccine only induces humoral immunity whereas the live virus vaccine induces both humoral and duodenal antibodies (see Figure 1.6).

In the 1960s, an adventious virus, simian virus 40 (SV40), which has been shown to cause tumors in rodents and can transform human tissue culture cells, was recognized in primary monkey kidney tissue cultures used to prepare some vaccines. It is estimated that up to 100 million Americans may have been exposed to SV40, which contaminated the inactivated

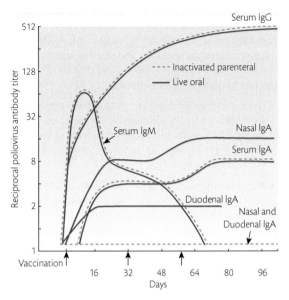

Figure 1.6 Serum and secretory antibody responses to orally administered, live attenuated polio vaccine and to intramuscular inoculation of inactivated polio vaccine. From Ogra PL, Fishant M, Gallagher MR (1980). Viral vaccination via mucosal routes. Review of Infectious Diseases 2(3); 352–369.

polio vaccine when it was first introduced. In addition, SV40 also contaminated the first oral polio vaccine, but that contaminated vaccine was only given to people during the original clinical trials. Furthermore, SV40 has been found as a contaminant of some of the adenovirus vaccines given to military recruits during that same period of time. Once the contamination was recognized, steps were taken to eliminate it from future vaccines; no vaccines licensed for use in the USA or other countries currently are contaminated with SV40.

The oral polio vaccine was inexpensive to produce, did not require trained health providers to administer with needle and syringe (as it was given to children on a lump of sugar), and protected a higher proportion of those immunized, as well as protecting those around them by community (or herd) immunity (see Chapter 18 for details on herd immunity). When used in outbreak settings, the live vaccine also stops the transmission of polioviruses (and other related enteroviruses) when a high proportion of individuals have been immunized, because this vaccine replicates in the human gastrointestinal tract blocking enteroviral replication.

Because SV40 causes tumors in rodents and can transform human cell cultures, it has been intensively studied, both in the laboratory and epidemiologically as a possible cause of human malignancies. This concern appears to have now been excluded:

- Newborn babies who received SV40 in polio vaccine were followed for 35 years and had no excess risk of cancer. This is particularly important because newborn animals are much more susceptible to SV40 tumors than older animals.

- A case-control study of cancers among Army veterans found no risk of brain tumor, mesothelioma, or non-Hodgkin's lymphoma associated with receipt of adenovirus vaccine that contained large amounts of SV40.

- People infected with human immunodeficiency virus (HIV) are at increased risk of developing non-Hodgkin's lymphoma. This risk was not increased if they had received SV40-contaminated polio vaccine compared to those who had not received it.

- Earlier studies reported that many people had antibodies against SV40, but those studies now appear to have detected cross-reacting antibodies to similar but different human viruses. Using new methods to test for SV40 antibody, recent studies have demonstrated a lack of SV40 antibody response in humans—in contrast to animals.

- Molecular tools frequently used to detect SV40 in cancerous tissues may have commonly detected SV40 contaminants in the laboratory when, in fact, it was not present in the cancer.

- Finally, if SV40 caused cancer in humans, the proteins it produces in animal tumor cells should be measurable in human cancers, which they have not.

Adapted from Myers MG and Pineda DI. Do Vaccines Cause That?! I4PH Press, 2008, with permission.

Unfortunately, while replicating in the gastrointestinal tract, viral strains are excreted and can be recovered in feces. Often these strains have reverted to a neurovirulent phenotype (that is, they are capable of causing paralytic disease) due to reversion of attenuating mutations found in the live vaccine strain to those found in wild-type poliovirus. This is a rare but important complication of the oral vaccine, called *vaccine-associated paralytic poliomyelitis* (VAPP). This can occur among those unimmunized persons in contact with immunized children due to the excretion of viruses in feces. In addition, persons with certain immunodeficiencies also may continue to shed vaccine virus in their feces for very long periods of time (years), severely complicating efforts to eradicate poliomyelitis.

Because of continuing cases of VAPP in the USA after the elimination of wild-type polioviruses, the USA and other countries began once again to employ the safer but less effective inactivated vaccine for routine use in 2000.

Measles

Measles is no longer an endemic disease in the USA. However, measles often arrives via infected travelers by airplane from other areas of the world, often spreading to susceptible persons before the classic symptoms become apparent. Due to its high transmissibility by aerosol, it is frequently transmitted in emergency rooms and medical offices from people who are seeking care during the early manifestations of measles infection.

Despite an effective live virus vaccine that was licensed in 1963, measles remains one of the leading causes of death in children younger than 5 years of age and kills approximately 400 children per day worldwide. Measles is a serious disease, which spreads rapidly to others in respiratory droplets from sneezing and coughing. It is one of the most contagious diseases known.

The global measles initiative to reduce measles mortality worldwide has had remarkable success at reducing deaths from measles from 733,000 in 2000 to 164,000 in 2008. Measles in the developing world has a much higher mortality rate than in developed countries because of complex interactions between malnutrition, age at infection, type and outcome of complications, crowding or intensity of exposure, and the availability of care.

Measles in the USA prior to the measles vaccine was estimated to cause 4,000,000 cases per year (equivalent to the entire birth cohort in the USA); virtually every person had measles virus infection by age 20. There were 150,000 cases with lower respiratory complications (such as bacterial or viral pneumonia, bronchitis, and croup); 150,000 cases of otitis media; 48,000 hospitalizations; and 4000 cases of encephalitis annually. Between 1989 and 1991, when the USA experienced renewed measles activity—prior to introducing a second dose of measles vaccine—there were 55,000 cases and more than 130 deaths.

Uncomplicated measles in developed countries begins 1 to 2 weeks after exposure. The illness begins with fever followed by cough, coryza (runny nose), and conjunctivitis, similar to many other respiratory infections; the infection is very contagious at this stage.

After several days the fever increases and the pathognomonic enanthem, Koplik spots appear (a rash on the inside of the cheek, which is often not observed). One to 2 days later (usually about day 14 after exposure) the characteristic erythematous maculopapular rash (see Figure 1.7) appears first on the face and then spreads down the body. Early on, the rash usually blanches on pressure, but as it begins to fade 3–5 days later it becomes brownish, also clearing first on the face and spreading down.

Infections of the middle ears, pneumonia, croup, and diarrhea are common complications of measles. Approximately 5% of children (500 out of 10,000) with measles will develop pneumonia. Measles encephalitis occurs in 1 per 1,000 cases of natural measles, and when it occurs it has a mortality of almost 50%; many of the survivors have permanent brain damage. This translates to 1 to 3 of every 1,000 children who get measles in the USA will die from the disease. Death occurs more commonly in infants, especially malnourished children, and among immunocompromised persons, including those with HIV infection and leukemia. These latter persons—who often cannot be immunized—can be protected by herd immunity if those around them are immune.

Subacute sclerosing panencephalitis (SSPE) is a rare fatal illness caused by ongoing measles virus infection of the brain. Symptoms of brain damage usually begin 7 to 10 years after infection. Death occurs 1 to 3 years after the onset of symptoms. Risk factors for developing SSPE include developing measles infection at a young age. The incidence of SSPE is estimated to be between 7 and 11 cases per 100,000 cases of measles. The measles vaccine virus has not been associated with SSPE.

The measles virus was first isolated in tissue culture in 1954, just as the polioviruses in the laboratory of John Enders. Vaccine development followed rapidly with licensure in the USA in 1963. The virus was passaged multiple times, first in human kidney cells and then in human amnion cells. It was then adapted to chick embryos and finally passaged in chick embryo cells. The initial live virus vaccine that was licensed prevented measles complications but was associated with high rates of fever and rash, leading to further attenuation of the vaccine.

The vaccine virus was found to be both temperature and light unstable, and required the addition of stabilizers. Even in the lyophilized form with the addition of stabilizers, it must be stored in the dark at 2–8°C. After reconstitution, the virus loses about 50% of its potency in 1 hour at room temperature.

The further attenuated live virus vaccine was combined in 1971 with mumps and rubella live virus vaccines into a single injection, the measles, mumps, and rubella vaccine (abbreviated MMR), and subsequently with varicella vaccine (MMRV) in 2005. Two doses of vaccine are recommended for all the vaccine components to ensure that more than 95% of the population be immune to measles, which is the threshold for maintaining community (herd) immunity.

A formalin-inactivated vaccine was also developed and licensed at the same time as the live virus vaccine

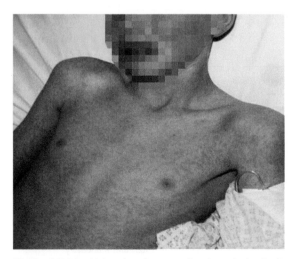

Figure 1.7 Measles in a boy demonstrating the typical rash of measles. © Martin G. Myers

but is no longer utilized because those who received that vaccine developed a new disease called "atypical measles," which resembled Rocky Mountain Spotted Fever (a tick-borne disease caused by the bacterium *Rickettsia rickettsia*), when they encountered live measles virus (either wild type or vaccine virus).

Following licensure of measles vaccine, rates of the disease in the USA fell dramatically. However, 95% or more of individuals must be immune to measles to prevent its transmission in communities. Because of this, most states in the 1970s instituted mandatory immunization of children as a condition of school entry. In 1991 a two-dose immunization strategy was instituted. This has resulted in elimination of endemic measles in the USA (see Figure 1.8).

Because of misinformation about measles vaccine safety in the United Kingdom, beginning in 1998, MMR vaccine coverage declined across Europe, resulting in outbreaks of measles and mumps in Europe, the USA, and Canada.

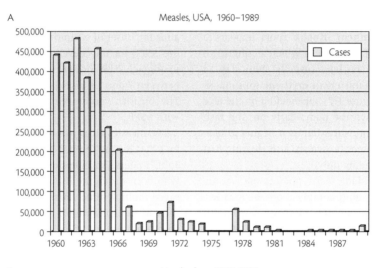

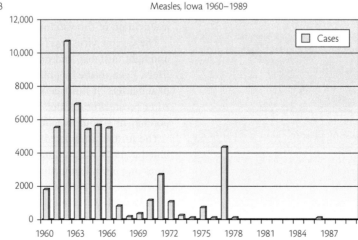

Figure 1.8 Measles in (A) the USA (Centers for Disease Control and Prevention, 1995) and (B) Iowa (Iowa Department of Health, 2007, www.idph.state.is.us/adper/pdf/cade/decades/pdf) 1960–1989. Measles vaccine was licensed in 1963, and mandatory immunization laws were enacted widely by states in the late 1960s and 1970s. Iowa enacted its immunization law in 1977 (Iowa Administrative Code, 1977). From chapter 17 in Myers & Pineda in Barrett & Stanberry (Elsevier).

There were 140 cases of measles in the USA in 2008; more than three quarters of these cases were linked to imported measles from another country, and most of the imported cases occurred among unimmunized American travelers.

Rubella

Rubella is caused by a virus that is transmitted from person to person in respiratory secretions. Rubella is a mild illness; indeed, it is often asymptomatic. When symptoms occur, they include low-grade fever and swollen lymph nodes in the back of the neck followed by a generalized erythematous rash. Conjunctivitis does not occur. Self-limited complications may include joint pain, a temporary decrease in platelet count, and, uncommonly, postinfectious encephalitis. Temporary arthritis may also occur not uncommonly, particularly in adolescent and adult women; although chronic arthritis has been reported to occur in adult women, the data are inconclusive.

In contrast, rubella in pregnant expectant women—who are often asymptomatic—frequently leads to congenital rubella syndrome (CRS) in the fetus (see Figure 1.9). This is a devastating disease characterized by microcephaly, small birth size for gestational age, deafness, mental retardation, cataracts and other eye defects, heart defects, and diseases of the liver and spleen that may result in a low platelet count with bleeding under the skin. The incidence and severity of congenital defects are greater if infection occurs during early gestation; as many as 85% of expectant mothers infected in the first trimester will have a miscarriage or deliver a baby with CRS. Once fetal infection is established, viral infection occurs in multiple organs with potential progressive damage.

In 1963–1964, before vaccine was available, there was a rubella outbreak in the USA during which 12 million people were infected. Because some who were infected were pregnant women, 11,000 fetuses died and 20,000 babies were born with permanent disabilities.

Several live attenuated virus vaccines were licensed in the USA and elsewhere in 1969–1971, but the RA27/3 strain—isolated from an infected fetus and propagated in human fetal cells—was adopted in the USA and most other countries because it induced consistent and persistent immunity, had a low rate of side effects, and because recipients developed resistance to reinfection with rubella virus. As stated in the measles vaccine section, rubella vaccine in the USA is given in combination with MMR and also sometimes with the addition of varicella vaccine (MMRV).

The number of cases of rubella fell very sharply once the rubella vaccine was licensed, and became widely used in the USA in 1969; in 2009 there were only two cases of CRS reported in the USA.

Since the introduction of rubella live virus vaccine, most CRS cases occur in developing countries, although it also continues to occur in developed countries among infants born to unimmunized mothers (see Table 1.4).

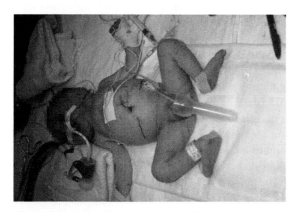

Figure 1.9 Newborn with congenial rubella syndrome, including hepatosplenomagly, cataracts, purpura, and microcephaly. © Martin G. Myers

Mumps

Mumps is also a viral respiratory infection. Before widespread vaccination, there were about 200,000 cases of mumps and 20 to 30 deaths reported each year in the USA. In 2009, there were fewer than 2000 cases.

Mumps usually begins with swelling and tenderness of one or more of the salivary glands. This lasts for about a week. In children, the infection is usually fairly mild although permanent hearing loss occurs in 1 out of 2000 cases, and aseptic meningitis occurs in about 15% of cases, but this is usually self-limited. Pancreatitis may occur in as many as 4% of cases but an association with diabetes mellitus has not been

Table 1.4 Rubella, Netherlands, September 2004–2005.

387 recognized cases
- 381 unvaccinated
  - Median age of females: 14 years
  - 32 cases in pregnancy
  - 29 recognized in pregnancy
  - 15 in first trimester
    - 2 intrauterine deaths
    - All live-born affected: deafness (all), congenital heart defect (62%), microcephaly and/or delay (77%)
  - 3 cases only recognized because of congenital rubella syndrome in the infant

From Hahné, S, Macey J, van Binnendijk R, et al. (2009). Rubella outbreak in the Netherlands, 2004–2005. Pediatric Infectious Disease Journal 28(9); 795–800.

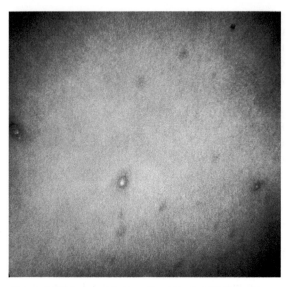

Figure 1.10 Early vesicle formation following VZV infection. © Martin G. Myers

demonstrated. Complications are more common in adults and include orchitis in 20–50% of postpubertal males, which is often associated with decreased fertility; mastitis in more than 30% of postpubertal females; and pelvic pain, possibly oophoritis, in as many as 5% of women. Brain involvement may involve aseptic meningitis or meningoencephalitis; encephalitis occurs uncommonly but accounts for most of the fatal cases.

Mumps infection has not been associated with problems during pregnancy, although there are some reports of an increase in fetal loss associated with mumps infection during the first trimester.

Multiple live mumps virus vaccines have been prepared but only one is licensed in the USA. It was attenuated in embryonated chicken eggs and further passaged in chick embryo cell culture. It is available as MMR and MMRV vaccines, and two doses seem to confer about 90% immunity to mumps.

Varicella zoster virus (VZV)

Chickenpox (varicella) is the initial infection with the herpesvirus varicella zoster virus (VZV), which then remains latent in dorsal root ganglia for life. Herpes zoster (shingles) is the consequence of reactivation of the VZV. The same vaccine—in different dosages—is used prophylactically to prevent chickenpox and as an immune booster to prevent zoster and its complications.

Varicella

Varicella is highly contagious caused by varicella zoster virus (VZV), although somewhat less so than measles. In households, most individuals who are susceptible will acquire infection, as will about one in six of those exposed in school. It is spread by the airborne route primarily from the skin vesicles. Viral replication initially occurs in the oropharynx, followed by a brief viremia. After an incubation period of 10–21 days (usually 14–16 days), the normal child may have malaise and fever for a day or two, but usually all symptoms start at about the same time with the typical rash (see Figure 1.10), which appears in crops starting as macules and papules. These quickly become vesicles and then pustules followed by crust formation. In the unimmunized child, the number of lesions usually numbers between 250 and 500.

The most common complication of varicella is bacterial skin infection in about 5%. These are usually self-limited when treated with antibiotics. However, some cases of secondary infection can be invasive and

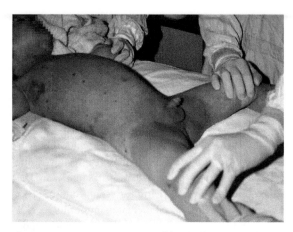

Figure 1.11 Group A streptococcal fasciitis in a previously normal child with varicella. © Martin G. Myers

are potentially fatal. For example, bacterial necrotizing fasciitis (e.g., Group A streptococcus [*Streptococcus pyogenes*] [see Figure 1.11]), is preceded by varicella in more than half the cases.

Cerebellar ataxia occurs in about 1 of 4000 cases of varicella in children but is usually self-limited. Reye's syndrome of liver failure and cerebral edema, a serious and not infrequently fatal complication of varicella or influenza B virus infections, has decreased substantially in frequency since medications that contain aspirin are no longer commonly given to children for fever.

Varicella in adults may be associated with viral pneumonia, especially among pregnant women in the third trimester of pregnancy in whom the pneumonia may be quite severe. In addition, varicella infection during pregnancy can damage the fetus, causing permanent scarring of the skin, abnormalities of the limbs, congenital cataracts, chorioretinitis, microphthalmia, mental retardation, and fetal loss.

Varicella in immunocompromised patients may cause progressive varicella. The greatest risk groups are children with leukemia, other malignant diseases on chemotherapy, those who are receiving high doses of corticosteroids (e.g., for asthma), and those with congenital cellular immunodeficiencies. As many as 30% may be affected, and 7% die if untreated with antiviral drugs. High titered human anti-varicella immunoglobulin (VZIG) given shortly after exposure of high risk individuals to VZV can prevent progressive varicella.

Multiple attempts to produce an attenuated varicella vaccine were initially unsuccessful at identifying a vaccine candidate of low reactogenicity that retained immunogenicity. However, the Japanese licensed Oka strain varicella vaccine in 1987, and it was licensed in the USA in 1995. It was prepared from an isolate of VZV obtained from a normal child with varicella. It was serially propagated in human embryo fibroblasts, fetal guinea pig cells (one of the few nonprimate cells lines that support the growth of VZV), and then in human fibroblast cultures. The Oka strain has proven to be safe and effective although it does establish latency in recipients (i.e., the virus remains dormant in dorsal root ganglia) with the potential to produce shingles (but at a reduced rate) later in life. In recent years molecular differences between the Oka strain and wild-type strains of VZV have been used to distinguish clinical isolates of VZV from vaccine strain.

In the USA, varicella vaccine is available as a monovalent vaccine and as a quadrivalent vaccine (MMRV). Because the varicella component was found to be inferior in initial studies of the early combination vaccine, the licensed MMRV vaccine contains a greater dose of VZV than the monovalent vaccine so as to be "noninferior," a regulatory requirement.

Prior to the introduction of varicella vaccine, there were 3 to 4 million cases of varicella in the USA each year. About 10,000 people were hospitalized with complications, and approximately 100 died. While only 5% of reported cases of varicella are in adults, adults accounted for 35% of the deaths from the disease. The varicella vaccine is 85% to 90% effective for the prevention of varicella and 100% effective for prevention of moderate or severe disease (defined as many skin lesions).

Children receiving varicella vaccine in pre-licensure trials in the USA were protected for 11 years. However, "breakthrough infection" (cases of chickenpox after vaccination) can occur in some who have been immunized; more recent studies have demonstrated waning immunity over time. Breakthrough varicella usually results in mild rather than full-blown varicella, although some school outbreaks have resulted in some vaccinated children having more lesions that were communicable. For these reasons, a second dose of a varicella vaccine is now recommended.

A majority of people who get varicella vaccine have no side effects. Of those who do have side effects, most will have only a mild reaction such as soreness and swelling where the shot was administered, and a mild rash. Pain and redness at the injection site occurs in about one in five children (and about one in three teenagers). About one in five may also have a few chickenpox-like lesions at the injection site. One to three weeks after vaccination, some may develop a few chickenpox-like lesions elsewhere on their bodies.

Although fever occurs in as many as 15% of children following administration of the varicella vaccine, it also occurred in children who had received the placebo in comparative trials. MMRV combination vaccine has comparable rates of reactions to children who received MMR and varicella vaccine at different sites on the same day—except that those that received MMRV vaccine more commonly experienced fever, a measles-like rash, and rash at the injection site. It has also been observed that children who received MMRV for the first dose of these vaccines had an increased risk of febrile seizures of about 1 child per 1000 when compared to children who received MMR and the varicella vaccine at different sites. For these reasons,

many health care professionals prefer to administer MMR and varicella vaccines as two injections at different sites for the first dose but prefer MMRV for the second dose to reduce injections.

Herpes zoster vaccine

Zoster (shingles) is an infection caused by the same virus that causes chickenpox. The VZV virus—which remains in the nerve cells for life after chickenpox or after the chickenpox vaccine—may reappear as shingles in later life (Figure 1.12), particularly in the elderly and those who are immunocompromised. This is because of declining cell mediated immunity to VZV (Figure 1.13).Thus, anyone who has had chickenpox or the chickenpox live virus vaccine can develop shingles. Although shingles can occur at any age, the risk increases dramatically as people get older.

When shingles develop, people often experience discomfort in a region that is followed by a rash with blisters, generally in the distribution of a dermatome (Figure 1.14). Because the rash contains virus, VZV can be transmitted to others who are susceptible to chickenpox, although the virus is much less communicable from shingles than varicella lesions.

Reactivation of VZV in sensory neurons can destroy the cell, causing debilitating pain, which sometimes lasts for months after the rash has healed. Like the occurrence of shingles, this postherpetic neuralgia

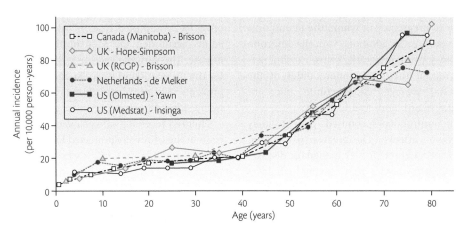

Figure 1.12 Age-specific incidence of herpes zoster as a function of age. From figure 39.2 in Levin M in Plotkin et al. (eds) Vaccines, 6th edition (with permission from J. Pellissier and M. Brisson, Merck & Co, Inc.).

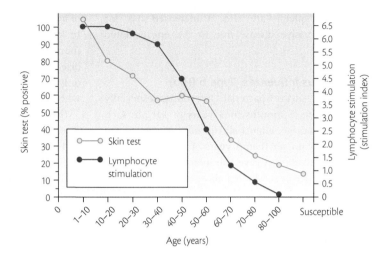

Figure 1.13 Age-related cellular immune response to varicella zoster virus. From figure 39.3 in Levin M in Plotkin et al (eds) Vaccines, 6th edition. Data from Burke et al.

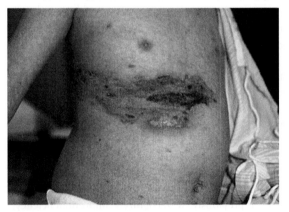

Figure 1.14 A child with leukemia and herpes zoster with the characteristic distribution of rash in the distribution of a dermatome. © Martin G. Myers

(PHN), occurs more commonly in older individuals, with age being the strongest prognostic factor. PHN occurs in 30% of people older than 59 years of age.

Herpes zoster vaccine is the first "therapeutic" vaccine (i.e., a vaccine given to someone who has had the disease). The intent is to boost cell-mediated immunity (CMI) to VZV. The shingles vaccine contains the same attenuated Oka strain of VZV as the varicella vaccine but at a greater dose, determined by CMI response titration assays. The vaccine given to those over 60 years of age both reduces the frequency of herpes zoster and, in those who develop shingles, reduces the frequency and severity of PHN.

Vaccines for polysaccharide encapsulated bacteria

The virulence of some bacterial pathogens is greatly enhanced by the elaboration of a polysaccharide that evades opsonization. B-cell receptors recognize polysaccharide antigens; however, because they are not presented to T cells in association with major histocompatability complex class II molecules, the immune response is T-cell independent, immunologic memory is not established, and an anamnestic response is not induced upon reexposure. Some polysaccharide vaccines for infants have proven effective in certain situations; however, because the immune systems of young infants are immature, they only respond with low titers of antibody after exposure to polysaccharide antigens. However, chemically conjugating polysaccharides to proteins was found to create a vaccine against the polysaccharide moiety that recruits T-cells, making the polysaccharide antigen immunogenic in infants younger than 6 months of age and inducing a booster response on reexposure. Indeed, the T-cell dependent B-cell immune response was initially recognized during the development of vaccines for *Haemophilus influenzae*, Type b (Hib) infections in young infants.

People with certain health problems—such as certain immune deficiencies and those who lack a functioning spleen—are also at increased risk for acquiring invasive disease due to the encapsulated bacteria.

Haemophilus influenzae, Type b (Hib)

Hib causes severe bacterial infections, especially among infants 3 months to 3 years of age. In fact, before the vaccine, almost all Hib infections occurred in children younger than 5 years of age. There were more than 20,000 invasive Hib infections in children in the USA per year, about half of whom developed bacterial meningitis. Hib meningitis was essentially always fatal prior to antibiotics. With antibiotic and other treatment, the mortality of Hib meningitis dropped to about 2% but then antibiotic resistance emerged. As many as 25–50% of the children who survived Hib meningitis had permanent brain damage.

In the 1930s, Hib was recognized to be encapsulated and that the lack of a bactericidal antibody appeared to explain why this age group was at increased risk (Figure 1.15). Infants are born with an antibody directed at the capsule of Hib, which is acquired from their mother, but this is lost at about 3 months of age. They begin to reacquire the bactericidal antibody at about 2 years of age. Children with invasive Hib infections, including those with Hib meningitis, were also observed to not respond immunologically to Hib.

In the 1970s, the capsule of Hib was recognized to be polyribosylribitol phosphate (PRP), antibody to which was bactericidal. In addition, PRP was shown to be immunogenic and safe in children over 2 years of age but was not immunogenic in younger children. In 1985, a PRP vaccine was licensed for children older than 18–24 months of age as a means to reduce Hib disease burden in children 2–5 years of age, but this only represented a small proportion of the children who were at risk.

These observations led to the recognition of the T-cell dependent B-cell immune response mechanism and that that pathway in young infants and children did not develop until they reached 18–24 months of age. After PRP was chemically conjugated to carrier proteins, the conjugated PRP was shown to also be immunogenic in young infants. Field trials quickly demonstrated the safety and efficacy of candidate conjugate vaccines leading to licensure in 1987.

The impact of Hib vaccines on Hib has been remarkable both because of its effectiveness at protecting infants and young children but also because of community (herd) immunity (Figure 1.16), which occurs because these vaccines also decrease the nasal carriage of Hib.

Unfortunately, misinformation about the safety of Hib vaccine in recent years has caused some parents to withhold vaccine from their children with serious consequences for their children and their communities. In Minnesota in 2008, for example, there were five cases of invasive Hib in young children, three of whom were unimmunized, and one of whom died. One other child was too young to have been fully immunized while the other had been immunized but had a previously unrecognized immunodeficiency;

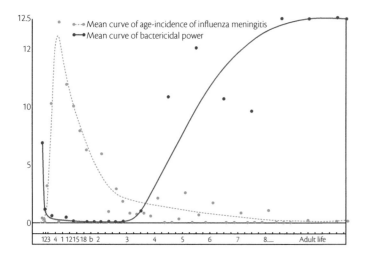

Figure 1.15 The relation of age incidence of influenzal meningitis to the bactericidal power of human blood at different ages against a smooth meningeal strain or *H. influenzae*. From Fothergill LD and Wright J (1933). Journal of Immunology 24, 273–284.

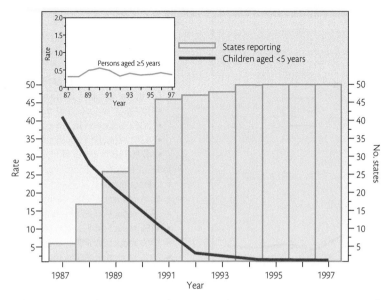

Figure 1.16 Incidence of *Haemophilus influenzae* invasive disease, United States, 1987–1997. From Centers for Disease Control and Prevention. (1998). Progress towards eliminating Haemophilus influenzae Type b disease among infants and children—United States, 1987–1997. Morbidity and Mortality Weekly Report 47(46), 993–998.

both of these latter two children should have been protected by community (herd) immunity.

Streptococcus pneumoniae

The *S. pneumoniae* are a large group of bacteria consisting of many serotypes that, like Hib, inhabit the nasopharynx of people of all ages. These bacteria (also collectively known as "pneumococci") are capable of causing infections of the middle ear and sinuses, bacterial pneumonia and meningitis, and bacteremia. They became the chief cause of bacterial pneumonia and bacterial meningitis once there was a vaccine against Hib.

Serious pneumococcal infections are most common in infants, toddlers, smokers, and the elderly, in addition to those with certain immunodeficiencies and those who lack a functioning spleen. African-American and Native American children also have higher rates of invasive pneumococcal disease than do white children.

A multivalent pneumococcal polysaccharide vaccine was licensed in 1977 based on the distribution of strains causing invasive pneumococcal infections in adults. This 23-valent pneumococcal polysaccharide vaccine (PPS23) induces a serotype-specific anticapsular antibody in individuals over 2 years of age and has been employed to immunize older adults who are at increased risk of invasive pneumococcal disease (IPD) and those with chronic medical conditions (such as those with immunodeficiencies, chronic lung disease, diabetes, chronic heart disease, following a splenectomy, or after renal transplantation). The antibody response wanes rapidly following primary immunization, and although revaccination does reinduce antibody, there is no "booster response" and antibody titers are lower than primary immunization due to immune tolerance. For these reasons, and because PPS23 is not effective at protecting young infants from IPD, a heptavalent pneumococcal conjugate vaccine (PCV7 vaccine), containing the seven most common pneumococcal serotypes that cause invasive infections in children in North America, was licensed in the USA and recommended for routine use in infants in 2000.

PCV7 given to young children dramatically reduced the rates of IPD, otitis media, and nasal carriage of the vaccine serotypes among all age groups, including the immunocompromised and older individuals (Figure

21

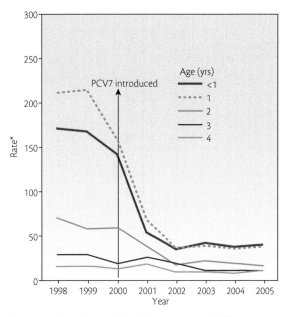

Figure 1.17 Incidence of invasive pneumococcal disease (IPD)/100,000 in children younger than 5 years of age. From Centers for Disease Control and Prevention. (2008). Invasive pneumococcal disease in children 5 years after conjugate vaccine introduction—Eight States, 1998–2005. Morbidity and Mortality Weekly Report 57(6), 144–148.

Table 1.5 Direct and Indirect Effects of 7-Valent Pneumococcal Conjugate Vaccine

- Direct effect, age <5 yrs:
  - 75% reduction in IPD (94% for vaccine serotypes)
  - For those <2 years of age
    - 17–28% reduction in frequent AOM
    - 20% reduction in tympanostomy tubes
    - 43% reduction in visits for AOM
    - 42% reduction in antibiotic prescriptions
- Indirect effects (2.2 fold more cases prevented than for direct effects):
  - 40% reduction IPD in those <90 days of age
  - 33% reduction IPD in those 5–17 yrs of age
  - 41% reduction IPD in those 18–39 yrs of age
  - 13% reduction IPD in those 40–64 yrs of age
  - 28% reduction IPD in those >64 yrs of age
  - 58% reduction in AOM visits in those <13 yrs of age
  - 20% increase cases of IPD due to non-PCV7 serotypes

IPD, invasive pneumococcal disease; AOM, acute otitis media; PCV7, 7-valent pneumococcal conjugate vaccine. From (1) Centers for Disease Control and Prevention. (2005). Direct and indirect effects of routine vaccination of children with 7-valent pneumococcal conjugate vaccine on incidence of invasive pneumococcal disease—United States, 1998–2003. Morbidity and Mortality Weekly Report 54(36), 893–7. (2) Poehling KA, Talbot TR, Griffin R, et al. (2006). Invasive pneumococcal disease among infants before and after introduction of pneumococcal conjugate vaccine. JAMA 296; 1668–74. (3) Rodgers GL, Arguedas R, Cohen R, Dagan R. (2009). Global serotype distribution among Streptococcus pneumoniae isolates causing otitis media in children: potential implications for pneumococcal vaccines. Vaccine 27; 3802–10.

1.17). The vaccine has also reduced the racial disparities in IPD.

PCV7 proved to be a cost-effective vaccine because of the disease it prevents in young children but also because it provided herd immunity protection to their family members and the communities in which they lived (Table 1.5). However, while the PCV7 vaccine reduced IPD caused by the seven most common types causing infection in children, there are additional pneumococcal types that can also cause serious infections in children. Indeed, surveillance suggested that there was starting to be an increase in disease among children aged younger than 5 years due to these nonvaccine serotypes, some of which were antibiotic resistant.

Because PCV7 immunization of children also protected their family members from those serotypes in the vaccine, broadening the coverage of serotypes in the vaccine became even more desirable.

In 2010, the FDA licensed a 13-valent pneumococcal conjugate vaccine (PCV13), and that vaccine was recommended as a replacement for PCV7 in young children. However, the PPS23 vaccine also continues to be used in adults and older children because it prevents infection from additional pneumococcal serotypes.

Neisseria meningitidis

Neisseria meningitidis, or the meningococcus, is a group of encapsulated bacteria that can cause life-threatening

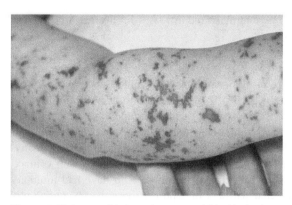

Figure 1.18 Purpura fulminans in a young child with shock due to meningococcal bacteremia. © Martin G. Myers

infections of the bloodstream, bacterial meningitis, or both. *N. meningitidis* can kill children, adolescents, and young adults within hours despite early diagnosis and the use of effective antibiotics. Serious complications occur in 11–19% of survivors, including deafness and other neurologic impairment as well as purpura and shock that may lead to gangrene and amputation of limbs (Figure 1.18). Because these bacteria are also communicable, the occurrence of a case of disease in schools is very upsetting to communities.

At least 13 serogroups of *N. meningitidis* have been identified, but almost all invasive disease is caused by 1 of 5 serogroups: A, B, C, Y, and W-135. The relative importance of each serogroup depends on the geographic location, as well as other factors, such as age and crowding. For example, serogroup A is a major cause of disease in sub-Saharan Africa but is rarely isolated in the USA, whereas serogroup C has been dominant in the UK and serogroup B in New Zealand.

Large outbreaks of meningococcal disease occur in sub-Saharan Africa during the dry season (December through June) and among travelers to Mecca during hajj. However, epidemics have not occurred in the USA since the 1940s, although outbreaks continue to occur sporadically. With major reductions in the frequency of Hib and pneumococcal infections, *N. meningitidis* has now become a major cause of invasive bacterial infections in the USA. Approximately 2,600 cases of meningococcal meningitis occur in children younger than 5 years old.

Meningococcal disease in the USA occurs most frequently among children younger than 2 years of age;

another disease peak occurs between 15 and 24 years of age. In addition, military recruits and first-year college students, especially those living in dormitories, also have an elevated risk for meningococcal disease. Finally, close contacts of a person with meningococcal infection have a higher risk of infection, sufficient to warrant that some of these persons may be given antibiotics to prevent infection, depending on the type of exposure.

The first monovalent (group C) polysaccharide vaccine was licensed in the USA in 1974, and a quadrivalent polysaccharide vaccine against serogroups A, C, Y, and W-135 (MPS4) was licensed in 1978, which was used for individuals who were at increased risk from invasive meningococcal disease.

A quadrivalent conjugate vaccine (MCV4) was licensed in the USA in 2005 and recommended for routine use among adolescents at 11–12 years of age with a booster dose at 16. The vaccine is also recommended for others at increased risk from meningococcal disease, including those who work with the organisms (such as clinical microbiologists), travelers to hyperendemic or epidemic areas, adolescents with HIV infection, and those with complement immunodeficiencies or functional or anatomic asplenia.

Prior to US licensure of the MCV4 vaccine for children ages 11 to 12, older adolescents, and young adults, the incidence of meningococcal disease was at its nadir of 0.35 per 100,000 in the USA, although it varied from 0.5 to 1.5 cases per 100,000 population over the preceding decades.

Unfortunately, there is no serogroup B vaccine in the USA, which is the most frequent etiology of meningococcal disease in young infants and children, because the structure of the polysaccharide is similar to that of human tissue. With the complete genome of multiple serogroup organisms now available, it is hoped that a vaccine may be feasible by identifying other unrecognized surface proteins that are highly conserved. Currently, one vaccine has been licensed in Europe and another is in phase III trials.

Vaccines for hepatitis viruses

Hepatitis is a generic term for liver inflammation. In the late 19th century, it was recognized that a form of hepatitis was transmissible in human lymph used in a smallpox campaign in Germany and blood products were recognized as a source of hepatitis during World

War II after yellow fever vaccine containing human serum as a stabilizer was given to US soldiers. These observations were confirmed by direct inoculation of volunteers. In the 1960s and 1970s two types of hepatitis were distinguished. One was transmissible by the fecal–oral route and had a shorter incubation period ("infectious hepatitis" or hepatitis A) and the other by the percutaneous route with a longer incubation period ("serum hepatitis" or hepatitis B). Presently, five viruses (hepatitis A to E) are recognized as causing hepatitis. There are vaccines available to prevent two in the USA and Europe, and a hepatitis E vaccine has recently been licensed in China.

Hepatitis B virus vaccine

Hepatitis B virus (HBV) infection causes subclinical infection, acute hepatitis, fulminant hepatitis, and chronic hepatitis. The age of the individual at acquisition of HBV infection is the single most important factor in determining the clinical manifestation of infection as well as the development of chronic infection. Younger individuals are the least likely to have clinical illness but have the greatest likelihood of chronic hepatitis B infection.

Persons with chronic HBV infection (also called "chronic carriers") are usually asymptomatic and often unaware that they are infected. About 5% of adults and 90% of newborns who are infected will develop chronic HBV infection. Approximately 25% of chronic HBV carriers die prematurely from chronic liver disease or hepatocellular carcinoma. Annually in the USA, 3000–4000 persons die from cirrhosis and another 1000–1500 from liver cancer due to HBV.

In the USA, HBV is transmitted most frequently by perinatal transmission from infected mothers to their newborns at birth, by sexual contact, by percutaneous exposure to body fluids (such as serum, saliva, semen, and vaginal fluid), or by nonsexual person-to-person contact.

The detection of an antigen in the blood of Australian aborigines in 1965—now known to have been a marker for hepatitis B surface antigen (HBsAg)—quickly led to initial trials of boiled serum as a potential vaccine. Initial plasma-derived vaccines, licensed in the USA in 1981, were quickly supplanted after the elucidation of the genomic sequence of HBV, including sequencing of the HBsAg. Recombinant HBsAg vaccine, manufactured in yeast, was licensed in the USA in 1986.

Initial HBV vaccine interventions in the USA between 1981 and 1991 targeted the highest risk groups of acquiring HBV infection by screening mothers for HBsAg (in order to begin immunization of their infants in the nursery and to give them hepatitis B immunoglobulin [HBIG]) and by attempting to identify those with risk factors. Unfortunately, many with risk factors (such as heterosexuals with contact with infected persons; those who have had multiple sexual partners or whose partner has had multiple sexual partners; intravenous drug users; and men who have sex with men) either did not know that they had a risk factor, were hard to reach, or denied having a risk factor.

In 1991, the vaccination recommendation was expanded to include immunization of all newborn infants for the following reasons:

• Universal immunization of children has proven to be the most effective immunization strategy
• Approximately 30% of people who get HBV infection do not have any identifiable risk factors, including children
• HBV infection of children of all ages leads to an increased risk to develop chronic HBV infection

In 2005, HBV vaccine recommendations were expanded further to include the following:

• Routine infant hepatitis B vaccination to begin at birth, before hospital discharge
• Implementation of enhanced programs to detect perinatal HBV infection
• Routine immunization of all previously unvaccinated children and adolescents
• Identification and vaccination of previously unvaccinated adults who were at increased risk for infection by virtue of being in settings where a high proportion of adults are likely to have a risk factor for HBV (such as incarcerated persons)

Many countries that have instituted routine HBV immunization of infants, children, and adolescents have begun reporting declines in HBV infections and declines in HBV-related liver disease. In the USA, a number of states have also begun to report similar outcomes.

Hepatitis A vaccine

Hepatitis A is caused by hepatitis A virus (HAV), a picornavirus that causes infection that is spread primarily by the fecal–oral route, particularly in regions with poor sanitary conditions. Children are the major sources of infection, being infected at an early age in developing countries. They usually have asymptomatic infection but they can shed the virus in their stool for long periods of time. Older children and adults usually develop symptoms that include fever, weakness, nausea, abdominal pain, dark urine, and yellow eyes and skin that lasts less than 2 months in most individuals, although as many as 10–15% will have illness lasting up to 6 months.

In the pre-vaccine era in the USA, there were 125,000–200,000 symptomatic cases and 70–100 died, most over the age of 40 years. About one third of the hepatitis A cases in the USA occurred in children 5 to 14 years of age. The lowest rate of infection was in adults older than 40 years of age.

In developed countries, outbreaks sometimes occur when many people have eaten from the same HAV-infected food source. In recent years, international travel has become a major source of HAV outbreaks.

However, almost half of people who acquire HAV infection have no identifiable risk factor.

In the USA, hepatitis A disease occurs in community-wide outbreaks, with infection being transmitted from person to person in households and extended family settings. Infected individuals are most likely to spread HAV during the 2-week period before they know they are infected. Since most infected preschool children show no symptoms of HAV infection, they often unknowingly spread the virus to others.

Before vaccine, an interesting observation was that the rates of HAV infection and disease were much greater in some areas of the country than others. As a consequence, the hepatitis A vaccine was introduced incrementally first for children living in communities with the highest rates of disease (1996) and then for children living in states or communities with consistently elevated rates of infection (1999). The impact of immunization with hepatitis A vaccine was a dramatic decline in the rates of disease and a sharp reduction in the groups with the highest risk of infection: American Indians and Alaska Natives. Rates of hepatitis A infection are now similar in most areas of the USA (Figure 1.19). As a consequence, hepatitis A vaccine

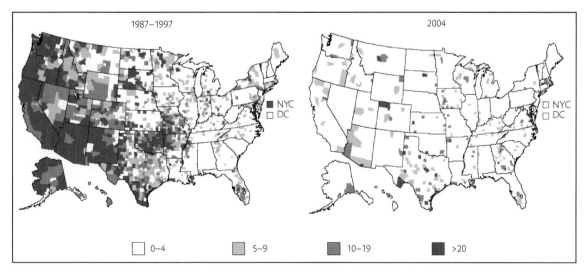

Figure 1.19 Rate of hepatitis A by county in the USA, 1987–1997 and 2004, per 100,000 population.. From Centers for Disease Control and Prevention. (2006). Prevention of Hepatitis A through active or passive immunization: recommendations of the Advisory Committee on Immunization Practices (ACIP). Morbidity and Mortality Weekly Report 55 (No. RR-7), 1–23.

has now been recommended for all children in the USA who are 12–23 months of age in order to eliminate HAV transmission nationally.

Because international travel represents such an important source of infection in the USA, families should be immunized against HAV 4 weeks before an internationally adopted child enters the household or before they embark on international travel, although travelers to Australia, Canada, western Europe, Japan, and New Zealand are at no increased risk than individuals residing in the USA. If there is insufficient time to assure immunity to HAV (at least 4 weeks), prospective parents should discuss with their health professional whether they and other family members should receive immunoglobulin prophylaxis.

Vaccines for human papillomaviruses

Human papillomaviruses (HPVs) are a group of more than 120 serologically different viruses (termed "types"). Some HPV types are spread by casual skin-to-skin contact with another person; for example, type 1 causes plantar warts on the feet and types 2 and 3 cause warts on the fingers. Others are acquired by intimate sexual contact. Approximately 40 HPV types are primarily sexually transmitted from person to person (for example, genital–genital contact, oral–genital contact, and sexual intercourse), infecting the oral, anal, or genital areas of both men and women. Genital HPV infections are very common: 25% of females have been infected with genital HPVs by 15–19 years of age, 45% by 20–24 years of age, and 70–80% by 50 years of age.

The US Centers for Disease Control and Prevention (CDC) estimates that 6.2 million Americans get a new genital HPV infection each year. Sexually active adolescents and young adults are most likely to acquire genital HPV infection. Genital HPV infections are often acquired within a few months after beginning sexual activity. The prevalence declines with age after 25 years, but increases again in women about the time of menopause. Genital infection with more than one type of HPV is common.

The vast majority of people recover from genital HPV infections uneventfully. Most genital HPV infections cause no symptoms and are cleared by the immune system within a few weeks or months. However, some people develop persistent genital HPV infection. Persistent infection with nononcogenic

types of genital HPV can lead to genital warts in some people. Thus, types 6 and 11 are responsible for more than 90% of the 250,000 cases of genital warts in the USA. While it is rare, these types may also spread from mother to infant during delivery and can cause warts in the upper respiratory tract (throat, larynx) of the child. Persistent infection with "high-risk," oncogenic genital types of HPV can lead to precancerous changes that, in turn, can lead to carcinoma *in situ*, which may progress to invasive cancer. Types 16 and 18 and other high-risk types may cause abnormal Pap tests and cervical cancer in women, as well as a number of other cancers in both men and women. Although there are a number of other risk factors for cervical cancer, being infected with a high-risk type HPV appears to be a necessary factor for cervical cancer development. High-risk HPV infections are also thought to cause 85% of anal cancers, 50% of other anogenital cancers, 20% of cancers of the throat and mouth, and 10% of cancers of the larynx and esophagus. Cancer registry data have shown an annual 1% increase in oropharyngel and a 3% increase in anal cancers that are genital HPV associated.

A quadrivalent HPV recombinant vaccine (HPV4) containing vaccine-like particles consisting of the L1 external protein from HPV types 6, 11, 16, 18 was licensed for use in females in 2006, and a similar bivalent vaccine containing HPV types 16 and 18 (HPV2) was licensed in 2009. In 2009, HPV4 was also licensed for the prevention of warts in males and, in 2010, for the prevention of anal cancers in both males and females. Both vaccines have proven effective at preventing HPV infections of the specific HPV types contained in the vaccines and, therefore, prevent precancers and cancers due to HPV types 16 and 18. HPV4 has also been shown to prevent genital warts due to HPV 6 and 11 in both males and females.

In 2011, routine vaccination with HPV4 was recommended for all children 11–12 years of age as a three-dose series, although the vaccination series can be started in children as young as 9 years of age. Catch-up HPV4 vaccination has also been recommended for males 13 through 21 years of age and for females 13–26 years of age. Men who have sex with men should be immunized through 26 years of age. The vaccine is also licensed for use in males through 26 years of age and women through 45 years of age.

Influenza

Widespread epidemics of respiratory disease—presumably influenza—have been documented for hundreds of years. In the 19th century it was mistakenly thought that influenza was caused by *Haemophilus influenzae* because of its detection in lungs of people who had died with pneumonia associated with these epidemics. However, when influenza viruses were isolated in the 1930s, it was correctly proven that these were the causative agents.

Influenza viruses are classified by the types of nucleoprotein and matrix protein. There are three major types of influenza virus, termed A, B, and C. Human infections are largely caused by influenza A and B viruses. Sporadic cases of influenza C, a pathogen largely of swine, occur but have not been associated with epidemics.

Influenza viruses replicate in ciliated columnar epithelial cells with destruction of the cells. Viremia is rarely demonstrable. Infection leads to both humoral and cellular immunity, but antibody titers to the

---

Seasonal Influenza

- Causes annual epidemics
- Is highly infectious with a 1–5 day incubation period
- Severity of illness depends on prior influenza virus immune experience, health, and age
- May cause no symptoms in 30–50% of those infected by the virus
- Symptomatic disease: abrupt onset of fever muscle aches, sore throat, cough and headache
- Many school days (and caregiver work days) lost
- Can trigger life-threatening complications:
  In an average year, 114,000 hospitalizations and approximately 20,000 deaths in the USA
- The most common vaccine preventable disease in the USA

---

surface glycoprotein, hemagglutinin (H), correlate with protection.

Most persons infected with influenza virus shed virus in their respiratory secretions for 4 or 5 days, although children—who shed more virus than adults—usually shed virus for up to 2 weeks; immunocompromised individuals may shed virus for months. Influenza virus is spread by coughing and sneezing but the hands are also an effective means of transmission person to person.

Influenza Virus Infections

Influenza A
- Moderate to severe illness
- Affects all age groups
- Infects animals and humans
- Associated with seasonal epidemics
- Associated with pandemics

Influenza B
- Similar illness
- Primarily affects children
- Infects humans only
- Aspirin-associated Reye's Syndrome*

Influenza C
- Similar illness
- Infects primarily pigs
- Humans infected sporadically

*An illness in children of encephalopathy and fatty degeneration of the liver, often fatal.

Influenza Complications

Most common among
- Older adults
- Those with chronic health problems such as asthma, lung disease (including smoking), obesity
- Children younger than 5 years of age (especially younger than 2)
- Pregnant women

Complications
- Bacterial pneumonia, sinusitis, otitis media
- Encephalitis in children
- Rhabdomyelitis in adults (rare)

27

Pandemic influenza

- An influenza pandemic is a sudden widespread outbreak of a new strain of influenza A
- Not every novel strain becomes pandemic
- Because the strain is new, virtually no one is immune
- Severity (the proportion who cannot work for 7–10 days, who have complications, and/or die) varies substantially

Children spread the virus rapidly both within families and among themselves. Because many people (30–50%) are asymptomatic—or because they work while ill—health providers also frequently transmit virus to the most vulnerable persons in society.

Influenza illness onset is abrupt with fever, myalgias, which often causes prostration; chills; anorexia; and cough; it usually lasts about 7 days. In very young children the degree of fever and the child's irritability will often lead to hospitalization. In people with medical problems and in those over 65 years of age serious complications—mostly bacterial pneumonia—occur more frequently and may be fatal. In the USA, influenza is the most common cause of vaccine-preventable deaths, accounting for an average of approximately 24,000 deaths per year, mostly among those greater than 65 years of age.

Influenza A viruses are further subtyped according to the antigenic properties of the surface proteins—there are 18 types of hemagglutinin (H) and 11 types of neuraminidase (N). Fortunately, not all types of H and N are capable of infecting humans. Presently, influenza A types H1N1, H1N2, H3N2, and influenza B viruses are circulating in the population. Human influenza viruses are customarily identified by region of isolation, the year of isolation and the isolate number as well—such as A/Perth/16/2009 (H3N2) and B/Brisbane/60/2008.

Influenza viruses, especially influenza A viruses, cause annual epidemics, which in temperate climates occur in the autumn and winter. They are "promiscuous" viruses in the sense that during mixed infection of the same cell by two different influenza viruses the segmented single-stranded RNA (8 segments) can rapidly reassort and—without DNA and an associated repair mechanism—the H, a very plastic molecule, can mutate, or "drift," in response to immunologic pressure. However, the virus is said to have "shifted" when the H of the viruses circulating in the community changes dramatically, for example, from A (H2N2) to (H3N2) as it did in 1967–1968,

Wild waterfowl, which usually do not become ill, are the natural reservoirs of influenza A, transmitting viruses to other animals, including domestic poultry (which may be rapidly killed) and mammals where they may recombine with mammalian influenza viruses to create new strains that may lead to antigenic shift.

When there has been a shift, most of the population is susceptible to infection and a pandemic may ensue, often involving different risk groups and which may occur at different times of the year. Many new strains emerge but pandemics only occur from time to time, usually three or four times a century. The occurrence of a pandemic requires the emergence of a strain to which most everyone is susceptible and a virus that transmits easily person to person. The severity of a pandemic is dependent on the virulence of the pathogen.

In 2009, a new influenza A strain emerged causing the best-studied pandemic in 2009–2010. Due to advances in molecular biology scientists were able to monitor the pandemic in "real-time." The novel virus contains gene segments from viruses circulating in swine, including the H derived from the 1918 pandemic as shown in Figure 1.20.

The ensuing pandemic caused a higher rate of hospitalizations and deaths among children, pregnant women, and young adults. Of the 99.6% of influenza isolates that year that were influenza A, 99.8% were the pandemic strain, whereas previously circulating seasonal strains accounted for the remainder.

Influenza vaccines

To prepare candidate virus strains for vaccine manufacture, various reassortant methods are utilized to rapidly create strains that contain the desirable H and N surface proteins while rendering the strain suitable for multiplication in embryonated chicken eggs to high titer.

Ideally, in the Northern hemisphere, people should receive their annual influenza vaccine from the beginning of October through November each year, prior to the influenza season, which generally peaks during

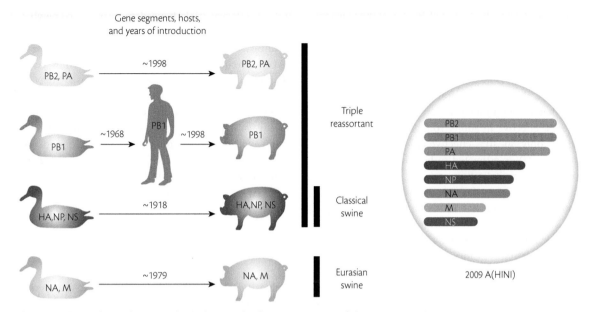

Figure 1.20 Host (avian, human and swine) origins for the gene segments of the 2009 A(H1N1) virus: PB2, polymerase basic 2; PB1, polymerase basic 1; PA, polymerase acidic; HA, hemagglutinin; NP, nucleoprotein; NA, neuraminidase; M, matrix gene; NS, nonstructural gene. Color of gene segment in circle indicates host. From Garten RJ, Davis CT, Russell CA, et al. (2009). Antigenic and genetic characteristics of swine-origin 2009 A(H1N1) influenza viruses circulating in humans. Science 325(5937), 197–201.

late December through March. However, vaccination later in the season is still considered worthwhile.

The effectiveness of influenza vaccines varies by how good the match is between the H contained in the vaccine and the strains that actually circulate in the population.

In 2010, in an attempt to reduce disease morbidity and mortality, the USA instituted a universal annual immunization policy for everyone older than 6 months of age. Because influenza vaccines are not effective in children younger than 6 months of age, immunization of their caregivers is particularly encouraged.

Inactivated influenza vaccines

Influenza vaccines were first licensed in the USA in 1945 as formalin-inactivated virus grown in the allantoic fluid of embryonated chicken eggs. Currently, all influenza vaccine candidate seed strains must be isolated in specific pathogen-free eggs under conditions of documented good laboratory practices. Although most inactivated influenza vaccines in the USA are still grown in eggs, there are several vaccines licensed that

have been prepared in cell cultures, either chick embryo fibroblasts or Madin–Darby canine kidney (MDCK) cells (depending on the country). Cell culture-derived vaccines will reduce the supply limitations imposed by the need for specific pathogen-free embryonated eggs.

Currently in the USA, following viral inactivation with either formalin or β-propriolactone, the virus particles are disrupted by a solvent in order to separate the H and N proteins from the matrix and nucleoproteins, greatly reducing the numbers of febrile and local vaccine reactions that occurred with inactivated whole cell vaccines.

Because of the rapid drifting of the H, a new vaccine must be formulated annually. Usually, the vaccines have been formulated to contain three virus strains (H1, H3, and B; trivalent) that are selected as those expected to be the most likely to affect the USA in the upcoming winter. For the 2009–2010 season, there was also a monovalent vaccine prepared that was deployed separately from the seasonal vaccine because the newly recognized pandemic strain appeared after it was too late to be included in the 2009 seasonal vaccine formulations. For 2013–2014, there is also a quadrivalent formulation containing two A and two B viruses.

With a good match between the vaccine components and the circulating influenza strains, the trivalent inactivated influenza vaccine (TIV) has been 70–90% effective in adults younger than 65 years of age but only 30–40% effective among older persons. However, TIV is estimated to be 50–60% effective at preventing hospitalization and 80% effective at preventing death (90% of deaths occurring in those older than 64 years of age).

In 2010, a new high-dose formulation of TIV became available for use in people 65 years of age or older that contained four times the amount of H and N in an attempt to induce a higher immune response in these older persons. This TIV vaccine appears to have slightly higher rates of local reactions but may afford greater protection.

TIV is given by the intramuscular route; its formulation differs according to the manufacturer. It cannot cause influenza—although they may cause mild "flulike" symptoms of fever, and myalgias as well as local reactions at the injection site—but they do prevent the complications of influenza.

Live attenuated influenza vaccine

Cold adaption of influenza viruses (i.e., adaptation in cell culture to multiply at low temperatures only so that the vaccine virus does not multiply at the body temperature [37°C]) was demonstrated to be attenuated for humans. Using genetic reassortants with master strains has permitted the selection of attenuated vaccine candidate strains that are attenuated containing the desirable H and N. In 2003, such a live, attenuated, cold-adapted, temperature-sensitive, trivalent influenza virus vaccine (LAIV) was licensed in the USA and Europe. LAIV is administered as a nasal spray and is the first nasally administered vaccine to be marketed in the USA, as well as the first live virus influenza vaccine approved in the USA. The temperature-sensitive strains of virus contained in LAIV replicate in the nasal passages but not in the lower respiratory tract.

The possible advantages of LAIV are that it is easy to administer and that it has the potential to induce broad mucosal and systemic immune responses.

Indeed, efficacy trials have demonstrated somewhat broader protection than TIV for influenza virus drift. Because of presumed viral interference, two doses of LAIV are required in children younger than 8 years of age to ensure serologic protection in 96% of recipients.

Because LAIV was associated with an increased risk among asthmatic children and has not been studied in others with medical problems or in older persons, LAIV is only administered to healthy persons 2–49 years of age, depending on the country.

In 2013, a quadrivalent live attenuated vaccine was licensed that contains two A viruses and two B viruses.

Rotavirus vaccines

Rotaviruses cause intestinal infection in many species of mammals, including humans, cows, and monkeys. The animal strains are antigenically distinct from those that cause human infection, and they rarely cause infection in humans.

Human rotaviruses infect virtually all children by 3 years of age. The incidence of clinical illness is highest among children 3 to 35 months of age, suggesting that maternal antibodies may initially be protective. Breast-fed infants also generally have less diarrheal disease than non-breast-fed infants.

Rotaviruses are the most common cause of severe diarrhea and dehydration in children. The illness also causes fever and vomiting, which may persist for a week or longer; it can cause persistent infection in immunocompromised people. The immune correlates of protection from rotavirus are poorly understood. However, recovery from rotavirus infection usually does not lead to permanent immunity, although the first infection is usually the most severe. After a single natural infection, most are protected against severe rotavirus diarrhea. Subsequent infections appear to confer progressively greater protection, although recurrent rotavirus infections affect persons of all ages, resulting in either asymptomatic infection or mild diarrhea that may be accompanied by vomiting and low-grade fever.

Most rotavirus infections are mild, but in about 1 in 50 cases, patients develop severe dehydration. Each year in the USA before vaccine, rotavirus infections resulted in 22.5 hospitalizations and 301 emergency

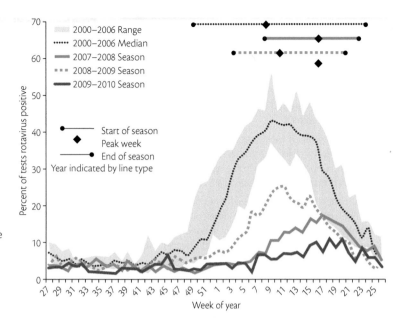

Figure 1.21 Percentage of positive rotavirus tests by week and year: USA 2000–2010. From panel A of figure 1, Tate JE, Mutuc JD, Panozzo CA, et al. (2011). Sustained decline in rotavirus detection in the United States following the introduction of rotavirus vaccine in 2006. Pediatric Infectious Diseases 30; S30–S34.

room visits per 10,000 children younger than 3 years of age. That translates to 1 in 150 children being hospitalized and another 1 in 11 who required medical attention in an emergency room or an outpatient clinic for rotavirus infection. Of those with severe rotavirus infection, loss of intestinal disaccharidases often causes secondary milk intolerance. Before vaccine, it was the cause of 20 to 40 deaths in the USA annually; in developing countries, rotavirus leads to an estimated 480,000 to 640,000 deaths each year.

An initial rotavirus vaccine, a tetravalent, reassortant rhesus–human rotavirus vaccine was licensed in 1998. However, after approximately 1 million children had been immunized with that vaccine, the CDC detected an unexpected increase in the number of children who developed intussusceptions—a potentially lethal bowel disease—after the first dose of vaccine, at a rate of approximately 1 case per 10,000 infants vaccinated (which is about three times more frequently than among unvaccinated children). That vaccine was withdrawn in 1999.

Two additional rotavirus vaccines, a pentavalent human–bovine reassortant vaccine and a monovalent naturally occurring less virulent human strain, were each extensively tested in more than 60,000 children before their licensure in 2006 and 2008, respectively, to be certain that they were not associated with intus-

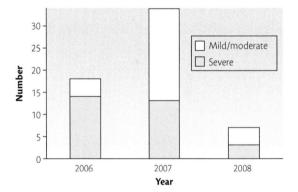

Figure 1.22 Number of children with mild/moderate and severe rotavirus diarrhea in Aracaju, 2006–2008. From Gurgel RG et al. (2009). Gastroenterology 137:1970–1975.

susceptions. In 2010 DNA fragments of porcine circovirus (a single-stranded DNA virus that naturally infects pigs) were detected in one vaccine and then the second vaccine. After extensive review, the FDA determined that it was safe to use both vaccines. Both vaccines are effective against rotavirus gastroenteritis of any severity and both have high efficacy against severe rotavirus gastroenteritis. The vaccines have impacted cases of rotavirus both in the USA (Figure 1.21) and in the developing world (Figure 1.22).

31

Summary

- The history of vaccine development is intimately linked to the evolution of the biologic and medical sciences. Initial vaccines were developed empirically, but as science has progressed so have the technologies used to develop vaccines.

- There have been great successes at the development of vaccines for childhood diseases, which have resulted in huge decreases in the number of cases, such that many of these diseases are rarely seen today.

- New understandings of diseases pathogenesis, modern technologies, and strategies for developing pathogenic insights suggest that the future of vaccinology will lead to new ways to prevent and treat diseases with vaccines.

Further reading

Plotkin SA and Plotkin SP (2011). The development of vaccines: how the past led to the future. Nature Reviews Microbiology 9, 889–893.

Vaccines, 6th edition (eds SA Plotkin, WA Orenstein, and PA Offit), New York: Academic Press, 2013.

2 The vaccine development pathway

David W.C. Beasley

Sealy Center for Vaccine Development, Galveston National Laboratory Regulatory Compliance Core, and Department of Microbiology & Immunology, University of Texas Medical Branch, Galveston, TX, USA

Abbreviations

BLA	Biologics License Application	ICH	International Conference on Harmonisation
CBER	Center for Biologics Evaluation and Research	IND	Investigational new drug
		NRA	National regulatory authority
CDC	US Centers for Disease Control and Prevention	OECD	Organisation for Economic Cooperation and Development
DSMB	Data safety monitoring board	TGA	Therapeutic Goods Administration
		US FDA	US Food and Drug Administration
EMA	European Medicines Agency	VAERS	Vaccine Adverse Event Reporting System
EUA	Emergency use authorization	VRBPAC	Vaccines and Related Biological Products Advisory Committee
GLP	Good laboratory practice		
GMP	Good manufacturing practice	WHO	World Health Organization

Introduction

Vaccines represent a relatively small proportion of the entire pharmaceuticals industry, but in the past decade there has been an increasing interest from both public and private sector groups in developing new vaccine products for a range of infectious and noninfectious diseases. Several new vaccines have achieved "blockbuster" status, with annual US sales in excess of $500 million. However, the time line for development and approval for most vaccines is long, usually in excess of 15 years, and it requires investments of hundreds of millions of dollars as the candidate vaccine moves toward regulatory approval. This chapter will provide a high level overview of the vaccine development process, each component of which will be covered in greater detail in subsequent chapters.

The primary considerations in the eventual approval of a vaccine product are safety, immunogenicity, and efficacy, meaning a relative freedom from harmful effect and a reasonable expectation that, when used correctly, the product will serve a clinically significant function in the treatment or prevention of disease. Throughout the history of vaccination the perceived importance of safety versus efficacy has varied, but at the present time the expectation of most vaccine recipients is for very high efficacy with essentially no risks to safety—a very challenging expectation for a complex biological product that mediates its effect via activation of multiple components of a host immune

Vaccinology: An Essential Guide, First Edition. Edited by Gregg N. Milligan and Alan D.T. Barrett.
© 2015 John Wiley & Sons, Ltd. Published 2015 by John Wiley & Sons, Ltd.

response. Unlike most drug products, which are given therapeutically to treat a sick person, vaccines are generally administered to otherwise healthy individuals, often children, to prevent disease (i.e., prophylactic vaccination). The challenge for manufacturers and regulators is to effectively balance the expectations for safety and for efficacy so as to permit the timely licensure of vaccine products without unnecessarily adding to the cost and duration of nonclinical and clinical testing. Note the term "nonclinical" was proposed by the World Health Organization (WHO) to describe all research undertake prior to studies in humans. Most countries have adopted this term. In the USA, the terms *preclinical* and *nonclinical* are both employed in describing aspects of development and testing not directly related to clinical trials. The term *nonclinical* is used in this chapter.

A schematic of the typical phases of vaccine development and approval is shown in Figure 2.1. The progression through basic discovery to nonclinical

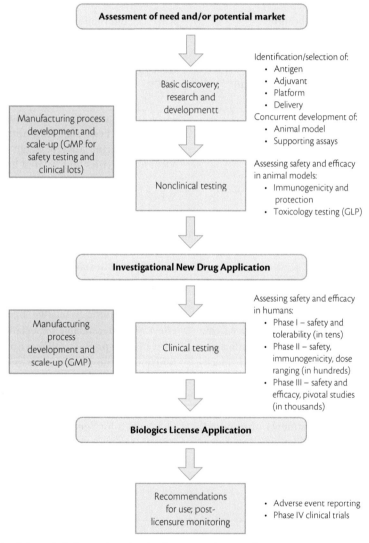

Figure 2.1 A schematic of the typical phases of vaccine development and approval.

testing and clinical trials involves increasingly greater investment on the part of the vaccine developer and is usually driven by progress at key development and regulatory decision points. Most of the vaccines currently licensed in the USA have their origins in academic or government research programs and were subsequently licensed to pharmaceutical companies for further development and testing. The costs of nonclinical development and the resources required for manufacturing of the vaccine product have traditionally required the involvement of a major pharmaceutical company, although in the past decade the role of government public health agencies and not-for-profit organizations in funding and directing the advanced development of vaccine products has increased, particularly for the development of biodefense-related vaccines and so-called poverty vaccines (vaccines where there is a need but no one to pay for the vaccine).

Key terms and definitions

Safety: Relative freedom from harmful effect.
Purity: Relative freedom from extraneous matter.
Potency: Specific ability/capacity of the product to affect a given result.
Efficacy: Reasonable expectation that when administered under adequate directions for use will serve a clinically significant function in diagnosis, cure, mitigation, treatment, or prevention of disease.
Immunogenicity: Ability of a vaccine to stimulate an immune response. Measurements of immunogenicity may include antigen-specific antibody titers, seroconversion rates, cellular immunity, cytokine responses, or other immune parameters.

The decision to develop a vaccine is usually based on some assessment of market need. The instigation of research on a new vaccine candidate is often via academic or government researchers funded by public health agencies or nongovernment organizations, whose perception of market need may be somewhat altruistic and focused on the relative public health importance or global incidence of a particular disease. However, the ultimate decision to progress a candidate

vaccine product through the development and testing process has invariably been based on financial considerations: Will the cost of development, manufacture, and distribution be exceeded by the anticipated revenue obtained by the licensed vaccine? In the case of infectious diseases more commonly found in the developing world, where individuals and governments may lack the financial resources to purchase a vaccine product, that new vaccine may still be considered worthwhile on the basis of potential markets among travelers or developed world governments that can afford to pay a premium price.

An exception to this typical process in the past decade has been the development of biodefense-related vaccines (such as vaccines for smallpox, anthrax, and hemorrhagic fever viruses such as Ebola) funded by governments primarily for inclusion in emergency stockpiles or for use by government agencies. This has been seen by some in the industry as utilizing resources that might be more effectively applied to development of vaccines for diseases that are prevalent and represent a current threat to human health. However, one positive outcome of this surge in vaccine-related research and development is an improved understanding of the economic and regulatory considerations associated with vaccine development among many basic science researchers. Coupled with the implementation of various quality system elements during early research, the overlap between research and development activities is likely to improve the quality of intellectual property associated with many public sector discoveries, minimize the amount of fundamental basic science work that needs to be repeated, and ease the transition of these candidate products into the industrial development process.

Regulation and approval of vaccines

Licensure of candidate vaccines, like other drug products, is typically the responsibility of a national regulatory authority (NRA). In the USA, this is the Food and Drug Administration (US FDA; http://www.fda.gov) and, more specifically, the Center for Biologics Evaluation and Research (CBER). This chapter will focus on vaccine development and approval processes as they currently exist in the USA. In the European

Union, products are licensed by the European Medicines Agency (EMA; http://www.ema.europa.eu), but there are numerous individual NRAs throughout the world that license products manufactured within their own countries or that may be imported by a multinational manufacturer (see Chapter 12). Regulatory agencies like the US FDA not only review vaccine licensing applications but also inspect facilities involved in all phases of vaccine development and manufacture to ensure compliance with the appropriate regulations covering each of those activities and can impose penalties on facilities and individuals for noncompliance.

Licensure of vaccines and other medical products is generally based on an assessment of the relative risks versus benefits for the product. For example, the Therapeutic Goods Administration (TGA; http://www.tga.gov.au), which licenses vaccines in Australia, employs a "risk management approach" to the regulation of therapeutic goods (http://www.tga.gov.au/industry/basics-regulation-risk-management.htm). This relies on (1) identifying, assessing, and evaluating risks posed by therapeutic goods, (2) applying necessary measures for treating those risks, and (3) monitoring and reviewing risks over time, before and after licensure. Those risks may be inherent to the vaccine product itself, or its manufacturing process, or the way it is used in the clinic. Risk assessment and risk management by the manufacturer and the regulatory authority assure that the potential clinical benefit of the vaccine outweighs the potential risks.

Because many vaccine products are likely to have global markets, approval by multiple NRAs is often a consideration for vaccine developers. Interactions between NRAs are facilitated by nondisclosure agreements, allowing them to share information on candidate products, and by the International Conference on Harmonisation of Technical Requirements for Registration of Pharmaceuticals for Human Use (ICH). ICH publishes guidance documents on acceptable processes to establish safety, efficacy, and quality for drug and biologics (e.g., vaccines) development, including recommendations for the conduct of nonclinical testing and clinical trials. In addition, the WHO Expert Committee on Biological Standards provides guidance to governments on acceptable standards for vaccine development. Many governments have adopted WHO's specifications as the basis for their own licensing requirements for vaccines. The WHO also plays an important role via prequalification of some vaccines for use by United Nations agencies.

Basic research and development

Initial development of a candidate vaccine requires an understanding of the target disease, the infectious or other agent responsible for the disease, and the basis of protective immunity. These fundamental studies are typically performed in basic research laboratories, and from these starting points the vaccine researcher can begin to evaluate candidate immunogens and address related issues such as evaluation of available adjuvants and stabilizers to be incorporated in the final product.

Early decision points will include the selection of the most appropriate vaccine platform(s) to be included in development. For instance, live attenuated vaccines are often highly efficacious but carry risks associated with reversion to virulence or may cause disease in a small proportion of recipients with underlying health issues, whereas inactivated or nonreplicating antigens are typically safer but less immunogenic, probably require multiple doses, and will require an adjuvant to boost the immune response. This basic research and development must also include assessment of the likely efficacy of the candidate vaccine. Typically this will involve development of animal models of disease and/or identification of immunological markers indicative of protection (e.g., neutralizing antibodies) that can be measured using *in vitro* assays. These models and assays will also undergo further refinement as the candidate vaccine moves through the development pipeline.

A key component of the nonclinical development of a candidate vaccine is the demonstration of safety in animals. Nonclinical safety and toxicology testing for products submitted for licensure in the USA must be performed in compliance with regulations for good laboratory practice (GLP), as defined in 21 CFR 58, which defines minimum standards for performance and documentation of nonclinical studies and is intended to ensure the quality and integrity of data generated in support of product licensure. Other international guidance documents for GLP have been prepared by the Organisation for Economic Cooperation and Development (OECD) and the ICH.

Safety and toxicology studies aim to assess any direct toxic effect of the vaccine or the induced immune response. Testing is often performed in two animal species, typically rodent and nonhuman primate, and will include single dose and repeat dose studies using the same lot(s) of vaccine formulation that are intended to be employed for phase I clinical trials or, if that is not practical, using nonclinical lots that are comparable to clinical lots and manufactured under cGMP standards. Vaccine will be delivered via the intended route and at escalating doses including exceeding the maximum dose, and maximum number of doses, planned for evaluation in clinical trials. These studies assess both toxicological and pharmacodynamic parameters related to the direct effects of the vaccine and the induced host immune response as measures of safety. Given that some vaccines may

potentially be used in pregnant women, developmental toxicity studies employing pregnant animals may also be warranted to assess the possible impact of the vaccine on maternal health and fetal development, and to assess differences in vaccine performance. Immunizations will be timed to allow assessment of responses at varying stages during fetal development and postpartum.

Manufacturing and process development

The nonclinical development of experimental vaccine candidates must also include examination of the manufacturing process and preparations for scale-up from "experimental" production in a laboratory setting to the eventual industrial process-based manufacture of the vaccine. The production process must be scalable to ensure that minimal re-testing and reformulation occurs during the entire development and approval process, and planning for scale-up should ideally occur early in development with involvement of both scientific and process engineering experts. The formulation and manufacturing of vaccine products is usually more complex than that of many small molecule drug compounds and may require sophisticated processes to confirm the identity and purity of each component and the final product. Development of the manufacturing process must be accompanied by the development and validation of appropriate analytical methods to assess the purity and potency of the manufactured vaccine product.

Nonclinical testing may include use of pilot lot materials, sometimes developed under GLP conditions, but materials prepared for nonclinical safety studies and for use in subsequent clinical trials must be manufactured in compliance with regulations for GMP, as described in 21 CFR 211 and applicable sections of 21 CFR 600-680 (for vaccines, primarily 600/601). GMP aims to ensure the ongoing production of vaccine lots with consistent safety, purity, and potency, and includes requirements covering personnel, equipment, and procedures used during manufacturing, and for testing or characterization of raw materials used during production and the final vaccine product. Significant emphasis is placed on the characterization of materials used in vaccine production, which will vary depending upon the type of vaccine product but will almost always include biological products. Potential sources of contamination must be identified, absence of adventitious agents in raw biological materials must be verified, and the identity and growth properties of cell substrates must be determined. Testing for identity/purity, stability, sterility, adventitious agents, and residual process contaminants (e.g., cellular proteins or nucleic acids) will be performed at multiple stages of the production process.

Investigational New Drug Application: the "IND"

In the USA, the investigational new drug (IND) application is a request for authorization from the US FDA to administer an investigational vaccine (or other regulated product) to human patients and is required prior to interstate shipment and administration of any unapproved product in the USA. The requirements for an IND are spelled out in 21 CFR 312, and the documentation submitted to the US FDA CBER for review should describe not only the results of nonclinical testing (pharmacology and toxicology from GLP safety studies) and manufacturing (identity, potency, purity, safety, quality, stability) of the candidate vaccine but must define the investigational plan for clinical evaluation of the product, and specifically present the clinical protocol(s) for proposed phase I clinical trials and information that will be provided to study investigators. This information is essential to allow assessment of the potential risks and benefits associated with use of the candidate vaccine in humans, and to ensure that study participants are not subjected to unreasonable risks. The US FDA has 30 days following submission to review the IND application and determine if the proposed trial(s) may proceed or be placed on "clinical hold" (see the following section).

Holders of approved INDs must report to the US FDA during the course of clinical trials and submit annual reports that summarize ongoing activities related to the IND. The IND itself is a "living document" that will be updated and amended throughout the course of clinical testing as new information is obtained. New clinical trials, inclusion of new investigators, and other significant changes must all be incorporated by amendments to the IND. All clinical trials initiated or ongoing since September 2007 that involve drugs, biological products, or devices subject to US FDA regulation are also required to be registered with and report updated information to the US National Institutes of Health's Clinical Trials database (http://www.clinicaltrials.gov). The EMA has a similar database (http://www.clinicaltrialsregister.eu)

Major phases of clinical trials

21 CFR Part 312 "Investigational New Drug Application" section 21 defines the following phases for clinical trials:

- **Phase I** includes the initial introduction of an investigational new drug into humans. Phase I studies are typically closely monitored and may be conducted in patients or normal volunteer subjects. These studies are designed to determine the metabolism and pharmacologic actions of the drug in humans, the side effects associated with increasing doses, and, if possible, to gain early evidence on effectiveness. During phase I, sufficient information about the drug's pharmacokinetics and pharmacological effects should be obtained to permit the design of well-controlled, scientifically valid, phase II studies. The total number of subjects and patients included in phase I studies varies with the drug, but is generally in the range of 20 to 80.

- **Phase II** includes the controlled clinical studies conducted to evaluate the effectiveness of the drug for a particular indication or indications in patients with the disease or condition under study and to determine the common short-term side effects and risks associated with the drug. Phase II studies are typically well controlled, closely monitored, and conducted in a relatively small number of patients, usually involving no more than several hundred subjects.

- **Phase III** studies are expanded controlled and uncontrolled trials. They are performed after preliminary evidence suggesting effectiveness of the drug has been obtained, and are intended to gather the additional information about effectiveness and safety that is needed to evaluate the overall benefit–risk relationship of the drug and to provide an adequate basis for physician labeling. Phase III studies usually include from several hundred to several thousand subjects.

Clinical trials

The clinical testing of a new vaccine is designed to assess the safety, immunogenicity, and efficacy of that product in human recipients. Clinical trials typically occur in a stepwise fashion and will include predefined end points for measurements of safety, immunogenicity, and efficacy. Those end points are product specific and may be a clinical end point (e.g., reduction of disease in vaccinated subjects versus controls) or an immunological end point (e.g., seroconversion rates or neutralizing antibody titers) if this has been established as a correlate of protection or efficacy and deemed acceptable by the particular NRA.

Clinical trials intended for submission to the US FDA must be performed in compliance with principles of GCP and regulations for protection of human subjects, according to 21 CFR 50 (Protection of Human Subjects) and 56 (Institutional Review Boards). These aim to ensure the protection and safety of human study participants and the quality of data generated from the studies. Clinical trials may occur outside the USA and may require additional approvals from local authorities. Every entity performing a clinical investigation of a vaccine (or other US FDA-regulated product) must have an institutional review board (IRB) that is registered with the US FDA. The IRB is responsible for reviewing and approving each clinical trial protocol included in the IND and is required to carry out continuing review of active protocols on at least an annual basis, or more frequently based on assessment of risk.

The IND holder must report any unexpected events, and serious adverse events must be reported to the US FDA within 7 days, with a written report to be subsequently submitted following further investigation and evaluation. Before or during clinical studies, the US FDA may initiate a clinical hold, which is an order to delay a proposed study or suspend an in-progress study, often on the basis of concerns regarding safety, suitability of the protocol and/or investigators, insufficient documentation, or an inability to meet the study objectives. Large clinical trials, especially multisite trials, will often have an independent data safety monitoring board (DSMB) comprising experts in multiple disciplines. The DSMB will periodically review blinded or unblinded data throughout the trial to identify potential safety concerns and may recommend ending a study if significant problems are identified.

Phase I trials are usually the "first in human" safety and tolerability studies. These are typically performed using a small number (tens) of healthy individuals and often will include some assessment of immunogenicity. These studies will evaluate the anticipated dose(s) and route(s) of vaccine delivery and are expected to identify any significant safety problems. Phase I studies may be performed under "open label" conditions but are often randomized, controlled, and double-blinded. If the target population for the vaccine candidate is not healthy adults (e.g., pediatric or geriatric individuals), then initial safety testing in healthy adults will be followed by stepwise testing in other age groups.

Phase II trials are larger studies, usually involving several hundreds of subjects, and are designed primarily to assess vaccine immunogenicity. These studies will also provide a more extensive assessment of common adverse events. Dose ranging—the determination of an optimal dose for greatest safety and efficacy—will be assessed in phase II if not already included in phase I testing. There is often significant overlap between phase I and II studies during vaccine development, and each phase may include multiple clinical trials as additional information becomes available to the sponsor and the US FDA.

Phase III trials represent the most significant investment of time and resources during the development process. These are large-scale studies involving thousands of subjects, which means they can also facilitate detection of lower frequency adverse events, intended to demonstrate clinical efficacy of the candidate vaccine. Although multiple phase III studies may be performed, generally a "pivotal" study is undertaken that is designed to demonstrate efficacy and safety for the dose and schedule of immunization determined through phases I and II. The size of these studies will be determined by the known epidemiology of the target disease and the expected level of protection conferred by vaccination. They are often multisite studies, sometimes including study sites in multiple countries, and are randomized, placebo controlled, and double blinded (i.e., study participants and investigators do not know who receives vaccine or who receives the control). Generally two trials are required, unless a single large trial generates clear evidence of efficacy.

The biologics license application

Assuming the candidate vaccine progresses through the phases of nonclinical and clinical testing with favorable safety and efficacy parameters, the sponsor will prepare and submit a Biologics License Application (BLA). The BLA includes detailed information on the performance of the candidate vaccine in nonclinical and clinical testing, on the manufacturing processes and facilities that will be used for commercial production, which must be in compliance with regulations covering GMP, and on the proposed labeling of the vaccine product. The US FDA requires that at least 1 month prior to submission, the sponsor should provide an executive summary of the clinical studies that were performed, a description of the proposed format of the BLA submission, information on any ongoing studies still in progress, and any other information the sponsor may believe is relevant to discussion and evaluation of the candidate vaccine. At the time of BLA submission, the manufacturing facility must be ready for inspection to assess GMP compliance.

The entire BLA submission is reviewed by an internal US FDA CBER panel comprising experts from multiple disciplines (e.g., physicians, microbiologists, biostatisticians) to evaluate the reported safety, efficacy, purity, and potency of the candidate vaccine product, along with the capability for consistent manufacturing of that product. The CBER may conduct additional testing on the candidate product or components and the manufacturing facility (or facilities) will be inspected. The CBER may also seek advice from their Vaccines and Related Biological Products Advisory Committee (VRBPAC), which is an independent committee of non-US FDA experts, and other consultants regarding the adequacy of data in the BLA to support the proposed use of the vaccine. Another significant consideration is the proposed labeling of the product, which must provide sufficient information for health care providers to understand the intended and proper use of the vaccine, and its potential risks and benefits.

Ultimately, the vaccine may be licensed, additional studies may be required prior to approval, approval

> ### Some US Food and Drug Administration guidance documents related to vaccine development
>
> - Guidance for Industry: Formal Meetings Between the FDA and Sponsors or Applicants
> - Guideline on the Preparation of Investigational New Drug Products (Human and Animal)
> - Guidance for Industry: cGMP for Phase I Investigational Drugs
> - Guidance for Industry: Bioanalytical Method Validation
> - Guidance for Industry: Characterization and Qualification of Cell Substrates and Other Biological Materials Used in the Production of Viral Vaccines for Infectious Disease Indications
> - Guidance for Industry: Considerations for Plasmid DNA Vaccines for Infectious Disease Indications
> - Guidance for Industry: Toxicity Grading Scale for Healthy Adult and Adolescent Volunteers Enrolled in Preventive Vaccine Clinical Trials
> - Guidance for Industry: Considerations for Developmental Toxicity Studies for Preventive and Therapeutic Vaccines for Infectious Disease Indications
> - Guidance for Industry: Content and Format of Chemistry, Manufacturing and Controls Information and Establishment Description Information for a Vaccine or Related Product
> - Guidance for Industry: How to Complete the Vaccine Adverse Event Reporting System Form (VAERS-1)
> - Guidance for Industry for the Evaluation of Combination Vaccines for Preventable Diseases: Production, Testing and Clinical Studies

may be contingent on the sponsor performing additional post-licensure "phase IV" studies, or it may be rejected.

Meetings with regulatory agencies

Throughout the vaccine development and approval process, sponsors of candidate vaccines are required to meet with regulatory agencies to ensure that the proposed nonclinical, clinical and post-licensure studies are adequate. The unique nature of most vaccine products means that the expectations for appropriate testing are likely to vary and therefore must be dis-

Drafts

- Guidance for Industry: Non-Inferiority Clinical Trials
- Draft Guidance for Industry: Early Clinical Trials With Live Biotherapeutic Products: Chemistry, Manufacturing, and Control Information
- Draft Guidance for Industry: Clinical Considerations for Therapeutic Cancer Vaccines
- Draft Guidance for Industry: Considerations for Plasmid DNA Vaccines for Infectious Disease Indications
- Draft Guidance for Industry: Postmarketing Safety Reporting for Human Drug and Biological Products Including Vaccines
- Draft Guidance for Industry: Considerations for Reproductive Toxicity Studies for Preventive Vaccines for Infectious Disease Indications

(Vaccine-related US FDA guidance documents are accessible at http://www.fda.gov/BiologicsBloodVaccines/GuidanceComplianceRegulatoryInformation/Guidances/Vaccines/default.htm)

cussed and evaluated with regulators throughout the development process. Critical meetings with the US FDA occur at specific phases of the development process: (1) prior to submission of an IND, to ensure adequacy of the nonclinical data; (2) after phase I and/or II clinical trials, to ensure adequate safety and/or efficacy has been demonstrated to warrant continuation to subsequent clinical trial phase(s) and agree on the design of those studies; and (3) prior to submission of the BLA to ensure that US FDA staff are aware of the proposed content of the BLA and can provide advice to the sponsor on effective preparation of the application. These meetings are all designed to resolve questions and issues, thereby streamlining the development and approval processes, and minimizing wasted time and resources, both for the sponsor and for the agency.

Post-licensure activities

Once a vaccine is licensed, manufacturing must be accompanied by ongoing lot release testing to ensure consistency of the manufactured product. This testing includes assessments of sterility, safety (in animal models), identity, purity, and potency. Samples of each lot are also submitted to the US FDA, which may perform its own testing. US FDA also conducts inspections of manufacturing facilities at least every 2 years to ensure continued GMP compliance. Any significant changes to the manufacturing process or requests for changes in the approved use of the vaccine will require additional post-licensure studies.

Manufacturers and government public health agencies conduct continued monitoring for adverse events and assessment of approved vaccine effectiveness in "real world" populations. In some cases this may be a condition of licensure. Given that vaccine clinical trials are generally performed on otherwise healthy individuals, or groups that meet particular eligibility criteria, the actual effectiveness of the vaccine in reducing disease and the rates of particular adverse events may be different to the safety and efficacy observed in a particular clinical trial population. Phase IV studies may be employed to assess ongoing performance of the vaccine over time. These post-licensure activities will also identify very rare serious adverse events. In the USA, post-licensure monitoring of vaccine safety is also facilitated via the Vaccine Adverse Event Reporting System (VAERS), which is jointly managed by the US FDA and the Centers for Disease Control and Prevention (CDC), and the CDC's Vaccine Safety Datalink. Health professionals and vaccine manufacturers report vaccine-associated adverse events to those agencies using these systems, which allows for identification of rare and serious safety problems after licensure.

Alternative pathways to licensure

In addition to the processes outlined above, the US FDA has established alternative mechanisms to facilitate approval of certain types of vaccine products. A "fast track" mechanism has been established to facilitate development of vaccines and other products for high priority, life-threatening diseases or conditions. Under this fast track, the sponsor is promised frequent and early communication to facilitate design of phase II and III clinical trials, and priority review of the BLA in 6 months, rather than the standard 10-month time frame. Likewise, to encourage development of vaccines and other products for rare and neglected diseases, the US FDA has a priority review voucher mechanism, whereby a sponsor who successfully

41

licenses a product for a neglected disease receives a priority review voucher that can be applied to any other product submission by that sponsor.

As of 2002, the US FDA amended regulations to allow, in cases where traditional efficacy trials were considered impractical or unethical, appropriate animal studies to provide evidence of the effectiveness of new drug and biological products used to reduce or prevent the toxicity of chemical, biological, radiological, or nuclear substances. Whereas historically the US FDA required products for use in humans to have been proven both safe and effective in clinical trials involving humans as a condition for approval, under the "Animal Rule" the US FDA can rely on evidence from animal studies to provide substantial evidence of product efficacy. Approval of a vaccine product would then be based on animal efficacy studies and demonstration of safety and immunogenicity in human clinical trials. Up to 2014, no vaccine has been approved under the Animal Rule.

The US FDA also has authority to issue an emergency use authorization (EUA) for the use of unapproved vaccines in prevention or treatment of life-threatening disease. This requires that an emergency has been declared by the Secretary of the Department of Health and Human Services, or other designated individuals, according to specific criteria. Any available data indicating that the product may be effective can then be evaluated, although it is recommended that an EUA submission should ideally include preclinical testing data for *in vitro* and animal toxicity, *in vitro* and animal data supporting effectiveness in preventing or treating the disease, data to support the proposed dosage, and any clinical data that may indicate safety and efficacy in humans. To date, the only vaccine-related EUA was issued for the use of anthrax vaccine adsorbed (AVA) in individuals at high risk for aerosol exposure to anthrax. This EUA was established in January 2005, extended once, and discontinued in January 2006. During the H1N1 "swine flu" outbreak of 2009, multiple EUAs were issued for use of antiviral drugs in unapproved populations and for new diagnostic assays, but H1N1 vaccines developed at that time were approved via the normal US FDA processes.

Summary

- Vaccine development is a complex, resource intensive, and highly regulated process that demands enormous investments of time and money to bring a licensed product to market.

- Development of vaccines has relied on interactions between academia, government researchers, and funding bodies, and industry to progress candidate products through the development and approval pipeline.

- Rapidly evolving technologies for bioinformatics and the potential for "personalized medicine" will only increase the complexity of these processes and require the continued education and training of both vaccinologists and regulators to ensure the cost-effective and timely delivery of the next generation of vaccines.

Further reading

Buckland BC (2005). The process development challenge for a new vaccine. Nature Medicine 11 4Suppl, S16–S19.

Francis DP (2010). Successes and failures: worldwide vaccine development and application. Biologicals: Journal of the International Association of Biological Standardization 38, 523–528.

Kanesa-thasan N, Shaw A, Stoddard JJ, and Vernon TM (2011). Ensuring the optimal safety of licensed vaccines: a perspective of the vaccine research, development, and manufacturing companies. Pediatrics 127 Suppl 1, S16–S22.

Kresse H and Shah M (2010). Strategic trends in the vaccine market. Nature Reviews Drug Discovery 9, 913–914.

Marshall V and Baylor NW (2011). Food and Drug Administration regulation and evaluation of vaccines. Pediatrics 127 Suppl 1, S23–S30.

Stevens AJ, Jensen JJ, Wyller K, Kilgore PC, Chatterjee S, and Rohrbaugh ML (2011). The role of public-sector research in the discovery of drugs and vaccines. New England Journal of Medicine 364, 535–541.

Weinberg GA and Szilagyi PG (2010). Vaccine epidemiology: efficacy, effectiveness, and the translational research roadmap. Journal of Infectious Diseases 201, 1607–1610.

3 Control and eradication of human and animal diseases by vaccination

Nigel Bourne and Gregg N. Milligan

Sealy Center for Vaccine Development, University of Texas Medical Branch, Galveston, TX, USA

Abbreviations

ACIP	Advisory Committee on Immunization Practices	OIE	Office of Internationale des Epizooties (also known as the World Organization for Animal Health)
AFP	Acute flaccid paralysis		
CDC	Centers for Disease Control and Prevention	OPV	Oral polio vaccine
		PARC	Pan African Rinderpest Campaign
DIVA	Differentiate infected from vaccinated animals	PCV7	Seven-valent pneumococcal conjugate vaccine
FAO	Food and Agriculture Organization of the United Nations	PPR	*Peste des Petits Ruminants*
		R_0	Basic reproductive number
FMD	Foot-and-mouth disease	SSPE	Subacute sclerosing panencephalitis
GREP	Global Rinderpest Eradication Program	UNICEF	United Nations Children's Fund
IPV	Inactivated polio vaccine	VAPP	Vaccine-associated paralytic polio
NID	National Immunization Days	WHA	World Health Assembly
NSP	Nonstructural proteins		

The control of diseases by vaccination

Vaccination has been described as one of the top 10 public health achievements of the past 100 years. Through the development and use of vaccines we are now able to control many important diseases that used to cause significant morbidity and mortality worldwide.

Due to the importance of vaccines in public health, many countries have developed an extensive infrastructure around their use. Initially this involves careful safety and efficacy testing for new vaccines before they are licensed for use. Following licensure, one major issue is to develop policy on who should

receive the vaccine and at what age. In the USA, the Advisory Committee on Immunization Practices (ACIP) of the Centers for Disease Control and Prevention (CDC) is responsible for making these recommendations. The ACIP meets regularly and develops vaccine policy based on scientific information. The ACIP is also responsible for generating the list of vaccines that are recommended for the Vaccines for Children Program, a federally funded program that provides vaccines at no cost to children who, for whatever reason, cannot pay.

Furthermore, monitoring continues in many countries once a vaccine has been approved for use. In the USA, the National Immunization Survey provides

Vaccinology: An Essential Guide, First Edition. Edited by Gregg N. Milligan and Alan D.T. Barrett.
© 2015 John Wiley & Sons, Ltd. Published 2015 by John Wiley & Sons, Ltd.

information on vaccine coverage rates in children and collects surveillance data to determine the impact of vaccines on morbidity and mortality, and, importantly, on vaccine safety. Such post-licensure testing is needed because pre-licensure phase I, II, and III clinical trials generate data on safety and efficacy from a limited population (usually fewer than 100,000 individuals) and the results are extrapolated to the vaccine target population (which is often in the millions). By careful post-licensure surveillance it is possible to determine whether or not safety and efficacy profiles used in licensing a vaccine are translated to the general population and to detect rare adverse events that may only be noticed once a vaccine is being used on a population level. This is sometimes referred to as phase IV studies.

Worldwide, rotavirus is the leading cause of severe diarrheal disease among infants and young children. A quadravalent live attenuated rotavirus vaccine, Rotashield®, was clinically tested and licensed in the USA. During the first year of widespread use, it was determined that vaccination with Rotashield was associated with an increased risk of intussusception, an invagination of a length of intestine resulting in an obstruction, and it was removed from the market. Due to the urgent need for a rotavirus vaccine, new efforts at rotavirus vaccine development were encouraged by the World Health Organization and the Global Alliance for Vaccines and Immunization that would include assessment for intussusception in the clinical testing phase of development. Two new live attenuated rotavirus vaccines, RotaTeq and Rotarix were vigorously tested in phase I–III trials in both developed and developing nations and shown to be safe and efficacious as a result of these efforts, and were subsequently licensed.

It is important to recognize that vaccines are licensed with the goal of disease control, i.e., reducing the incidence of the disease to a level that is determined to be acceptable in the population. Using this approach, a large number of what were once common infectious diseases have now been controlled in many countries and in some cases (e.g., poliomyelitis) are rarely seen. In general, while it would be desirable, it is not expected that the introduction of a vaccine will result in elimination or eradication of a disease. As we shall see in this chapter there are a number of reasons for this. Some are biological: for example, certain pathogens, such as the yellow fever virus, have a complex life cycle in which the virus is propagated in mammalian and nonmammalian species and exists in animal reservoirs, or in which a pathogen, such as herpes simplex virus, exists in a relatively nonaccessible stage, such as in latent infections. Other pathogens, such as influenza virus, are maintained in animal hosts and exposed to immunological or biological pressures that periodically select mutated forms of the pathogen in which the amino acid sequence of important surface-exposed molecules is altered, changing the antigens and necessitating the development of new vaccines. Nonetheless, some pathogens do have biological characteristics that make eradication feasible. These features include the lack of an animal reservoir of the infection, in which the pathogen infects only one or a limited number of species; no latent, persistent, or chronic infection of humans (or veterinary animals); infection results in an easily diagnosed disease; and there is an effective, inexpensive treatment or vaccine that elicits strong, long-lasting protective immune responses. However, even in cases where the biological characteristics are favorable there are multiple additional factors that contribute to determining whether or not a regional elimination or global eradication program is feasible. These include determination of whether the burden of morbidity and mortality associated with the disease is sufficient to warrant such efforts and will provide the sustained political will to achieve the goals of the program and the ability to obtain sufficient funding to support the public health infrastructure required for the program. This infrastructure includes disease surveillance and diagnostics, the production of the required amount of well-characterized vaccine stocks, the capacity to distribute and administer vaccines, and a certification procedure to confirm when countries become disease free.

Definitions

Cold chain: The process where a vaccine must be transported and stored at reduced temperatures that maintain the viability of the vaccine. This is particularly important for live attenuated vaccines.

Control: Reduction of disease incidence, prevalence, and morbidity and mortality to locally acceptable levels as a result of deliberate efforts.
Elimination: Reduction to zero in the incidence of a disease in a defined geographical area.
Eradication: Permanent reduction to zero of the worldwide incidence of infection caused by a specific agent.
Extinction: The specific agent no longer exists in nature or the laboratory.
Herd immunity: The proportion of a population that must be immunized with a vaccine for a particular infectious disease to ensure that an entire population is protected from a specific infectious disease.

In the sections below we will examine some to the factors that are important in attempts to control and eradicate diseases through vaccination and discuss efforts with a number of specific human and veterinary diseases.

Herd immunity

Vaccination results in both direct and indirect protective effects against infectious diseases. The direct effects are obtained only by the immunized individual and are manifested as direct resistance to infection following exposure to the pathogen. However, it has been recognized that for pathogens that are easily transmitted by person-to-person contact, the presence of immune individuals in a population provides a level of protection for unimmunized individuals through an interruption in disease transmission. This phenomenon is referred to as *herd immunity* and is discussed in more detail elsewhere in this book. It has come to be associated with a variety of meanings in the world of vaccinology, but in its simplest form it refers to the proportion of a population that must be immunized with a vaccine for a particular infectious disease to ensure that an entire population is protected from the specific infectious disease. As will be discussed in more detail later in this chapter, the concept of herd immunity plays a critical role in strategies to eradicate human and veterinary pathogens.

From a theoretical standpoint, individuals infected with a given pathogen and mixing randomly in a population would transmit the pathogen to a given number of other individuals. The basic reproductive number (R_0) describes this phenomenon and is defined as the average number of transmissions from an index case introduced into a totally susceptible population. The higher this number is, the greater the likelihood that the pathogen will be transmitted to new individuals. The introduction of individuals fully immune to the pathogen into the population would result in an interruption in transmission of the pathogen to non-immune individuals, and if the number of immune individuals was increased to some threshold number, the incidence of infection in the population would begin to decline and disappear altogether. The application of this idea to vaccinology is that effective vaccines can be used to make individuals immune, significantly interfere with disease transmission, and provide protection in this indirect way to nonimmune individuals. The herd immunity threshold that must be reached depends to a large extent on the transmissibility of infection. From a control and eradication perspective the higher this R_0 is, the greater the vaccine coverage required in a population (threshold) to eliminate the infection. Although there are many variables that determine the R_0 value, it can be used to estimate the number of individuals that must be protected by vaccination in order to control or eradicate a pathogen.

From a practical standpoint, the important aspects of herd immunity include indirect protection, where selective vaccination of particular groups are utilized to reduce transmission to other groups, as, for example, the immunization of children against influenza to reduce morbidity and mortality in the elderly. Perhaps the most widely used example of herd immunity in the use of vaccines to control diseases has been the example of bacterial conjugate vaccines.

Bacteria such as *Streptococcus pneumoniae*, *Haemophilus influenze* type b, and *Neisseria meningitidis* colonize the nasopharynx. Effective vaccines such as polysaccharide conjugate vaccines directly impact colonization and thus diminish transmission. As a result of immunization programs in Canada it was determined that beyond the direct protection of immunizing individuals under 20 years of age with a meningococcal conjugate vaccine, a drop in the incidence of infection by meningococcal serogroup C organisms was noted in

(Continued)

individuals older than 20 years of age although these individuals had not been targeted with the vaccine. Similarly, the introduction of a seven-valent pneumococcal conjugate vaccine (PCV7) in the UK in 2006 significantly diminished disease caused by the seven serotypes covered by the vaccine in immunized infants and also in unimmunized individuals of age 65 or older.

Smallpox

Any discussion of the use of vaccination for the control and eradication of disease necessarily begins with smallpox. Smallpox was a severe acute disease caused by variola virus, a member of the genus *orthopoxvirus* within the *Poxviridae* family. The virus was transmitted directly from person to person usually by droplet spread through the respiratory tract. In variola major, the most historically significant form of the disease, following virus infection there was an asymptomatic incubation period that lasted approximately 2 weeks, followed by the rapid onset of the early symptoms indicating the onset of disease (the prodrome) that consisted of a fever lasting several days, accompanied by headache, fatigue, and back pain. As the fever subsided, the characteristic rash began to develop. This rash typically had a centrifugal distribution beginning on the face and extremities and then spreading to include the rest of the body (Figure 3.1). The lesions began as small red macules that progressed to become papules, vesicles, and then pustules. As the pustules scabbed over and the scabs detached, they left the characteristic depressed depigmented scars known as pockmarks. The disease had a mortality rate of approximately 30%. Among those who survived the disease, blindness was a common complication and most had characteristic pockmark scarring, which could be extensive over the body. A second much milder form of the disease known as variola minor, with a similar but less severe rash and significantly lower mortality rate, developed in the 19th century in Africa and the Americas.

The origins of smallpox are unclear, but evidence of the disease can be found dating back several thousand years, and it remained one of the most medically important diseases in many parts of the world throughout history. By the Middle Ages it was endemic and

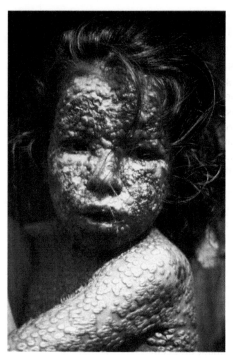

Figure 3.1 Photograph showing a young girl with severe rash characteristic of smallpox. Photograph from James Hicks/ Center for Disease Control and Prevention.

caused periodic epidemics in many regions of the world, including Europe, Africa, and Asia. It is widely reported to have been introduced to the New World by the conquistadors and is believed to have been a contributing factor to the fall of the Aztec empire, whose inhabitants had no natural immunity.

The high mortality and severe sequelae produced by smallpox combined with the observation that those who survived the disease did not become reinfected (what we now term *lifelong immunity*) led to attempts to produce a mild disease in people so that they would be protected. Historically, this was done either by grinding material from a smallpox scab into powder and blowing it into the nose (a process known as *insufflation*) or taking dried pus from a smallpox lesion and scratching it into the skin. These techniques, which are referred to as *variolation*, were generally successful in producing a milder illness, although occasionally fully virulent smallpox developed. Even with this concern, the case fatality ratio from variolation was approximately tenfold lower than that seen with natural infection, which led to the technique being used in many areas of the world. Although historical records show that a number of individuals in a similar time period were testing regimens to control smallpox, the great step forward in protection against the disease is credited to Edward Jenner, an English country physician, who observed that milkmaids who were exposed to cowpox as an occupational hazard did not develop smallpox. In 1796 Jenner introduced material from a cowpox lesion on the hand of a local milkmaid into the arm of a young orphan named Benjamin Phipps and later showed that Phipps was protected from developing the scar characteristic of variolation when he was inoculated with material from an active smallpox lesion. This procedure, which subsequently came to be known as *vaccination* is generally regarded as the beginning of the field of vaccinology. Jenner's use of an infectious agent from an animal species that is closely related to an agent that causes disease in humans is still used today as one approach in developing live attenuated vaccines. Another similar approach is to adapt an agent that causes disease in humans to grow in a nonhuman host species so that when it is reintroduced into humans it is weakened and no longer causes disease.

Interestingly, as well as being considered the "father of vaccinology," Edward Jenner is also credited with being the first to propose the idea that vaccination had the potential to eradicate a disease, stating that "the annihilation of the Smallpox, the most dreadful scourge of the human species must be the final result of this practice." While history was to eventually prove him correct, the road was a long and not always smooth one.

The potential of vaccination to protect against smallpox was quickly recognized, and its use spread rapidly throughout Europe as well as to the USA where it was used to combat an outbreak of smallpox in Boston as early as 1800. Unfortunately, at first the process required the use of fresh material from active lesions. Initially this was accomplished by taking material from the arm of one individual and using it to infect the arm of another individual. Orphaned children were often used as the stock source for this material. Clearly, the need for fresh lesions to provide vaccine material resulted in difficulties in transporting the vaccine to new areas and in producing adequate amounts of material for vaccination of large numbers of people. It

also resulted in other complications such as transmission of secondary infections due to transfer of material from individuals who added preexisting infections, including leprosy and syphilis, to vaccine recipients. Attempts to improve supply and transport by drying the lesion material produced highly variable results and was not widely used. However, a major breakthrough came with the discovery that the vaccine could be propagated on the flanks of cows, which provided a larger and more readily available source of material. The replacement of cowpox virus in the vaccine with the related but genetically distinct vaccinia virus occurred at some point after cows became the major source of vaccine production, although exactly how and when this happened remains unknown.

As the use of vaccination against smallpox became more widespread, an important observation was made that has since proven to be widely applicable in vaccinology: It soon became apparent that although natural infection with smallpox resulted in lifelong protective immunity in survivors, vaccination only provided protection for a few years, resulting in the recognition that periodic boost vaccination was needed to maintain protective immunity.

The availability of increased supplies of vaccine allowed smallpox to be brought under control in many industrialized countries. However, it was not until after the World War I that much of Europe became smallpox-free, and it took until the middle of the 20th century for transmission to be completely interrupted throughout Europe and North America. A significant problem with the vaccine was that since it was a live attenuated vaccine it only remained viable for a short period of time, particularly in tropical countries with high ambient temperatures. This contributed to the understanding of the need for a "cold chain" for the vaccine, i.e., that the vaccine must be transported and stored at temperatures that maintained the viability of the vaccine; this has become a critical issue in the development of a vaccine today. A major step forward for smallpox vaccines came in the 1940s when Leslie Collier, a British scientist, developed a process that allowed large-scale freeze-drying of the vaccine, enabling mass vaccination campaigns to be initiated in countries where it had previously been impossible. One of the first mass vaccination campaigns undertaken with freeze-dried vaccine was launched by the Pan American Sanitary Organization (later renamed the Pan American Health Organization) in 1950 using the newly available freeze-dried vaccine to eliminate smallpox from the Americas.

In 1958 the Union of Soviet and Socialist Republics proposed to the World Health Assembly (WHA) that global smallpox eradication was possible. The WHA ratified the resolution, and over the next 7 years a number of mass vaccination campaigns were undertaken with smallpox being eliminated from several countries, including China. Overall, however, the results of these efforts were disappointing. Recognizing the relative lack of progress, the WHA launched the intensified smallpox eradication program in 1966, allocating annual funding of $2.4 million with the goal of eradicating the disease within 10 years. At the time that the intensified program was launched, there were 10 million to 15 million cases of smallpox annually worldwide, and the disease remained endemic in more than 30 countries, with major reservoirs in Africa, Asia, Indonesia, and Brazil. The intensified eradication campaign was built on the use of well-characterized freeze-dried vaccines of ensured potency and stability in mass vaccination campaigns that aimed to reach at least 80% of the population throughout endemic areas. A second feature that became increasingly important as the number of smallpox cases decreased was the development of effective surveillance systems in endemic countries that allowed smallpox cases to be rapidly identified and focused containment responses to be mounted. A mainstay of this response was that any identified smallpox case was quickly isolated. All of the infected individual's known contacts were then vaccinated and closely observed for signs of disease. To provide a further protection, any persons known to have been exposed to the direct contacts were then also identified and vaccinated. In this way transmission of the disease was prevented by using vaccination to provide a ring of immunity around the case. Thus, the technique became known as *ring vaccination*.

Although the intensified eradication program encountered numerous problems, which included organizational difficulties, political instability (including civil war in some of the areas), famine, opposition to vaccination due to cultural beliefs, and lack of funding, it was ultimately successful. The last naturally occurring case of smallpox was reported in Somalia in 1977. A year later, two cases occurred following a laboratory exposure in Birmingham, England. Finally on May 8, 1980, the WHA declared that smallpox had been eradicated. It is important to note here that although smallpox has been eradicated as a disease, the virus is not extinct. Laboratory stocks of smallpox are currently maintained in two biosafety level four laboratories only: the CDC in Atlanta, GA, USA, and the State Research Center of Virology and Biotechnology (known as the VECTOR Institute) near Novosibirsk, Russia.

The fate of these virus stocks is the source of considerable ongoing debate. Some scientists believe that continued research on the virus is important while others believe that they represent a final reservoir from which the disease could potentially reemerge by accidental or deliberate release. Others argue that if there are other currently unknown stocks of the virus that could potentially be released, these known stocks could be invaluable in developing new vaccines or therapeutics. Interestingly, ring vaccination remains a key component of the public health plans to respond if there should ever be another smallpox outbreak.

A number of factors contributed to make smallpox eradication feasible. The disease was acute, with no chronic or carrier state, and the virus was spread directly between humans with no animal reservoir. The disease was highly distinctive and so easily recognizable, and victims became infectious at a time in the course of disease when the symptoms were usually severe enough to prevent widespread movement, thereby limiting the potential number of contacts. There was an effective vaccine available and the cost-benefit ratio of eradication in the endemic countries centered on patient care costs. Although smallpox was no longer endemic in most industrialized countries, these countries still expended considerable funds and resources on maintaining population-wide immunity. Thus the largest financial benefits were to be gained in countries in which the disease was still endemic, but it was clear that there were still considerable financial benefits to most industrialized countries if eradication could be achieved, as vaccination would no longer be needed.

The successful control and eventual eradication of smallpox stands as proof that eradication is possible. In the afterglow of the smallpox success story, a number of infectious diseases that are major public health problems and have no animal reservoir (i.e., infect only humans) were targeted for eradication. Measles and poliomyelitis are often cited as targets for eradication (see below). However, this process has proven more difficult than many imagined, and for some time it seemed possible that smallpox truly represented a unique case. However, a second success story has recently been completed, not among human diseases, but with an animal disease (rinderpest) that among cattle has proven as devastating as smallpox in humans.

Rinderpest

The genus *Morbillivirus* within the family *Paramyxoviridae* contains the viruses responsible for a number of important human and animal diseases, including human measles, canine distemper (a severe, often fatal, disease in dogs), *pestis des petites ruminants* (a significant disease in sheep and goats) and rinderpest (cattle plague). Rinderpest virus can infect most cloven-hoofed animals; however, cattle, water buffalo, yaks, and certain wildlife species, including African buffalo, giraffe, and warthogs, are particularly susceptible. Although a number of wildlife species are susceptible to infection, they did not provide a major reservoir, and it was domesticated cattle that were the most important maintenance host. In cattle, the disease could take multiple forms (acute, peracute, subacute, and inapparent). Of these, the classic or acute form of the disease was most important. In acute disease, virus infection started with a short incubation period (typically 4–5 days) and then a prodrome during which the animal experienced rapid onset fever, depression, and ocular and nasal discharge with reduced appetite and milk yield. This was followed after 2–5 days by the distinctive erosive mucosal phase during which the animal developed epithelial lesions on the lips, gums, tongue, and nasal and urogenital mucosal surfaces. The lesions were initially small but rapidly enlarged and became necrotic with sloughing of the epithelial layers. At the same time the ocular and nasal secretions become laden with mucous and pus (mucopurulent) and the animals become anorexic. A few days later the fever began to fall but the disease entered the diarrheal phase during which the animal experienced profuse watery diarrhea containing excess mucous, blood, and shreds of epithelial tissue described as having an unpleasantly sweet fetid smell. During this phase of the disease, the animal also typically showed increasing respiratory distress and rapidly developed dehydration. In cases of fatal disease, the diarrhea worsened and the animal became progressively weaker and more dehydrated until it collapsed and died. In nonfatal cases, the diarrhea gradually stopped, and the animal slowly began to recover. However, in animals that recovered there was a long period of convalescence during which they remained at increased risk of developing secondary infections. The disease was highly contagious and was spread by close contact with infected animals, with virus being shed in multiple secretions and excretions from late in the incubation period through the first week of clinical signs.

In areas where rinderpest was endemic, maternal transfer of antibodies provided young animals with protection during early life; however, this protection waned at approximately 6–11 months of age so that the disease was mainly seen in animals of this age. Nevertheless, the disease was most devastating when introduced to a new area (or reintroduced after a period of absence) with large numbers of susceptible animals. One of the most significant examples was its introduction into Africa in 1887 following importation of infected cattle from India. The disease spread rapidly across the continent in what became known as the Great African Pandemic. It is estimated that approximately 90% of all cattle in sub-Saharan Africa died during this pandemic, as well as large numbers of wild animals and other domesticated stock (Figure 3.2). The loss of food cattle and draft animals triggered a massive famine that resulted in widespread loss of human life. It also established a number of long-lasting reservoirs of infection in Africa.

Due to its importance as a disease of cattle, and consequently the loss of a source of food for humans, efforts to control rinderpest began before the development of vaccines. The disease was eliminated from most of Europe by the beginning of the 20th century, largely by the use of strict control measures that included restrictions on animal movement, and the slaughter and disposal of infected animals. However, global control of the disease and its eventual eradication was based on the development of effective vaccines. One of the first important methods of vaccination was a procedure somewhat similar to variolation against smallpox in which naïve animals were

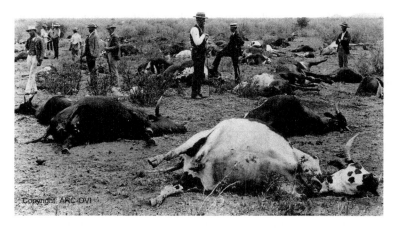

Figure 3.2 Introduction of rinderpest into Africa resulted in a massive pandemic with huge livestock losses due to the disease and associated "stamping-out" policy initiated to stop its spread as shown in this photograph. Photograph from Agricultural Research Council: Onderstepoort Veterinary Institute.

injected with serum from an animal that had recovered from rinderpest (i.e., serum containing anti-rinderpest antibodies) and, at the same time, with blood containing virus from actively infected animals. This "serum-simultaneous procedure" elicited lifelong immunity, and despite the inherent risk of the animal developing severe disease it was used extensively until safer effective vaccines became available. Among the first true vaccine candidates were a number of chemically inactivated vaccines; however, their impact on control and eradication of the disease was limited because they elicited only short-term protection, which required animals to undergo repeated immunizations. It was the development of live attenuated vaccines that was to prove crucial. One method for generating live attenuated vaccines is to adapt the infectious agent to a new host by multiple passages in that host species with the goal of adaptation giving rise to a variant that multiplies to induce a protective immune response but no longer causes disease in the original host. Thus, the first such vaccines were produced by serial passage of rinderpest virus in goats or rabbits. A number of successful vaccines were developed in this way that elicited long-lasting immunity. However, they tended to produce some mild clinical signs of disease in cattle. A significant breakthrough came with the advent of tissue culture techniques for virus culture. British scientist Walter Plowright and colleagues developed a tissue culture attenuated vaccine by performing 90 serial passages of rinderpest virus in primary calf kidney cells. The Plowright vaccine elicited long-lasting protective immunity

without causing any clinical signs of disease in cattle of all ages. It became the mainstay of rinderpest control and elimination programs until the 1980s, when US scientist Jeffrey Mariner and colleagues adapted the virus for growth in monkey kidney Vero cells. This made production easier and improved the chemical stabilization and freeze-drying techniques, resulting in a more thermostable vaccine known as Thermovax, which proved better suited for use in tropical areas of the world during the final stages of eradication.

As with smallpox, much of the progress toward global control of rinderpest was undertaken by individual countries or by regional groups of countries. For example, India launched an initiative to eliminate the disease in 1954 based on the use of mass vaccination aimed at covering 80% of cattle and buffalo within 5 years, with the remaining 20% of animals being immunized in the follow-up period during annual campaigns in which all calves would be immunized. While this campaign had some success and endemic disease was eliminated from a number of Indian states, it ultimately failed to eliminate the disease nationwide due largely to the fact that the initiative was implemented on a state-by-state basis rather than being a centralized, coordinated national effort. Subsequently, a second major initiative was launched in India in 1983 for states where the disease remained endemic. This initiative was based on mass vaccination to achieve 90% coverage within 3 years, while in states where rinderpest was no longer endemic, the effort focused on vaccinations around disease outbreaks. Vaccination efforts were also coupled with the introduction of strict controls on cattle movements. Ultimately these efforts were successful with rinderpest being eliminated in India in 1995.

The Joint Program 15 was a large regional effort designed to eliminate rinderpest from a number of countries in Africa by coordinated mass vaccination. Initially, the program was highly successful, greatly reducing the burden of disease throughout the region. However, it failed to clear a small number of persistent reservoirs of infection and as funding for the project ran down and the sustained vaccination effort was lost, the disease reemerged from these reservoirs and spread rapidly across sub-Saharan Africa, resulting in what is known as the Second Great African Pandemic in the early 1980s. The extent of this pandemic and the resultant loss of livestock led to the organization of the Pan African Rinderpest Campaign (PARC) involving 34 African countries. PARC relied largely on a combination of disease surveillance and mass vaccination, and was highly successful in again reducing the burden of rinderpest across the continent and limiting the disease to a small number of reservoir areas.

The final push came in 1994 with the launch of the Global Rinderpest Eradication Program (GREP), which was established with the time-dependent goal of eradicating rinderpest by 2010. At the time GREP was launched, control efforts had contained rinderpest to six areas: four within Asia and two in Africa. Similar to the strategic action program for smallpox eradication, GREP was a collaborative effort involving multiple international and regional agencies, including the Food and Agriculture Organization of the United Nations (FAO), the Office of Internationale des Epizooties (OIE; also known as the World Organization for Animal Health) and the International Atomic Energy Agency. Another similarity to the smallpox eradication program was that GREP was based on a number of core strategies. Initially mass vaccination campaigns were used to protect cattle and buffalo in areas were the disease was still present. However, GREP also included developing an increased understanding of disease epidemiology and improved surveillance techniques. This proved important in helping to identify exactly where rinderpest remained and how it was being maintained, allowing for more focused vaccination efforts. As the number of rinderpest cases decreased, GREP also assisted national veterinary services in halting vaccination and maintaining sustained surveillance programs that allowed them to conform to the OIE guidelines for declaration of freedom from disease and infection. The last rinderpest outbreak occurred in Kenya in 2001 and the last vaccinations against the disease were administered in 2006. On May 25, 2011, the OIE world assembly declared rinderpest had been eradicated; this was followed by the official proclamation by the FAO on June 28, 2011.

Again, like smallpox, rinderpest eradication does not mean that the virus is extinct. The GREP includes a posteradication strategy to minimize the chance of an accidental or deliberate reintroduction of the disease by maintaining samples of the virus and vaccines only in certain agreed-upon laboratories, with stocks in all other locations being destroyed.

There were a number of important similarities between rinderpest and smallpox in regards to control and eradication. First, there was a single serotype of the virus worldwide (although there were three distinct genetic lineages) so that a single vaccine provided protection against the disease, and animals that survived infection developed lifelong immunity. Although wildlife provided minor virus reservoirs, the major reservoir was domestic cattle, which greatly simplified vaccination efforts. In addition, as with smallpox, rinderpest had a long history as a devastating disease of livestock, which provided a strong economic incentive that helped to sustain the eradication efforts.

Poliomyelitis

In 1988 the WHA proposed that poliomyelitis become the second human viral disease targeted for eradication using a strategy based on vaccination. Poliomyelitis is caused by three distinct serotypes of poliovirus that are members of the genus *Enterovirus* within the *Picornaviridae* family. The viruses enter cells using a receptor found only in humans (and a small number of ape species), and so like smallpox, poliomyelitis is a human disease without an animal reservoir. Infection with poliovirus normally occurs by oral–oral or fecal–oral transmission. After replicating in the gastrointestinal tract, the virus can then spread, causing a viremia, and in some cases invade the central nervous system, in particular the anterior horn cells of the spinal cord and brain stem cells that innervate the muscles controlling respiration. The vast majority of cases of polio infection are asymptomatic. However, even those who are asymptomatically infected can shed the virus in their feces and transmit the virus to others. Among those who do develop a symptomatic infection, the majority experience only a mild illness with fever, malaise, and vomiting. A much smaller percentage of symptomatic infections result in a non-paralytic poliomyelitis with aseptic meningitis. Finally, a very small minority of those who become infected develop paralytic poliomyelitis, often referred to acute flaccid paralysis (AFP). The paralysis is more common in the legs than the arms and is often asymmetric. In addition, bulbar polio is seen when the cells of the motor respiratory centers are involved. Because central nervous system tissue does not regenerate, the damaged tissue does not repair and individuals can be paralyzed for life; however, in many cases the body compensates and allows a partial or full recovery.

The origins of poliomyelitis, like those of smallpox, can be traced back into antiquity with Egyptian mummies showing deformities consistent with paralytic poliomyelitis. The first clinical description of the disease was provided in 1790 by Michael Underwood, an English physician. Poliomyelitis remained predominantly an endemic disease in many countries. However, toward the end of the 19th century, the epidemiology of the disease began to change in a number of temperate countries, most notably the USA and Scandinavia, from a predominantly endemic disease to one where there were periodic epidemics. The first of these in the USA was in 1894 in Vermont.

Subsequently, the first large epidemic was seen in 1916 with 27,000 cases and 6,000 deaths. In the USA, one direct result of the public health concern about polio was the establishment of the National Foundation for Infantile Paralysis in 1938. This grassroots program was characterized by large numbers of people giving small amounts of money, leading to its popular name—the March of Dimes—which still continues today. It supported both care of those with polio and research to develop an effective vaccine.

The first such vaccine to become available was the inactivated polio vaccine (IPV) developed by Jonas Salk. IPV contains chemically inactivated forms of all three serotypes of poliovirus. The viruses were originally grown in primary monkey kidney cells and then chemically inactivated using formaldehyde. The vaccine was licensed in the USA in 1955 and has been remarkably successful, remaining in use today. Because it is an inactivated virus vaccine it has an excellent safety record, with the only major adverse event occurring shortly after licensure in 1955 in what is known as the Cutter Incident, when 204 cases of poliomyelitis were traced to batches of incompletely inactivated vaccine produced by Cutter Laboratories. As a killed vaccine, multiple doses are required to generate protective immunity, and booster doses are required to maintain immunity. Since its licensure, improved manufacturing processes have helped improve the immunity elicited by the vaccine, including the use of continuous cell culture for antigen production and better antigen concentration procedures.

A second polio vaccine was developed by Albert Sabin and licensed for use in humans initially as a monovalent vaccine in 1961 and as a trivalent 2 years later. Known as the oral polio vaccine (OPV) it is a live virus vaccine in which the original wild-type viruses were attenuated by sequential tissue culture passage with periodic testing in animals to determine when the virus had lost neurovirulence. The licensure of IPV and OPV resulted in a rapid and dramatic reduction in the number of cases of paralytic poliomyelitis. The public demand for the polio vaccination was high (Figure 3.3). Because OPV is a live attenuated virus vaccine it does not need to be administered as frequently as IPV to elicit protective immunity, and it is better able to protect against infection compared to IPV because it replicates in the intestine, producing extended exposure to antigens and inducing good mucosal immunity. In addition, because OPV replicates in the intestines of recipients and, like wild-type polio virus, is shed in feces, it can be transmitted to close contacts, allowing people not directly given the vaccine to be passively vaccinated. The importance of this indirect immunization effect in elimination campaigns was recognized because it reduced the number of people who had to be actively vaccinated. However, the live vaccine virus can occasionally revert to wild-type phenotype due to accumulation of mutations during replication in the gut. Disease caused by vaccine virus reverting to the neurovirulent wild type is termed *vaccine associated paralytic polio* (VAPP). It has been seen both in primary vaccinees and in close contacts who were exposed to revertant virus shed by the vaccinee. Concerns about VAPP have resulted in a

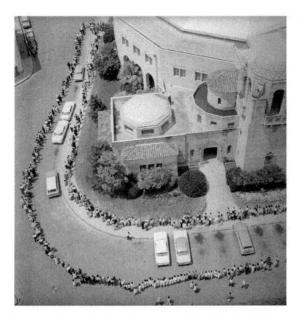

Figure 3.3 This photograph shows people waiting in line to receive polio vaccination in San Antonio, Texas (1962), illustrating the public demand for this vaccine. Photograph from Mr. Stafford Smith/ Centers for Disease Control and Prevention.

number of countries in which poliomyelitis has been eliminated or where it is extremely rare stopping the use of OPV and returning to IPV vaccination.

In 1962 Cuba successfully eliminated polio using a strategy that involved simultaneous immunization of large numbers of children in a short space of time in what was termed *national immunization days* (NIDs). These were an important part of the strategy that was targeted in the winter when the natural transmission of polio was at its lowest and became the best strategy for breaking the transmission cycle. The last case of polio caused by a wild-type virus in the USA was in 1979.

In 1985 the Pan American Health Organization used an initiative based on the use of NIDs to supplement routine childhood vaccination and also used surveillance to rapidly identify and target cases of AFP to eliminate poliomyelitis from the Americas. The last case of polio in the Americas was seen in Peru in 1991, and the Americas were certified as polio-free in 1994.

The success of this program, coupled with the success of the smallpox eradication program, led to the WHA Global Polio Eradication Program in 1988. At that time, polio remained endemic in 125 countries, and worldwide there were approximately 1000 cases of paralytic polio each day. The target was to eradicate poliomyelitis by the year 2000 using a strategy based on reaching and maintaining high routine OPV coverage in children younger than 1 year of age with a three-dose regimen. Routine coverage was to be supplemented with OPV immunization of children younger than 5 years old in NIDs to interrupt transmission. There was also to be house-to-house follow-up vaccinations campaigns in high-risk areas where transmission was believed likely to persist at low levels and where surveillance for AFP would indicate the need for targeted vaccination efforts.

Overall, the WHA polio eradication program has been of great public health benefit. Since its inception, the global incidence of poliomyelitis has decreased by over 99%. Wild-type poliovirus serotype 2 has not been isolated since 2009 and is believed to have been potentially eradicated. In January 2012, India was declared wild-type poliovirus-free for 1 year. However, we are over a decade past the original target date for polio eradication, and approximately $7 billion have been expended. The disease remains endemic in a number of countries (e.g., Afghanistan, Nigeria, and Pakistan), transmission has been reestablished in a number of other countries in Africa, and there have also been periodic cases of imported polio in several other countries. Currently there are real concerns that a lack of sustained political and financial commitment to the process will ultimately lead to the failure of efforts to eradicate polio and ultimately to a marked resurgence in the incidence of disease. However, there are moves to enhance the eradication program through increased efforts of nongovernmental organizations such as the Bill and Melinda Gates Foundation.

Measles

Measles is a highly contagious disease with one of the largest R_0 values known for a human disease. It is caused by a member of the genus *Morbillivirus* within the family *Paramyxoviridae*. Measles virus has one serotype and is closely related to rinderpest virus. As with the other human viruses targeted for eradication, measles virus is highly host-species restricted, infecting only humans and a few nonhuman primate species.

Measles infection typically occurs when small droplets containing the virus are inhaled. Infection is followed by a 10- to 12-day incubation period during which the virus replicates and spreads throughout the body. The prodromal illness normally includes fever, cough, coryza (runny nose), and conjunctivitis. In addition, during the prodrome, small white-blue spots develop in the mouth. These spots, known as Koplik's spots, are highly diagnostic of measles. Several days after the onset of symptoms, the fever increases and a maculopapular rash develops, characteristically starting on the face and neck and spreading downward and outward to include the trunk and extremities. The rash normally lasts 5–6 days, and in uncomplicated cases of measles, recovery begins soon after it appears. However, complications are seen in about 30–40% of measles cases and are most common in young children (<5 years old) and adults. The most frequently seen complications are diarrhea, pneumonia (which can be caused by the measles virus or by secondary bacterial infection and which is the major cause of death in measles infections), and ear infections. An uncommon but serious complication is acute encephalitis, which is seen in about 1 in 1000 measles cases.

In addition, a second severe neurologic complication of measles infection is subacute sclerosing panencephalitis (SSPE). This is a rare (approximately 1 in 10,000–100,000 measles cases) fatal neurodegenerative disease that develops years after the initial infection and is believed to be the result of persistent virus infection in the brain. As noted above, the ability of a virus to establish a persistent infection is normally regarded as an unwanted feature in eradication efforts. However, studies have shown that in SSPE virus assembly and budding is defective so that no infectious virus is present in this condition.

The presence of Koplik's spots is considered diagnostic of measles infection although other tests have been developed for a definitive diagnosis. Serological tests that measure the presence of measles-specific IgM antibodies in serum or oral fluid also provides valid diagnosis of measles infection as does isolation of measles virus from nasopharyngeal and conjunctival swabs, blood, or urine. Measles infection can also be detected by reverse transcriptase–polymerase chain reactions (RT-PCR) from these clinical specimens. Thus, several valid diagnostic tests are available for detection of measles infection.

Measles virus was isolated in tissue culture by Enders and Peebles in 1954. To develop an attenuated vaccine, the virus was passaged multiple times in tissue culture using human cells. It was then adapted to grow in chick embryos and then underwent additional tissue culture passages in chick embryo fibroblast cells. The resultant Edmonston B virus vaccine strain was licensed in the USA in 1963. This vaccine proved to be highly protective and rapidly reduced the number of measles cases seen in the USA. However, the vaccine produced a fever and mild rash in a significant number of vaccinated children. This led to the development of a further attenuated, less reactogenic strain known as the Moraten strain, which became available in 1968.

The measles vaccine has been shown to be safe, effective, and provides long-lasting protection. The overall effectiveness is estimated at 90%, with a slightly lower rate of 77% for infants aged 9–11 months, and 92% for children older than 12 months. Vaccine effectiveness is believed to be low for children under the age of 9 months due to the presence of measles-specific maternal antibodies. The highly contagious nature of measles means that extremely high vaccination rates are required in order to interrupt transmission of the disease. It has been estimated that at least 95% of the population must be covered by vaccine protection to interrupt measles virus transmission. Although a single dose of vaccine protects the individual against measles disease, two doses are required to achieve a 95% population coverage required to impact transmission. Thus, the measles vaccine represents a very effective intervention strategy for achieving eradication.

Before widespread immunization programs, millions of people died annually following measles infection. Even after the global implementation of vaccination with a single dose of measles vaccine, an estimated 1 million deaths per year resulted from measles infection. The implementation of a two-dose vaccination program resulted in the elimination of measles in the USA in 2000 and in the WHO Americas Region in 2002. A strategy for global utilization of a two-dose vaccination program was developed in 2001 by the WHO and the United Nations Children's Fund (UNICEF). Subsequent to the implementation of this strategy, worldwide deaths due to measles declined dramatically. In 2010, the Global Consultation on the

Feasibility of Measles Eradication determined that measles could be eradicated and set the eradication by 2020 as a feasible goal. The WHO Strategic Advisory Group of Experts on Immunization agreed with the conclusion that measles could be eradicated but did not set a timetable for eradiation to be achieved. As a step toward this goal, member states agreed to accelerate control targets for increasing vaccine coverage. However, despite this progress, measles infections have begun to increase globally since 2009. This is due to a number of factors including loss of financial and political support for the vaccination programs and the failure of routine immunization and supplemental immunization campaigns to reach and sustain the required high vaccine coverage.

Foot-and-mouth disease

Foot-and-mouth disease (FMD) is a severe disease of cloven-hooved livestock and wildlife species. Worldwide it is one of the most economically significant veterinary diseases, and this has led to calls for it to be targeted for eradication. FMD is caused by a virus of the genus *Apthovirus* within the *Picornaviridae* family. It is highly contagious, and the virus can be transmitted between animals by a variety of mechanisms including inhalation, direct contact with mucous membranes and skin abrasions, and ingestion. The disease is characterized by a short incubation period (2–12 days) followed by fever and the development of viral vesicles at multiple sites including the mouth and tongue, snout, muzzle, nostrils, teats, and feet. These vesicles can become eroded as the disease progresses. Animals with vesicles around the mouth and nostrils often develop excess salivation with drooling and nasal discharge (a common feature of the disease in cattle), while lesions on the hooves result in lameness (the most common sign of the disease in pigs). Although most cloven-hooved animals are susceptible to FMD, there is considerable variability in disease severity between species. Among livestock species, cattle and pigs experience severe disease while sheep and goats tend to experience mild disease and may not show clinical signs. They can, however, serve as a source of transmission to other species. Although this is rare, foot-and-mouth disease virus (FMDV) can infect humans through contact with infected animals. Symptoms in humans include fever, malaise, vomit-ing, ulcerative lesions of oral tissues, and vesicular lesions of the skin.

Although mortality from FMD can be high in young animals, it is generally low in adults. However, the disease is highly debilitating, resulting in weight loss, reduced milk yield, and decreased draft power that can persist for a considerable time and which contribute to the economic impact of the disease. In addition, as many as 50% of animals that become infected do not clear the virus and develop a persistent asymptomatic infection, which is known as the *carrier state*. Whether these carrier animals play an important role in the spread of the disease is not well understood.

The vaccines used currently against FMD are inactivated virus vaccines. These vaccines were originally produced by growing virus on cultured tongue epithelium obtained from healthy slaughtered cows and inactivating it with formaldehyde. Production was greatly increased in the 1960s when cell culture replaced the use of tongue epithelium. Today the FMDV is grown on baby hamster kidney cells and inactivated with binary ethyleneimine prior to mixing with adjuvant. Because the process requires virulent virus, the vaccine must be manufactured under biosecure conditions to prevent accidental virus release into the environment. Vaccine production efforts are further complicated by the fact that worldwide there are seven distinct serotypes of FMDV with multiple subtypes within each serotype. Vaccination against one serotype may provide variable protection against subtypes within that serotype but does not protect against other serotypes. The distribution of the different serotypes differs geographically, and in endemic countries there is frequently more than one viral serotype circulating. Consequently, FMDV vaccines often consist of a mixture of several virus serotypes tailored to the particular country in which they are to be used. Like many others vaccines, those for FMD have a very limited shelf life and require cold chain maintenance, which complicates distribution and storage in developing countries. Although vaccination elicits protective immunity, the response is relatively slow (taking at least 7 days), and the resulting protection is short-lived. For this reason, large-scale prophylactic vaccination programs must be undertaken in endemic countries as often as every 6 months to control the disease. A further major problem with current inactivated FMD vaccines is that although they prevent disease they do not prevent infection, and immunized animals that become infected can become asymptomatic carriers similar to naturally infected animals. Despite these limitations, use of the current vaccines in conjunction with the slaughter of infected and contact animals has enabled a number of countries to successfully eliminate FMD. Currently, FMD-free countries include the USA, Canada, Australia, New Zealand, most of Europe, and many parts of South America. However, FMD remains endemic in parts of Africa, Asia, the Middle East, and South America. Some FMD-free countries use routine vaccination to maintain their disease-free status. However, most do not vaccinate as there is controversy about the effectiveness of the serologic assays that are used to differentiate infected from vaccinated animals (known as "DIVA" assays) for FMD. Thus, many countries have implemented strategies based on surveillance and impose strict controls on the import and movement of animals and animal products to maintain their FMD-free status. Sporadic outbreaks of FMD have occurred in a number of disease-free countries, including Taiwan (1997), the UK (1967, 2001, 2007), and the Netherlands (2001). These outbreaks have been controlled by mass slaughter of infected and in contact-susceptible animals. In some cases emergency vaccination has been used during outbreaks (such as the Netherlands in 2001) to help control the spread of the disease, but vaccinated animals have subsequently been culled in a process known as "vaccinate-to-kill" to ensure that the country can rapidly regain its FMD-free status.

However, the large-scale slaughter of uninfected animals in attempts to control recent outbreaks in the UK and the Netherlands has led to widespread public outcry and demands for changes in this policy (Figure 3.4). An alternative known as "vaccinate-to-live" has been proposed. Using this approach, following discovery of a FMD outbreak, susceptible animals in the surrounding area would be vaccinated during a short period of emergency vaccination to control spread of the disease. Subsequently there would be a follow-up period during which the vaccinated animals would be monitored, and only those that became infected would be culled. In support of this approach, the OIE and European Union have recently changed their regulations to shorten the time taken to regain FMD-free status in countries that use this approach. A mainstay

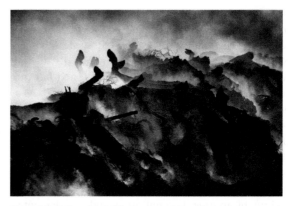

Figure 3.4 Slaughtered livestock are burned to prevent spread of foot-and-mouth disease during the outbreak in the United Kingdom in 2001. The large number of uninfected animals slaughtered during recent outbreaks had led to demands for changes in strategy to control outbreaks. Photograph by Murdo Macleod.

of this approach is the availability of DIVA assays. These are generally based on the detection of antibodies to viral nonstructural proteins (NSPs), which are found in infected animals but do not develop following vaccination with inactivated vaccines. One concern is that the vaccines produced in some areas of the world still contain traces of NSPs that could elicit antibody responses, particularly in animals that have been administered multiple vaccinations, resulting in the mistaken identification of these animals as being infected.

An FMDV outbreak occurred in the UK in 2001 as a result of the improper processing of animal feed. The infection was not recognized immediately and the delay in action most likely led to escape of the virus to neighboring flocks of sheep. Transport of these animals with unrecognized disease resulted in dissemination of the virus throughout Britain. Once recognized, the outbreak was contained by strict transportation restrictions, zoo-sanitation measures, and extensive culling of potentially infected animals. Approximately 7 million sheep and cattle were culled, resulting in difficulties in transportation through infected areas and elimination of carcasses. Vaccination was not employed to halt the outbreak due to concerns that the ability to screen for ultimate control of the outbreak would be compromised. The outbreak was estimated to have cost Britain approximately $16 billion.

Globally, the burden of disease associated with endemic FMD and periodic outbreaks and the costs associated with routine vaccination, surveillance, and outbreak response make FMD a leading candidate for eradication efforts among veterinary diseases. However, the situation is complicated by the considerable genetic diversity of the virus, which prevents the use of a single standardized vaccine and the fact that current vaccines are suboptimal both in terms of the short duration of protection provided and the inability to prevent infection rather than just disease. Many different approaches have been pursued in efforts to develop an improved FMDV vaccine. Ideally, an optimized vaccine could be given orally and would stop viral replication and transmission soon after immunization. Live attenuated vaccines have been tested, but reversion to virulence has been problematic. A variety of subunit vaccines have been proposed, but the immune response is limited to a single candidate, and the resulting immune response is often limited. DNA vaccines alone or in prime-boost regimens have been tested as have replication-defective human adenovirus vectors. More recent approaches have involved production of empty capsid vaccines that contain the immunogenic sites of the virus but lack the viral genetic material, and production of baculovirus-expressed FMDV capsid pentamers. While these approaches are promising for the eventual development of more effective vaccines, currently it is difficult to envisage that a successful eradication campaign could be undertaken, particularly since many of the countries that would be central to the effort have limited resources and may not view FMD as among their highest priorities.

Other potentially eradicable diseases

A number of other diseases have been suggested as candidates for eradication by vaccination (see box). Among veterinary diseases, eradication of FMD would probably be of the greatest worldwide benefit; however, as described previously, such an effort does not appear feasible with current vaccines. The successful eradication of rinderpest is suggestive that the closely related *peste des petits ruminants* (PPR) virus could be eradicable, but in this instance it is unclear that the disease is of sufficient global importance to provide the needed impetus for the efforts that would be needed. Among the human diseases, measles is

perhaps the most attractive target particularly since the availability of combined measles, mumps, and rubella vaccines theoretically would allow the combination of efforts to eradicate all three diseases. However, despite the success in eliminating smallpox, the continuing struggle in attempts to eradicate poliomyelitis clearly demonstrates the complexity of undertaking eradication programs.

Other possible disease targets for eradication by vaccination

- Measles
- Mumps
- Rubella
- Hepatitis A
- Hepatitis B
- *Peste des Petits Ruminants* (PPR)

One major issue in this regard is that vaccines are given on a semivoluntary basis where there are a number of opportunities to opt out of vaccinations. In the 20th century we were very successful at reducing childhood infectious diseases due to vaccinations, and in the early 21st century many of the scourges of the 20th century have nearly disappeared, including polio and measles. Accordingly, people are starting to question why they need to vaccinated if there is no disease, and in many resource poor countries there are higher health care priorities.

Summary

- Pathogens that are candidates for eradication have the following characteristics: infect one or only a limited number of species, do not result in a persistent infection, result in an infection that can easily be diagnosed, and an effective, inexpensive vaccine exists.
- Vaccination results in direct beneficial effects for the immunized individual and indirect effects at the population level.

(Continued)

- The biological characteristics of individual diseases are important in determining the proportion of the population that must be vaccinated to achieve disease control.
- Development of herd immunity is important for control of many diseases caused by colonizing bacteria, as well as in the eradication of the viral pathogens smallpox and rinderpest virus.
- A long-term, concerted effort mediated through many international health agencies is required for the global eradication of a pathogen.

Further reading

Dowdle WR and Cochi SL (2011). The principles and feasibility of disease eradication. Vaccine 29S, D70–D73.

Fine P, Eames K, and Heyman DL (2011). "Herd Immunity": a rough guide. Clinical Infectious Diseases 54, 911–916.

Henderson DA (2011). The eradication of smallpox-An overview of the past, present and future. Vaccine 29S, D7–D9.

Minor PD (2012). The polio-eradication programme and issues of the end game. Journal of General Virology 93, 457–474.

Moore ZS, Seward J, and Lane JM (2006). Smallpox. Lancet 367, 425–435.

Moss WJ and Strebel PJ (2011). Biological feasibility of measles eradication. Infectious Diseases 204, S47–S53.

Nathanson N and Kew OM (2010). From emergence to eradication: the epidemiology of poliomyelitis deconstructed. American Journal of Epidemiology 172, 1213–1229.

Parida S (2009). Vaccination against foot-and-mouth disease virus: strategies and effectiveness. Expert Review of Vaccines 8, 347–365.

Rodriguez LL and Gay CG (2011). Development of vaccines towards the global control and eradication of foot-and-mouth disease. Expert Review of Vaccines 10, 377–387.

Roeder P (2011). Rinderpest: the end of cattle plague. Preventive Veterinary Medicine 102, 98–106.

4 Pathogenesis of infectious diseases and mechanisms of immunity

Jere W. McBride and David H. Walker

Department of Pathology, Sealy Center for Vaccine Development, University of Texas Medical Branch, Galveston, TX, USA

Abbreviations

CNS	Central nervous system	HIV	Human immunodeficiency virus
Fc	Fragment crystalline of antibody molecule	NADPH	Reduced form of nicotinamide adenine dinucleotide phosphate
HBsAg	Hepatitis B surface antigen	PAMPs	Pathogen-associated molecular patterns
HBV	Hepatitis B virus	RSV	Respiratory syncytial virus

Introduction

Infectious diseases are caused by a great variety of agents, ranging from viruses and bacteria to fungi, protozoa, and worms. The sequence of steps in the disease process and the mechanisms mediating injury of cells, tissues, and organs are known as *pathogenesis*. The general concepts that comprise pathogenesis of infections are transmission of the agent, portal of entry into the body, routes of spread within the body, target organs or cells, and mechanisms of evading host defenses and damage to the cells, tissues, and organs. Transmission of communicable diseases occurs mainly through portals of entry including respiratory, gastrointestinal, or urogenital tracts. Transmission through damage to the skin barrier, introduction by arthropods, or mechanical inoculation (e.g., needlestick) is also a major mode of microbe transmission. Some pathogens replicate at the epithelial surface without spreading throughout the body, while others spread through the body via the bloodstream or lymphatics, infecting susceptible cells or organs. Infection by pathogenic microorganisms involves pathogen-specific virulence mechanisms that include attachment and invasion mechanisms, and mechanisms to evade innate and/or adaptive host defenses. A compromised natural barrier or an immunocompromised host can lead to the entry of microbes that cause disease only in these altered circumstances and thus are considered opportunistic pathogens. Once inside the host, microbes must be able to replicate by avoiding host defense mechanisms in extracellular or intracellular environments and may spread throughout the body. In the case of bacteria, systems that allow the extracellular secretion of virulence factors such as toxins that kill host cells, or effector proteins that alter cellular processes and function are important characteristics of these microbes that distinguish them from their nonpathogenic counterparts. In a naïve host, these characteristics allow microbes to evade innate immune defenses that are critical in the early stages of infection before adaptive immune responses are well developed. Survival in the host in order to complete the replication cycle usually involves evasion of

Vaccinology: An Essential Guide, First Edition. Edited by Gregg N. Milligan and Alan D.T. Barrett.
© 2015 John Wiley & Sons, Ltd. Published 2015 by John Wiley & Sons, Ltd.

adaptive immune responses and ultimately leads to host tissue damage through mechanisms that may involve microbial toxins, direct cell lysis or programmed cell death, or be a result of host inflammatory or immune responses initiated to eliminate the microbe. This chapter will provide an overview of microbial pathogenesis and provide specific examples to illustrate the concepts involved in this process and how vaccines prevent the associated pathologic outcomes.

Definitions: colonization, infection, disease, signs, symptoms

Infection is defined as the presence of an organism in an ordinarily sterile body site or an organism other than normal flora on a body surface. The presence of an organism on a nonsterile body surface such as skin or mucosa of the mouth, nasopharynx, large intestine, or vagina is defined as *colonization*. The presence of a pathogenic agent on such a nonsterile body surface in the absence of disease is also colonization. If such an organism on a body surface produces a toxin that damages the tissue or enters the body and causes distant injury or if the organism invades normally sterile tissue, the condition has progressed to become an *infection*. Not all infections cause illness. For example, a low transient content of virus in blood may not result in any clinical manifestations. These are referred to as *subclinical infections*. *Infectious diseases* occur when the patient develops symptoms and signs. *Symptoms* are the clinical manifestations that the patient describes, such as headache, muscle ache, nausea, loss of appetite, or fatigue. *Signs* are objective observations that a physician observes, such as fever, cough, rash, paralysis, seizure, or rapid breathing. Use of these terms appropriately enables accurate understanding of the pathogenesis of infections.

Transmission and portal of entry

Transmission is the transfer of an infectious agent from its source to the patient. Pathogens' niches in nature or *reservoirs* include another person, an animal, water, and soil. Infections that are passed from one person to another are *communicable*. Person-to-person transmission of respiratory infections occurs by inhalation of infectious aerosol particles of 5 micrometers diameter or less or by transfer of infectious respiratory droplets, often from an infected nose-to-hand-to-recipient's hand-to-nose, eye, or mouth. Other person-to-person transmission occurs by contact of skin or mucous membranes (e.g., sexual transmission). Transmission through the skin may occur by the bite or feces of an arthropod (e.g., mosquito, tick, flea, louse) or animal (e.g., rabid dog) or by needle inoculation (e.g., hepatitis C virus from a drug addict's needle during sharing). Ingestion of an infectious agent in food or water usually enters nonsterile tissue through the wall of the small intestine.

Microbes infect the host through direct interactions with cells at portals of entry including the respiratory tract mucosa and lung, conjunctiva, alimentary tract, and the urogenital tract (Figure 4.1; Table 4.1). Microbes are also transmitted by arthropod vectors that bypass the physical barrier of the skin to access the blood supply or through breaks or mechanical intrusion (e.g., needle inoculation) and allow microbes to gain access to the blood stream of the host.

Routes of spread in the body

Some infectious agents replicate in epithelial cells at the portal of entry where they spread and cause damage to the epithelium. Respiratory and gastrointestinal viruses (rhinoviruses and rotavirus), gastrointestinal infections, such as with *Vibrio cholerae*, or epithelial skin infections caused by the human papilloma virus are examples of infections limited to the epithelium. However, many infectious agents may invade beyond the portal of entry by direct extension (e.g., streptococcal bacteria spread from a skin wound into the surrounding tissue). These pathogens typically spread after crossing the epithelium and accessing the blood stream or lymphatics where they can be transported throughout the body, infecting target cells such as leukocytes or specific organs (Figure 4.2). Examples of infections that extend beyond the epithelium include infection of a peripheral nerve that results in viral spread to another part of the nervous system including the brain, such as with herpes infections; or spread of bacteria upstream via the urethra to the urinary bladder that results in cystitis,

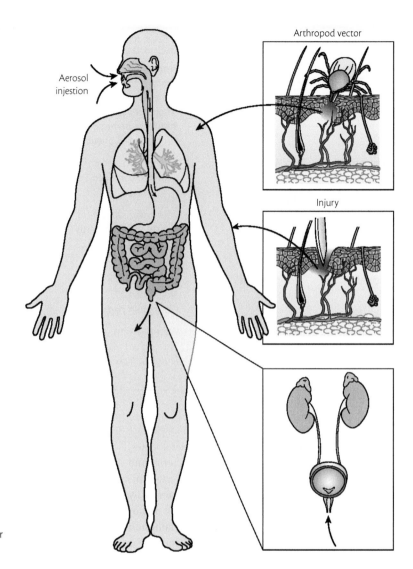

Aerosol injestion

Arthropod vector

Injury

Figure 4.1 Portals of entry/shedding for pathogenic microbes.

and subsequent retrograde spread up the ureters leading to kidney infection; or widespread infection of the endothelium lining blood vessels by *Rickettsiae* following a tick bite. Microbes can enter and invade through the respiratory tract or bloodstream and spread over the surface of the pleural, pericardial, or peritoneal cavity, resulting in empyema, pericarditis, and peritonitis, respectively. Meningococcal bacteria colonize the oropharynx but under certain conditions can invade the epithelium, spread through the bloodstream, and enter the cerebrospinal fluid in the ventricles and subarachnoid space.

Target organs and cells

Infectious agents may have a tropism to enter, replicate, and damage particular organs, which often lend their names to the agent. The liver is the target organ of hepatitis A, B, C, delta, and E viruses. The brain and spinal cord are targets of Japanese encephalitis virus, eastern and western equine encephalitis viruses, and poliovirus. Respiratory viruses target the epithelial lining of the nasopharynx, trachea, bronchi, bronchioles, and/or alveoli. Obligately intracellular bacteria such as *Rickettsiae* and *Ehrlichiae* target endothelium

Table 4.1 Portals of Entry for Bacterial and Viral Pathogens

Entry Site	Mode of Transmission	Pathogens	Disease
Respiratory tract	Aerosol	Influenza virus Respiratory syncytial virus *Bordetella pertussis* *Streptococcus pneumoniae*	Influenza Interstitial pneumonia/bronchiolitis Whooping cough Lobar pneumonia
Gastrointestinal	Food/water	*Campylobacter jejuni, Vibrio cholerae,* rotavirus, pathogenic *E. coli*	Diarrhea
Urogenital	Physical contact	HIV *Chlamydia trachomatis* Human papilloma virus	Acquired immune deficiency syndrome (AIDS) Pelvic inflammatory disease, urethritis Genital warts and cervical cancer
Wound	Compromised cutaneous barrier	*Staphlococcus,* *Steptococcus,* *Clostridium perfringens*	Necrotizing fasciitis Gas gangrene, cellulitis
Vectors	Mosquitoes Ticks	West Nile virus, dengue virus *Plasmodium falciparum* *Ehrlichia, Rickettsia, Borrelia*	West Nile encephalitis, dengue fever, malaria, ehrlichiosis, Rocky Mountain spotted fever, Lyme disease

lining the blood vessels of all organs or leukocytes, respectively. Viruses and intracellular bacteria and protozoa must gain entry into their target cells. Initially they attach to a host cell surface receptor(s) by a specialized surface protein (adhesin), which is analogous to the interaction of a lock and key. The adhesion to the cell triggers a series of cellular and molecular events that lead to entry of the infectious agent into the cell and replication in the host cell either in a modified endosome, or in the cytosol after phagosomal escape, or in the case of a virus, uncoating. Many microbes have evolved mechanisms to subvert innate immune defenses of the cell in order to survive, e.g., viral inhibition of interferon α/β. Some pathogens inhibit apoptosis and/or modulate the cell cycle of the host cell, allowing replication of the agent to proceed to the production of a larger population of infectious organisms. Many pathogens hijack other host cell processes to ensure survival, including modulation of the host cytoskeleton, immune signaling, and other immune subversion mechanisms such as chromatin manipulation and inflammasome activation. Finally,

the infectious agents manipulate the cell to achieve their release from the cell in order to spread to other cells or to be shed from the body in a manner that leads to transmission to another person or animal. In some circumstances, shedding of a live vaccine agent can lead to disease in contacts. For example, live attenuated poliovirus vaccine may mutate to a pathogenic genotype that is shed in the feces of the immunized person, (e.g., an infant in diapers could infect an unimmunized parent.)

Mechanisms of tissue injury and disease

In general, damage that occurs as a consequence of infection is caused by toxic products of the infectious agent or deleterious effects of the host's inflammatory and immune responses to the pathogen (Figure 4.3). Toxins produced by *Clostridium tetani, Corynebacterium diphtheriae,* and *Bordetella pertussis* cause cell dysfunction and tissue injury that underlie the clinical signs and symptoms of tetanus, diphtheria, and whooping

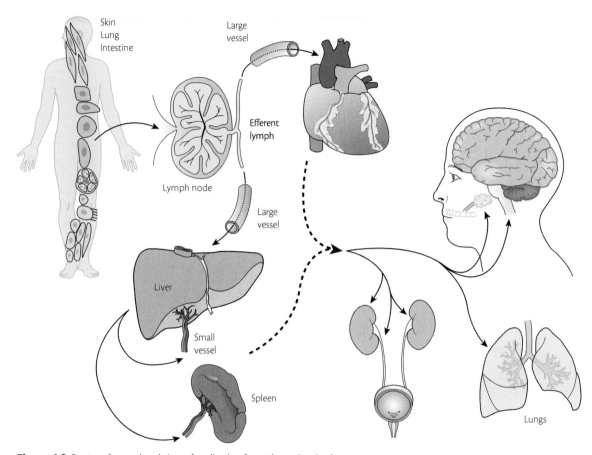

Figure 4.2 Routes of spread and sites of replication for pathogenic microbes.

cough, respectively. Inflammation characterized by the influx of neutrophilic polymorphonuclear leukocytes can cause organ dysfunction owing to its mere presence, such as airspaces in the lung filled with inflammatory exudates that prevent the entry of air, the absorption of oxygen into the red blood cells in alveolar capillaries, and the exchange of carbon dioxide. Abscesses are accumulations of pus, neutrophils that infiltrate a focus of infection to combat the pathogen, die, and release their enzymes such as proteases that damage and digest nearby tissues. While an abscess in the skin that corrals a bacterial infection and prevents its spread may be only a minor concern, an enlarging abscess in the brain not only destroys a part of this vital organ but is also a space-occupying lesion that exerts pressure on the rest of the brain that may impede the blood flow into the cranium and even

squeeze the brain out of the cranial vault, compress the brainstem, and disrupt its vital functions.

The host defenses that are effective in destroying pathogens when appropriately activated can cause severe disease when overactivated. Important elements of the humoral host defenses include cytokines, which are products secreted by cells such as lymphocytes, macrophages, and dendritic cells. Critical cytokines include interferons, interleukins, and tumor necrosis factor. Many of the common manifestations of infection such as fever and muscle aches are mediated by cytokines (Figure 4.4). Sepsis is a grave clinical condition mediated by an excess concentration of cytokines, most notably tumor necrosis factor alpha. Associated frequently with bloodstream infection by Gram-negative bacillary bacteria, sepsis is the exaggerated response of the host, including triggering of

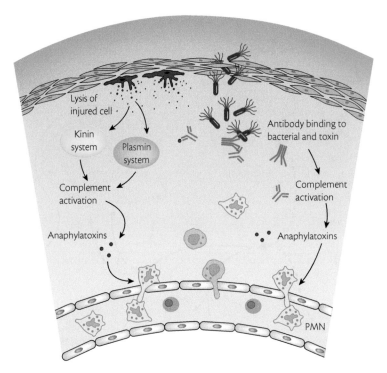

Figure 4.3 Inflammation at the site of infection initiated by complement activation.

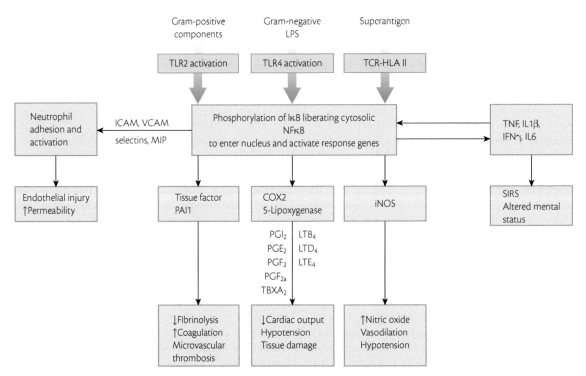

Figure 4.4 During sepsis bacterial components trigger generation of inflammatory mediators and an inflammatory cascade.

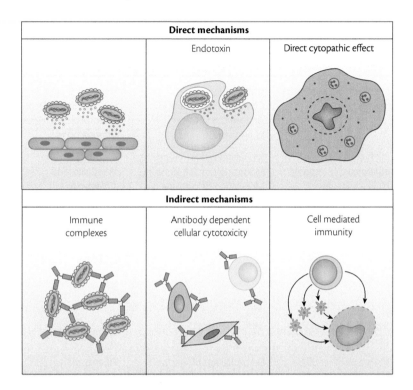

Figure 4.5 Pathogen (direct) and host response (indirect) mediated tissue damage during infection.

Toll-like receptor 4 by bacterial lipopolysaccharide. The most severe result is hypotensive shock (failure to perfuse the organs) and disseminated intravascular coagulation (uncontrolled deposition of fibrin thrombi in otherwise normal blood vessels) that can cause tissue death owing to lack of blood circulation.

Furthermore, the adaptive immune response that recognizes and responds to specific antigens of the pathogen and, in general, mediates clearance of the invaders can also cause injury that may be a minor by-product or occasionally a significant feature of the disease (Figure 4.5). Antibodies that opsonize (coat the surface of) pathogens, rendering them more susceptible to engulfment and destruction by phago-cytes, can, when present in particular ratios with their corresponding antigens, form antigen–antibody complexes that are deposited in tissues such as renal glomeruli. There, they activate the cascade of com-plement proteins and attract inflammatory cells that exert severe bystander injury to the involved tissue, e.g., glomerulonephritis and renal failure. Cellular immunity may also act as a double-edged sword, causing damage as it holds the pathogen in check, e.g.,

granulomas comprising activated macrophages that restrict the growth and spread of *Mycobacterium tuber-culosis*, or eliminate virus-producing host cells, e.g., cytotoxic T lymphocytes inducing apoptotic cell death in hepatitis B virus-infected liver cells.

Pathogen evasion of host defenses

Evasion of host defenses begins with the pathogen adhering to the epithelial surfaces of the mucosa and overcoming the protective physical mechanisms such as the mucociliary escalator of the respiratory tract that is designed to trap potentially harmful microbes in mucus and cilia to propel them up the bronchus for removal (Table 4.2). In the intestine, the flow of luminal contents and mucus plays a role in con-trolling microbial colonization; in the mouth, saliva plays a role in removing and inactivating microbes. Many pathogens establish infection by adherence to a mucosal surface through a molecular interaction between surface proteins on the pathogen and surface receptors on the host cell. The proteins expressed on

Table 4.2 Host Defense Subversion Strategies by Pathogenic Bacteria and Viruses

Target	Strategy	Pathogen	Effect
Inhibition of humoral immunity	Glycan shield Complement resistance Antigenic variation Ig proteases	Hepatitis C virus HIV and *Staphylococcus* *Streptococcus; Neisseria* *Streptococcus*	Prevents antibody binding Inactivation of complement Prevents antibody recognition Inactivate antibody
Inhibition of inflammatory response/ block of innate immune sensing or cytokine effect	Modulation of NF-κB activity Modulation of TLR signaling Modulation of cytokine signalling	Cytomegalovirus West Nile virus *Chlamydia* *E.coli* *Shigella* Vaccinia virus Hepatitis C virus *Ehrlichia*	Targets NF-κB to autophagosome Inhibits NF-κB translocation Deubiquitinates IκBα; blocks IκBα ubiquitination Ubiquitinates NF-κB essential modulator (NEMO) Blocks TLR TIR domain interaction with MyD88 Blocks IRAK and MyD88 interaction Blocks Jak/Stat pathway
Block antigen presentation	MHC-I transport	HIV	Impairs immune recognition
Inhibition of reactive oxygen	Detoxification of reactive oxygen species and degradation and altered trafficking of NADPH components	*Anaplasma* *Ehrlichia* *Salmonella*	Impairs oxygen mediated killing mechanisms
Inhibition of apoptosis	Various mechanisms	*Chlamydia* *Anaplasma* Hepatitis C virus	Prolong host cell and pathogen survival

the surface of a pathogen that mediate adhesion to a host cell receptor are called *adhesins*. In many cases, pathogens have multiple adhesins that allow interactions with different target cells and are determined by the molecular domains of the adhesin. Receptors can be proteins or sugars that decorate proteins (glycoproteins), and many of the host cell receptors that interact with pathogens are signaling molecules. Interactions between these receptors and the pathogen can trigger cellular events that result in receptor-mediated endocytosis or downregulation of host cell defenses. Many of the natural host cell defenses can be compromised by prior infection with a pathogen, creating an environment where other microbes can colonize and cause secondary infections. For example, many upper respiratory viruses cause damage to the ciliated cells of the respiratory tract, which allows a bacterial pathogen to colonize the mucosal surface. Infections of the sinuses and lung with opportunistic bacteria are common after primary viral infections.

Microbes have also evolved mechanisms that allow them to evade a diverse array of innate and adaptive host defense mechanisms. These organisms often accomplish this feat by producing virulence factors that enable them to circumvent host defenses. Escaping phagocytosis is one strategy that is utilized by many extracellular bacteria to survive longer in the host. A common virulence factor is a surface polysaccharide layer, or capsule, that enables bacteria to avoid engulfment by phagocytes such as macrophages.

Examples of such organisms that cause common infections in humans include *Staphylococcus* and *Streptococcus* spp. Intracellular bacteria use a variety of approaches to evade innate immune responses. Some intracellular bacteria such as *Ehrlichia* spp. lack pathogen-associated molecular patterns (PAMPs), the molecules that are recognized by Toll-like receptors that are strong stimulators of the innate immune response. Similarly, viruses have developed mechanisms to prevent recognition by innate immune receptors and possess interferon α/β antagonists such as NS1 of influenza virus that prevents the antiviral effects or NS3/4A of hepatitis virus C that counteracts the RIG-I innate immune sensing pathway. Other mechanisms utilized by intracellular bacteria include prevention of lysosomal fusion, inhibition of nicotinamide adenine dinucleotide phosphate (NADPH), oxygen-dependent killing, and escape from the phagosome.

Evasion of adaptive host defenses involves overcoming antibody and cellular immune responses. Extracellular microbes evade adaptive immune responses by altering surface proteins that are recognized by antibody, which would mediate the elimination of the pathogen. Microbes such as seasonal influenza A virus, streptococcus and *Anaplasma* spp. utilize antigenic variation to avoid protective antibodies. Other pathogens produce proteases that cleave antibody, such as IgA protease produced by *Neisseria*, *Streptococcus*, and *Haemophilus* spp., inactivate, complement, or decorate their surface with proteins that bind the Fc portion of the antibody molecule and prevent specific antibodies from recognizing surface epitopes and thereby neutralizing the pathogen. Other pathogens produce proteases that cleave antibody, such as IgA protease produced by *Neisseria*, *Streptococcus*, and *Haemophilus* spp., inactivate, complement, or decorate their surface with proteins that bind the Fc portion of the antibody molecule and prevent specific antibodies from recognizing surface epitopes, and neutralizing the pathogen. Some extracellular bacteria secrete toxins or effector proteins that kill phagocytes such as *Bacillus anthracis* lethal toxin or *Yersinia pestis* Yop effectors. Occasionally, microbes use the antibody response as a mechanism to enter the host cell, such as dengue virus, for which non-neutralizing antiviral antibody enhances host cell entry though Fc receptor-mediated uptake. In many cases, microbes evade the immune response by seeking an intracellular niche that protects them from circulating antibodies and extracellular innate immune defense proteins including complement.

Cellular immune mechanisms are often targeted by microbes by interfering with antigen presentation or by modulation of cytokines that drive T-cell responses. This approach is utilized by many intracellular microbes to survive and replicate in immune cells such as phagocytes, antigen presenting cells, or T cells. In the case of the human immunodeficiency virus (HIV), a virus encoded protein, Nef, interacts with major histocompatibility complex class I (MHC-I) proteins altering their transport to the cell surface and resulting in reduced T-cell recognition of the pathogen's antigens. In addition, downregulation of MHC-I expression has been associated with other viral infections, including herpes and papilloma viruses and intracellular bacteria such as *Chlamydia* and *Ehrlichia*. Other intracellular bacteria modulate expression of important cytokines and inhibit induction of the immune response by blocking the effects of IFN-γ during infection of the macrophage by *Ehrlichia* spp. By avoiding innate immune defenses of the macrophage and modulating the response of the macrophage to T-cell–produced IFN-γ, *Ehrlichia* are able to successfully avoid both innate and adaptive immune responses.

Vaccines for infectious diseases and mechanisms of vaccine-induced immunity

Vaccines often do not prevent entry of the pathogen and its growth for a short time but they do stimulate a host immune response that blocks the pathogenic mechanism or inhibits the growth and survival of the pathogen prior to the occurrence of sufficient damage and organ dysfunction that would reach the threshold of clinical disease (Figure 4.6). Indeed, a vaccine that fails to prevent disease but effectively prevents death would represent an advance for an ordinarily highly lethal infection. The four types of vaccines are toxoids (modified forms of the toxin that are not toxic themselves) but do stimulate antibodies that block the toxin's effect; killed viruses or bacteria; live attenuated

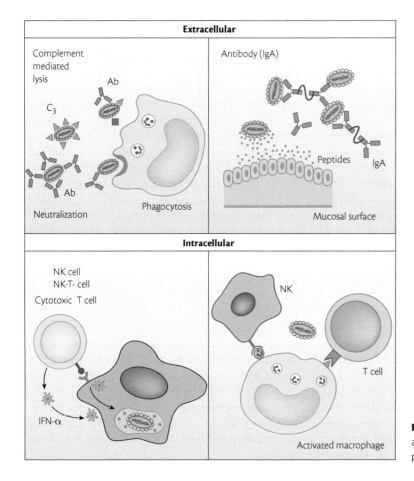

Figure 4.6 Primary immune mechanisms against extracellular and intracellular pathogens.

organisms (weakened but capable of stimulating immunity); and subunit vaccines.

Toxin-mediated diseases

Tetanus

Clostridium tetani resides in the soil and can be introduced through the skin by a traumatic puncture wound. The bacterial spores introduced deep into damaged tissue germinate, replicate by binary fission, and secrete a protein toxin, tetanospasmin (a zinc-dependent matrix metalloproteinase) (Figure 4.7). The toxin's heavy chain binds to a neuronal cell surface receptor that transports the protein that mediates the toxin's entry into the presynaptic terminals of lower motor neurons. Subsequently, the toxin spreads by retrograde axonal transport to neurons of the spinal cord and brainstem. The toxin diffuses to terminals of central nervous system (CNS) inhibitory neurons where it degrades synaptobrevin, a protein that is necessary for docking neurotransmitter vesicles with their release site on the presynaptic membrane. The prevention of neurotransmitter release blocks the action of inhibitory neurons on motor neurons, leading to motor neuron overactivity and muscular spasms, e.g., lockjaw. A toxoid of tetanospasmin stimulates the production of antibodies that bind to the toxin and prevent its entry into peripheral neurons.

Diphtheria

Corynebacterium diphtheriae contains a phage that encodes the toxin and integrates into the bacterial chromosome. Synthesis of the toxin depends on the availability of iron. The bacteria are transmitted from

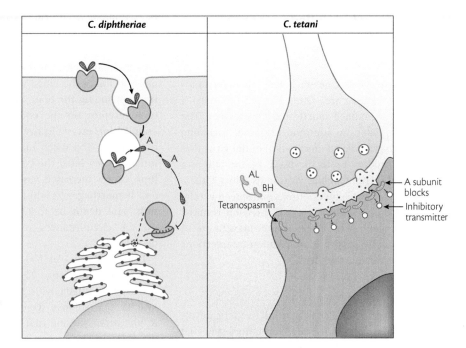

Figure 4.7 Mechanisms of bacterial toxin mediated damage.

person to person by respiratory droplets and colonize but do not invade beyond the respiratory mucosal epithelium. The toxin binds to a cell receptor and is cleaved followed by entry of a particular component into the cell (Figure 4.7). The toxic moiety catalyzes inactivation of transfer RNA translocase (elongation factor 2), blocking the addition of amino acids to developing polypeptides. The locally affected cells die, forming a necrotic pseudomembrane in the throat, and the toxin spreads through the bloodstream to cause damage to myocardial cells and the brain. Formalin-inactivated toxoid stimulates the production of antibodies that bind the toxin and prevent its entry into cells.

Anthrax

Bacillus anthracis resides in the soil as a spore. Anthrax is a disease of grazing animals that ingest soil with closely cropped vegetation as occurs during periods of drought. Dying animals with high concentrations of bacteria in their blood release bloody fluids from all orifices. The released bacteria sporulate, and spores remain in the soil for a very long time. Humans become infected when introducing spores into the skin while butchering an ill or dead animal or process-

ing its hide or wool. Gastrointestinal or inhalational anthrax occurs after ingestion of contaminated meat or inhalation of spores, respectively. The spores are engulfed by phagocytes such as dendritic cells; the phagocytes transport the spores through lymphatic vessels to regional lymph nodes where the spores germinate and produce three plasmid-encoded proteins: protective antigen, lethal factor, and edema factor. Protective antigen binds to host cell membrane receptors and is arranged into a heptamer, which binds lethal factor and/or edema factor and mediates their transfer into the cell. Lethal toxin inactivates particular signal transduction proteins, and edema toxin is an adenyl cyclase. The damage from these events results in edema, necrosis, hemorrhage, and in some situations dissemination by the bloodstream to the meninges and other organs. Immunization with protective antigen stimulates the production of antibodies that bind it and prevent the entry of lethal factor and edema factor into cells, consequent damage to the cells, and subsequent invasion of the blood. A veterinary vaccine against anthrax is a live bacterium that produces toxins that stimulate antibodies but lacks the capsule, resulting in bacterial clearance before disease ensues.

69

Diseases for which killed pathogen vaccines were developed

Rabies

At the dawn of the vaccine era, before the understanding of what viruses are, Louis Pasteur produced a vaccine that contained inactivated rabies virus. The vaccine stimulated an immune response, including antibodies that mediated inactivation of the virus that had been introduced into the tissue by the bite of a rabid animal secreting rabies virus in its saliva. Otherwise the virus would enter neurons and spread via the axons to the CNS where neuronal infection resulted in rabies encephalitis. Postexposure prevention of disease occurs by passive immunization by injections of antibodies against the virus.

Respiratory syncytial virus

A tragic chapter of vaccine history followed the development of a formalin-inactivated respiratory syncytial virus (RSV) vaccine. RSV infection is a major cause of lower respiratory infection in infants. The infection does not stimulate long-lasting immunity, and recurrent infections occur throughout life. Infection is transmitted from person to person via respiratory droplets that can infect respiratory epithelial cells from the nasopharynx, trachea, and bronchi to the bronchioles and alveoli. The most important clinical manifestation is bronchiolitis in infants. Adults even into old age suffer reinfection and inflammation of the upper respiratory tract.

The formalin-inactivated vaccine enhances hyperresponsive constriction of airway smooth muscle cells and fails to stimulate virus-neutralizing antibodies and to reduce viral replication. Some of the children who received the inactivated virus vaccine had enhanced severity of the lower respiratory tract disease, occasionally with a fatal outcome.

Epidemic louse-borne typhus

Rickettsia prowazekii is spread from person to person by body lice, which are infected by feeding on a bacteremic person. Lice leave the body of a febrile person to escape the excessively warm temperature and seek another human host. After approximately a week, the lice begin to shed *Rickettsiae* in their feces, which are deposited on the skin of the new host during the louse's blood meal. The bacteria are scratched into the person's skin and spread throughout the body in the blood. These bacteria cannot grow unless they are inside host cells, which in humans are the endothelial cells lining the blood vessel walls throughout the body, including the brain and lungs. *Rickettsiae* attach to a receptor on the endothelial cell, trigger their engulfment, escape from the phagosome, replicate in the cytosol, and when massive numbers have accumulated they burst the cell. Destruction of endothelium causes increased vascular permeability, edema, and hemorrhages, resulting in encephalitis, pneumonitis, and death in 15–60% of patients depending on the circumstances (e.g., famine, war, natural disasters).

During World War I and the Russian Revolution, and their aftermath, 25 million cases of typhus occurred in Russia with 3 million deaths. In World War II, U.S. soldiers were immunized with a killed *R. prowazekii* vaccine that contained rickettsial outer membrane protein B, a rickettsial adhesin, and invasin. There were no deaths among vaccinated soldiers, although in civilian populations in the same geographic regions there were epidemics and many deaths. As is frequently the case with killed bacterial vaccines, immunity did not always prevent infection and disease.

Live attenuated pathogen vaccines

Epidemic louse-borne typhus

Also during an epidemic of typhus in Spain in World War II, an isolate of *R. prowazekii* was made in a laboratory and passaged by inoculation of the yolk sac of embryonated chicken eggs through more than 250 passages. A spontaneous mutation occurred that weakened the virulence of the organism. Subsequently during the 1950s and 1960s, the mutant Madrid E strain was evaluated as a vaccine and demonstrated to be very effective. Later it was noted that 14% of vaccinees developed a generally mild illness and that passage of the vaccine organisms in experimental animals resulted in reversion to the virulent state. The vaccine was abandoned. Recently, we determined that attenuation was due to a single point mutation of a methyltransferase gene. When genetic manipulation systems are developed for these obligately intracellular bacteria, knockout of this gene would yield an excellent vaccine candidate.

Yellow fever

Yellow fever virus occurs in sylvatic zoonotic cycles with transmission among nonhuman primates and mosquitoes. Humans who enter a location where such a cycle is occurring can also be infected by a virus-carrying mosquito. More threatening are urban yellow fever epidemics, spread from infected person to an uninfected person by *Aedes aegypti* mosquitoes. After introduction of the virus into a person's skin via the saliva of the feeding mosquito, the virus spreads hematogenously with its most notable target organ being the liver. Severe hepatocellular necrosis results in jaundice and coagulopathy owing to inadequate hepatic synthesis of coagulation factors. The vaccine is a live yellow fever virus that underwent spontaneous attenuating mutation during laboratory passage long ago. Vaccination results in the production of neutralizing antibodies that prevent yellow fever for at least 10 years.

Childhood viral infections

Measles, mumps, and rubella have been controlled by the administration of a vaccine that contains all three of these live attenuated viruses. In general, viral infections are believed to be controlled mainly by neutralizing antibodies. However, live attenuated vaccines also stimulate cellular immunity, which may also contribute to vaccine-associated protective immunity.

Subunit vaccines

Hepatitis B

Hepatitis B virus (HBV) vaccine contains hepatitis B surface antigen (HBsAg) that stimulates the production of antibodies that prevent disease associated with hepatocellular infection. HBV can be transmitted by inoculation of contaminated blood such as occurred with blood transfusions prior to the identification of HBV and the development of assays to test blood for safety before transfusion. The most important means of transmission is perinatal, from mother to offspring. Infections acquired perinatally are more likely to result in a persistent carrier state.

Neisseria meningitidis

Meningococcal meningitis occurs when the nasopharynx is colonized by encapsulated *N. meningitidis*. In some persons, invasive infection of the bloodstream occurs with spread to the brain and throughout the subarachnoid space. Vaccination with capsular antigen stimulates the production of antibodies that mediate opsonophagocytosis of the bacteria, preventing the disease.

Streptococcus pneumoniae

Aging is associated with less robust immune responses and increased susceptibility to pneumococcal pneumonia. *Streptococcus pneumoniae* are encapsulated Gram-positive bacteria that colonize the nasopharynx. Following inhalation of the bacteria in a susceptible person, the organisms grow in the pulmonary alveoli and stimulate an influx of inflammation that compromises respiratory function. Vaccines containing antigens of the capsules of the 23 types that most commonly cause pneumonia stimulate antibodies that are protective, presumably by opsonophagocytosis and removal of bacteria before a sufficient quantity have grown to cause illness.

Summary

- Infectious diseases are caused by a great variety of agents, ranging from viruses and bacteria to fungi, protozoa, and worms. The sequence of steps in the disease process and the mechanisms mediating injury of cells, tissues, and organs are known as *pathogenesis*.

- *Infection* is defined as the presence of an organism in an ordinarily sterile body site or an organism other than normal flora on a body surface. The presence of an organism on a nonsterile body surface such as skin or mucosa of the mouth, nasopharynx, large intestine, or vagina is defined as *colonization*.

- In general, damage that occurs as a consequence of infection is caused by toxic products of the infectious agent or deleterious effects of the host's inflammatory and immune responses to the pathogen.

- The adaptive immune response that recognizes and responds to specific antigens of the pathogen and, in general, mediates clearance of the invaders can also

(Continued)

cause injury that may be a minor by-product or occasionally a significant feature of the disease.

- Evasion of host defense begins with the pathogen adhering to the epithelial surfaces of the mucosa and overcoming protective physical mechanisms. Microbes have also evolved mechanisms that allow them to evade a diverse array of innate and adaptive host defense mechanisms.

- Vaccines often do not prevent entry of the pathogen and its growth for a short time but they do stimulate a host immune response that blocks the pathogenic mechanism or inhibits the growth and survival of the pathogen prior to the occurrence of sufficient damage and organ dysfunction that would reach the threshold of clinical disease.

Further reading

Bounaguro L, Wang E, Tornesello ML, Buonaguro FM, and Marincola FM (2011). Systems biology approach to vaccine and immunotherapy development. BMC Systems Biology 5, 146.

Cheng AG, DeDent AC, Schneewind O, and Missiakas D (2011). A play in four acts: *Staphlyococcus aureus* abscess formation. Trends in Microbiology 19, 225–232.

Cole JN, Barnett TC, Nizet V, and Walker MJ (2011). Molecular insight into group A streptococcal disease. Nature Reviews. Microbiology 9, 724–736.

Gerber J and Nau R (2011). Mechanisms of injury in bacterial meningitis. Current Opinion in Neurology 23, 312–318.

Horst D, Verweij MC, Davison AJ, Ressing ME, and Wiertz EJ (2011). Viral evasion of T cell immunity: ancient mechanisms offering new applications. Current Opinion in Immunology 23, 96–103.

Kim HK, Thammavongsa V, Schneewind O, and Missiakas D (2012). Recurrent infections and immune evasion strategies of *Staphylococcus aureus*. Current Opinion in Microbiology 15, 92–99.

Manel N and Littman DR (2011). Hiding in plain sight: how HIV evades innate immune responses. Cell 147, 271–274.

McBride JW and Walker DH (2010). Progress and obstacles in vaccine development for the ehrlichioses. Expert Review of Vaccines 9, 1071–1082.

5 The host immune response, protective immunity, and correlates of protection

Gregg N. Milligan

Sealy Center for Vaccine Development, University of Texas Medical Branch, Galveston, TX, USA

Introduction

The utilization of vaccines for protection of humans against infectious disease is generally thought to have originated with Edward Jenner through his use of a cowpox "vaccine" to protect humans against smallpox. Since this event, vaccines designed to protect against a wide variety of bacteria, bacterial toxins, and viruses have been developed and approved for use in most countries around the world. These vaccines activate a diverse set of immune cells that yield a variety of immune mechanisms responsible for protection against these agents. The development of protective immunity represents the culmination of a series of complex events that are initiated very quickly after introduction of the vaccine into an individual.

The adaptive immune system is comprised of B and T lymphocytes that recognize pathogens in an antigen-specific manner. This arm of the immune system is responsible for production of pathogen-specific antibodies or expression of cellular effector immune functions such as cytolysis or cytokine production. These immune mechanisms are directly responsible for preventing or limiting infection and preventing disease by killing invading pathogens, neutralizing disease-causing pathogen products, or lysing pathogen-infected cells. The goal of vaccines is to induce adaptive immunity specific for vaccine antigens, and more specifically, to initiate the development of persistent antibody and

memory B- and T-cell responses that will protect the immunized individual upon subsequent contact with

Definitions

PAMP: Pathogen-associated molecular pattern. Highly conserved, molecular structures or patterns preferentially expressed by viral, bacterial, or parasitic pathogens that are recognized by extracellular and intracellular receptors of host cells. Examples of PAMPs include lipopolysaccharide, double-stranded RNA, flagellin, and unmethylated DNA oligonucleotides containing the CpG motif.

PRR: Pattern recognition receptor. These receptors include several groups of host receptor molecules that recognize specific PAMPs. Signal cascades resulting from PAMP ligand binding to PRRs result in release of type I interferon, proinflammatory cytokines, and induction of antimicrobial gene programs. Examples of PRRs include: Toll-like receptors (TLRs), RIG-I, MDA-5, and C-type lectin receptors.

TLR: Toll-like receptor. TLRs are a family of receptor molecules that recognize evolutionarily conserved pathogen-associated molecular patterns. These receptors are expressed primarily on the cell surface or in endosomal compartments.

CpG motif: Unmethylated cytosine-phosphate-guanine. Oligonucleotides containing unmethylated CpG dinucleotide sequences, found primarily in DNA of microbial origin, are recognized by the TLR-9 PRR.

Vaccinology: An Essential Guide, First Edition. Edited by Gregg N. Milligan and Alan D.T. Barrett.
© 2015 John Wiley & Sons, Ltd. Published 2015 by John Wiley & Sons, Ltd.

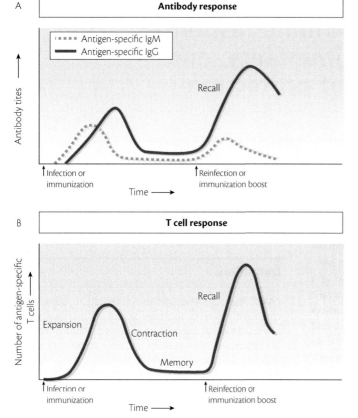

A

Antibody response

- ••••• Antigen-specific IgM
- —— Antigen-specific IgG

Antibody tites

Recall

Infection or
immunization

Time ⟶

Reinfection or
immunization boost

B

T cell response

Number of antigen-specific
T cells

Recall

Expansion

Contraction

Memory

Infection or
immunization

Time ⟶

Reinfection or
immunization boost

Figure 5.1 Primary and secondary immune responses to pathogens or vaccine antigens. Primary exposure of naïve T and B cells to pathogen or vaccine antigen results in a rapid increase in antigen-specific cell number. As the pathogen is cleared, a rapid contraction of the population due to cell death ensues. However, a portion of the antigen-specific population survives and is maintained for long periods of time as memory cells such that an increased frequency of antigen-specific cells is present in secondary lymphoid tissues and peripheral tissues. These populations rapidly expand following reexposure to antigen and are capable of providing protection and rapidly clearing the pathogen from the site of infection.

the virulent pathogen (Figure 5.1). Importantly, in most cases these responses do not prevent infection with the pathogen (i.e., sterilizing immunity), but do prevent manifestation of disease symptoms. We now realize that the process of inducing protective adaptive immune responses begins with successful engagement of the innate immune system by vaccine components. Our understanding of how immune responses are initiated and the role of specific cells and immune molecules in shaping the type, magnitude, and duration of these memory responses is currently being utilized to develop new vaccines as well as improve the protective efficacy of existing vaccines.

Induction of innate immunity

The innate immune system is responsible for the initial recognition of the presence of microorganisms

or their products, providing for the initial resistance against invading pathogens, and in initiating and driving the activation and differentiation of the adaptive immune response. Unlike the antigen receptors of the adaptive immune cells, innate immune cells recognize the presence of pathogens through a number of distinct, genetically conserved receptors that recognize specific, conserved molecular patterns expressed preferentially by pathogens. These pattern recognition receptors (PRRs) recognize and respond to specific types of pathogen-associated molecular patterns (PAMPs). The result of this recognition event is the activation of antigen-nonspecific immune mechanisms important in the initial resistance to pathogens and the mustering of additional innate immune cells to the site of PAMP exposure. Further, these initial innate immune cell products and activities drive the activation and differentiation of the antigen-specific adaptive immune response.

Toll-like receptors

Toll-like receptors (TLRs) are an important family of PRRs that recognize a variety of conserved microbial patterns. There are 10 TLRs that have been identified in humans and different sets of these receptors are expressed at different locations within and on cells. For example, TLR1, TLR2, TLR4, TLR5, TLR6, and perhaps TLR10 are present as membrane-bound proteins on the cell surface whereas TLR3, TL7, TLR8, and TLR9 are located intracellularly and primarily in the endoplasmic reticulum and endosomes. The expression of these receptors is also cell-type–specific. For example, TLR2 and TLR4 are expressed on macrophages, myeloid dendritic cells, B cells (mice not humans), granulocytes, natural killer (NK) cells, T cells, fibroblasts, and epithelial cells whereas TLR 7 and TLR 9 are expressed primarily at high levels in plasmacytoid dendritic cells. A diverse set of microbial products are recognized by TLRs, with each individual TLR recognizing distinct types of ligands (Table 5.1).

For example, TLR1, TLR2, and TLR6 recognize lipoproteins, whereas TLR4 detects bacterial lipopolysaccharides (LPS). TLR5 recognizes flagellin, a subunit of bacterial flagellar structures. Several TLRs detect different nucleic acids. TLR3 recognizes double-stranded RNA while TLR7 and TLR8 recognize single-stranded RNA. TLR9 has been shown to recognize CpG motifs of unmethylated DNA. The TLR-specificity for ligands is linked with its cellular localization such that the appropriate milieu is sampled for the presence of relevant PAMPs.

Following ligand binding to the TLRs, activation signals are transduced from the receptor to the nucleus by engagement of specific signal pathways. The TLR family members are type I integral membrane glycoproteins containing a cytoplasmic domain, the Toll-interleukin (IL)-1 receptor domain that associates with adaptor proteins. These proteins couple the receptors to downstream signal pathway proteins involved in activation of nuclear transcription factors.

Table 5.1 Pattern Recognition Receptors

	Ligand	Adaptor Molecule	Location
TLR			
1, 2	Triacyl lipopeptides	MyD88	Cell surface
2, 6	Diacyl lipopeptides	MyD88	Cell surface
3	dsRNA	TRIF	Endosome
4	LPS	MyD88, TRIF	Cell surface
5	Flagellin	MyD88	Cell surface
7	ssRNA	MyD88	Endosome
	Imiquimod and derivatives		
8	ssRNA	MyD88	Endosome
9	Unmethylated DNA	MyD88	Endosome
	CpG motifs		
10	Unknown	MyD88	Cell surface
RLR			
RIG-I	dsRNA	TRIF	Cytoplasm
MDA5	dsRNA	TRIF	Cytoplasm
NLR			
NOD1	Peptidoglycan	—	Cytoplasm
NOD2	Muramyldipeptide	—	Cytoplasm
NALP3 inflammasome	Muramyldipeptide	—	Cytoplasm
	Uric acid crystals		
NAIP, NLRC4	Flagellin	—	Cytoplasm

All TLRs utilize the myeloid differentiation primary response protein 88 (MyD88) adaptor protein except TLR3, which utilizes the Toll/IL-1R resistance (TIR)-domain-containing adaptor protein inducing interferon (IFN)-β (TRIF). The end result of TLR signaling is the activation of nuclear transcription factors that migrate to the nucleus and bind to specific promoter regions that drive the production of proinflammatory cytokines and type I IFN. These proteins then exert profound effects on innate immune cells and direct the differentiation of the adaptive immune response.

Definitions

RIG-I: Retinoic acid-inducible gene I. This is a protein expressed in the cytoplasm of cells that recognizes double-stranded RNA. Downstream signaling events from stimulation of this receptor lead to production of type I IFNs and proinflammatory cytokines.

MyD88: Myeloid differentiation primary response protein 88. This adapter protein is recruited to Toll-like receptors (TLRs) 1, 2, 4, 5, 6, 7, 9, and 11 following binding of the TLR ligand. Recruitment of MyD88 results in a signal cascade that activates the transcription factors, NF-κB and IRFs and ultimately leads to production of type I interferons and proinflammatory cytokines.

TRIF: Toll/IL-1 receptor-domain-containing adaptor protein inducing interferon (IFN)-β. This adapter protein is recruited to TLRs 3 and 4 following ligand binding. TRIF links ligand binding with downstream signal proteins resulting in activation of NF-κB and IRFs, and ultimately to the production of type I interferons and proinflammatory cytokines.

MDA5: Melanoma differentiation-associated gene 5. This molecule is a RIG-I-like receptor molecule expressed in the cytoplasm of cells that recognizes double-strand RNA. Signaling events downstream of this receptor result in production of type I IFNs.

NLR: Nucleotide-binding, oligomerizaton domain-like (NOD-like) receptors. The NLR family is a group of PRRs that contain a nucleotide-binding domain and a leucine-rich repeat region. NLRs are involved in the initiation of immune responses against microbes.

RIG-I-like receptors

Similar pathogen-sensing functions are provided by the cytoplasmic proteins retinoic acid-inducible gene I (RIG-I) and melanoma differentiation-associated gene 5 (MDA5). These proteins are triggered primarily by virus infection and recognize slightly different types of double-stranded RNA structures. RIG-I detects triphosphate RNA and is important in protection against influenza virus, paramyxoviruses, and Japanese encephalitis virus. Both receptors recognize the synthetic RNA ligand, poly inosine:cytosine (poly I:C); however, RIG-I seems to preferentially recognize short segments of the ligand whereas longer RNA segments preferentially lead to activation through MDA5. MDA5 plays an important role in defense against picornaviruses and measles virus. Binding of RNA ligands by these receptors results in expression of proinflammatory cytokines and type I IFN.

Definitions

NF-κB: A nuclear transcription factor required for initiation of a number of immunological events such as cytokine production.

ASC: Apoptosis-associated speck-like protein. ASC is an adaptor protein involved in the activation of the NALP3 inflammasome.

IL: Interleukin. A descriptive term for the group of molecules (cytokines) produced by lymphocytes.

DC-SIGN: Dendritic Cell-specific Intercellular Adhesion Molecule-3-Grabbing Non-integrin, also called CD209. This C-type lectin is expressed only on dendritic cells and functions as an adhesion molecule that binds to intracellular adhesion molecules on endothelial cells and T lymphocytes, a binding molecule for many glycosylated antigens, and as an activator of signal transduction pathways that ultimately guides DC function.

NOD-like receptors (NLRs)

The nucleotide-binding oligomerization domain (NOD)-like receptors (NLRs) comprise a family of cytoplasmic proteins that recognize PAMPs such as bacterial cell wall components or danger signals released from damaged host cells such as extracellular ATP and hyaluronan. The NOD1 and NOD2 NLRs recognize different components of peptidoglycan. NOD1 recognizes the meso-diaminopimelic acid component of peptidoglycan, which is found in both Gram-negative and Gram-positive bacteria, while NOD2 recognizes muramyl dipeptide. Interestingly, other NLR members NLRC4 (NOD-like receptor containing a caspase-associated recruitment domain [CARD]) and NAIP5 (NLR family, apoptosis inhibitory protein 5) are involved in recognition of intracellular flagellin. Based on this ligand-recognition profile, it has been suggested that NLRs may play a role in immune protection against intracellular bacteria. Signaling via NLRs commonly results in the activation of NF-κB and subsequent production of proinflammatory cytokines.

Recent interest has focused on the NLR proteins NALP1, 2, and 3, which can act as a components of a multiprotein complex referred to as the inflammasome complex. Once activated, the inflammasome induces activation of the protease caspase 1 that matures proinflammatory cytokines such as interleukin (IL)-1β and IL-18. The activation process begins with recognition of ligand by the leucine-rich repeat domain in the C-terminus of the NALP protein, which initiates a self-oligomerization process. The adapter protein, apoptosis-associated speck-like protein (ASC), then associates with the complex. Procaspase-1 is then recruited to the complex where it is auto-cleaved and activated. The activation of caspase-1 results in the processing and release of proteins such as IL-1β and IL-18 that play a role in inflammation as well as other proteins directly involved with tissue repair. Interestingly, a number of ligands have been identified for the NALP3 protein including extracellular ATP, amyloid-β fibrils, monosodium urate and calcium pyrophosphate dehydrate crystals, silica, and asbestos. Recent reports have suggested that aluminum hydroxide used in aluminum salt adjuvants is capable of activating the inflammasome complex and may play a role in the mechanism of action for alum adjuvants.

C-type lectin receptors

C-type lectin receptors represent a family of approximately 120 proteins that are primarily expressed on the cell surface of professional antigen-presenting cells. These proteins are involved in a number of cellular processes including cell adhesion and migration and may be involved in maintaining immune tolerance. Beyond these activities, C-type lectin receptors bind carbohydrate moieties from a number of different bacteria, viruses, and fungi, and may be useful for vaccine purposes for targeting vaccine antigens to professional antigen-presenting cells. Examples of C-type lectins include dendritic cell-specific intercellular adhesion molecule-3-grabbing non-integrin (DC-SIGN), the mannose receptor, Dectin-1, Langerhan cell-specific C-type lectin or Langerin, and DEC205.

Definitions

MHC: Major histocompatibility complex. These polymorphic gene products are expressed on the cell surface and are involved in antigen presentation and signaling events between antigen-presenting cells and T lymphocytes. Processed antigen peptides associated with class I MHC molecules are recognized by CD8+ T cells while peptides associated with class II MHC molecules are recognized by CD4+ T cells.

CCR7: The receptor for the CCL21 chemokine. This chemokine receptor is involved in homing of immune cells to secondary lymphoid tissue in response to the presence of the chemokine CCL21, which is constitutively produced by these lymphoid tissues.

DC: Dendritic cell. Bone marrow derived cells of lymphoid or mononuclear cell origin that play an important role in antigen uptake and presentation to T lymphocytes.

B7-1 (also called CD80) and **B7-2** (also called CD86): Cell surface molecules expressed by antigen-presenting cells that act as co-stimulatory molecules required for activation of naïve T cells.

Bridging innate and adaptive immunity

Dendritic cells (DCs) serve as important mediators of innate immunity and also link the recognition of pathogens or their products with the development of an antigen-specific, adaptive immune response. Bone marrow progenitor cells differentiate into DC precursors that migrate through the blood and populate body tissues. Following arrival in the various body tissues, they further differentiate to become immature DCs. These cells are very good at internalizing microorganisms, microbial products, or host cell products that they then degrade and display in association with major histocompatibility complex (MHC) proteins for recognition by T lymphocytes. Importantly, in the immature or inactivated state, these DC do not express many MHC molecules or the important co-stimulatory molecules required for efficient activation of antigen-specific T cells and thus cannot initiate and maintain T-cell activation. Therefore, while immature or inactivated DCs migrate constitutively to secondary lymphoid tissues at low levels in the absence of infection or inflammatory event, they are unable to help induce a T-cell response to antigens they may be displaying. It is thought that this constitutive migration of inactivated DCs that display predominantly processed host cell antigens may be involved in maintenance of self-tolerance.

A very different scenario occurs when immature tissue DCs come in contact with microbes or microbial products. Under these conditions, PAMP-containing microbial products such as proteins with repeating subunits, lipoproteins, or nucleic acid components of pathogens activate DCs by binding to the PRRs discussed previously. Upon recognition of a PAMP via the appropriate PRR, the immature DC begins a maturation process characterized by increased uptake and processing of pathogen-derived antigens. The chemokine receptor CCR7, which is necessary for homing to the T-cell zone of secondary lymphoid tissues, is also expressed, resulting in the movement of DCs that carry immunogenic pathogen molecules from the site of infection to the site of immune response induction. Additionally, maturing DCs express higher levels of MHC molecules and important co-stimulatory molecules such as B7-1, B7-2, and CD40 ligand on their surface, which promotes their ability to activate naïve T cells. The maturing DCs migrate in a CCR7-dependent fashion through the lymphatic vessels and into the T-cell area of the regional lymph node. Here, naïve T cells scan the surface of newly arriving DCs for the presence of foreign antigens/MHC complexes capable of binding to their antigen receptor. As discussed in the next section, once a specific antigen recognition event occurs, the T cell becomes activated and a program of T-cell proliferation and differentiation is initiated. DCs also respond to PRR signaling with the production and release of proinflammatory cytokines and type I IFNs. The specific types and amounts of each these products are determined to a large degree by the types of PRRs stimulated by the pathogen (or vaccine). This cytokine milieu, released at the site of infection and in the draining lymph node at the site of T-cell activation, is instrumental in guiding the activation and development of particular types of T-cell immunity.

Definitions

TCR: T-cell receptor. The cell surface-expressed T-cell antigen receptor. The TCR can exist as a heterodimer composed of α and β or of γ and δ chains. The TCR recognizes antigenic peptide/MHC protein complexes on the surface of antigen-presenting cells.
LFA-1: Leukocyte functional antigen-1. This β2 integrin protein is involved in cell–cell adhesion events.
TGFβ: Transforming growth factor-beta. A cytokine molecule that has immunosuppressive functions in addition to its ability to stimulate growth of fibroblasts.
Th-17: A subset of CD4$^+$ T lymphocytes characterized by production of IL-17. Th-17 cells are thought to be involved primarily in protection against bacterial infections.

Development of adaptive immune responses

The adaptive immune system comprises antigen-specific B and T lymphocytes that react specifically with antigen via antigen-binding domains of surface membrane receptors. Unlike the innate immune cells, which respond to PAMPs via a number of different and relatively conserved PRRs, B and T lymphocytes express many copies of a unique antigen receptor capable of interacting with a specific region of a pathogen-derived molecule. The antigen-recognition domains of these receptors are highly polymorphic due to a series of gene rearrangements during B- and T-cell development. Once rearrangement results in expression of a functional receptor, the rearrangement process is terminated and only copies of the functional receptor from this successful rearrangement are expressed by the cell. This process occurs in all immature B and T lymphocytes, resulting in expression of antigen receptors capable of recognizing nearly any antigen in the total lymphocyte population. Therefore, while each individual B or T lymphocyte expresses a unique receptor with a single binding specificity, the lymphocyte population of the individual as a whole expresses a huge and diverse repertoire of receptors capable of binding a variety of different antigens.

T and B lymphocytes also differ in the nature of the interaction between their antigen receptors and antigen. T lymphocytes recognize small peptide fragments derived from degraded proteins that become physically associated with the antigen-presenting cell's MHC molecules. Innate immune cells such as DCs or macrophages act as antigen-presenting cells and either ingest exogenous foreign proteins by endocytosis or express foreign proteins endogenously as a result of direct infection. In the case of endogenously expressed antigens, these proteins are degraded by proteasomes and gain access to Class I MHC molecules in the endoplasmic reticulum. Following peptide binding, the antigen-loaded MHC molecule is transported to the cell surface for recognition by CD8$^+$ T lymphocytes. Antigens obtained exogenously by phagocytosis or pinocytosis are degraded within the endosomal compartment, and processed peptides are loaded onto Class II MHC molecules, which colocalize to this cellular compartment. Once loaded with antigenic peptide, the loaded Class II MHC molecule then is transported to the cell surface for recognition by CD4$^+$ T lymphocytes. In contrast to antigen recognition by T cells, there is no requirement for antigen processing for recognition of antigen by B lymphocytes, and antigen can be recognized in an extracellular form. The antigen receptor for B lymphocytes can recognize linear sequences of amino acids or clusters of nonsequential amino acids brought into close proximity by the natural folding of the protein molecules. An additional difference is that once T-cell receptor (TCR) genes have successfully rearranged into a functional receptor, further rearrangement does not occur. However, the B-cell genes encoding immunoglobulin can undergo further rearrangement upon exposure to antigen, as discussed below, leading to an increase in binding affinity for the recognized antigen or expression of a specific heavy chain, which confers specific biological functions to the molecule. Thus, of importance to vaccinologists is the nature of the vaccine antigen and the manner in which it is presented to the adaptive immune system, which will dictate the type of cellular response and the type of antigens recognized by adaptive immune cells.

T lymphocyte immunity

T lymphocytes arise from progenitor cells in the bone marrow and begin their differentiation process in the thymus. At this site they begin expressing low levels

of a rearranged TCR as well as both the CD4 and CD8 co-receptor molecules and undergo a selection process in which cells with the ability to respond to MHC/self-peptide complexes are rescued from programmed cell death. These survivors then begin expressing high levels of the TCR and undergo a negative selection process in which the majority of T cells capable of responding to MHC/self-peptides are deleted to remove self-reactive cells from the T-cell repertoire. At this stage, the cells lose expression of one of the co-receptor molecules and express either the CD4 or CD8 surface markers that delineate the two major T-cell subsets. Naïve T cells leave the thymus and migrate through the blood to take up residence in the T-cell zone of secondary lymphoid tissues where they scan incoming DCs for the MHC/peptide complex for which they are specific. The T-cell recognition of a peptide/MHC complex on DCs results in a rearrangement of surface proteins on both cells such that an immunological synapse is formed. This structure is composed of an inner area, referred to as the *central supramolecular activation cluster*, which contains the TCR and numerous molecules involved in signaling such as CD2, CD28, Lck, Fyn, CD4, or CD8. This inner structure is surrounded by an outer area containing molecules such as LFA-1 and CD45 that are involved in strengthening the DC–T-cell interaction. The strength of the signals sent and duration of this interaction greatly influences the magnitude of the ensuing T-cell response. Following these signaling events, the T cell begins an extended period of intense proliferation. Naïve T cells specific for a given epitope are present in the body at very low frequencies prior to exposure to antigen. However, as a result of this rapid, antigen-specific expansion phase, the frequency of antigen-specific T cells may increase up to 100,000-fold. These T cells differentiate under the influence of the cytokine milieu present in the microenvironment of the DC–T-cell interactions to acquire specific immune effector functions that allow them to defend against the invading pathogen. For CD8$^+$ T lymphocytes, the presence of type I interferons and IL-12 is thought to facilitate differentiation of effector cells to become memory T cells. For CD4$^+$ T lymphocytes, the effect of this cytokine milieu on differentiation is even more apparent. CD4$^+$ T cells activated in the presence of IL-12 are driven to become Th1 cells, which produce IFN-γ and express cytolytic activity required for defense against intracellular pathogens. The activation of CD4$^+$ T cells in the presence of IL-4 results in development of Th2 type effector cells. These effector cells produce IL-4 and other cytokines necessary for the development of strong antibody responses and defense against many helminths. Transforming growth factor-beta (TGF-β) drives differentiation of regulatory T cells, which are required for modifying the strength and duration of cell-mediated immune responses. However, TGF-β in the presence of IL-6 drives production of IL-17 producing CD4$^+$ T cells (Th17) that are responsible for inducing the migration of granulocytes required for protection against extracellular bacterial pathogens.

Effector lymphocytes leave the lymphoid site of immune induction and migrate through the blood to the site of infection or inflammation. Upon entry into the inflamed tissue, effector T lymphocytes recognize their specific antigen, which has been internalized and processed by local DCs or on infected somatic cells at the site of infection, and exert their effector function to resolve the infection. As the infection is resolved, effector lymphocytes undergo a rapid contraction phase in which the number of effector lymphocytes is rapidly reduced. During this process, selected antigen-specific T cells survive the contraction process and are maintained long-term in the host as memory T cells (Figure 5.1). We know now that the maintenance of memory involves periodic stimulation of memory T cells with constitutively produced cytokines such as IL-7 and IL-15. Importantly, the remaining antigen-specific memory T cells are maintained at frequencies higher than that of the original antigen-specific naïve T cells. Populations of memory T cells have less stringent signaling requirements for their activation such that a more rapid response occurs upon subsequent reexposure to the antigen.

Several populations of memory T cells with very different properties have been identified that ultimately play different roles upon reexposure to antigen. A commonly used paradigm classifies these cells as effector memory and central memory cells based on the expression of cell surface molecules and tissue residence. Effector memory cells normally are maintained in peripheral tissues, replicate poorly to subsequent exposure to antigen, and exhibit rapid expression of effector functions on subsequent rechallenge. Based

on these properties, it is thought these cells provide rapid protection in the periphery against pathogen challenge. In contrast, central memory cells normally reside in secondary lymphoid tissues and proliferate strongly, but exhibit effect function in a delayed fashion following antigen reexposure. How these subsets develop, how they are related, and their exact roles in providing protection are areas of intense continuing research. The induction of a population of memory T lymphocytes represents one of the goals of immunization. Understanding how to elicit a vigorous memory T-cell response capable of effector functions appropriate for the specific pathogen and that can be maintained for long periods of time is an important avenue of immunological research directly relevant to vaccine development.

B lymphocyte immunity

B cells arise from hemopoietic stem cells in bone marrow and differentiate at this site to become immature B cells. It is at this stage that the genes encoding immunoglobulin are rearranged. After the immature B cells exit the marrow, they begin to express IgD and IgM molecules on their surface that serve as antigen receptors in the B-cell receptor (BCR) complex. B cells can be divided into two main populations, B1 and B2 B cells. B1 B cells produce antibody molecules that are polyspecific and bind with low affinity to a number of environmental antigens, microbes, or microbial products. This B1 B cell-produced antibody is thought to provide some level of immediate resistance against infection by a wide range of pathogens. B2 B cells, or conventional B cells, represent the majority of all B cells and are the population targeted for activation and expansion by immunization. Currently licensed vaccines generally induce vigorous antibody responses, and for nearly all approved vaccines, vaccine-specific antibodies are responsible for protection against the targeted pathogen or toxin. Recent advances in our understanding of the mechanisms of B cell activation and differentiation are being used to refine approaches to induce B cell responses of sufficient magnitude with the appropriate antigen specificity and response durability to provide immune protection against a wide variety of pathogens.

Definitions

BCR: B-cell receptor. The cell surface-expressed immunoglobulin molecules that serve as the antigen receptor for B lymphocytes.

B1 B cells: A B-cell subset that arises early during ontogeny that is found mainly in the peritoneum and pleural cavity fluid. Autoantigens and commonly encountered environmental antigens are responsible for the expansion and maintenance of this population. B1 B cells express a limited receptor repertoire and are thought to play a role in the early phase of adaptive protection against infection.

B2 B cells: The subset of "conventional" B cells that comprises ~95% of total B cells. The B2 B cell population expresses an extensive repertoire of receptors for antigen due in part to extensive mutagenesis of receptor genes. They can express all immunoglobulin isotypes and are primarily responsible for the antigen-specific antibody response to vaccines.

BLIMP-1: B-Lymphocyte Induced Maturation Protein-1. A transcriptional repressor protein that aids in differentiation of plasmablasts into plasma cells.

BAFF: B-cell activating factor. This member of the tumor necrosis factor (TNF) family acts as a survival factor for memory B cells and plasma cells.

APRIL: A Proliferation-Inducing Ligand. This cytokine is a member of the TNF family and is involved in mediating survival signals to plasma cells.

T cell-dependent B-cell responses

Naïve conventional B cells migrate through the blood and concentrate in the cortex of secondary lymphoid tissues (Figure 5.2). Here they may encounter an antigen for which their BCR is specific. The antigen may be in a cell-associated or freely diffusible form or may exist as antigen trapped in an immune complex composed of a meshwork of antibody-bound antigen. The binding of specific antigen to the BCR induces expression of the chemokine receptor CCR7, resulting in the homing of the antigen-specific B cell to the outer margin of the T-cell zone. The B cell also internalizes antigen bound to the BCR and processes it into peptides that become associated with class II MHC molecules for expression on the B cell surface. This peptide/MHC complex can be recognized by $CD4^+$ T cells that are also specific for the same antigen. While

at this site, the newly activated B cell interacts primarily through this mechanism with recently activated antigen-specific $CD4^+$ T cells and receives critical activation signals conveyed by the engagement of T cell-expressed CD40 ligand by B cell-expressed CD40. Some of the activated B cells stay in the extrafollicular region where they produce relatively low-affinity antibody and remain viable only a few days. It is thought this very early, low-affinity antibody response may provide a rapid resistance to pathogen challenge. The remainder of the recently activated B cells enter the B-cell follicle and establish a germinal center reaction. It is the establishment of this reaction process that is responsible for providing the memory B cells and long-lasting, high-affinity antibody response elicited by vaccines. The germinal center is composed of a dark zone in which vigorous B-cell proliferation occurs and a light zone characterized by the presence of follicular T helper cells and antigen-bearing follicular dendritic cells. During proliferation in the dark zone, the antigen-specific B cells undergo class switching under the influence of T cell-derived cytokines and express different immunoglobulin classes. As a result, the potential for different biological activities (for example, the ability to fix complement or to bind to certain IgG Fc receptors) is conferred on the antibody molecule. The immunoglobulin gene segments involved in antigen binding also undergo somatic hypermutation in the dark zone by a process involving nucleotide substitution in the variable region genes by uracil nucleoside glycosylase and activation-induced cytidine deaminase enzymes. These nucleotide substitutions may alter the antigen binding of the BCR either positively or negatively, which ultimately influences the ability of the B cell to survive. Germinal center B cells leaving the dark zone migrate to the light zone where they interact with antigen associated with follicular dendritic cells and receive important activation and survival signals from follicular T helper cells. Those B-cell populations expressing BCRs capable of high-affinity interactions with antigen survive, while those capable of lower affinity interactions do not compete well for access to antigen and undergo apoptosis. In this way, B cells with the highest affinity for antigen are selected for ultimate differentiation into antibody-producing plasma cells or antigen-specific memory B cells.

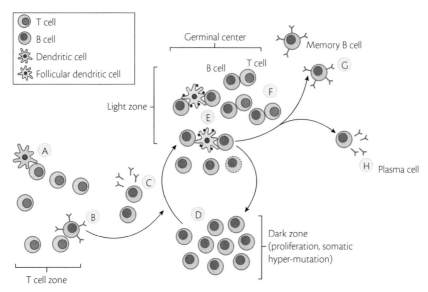

Figure 5.2 T cell-dependent B-cell responses. Antigen is presented to naïve T cells in the T-cell zone of secondary lymphoid tissue (A). Antigen also binds to the BCR of antigen-specific B cells, which then also migrate to the T-cell zone. Activated T cells provide help to the recently activated B cells (B). The B cells then either produce antibody outside of the B-cell follicle (C) or enter the follicle and cycle between an area of intense B cell proliferation and somatic hypermutation of BCR genes, the Dark zone (D), and an area where antigen selection and class switch occur, the Light zone (E). B cells that successfully compete for antigen depots on follicular dendritic cells and receive survival signals from follicular T cells (F) may undergo further rounds of proliferation and selection or exit the germinal center to become memory B cells (G) or antibody-secreting plasma cells (H).

Persistent production of vaccine-specific antibody and B-cell memory

Further differentiation of the antigen-activated B cells is provided by cytokines and differentiation factors produced by follicular dendritic cells. For example, the development and maintenance of antibody-secreting plasma cells is greatly influenced by the presence of the factors BLIMP-1 (B-lymphocyte induced maturation protein-1) and APRIL (a proliferation-inducing ligand). Germinal center B cells are either driven to become antibody-secreting plasma cells or memory B cells. Antibody-secreting cells generally have a life span of only a few days. However, plasma cells expressing the chemokine receptor CXCR4 exit the germinal center and migrate via the blood stream to the bone marrow by recognition of the chemokine CXCL12, which is constitutively produced by bone marrow stromal cells. CXCR4-expressing plasma cells follow the chemokine gradient to the source of its production in the bone marrow. Once in the bone marrow, the

plasma cell establishes a long-term interaction with these stromal cells and becomes fully dependent on survival-inducing molecules such as CXCL12, IL-6, IL-5, BAFF (B-cell activating factor), and APRIL produced by the stromal cells. Antigen-specific plasma cells can be detected in these survival niches in the bone marrow for many years after the primary antibody response. While it is not certain if these plasma cells enjoy an inherently long life span or if they are sporadically replenished from plasma cells generated during the occasional reactivation of memory B cells, there is much evidence for the first possibility. In fact, survival times for long-lived plasma cells have been estimated to range from several years to many decades depending on the nature of the antigen that first elicited the response. It is currently thought that the constant release of antigen-specific antibodies by these cells is responsible for the long-term presence of antigen-specific serum antibodies induced by immunization. The presence of a high titer of antigen-specific serum antibodies obviously provides immediate protection against exposure to the vaccine-targeted pathogen and periodic booster immunizations with some vaccines may be required to maintain protective levels of serum antibodies.

In contrast, memory B cells produced in the germinal center reactions migrate to extrafollicular areas of secondary lymphoid tissues and remain there for extended periods of time. Memory B cells are quiescent and do not release antibody unless restimulated with the original antigen (Figure 5.1 and Figure 5.3). Once restimulated, they rapidly proliferate and differentiate into plasma cells, which secrete antigen-specific antibody, or into replacement memory B cells. This anamnestic B-cell response of memory B cells to antigen is more rapid, of higher magnitude, and includes antibody of much higher affinity than that produced during a primary antibody response. It is thought that this type of antibody response would be needed for protection under circumstances in which the pathogen overwhelms any preexisting serum antibodies.

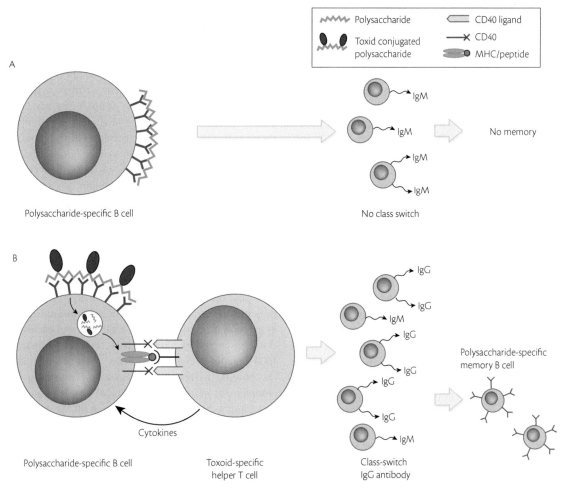

Figure 5.3 Induction of antibody responses using polysaccharide-protein conjugate vaccines. (A) Cross-linking of BCR on polysaccharide-specific B cell results in activation, proliferation, and production of IgM antibody. In the absence of T-cell help, the class switch to IgG antibody production and differentiation of memory B cells is extremely limited. (B) Conjugation of a protein molecule such as diphtheria toxoid to the polysaccharide results in binding to polysaccharide-specific BCR on the B cell surface, internalization and processing of the toxoid molecule, and presentation on class II MHC molecules. Recognition of the complex by toxoid-specific helper T cells results in delivery of critical co-stimulatory signals (CD40–CD40 ligand) and cytokines necessary for induction of class switch and differentiation of polysaccharide-specific memory B cells.

T cell-independent B-cell responses

Some types of antigens are capable of inducing an antibody response without the requirement for T lymphocytes. These antigens are referred to as *T cell-independent antigens* and generally contain repeating structural units that can bind and cross-link multiple surface immunoglobulin molecules. This binding results in delivery of a sufficient signal to activate the B cell and initiate IgM production, but is inadequate to induce optimal class switching or differentiation of memory B cells. Since T cell-independent antigens are quite often composed of carbohydrates that are not recognized by T cells, such as the capsular polysaccharides of *Streptococcus pneumoniae*, *Haemophilus influenzae*, and *Neisseria meningitidis*, cognate T cell–B cell interactions fail to occur, including signaling via CD40-CD40 ligand interactions, and therefore the class switch to IgG and induction of memory B cells does not occur. These encapsulated bacteria are important pathogens in young children, and early vaccines prepared with the purified capsular polysaccharides from these organisms were poorly immunogenic in children; immunization did not always result in a highly protective antibody response. In order to elicit higher affinity IgG antibodies and a memory B-cell component, the polysaccharide antigens have been coupled to a carrier protein, such as tetanus toxoid or diphtheria toxoid, which essentially converts the T cell-independent antigen into a T cell-dependent antigen (Figure 5.3). T cells specific for the protein carrier are thought to interact with capsular polysaccharide B cells that present the protein carrier antigens to protein-specific T cells. The resulting cognate T cell–B cell interaction results in delivery of the T-cell signals that drive the development of the germinal center reaction and ultimately the production of high affinity antibody and polysaccharide-specific memory B cells. Utilization of this vaccine approach has been hugely successful in preventing pediatric disease caused by these polysaccharide-encapsulated pathogens.

Mechanisms of antibody-mediated protection

There are five main classes of antibodies that can be produced by rearrangement of the immunoglobulin heavy chain genes following antigen exposure (Table 5.2). IgD and IgM antibody are expressed on the surface of naïve B cells and play a role in BCR-signaling events. IgD expression is usually lost upon antigen stimulation, and this antibody class is found only in extremely low levels in serum. IgM antibody is produced first following antigen activation and is secreted by activated plasmablasts. Normally, IgM has not undergone somatic hypermutation and is generally of low avidity. However, IgM monomers are bound together by a J chain and expressed as a pentamer such that each IgM molecule contains 10 antigen-binding sites. IgM antibodies can be transported across epithelial surfaces by the polymeric immunoglobulin receptor (pIgR); however, it diffuses poorly into tissues and is found predominantly in the bloodstream. It can bind to and neutralize pathogens or their toxins by preventing their attachment to or uptake by host cells. It is also extremely effective at activating the complement pathway, which can result in direct lysis of infected cells, or enhance uptake of IgM antibody–pathogen complexes by phagocytic cells. Activated B cells that undergo immunoglobulin class switch express IgA, IgE, or IgG heavy chain genes, of which IgA and IgG are the most relevant for vaccines. The IgG class of antibody exists in a monomeric form, diffuses easily into tissues, and represents the most abundant antibody class present in serum. In humans, there are four subclasses of IgG antibody: IgG1, IgG2, IgG3, and IgG4. As mentioned previously, the cytokine milieu present during B-cell activation influences the expression of particular IgG subclasses, and each subclass has a somewhat different biological function. IgG1 and IgG2 are exceptionally good at enhancing the binding to IgG Fc receptors and activating the complement system. The ability of the Fc region of these antibody subclasses to bind specific Fc receptors on the surface of innate effector cells such as neutrophils, macrophages, or natural killer cells facilitates the removal of antigens or pathogens by phagocytosis or destruction of pathogens or pathogen-infected cells by antibody-dependent cell-mediated cytotoxicity. These IgG subclass antibodies also are transported very well across the placenta by the neonatal IgG receptor, FcγRn, and can transfer antibody-mediated protection from mother to infant. As will be discussed in the next section, the IgA antibody class is well adapted for protection of mucosal surfaces. Two IgA monomers

Table 5.2 Characteristics of Human Immunoglobulins

Immuno-globulin	Heavy Chain	Structure	Molecular Weight (kDa)	Valency	Synthetic Rate (mg/kg/day)	% of Serum	Serum Half-Life (days)	Function
IgA$_1$	$\alpha 1$	Monomer (m)/dimer (d)	160(m)/300(d)	2(m)/4(d)	19–29	11–14	5–7	Secretory antibody, binds pIgR
IgA$_2$	$\alpha 1$	m/d	160(m)/350(d)	2(m)/4(d)	3.3–5.3	1–4	4–6	Secretory antibody, binds pIgR
IgD	δ	m	175	2	0.2	0.2	2–8	Mature B cell marker, homeostasis
IgE	ϵ	m	190	2	0.002	0.004	1–5	Binds FcεR on mast cells and basophils, defense against helminthic parasites
IgG$_1$	$\gamma 1$	m	150	2	33	45–53	21–24	Secondary response, cross placenta, binds to FcγR, fixes complement (IgG4 poorly), enhances phagocytosis, neutralization
IgG$_2$	$\gamma 2$	m	150	2	33	11–15	21–24	
IgG$_3$	$\gamma 3$	m	160	2	33	3–6	7–8	
IgG$_4$	$\gamma 4$	m	150	2	33	1–4	21–24	
IgM	μ	Pentamer (p)	950(p)	up to 10	3.3	10	5–10	Primary response, complement activation, neutralization

Compiled with information from Schroder HW and Cavacini L (2010). Structure and Functions of Immunoglobulins. J Allergy Clin Immunol 125(2), S41–S51.

are joined by a J chain into a dimeric molecule. IgA dimers produced by plasma cells residing in the intestinal *lamina propria* bind very efficiently to the pIgR found on the basolateral surfaces of many mucosal epithelial surfaces. The antibody is internalized and is carried by in endosomes to the apical surface. During transcytosis, the polymeric immunoglobulin receptor is cleaved and the IgA dimer is released at the apical cell surface into the mucosal lumen. In humans, the IgA1 subclass is found predominantly in serum whereas the IgA2 subclass is found at high concentrations in most mucosal secretions. The hinge region of IgA2 is truncated relative to IgA1 and is resistant to cleavage by many of the bacterial proteases that are prominent at mucosal surfaces. The protective function of IgA is manifested mainly through neutralization of pathogens or their toxins and formation of large antigen/IgA complexes that are readily trapped in mucosal secretions and excluded from the mucosal surface. IgA can also entrap organisms that have penetrated the epithelial barrier then transport them back across this barrier by binding them to the polymeric immunoglobulin receptor, followed by active transcytosis for release back into the lumen. IgA can also neutralize viral pathogens intracellularly when endosomes that ferry basolateral-bound virus fuse with apical surface-bound endosomes containing pIgR-bound IgA.

Development of immunity at mucosal sites

With a total surface area of approximately 400 m², mucosal surfaces represent the largest body surface available as a site of entry for pathogens. Not surprisingly, many human pathogens make first contact with their host through mucosal epithelial cells. The immune system must be able to protect against organisms such as *Escherichia coli*, *Vibrio cholera*, and *Shigella sp.* that attach to epithelia and produce enterotoxins or exotoxins. It must also protect against organisms such as rotavirus, or *Shigella sp.* that infect mucosal tissues locally, or organisms such as *Salmonella sp.* that invade systemically after penetration of the mucosal epithelium. Local immune responses including pathogen-specific CD4+ and CD8+ T cells and secretory IgA responses induced by mucosal infection or mucosal immunization with live attenuated organisms generally provide excellent protection against mucosal pathogens. While there is evidence that parenterally administered vaccines can provide some protection for mucosal sites, systemic immunization rarely induces a strong secretory IgA response. Therefore, there is currently a great deal of interest in improving protection of mucosal sites by direct immunization of mucosal tissues. Examples of success of this vaccine strategy include the Sabin attenuated live oral polio vaccine, the live attenuated influenza vaccine FluMist® or Fluenz®, the live attenuated rotavirus vaccines Rotarix® and Rotateq®, and the Ty21a live oral typhoid vaccine.

Definitions

pIgR: Polymeric immunoglobulin receptor. This receptor binds polymeric immunoglobulins and is involved in transport of the Ig from the basolateral surface of the cell to the apical surface of the cell.

MadCAM-1: Mucosal addressin Cell Adhesion Molecule-1. This molecule is a mucosal vascular addressin found on the endothelial walls of gut mucosal blood vessels. It is involved in proper homing of lymphocytes expressing the α4β7 integrin to the gut mucosa.

M cells: Microfold cells. These are specialized cells on the surface of gut-associated lymphoid tissue that function to internalize antigen and pathogens from the gut lumen and transcytose this material to underlying immune cells.

Induction of vaccine-specific immune responses with inactivated or recombinant antigens is complicated by the challenging environmental conditions of many mucosal sites and by the way that antigen applied at a given mucosal surface gains access to immune inductive sites. The various mucosal surfaces differ in the manner in which antigen exposure results in induction of adaptive immune responses. Perhaps the mucosal tissue that is best studied in terms of how adaptive immune responses are induced is the gastrointestinal mucosa. The immune response at the intestinal epithelium is highly regulated so as to prevent chronic inflammatory responses to commensal organisms and food antigens. The gut epithelium is covered by a simple columnar epithelial cell layer in which the gut antigens are normally physically excluded by the tight junctions between cells. Additionally, the intestinal epithelium is covered with a mucous layer that also serves as a physical barrier to commensal organisms, pathogens, and antigens. However, specialized sites referred to as Peyer's patches provide antigen-presenting cell access to lumenal antigens for the induction of adaptive immune responses (Figure 5.4). These immune inductive sites are covered with specialized microfold or M cells, which actively take up antigen from the lumen and transport it to pockets of DCs and macrophages at the basolateral surface. These cells are part of a larger mucosal-associated lymphoid tissue containing areas enriched

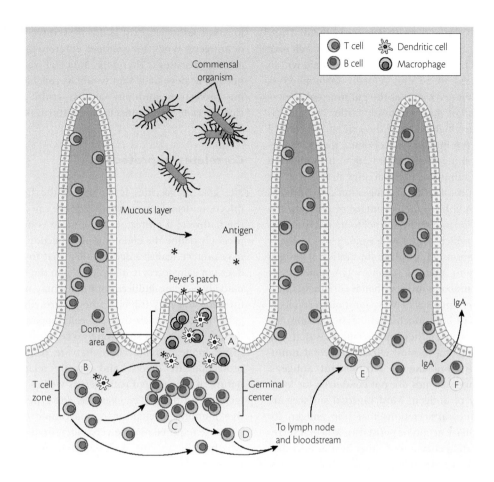

Figure 5.4 Development and retention of adaptive immune responses in the gut mucosa (A). Macrophages and dendritic cells in the dome region take up antigen that has transcytosed from the gut lumen through M cells and deliver it to the T-cell area of the mucosal associated lymphoid tissue (B). Antigen is presented to T cells, which become activated and migrate to the germinal center (C) and provide help for antigen-specific B cells. Activated, antigen-specific B and T cells migrate to the lymph node (D) and ultimately enter the bloodstream. As these cells circulate and pass through mucosal capillaries in the lamina propria region (E), they bind to the endothelial cells by a mechanism involving a MadCAM-1/α4β7 integrin interaction. T cells may stay in the lamina propria or further migrate to sites between the gut epithelial cells. IgA antibody secreted by lamina propria plasma cells binds to the pIgR on mucosal epithelial cells (F), is internalized, and is transported to the gut lumen.

for naïve T cells and naïve B cells. The antigen-containing DCs can then aid in the induction of antigen-specific B- and T-cell responses. Moreover, the DCs of the gastrointestinal tract induce the expression of the α4β7 integrin on the surface of the newly activated B and T cells, which imprints them with the ability to preferentially home back to and reside in mucosal tissues. In this process, the antigen-specific B and T cells leave the Peyer's patches and enter the circulatory system. Upon reaching the capillaries that feed the lamina propria region of the gastrointestinal tract, the α4β7 integrin on the lymphocyte surface binds to the MadCAM-1–expressing endothelial cells of the gut lamina propria. (MadCAM-1 stands for *mucosal addressin cell adhesion molecule-1*.) After extravasation, the new cell arrivals respond further to chemokine signals produced by the gut epithelium, leading some of the cells to take up residence between epithelial cells as intraepithelial lymphocytes. These cells act as sentinels and provide a very rapid response to reexposure to the antigen that induced them. Thus, mechanisms are in place that allow the adaptive immune cells induced by antigens encountered within the gut mucosa to be preferentially maintained as effector or memory T cells at the gut mucosal site.

The promise of mucosal immunization is that it is likely to induce high levels of the appropriate type of immunity at the mucosal site of entry, therefore preventing or limiting the initial infection. It should also be easier to administer the vaccines if they can be applied to mucosal tissues by ingestion or by inhalation. This would have the advantage of reducing the requirement for trained personnel to deliver vaccines by injection, which would be advantageous in many developing nations. Mucosal administration of antigen is more likely to induce a secretory IgA response for protection of mucosal surfaces than is parenteral injection. Moreover, mucosal delivery most often results in development of both mucosal and systemic immune responses. However, there are challenges that will need to be overcome to allow effective mucosal immunization with nonliving or recombinant antigens. First, most mucosal sites are not conducive for long-term stability of antigen. Most mucosal surfaces are bathed in mucosal secretions that trap antigen for removal by ciliary action or peristalsis. Mucosal secretions may contain enzymes of either host or microbial origin capable of degrading or digesting vaccines. Mucosal sites such as the gastrointestinal tract may also contain regions of extreme acid or alkaline pH. Delivery of nonliving or recombinant vaccine antigens will require development of new adjuvants, as most adjuvants used for currently licensed vaccines that are delivered parenterally do not work well when given via the mucosal route. Currently tested adjuvants include cholera toxin or *E. coli* enterotoxin that have been genetically altered to reduce toxicity while maintaining adjuvanticity. Although these adjuvants can help elicit strong antibody and cell-mediated responses, the interaction of these candidate mucosal adjuvants with olfactory nerves following intranasal delivery suggests that further development and refinement of this approach is needed to avoid undesirable interactions with the CNS. Mucosal adjuvant development will also need to be tempered by the need to selectively induce appropriate types and levels of immunity in an environment in which an overall noninflammatory environment must be maintained. Finally, some mucosal pathogens exist as diverse serotypes (*Shigella*) or antigenic types (for example, enterotoxigenic *E. coli* and noroviruses). Therefore, mucosal vaccines will need to be developed that would be capable of inducing protective immunity against entire groups of closely related, but antigenically distinct, pathogens.

Correlates of protection

The goal of vaccines is to protect the host against infectious disease; however, before we can understand the nature of a protective response, it is necessary to precisely define the end point of protection. A vaccine may protect against infection such that the pathogen does not gain access to and replicate in the host. Alternatively, vaccine-induced immunity may not prevent infection but may inhibit pathogen growth or pathogenic processes such that clinically apparent disease does not occur. Not surprisingly, the immune mechanisms induced by vaccines that are responsible for protection are diverse and directly related to the nature of the targeted pathogen as well as to the protection end point. For example, the type of protective immune mechanism or magnitude of immune response required may be very different depending on whether the vaccine is designed to protect against infection, disease, or mortality. Further, these vaccine response parameters may also vary according to whether the vaccine provides protection against a toxin (for example, diphtheria, tetanus, cholera, pertussis), viremia/bacteremia (e.g., smallpox, mumps, measles, yellow fever, *Haemophilus influenzae type b*), infection of neurons (e.g., rabies), reactivation from neurons (e.g., varicella virus), or mucosal replication (e.g., influenza, rotavirus, *Bordetella pertussis*). The human papillomavirus (HPV) vaccine is licensed as a cancer vaccine, and efficacy is based on a clinical end point of protection from HPV-induced cancer (cervical carcinoma in women).

While different types of adaptive immune responses might be induced by vaccination, it is important to understand which of these responses are correlated with protection and the magnitude of the critical response that is required to ensure protection against a particular pathogen. This concept of a "correlate of protection" is critical for measuring vaccine efficacy and guiding future vaccine improvement. The correlate of protection is the specific immune response elicited by a vaccine that can be shown to be associated with protection against a specific aspect of pathogenesis.

Definitions

Correlate of Protection: An immune response that is associated with protection against a defined element of pathogenesis. The correlate may be absolute, that is, the immune correlate is protective in nearly all cases, or relative, in which the immune correlate is protective in many but not all cases.

Co-correlate of Protection: An immune response that acts with another distinct type of response to achieve a desired type of protection

Surrogate of Protection: A substitute measurement for the true correlate of immunity when the true correlate is unknown or has not been measured.

Correlates of protection have been defined for many of the currently licensed vaccines and have been determined through the use of relevant animal models of infection, clinical observations of natural disease, and clinical trials of vaccines. For many of the currently licensed vaccines against bacterial toxins and invariant viruses, protection is mediated mostly, if not exclusively, by antibody, and the correlate of protection is represented by an identified concentration of serum antibody. It is important to note that in many instances the correlate of protection is defined in terms of a particular functional measurement of antibody (e.g., neutralization or opsonophagocytosis), which in most cases represents the functional mechanism responsible for protection. The identification of antibody correlates of protection is aided somewhat by the relative ease in detecting and measuring serum antibody concentrations and the availability of standard methods and reagents to quantify antibody effector functions. However, it is also important to recognize that vaccine-mediated protection may reflect the actions of both T and B cells rather than "either B cells or T cells." For some of the pathogens for which licensed vaccines exist, T cell-mediated immunity may play a role in protection, but the protective roles of T cells are much more difficult to identify and quantify. The T-cell epitopes recognized within a human popu-

lation are very diverse because multiple alleles of MHC antigens are expressed by humans. Since these epitopes are commonly required in T-cell assays to measure the vaccine-induced response, this response heterogeneity results in complications in assessing T-cell function and quantity. Unlike serologic assays to quantify vaccine-specific antibody and function, standardized methods and reagents for many T-cell assays are lacking, and methods for obtaining and storing cells are more cumbersome than for obtaining and maintaining serum samples for antibody detection. Moreover, the particular T-cell effector function associated with protection is not always clearly known, making it more difficult to ensure that the appropriate assay to measure the relevant T-cell effector functions will be performed. For pathogens with complicated life cycles or pathogenesis, or for pathogens capable of rapidly altering epitopes recognized by neutralizing antibody, T cell-mediated protection most likely plays an important role. An understanding of the type of T-cell response and how the cell-mediated response interacts with antibody-mediated immunity will likely be important for rational development of effective vaccines to these types of pathogens.

Benefits of identifying a vaccine correlate of protection

The establishment of a defined correlate of protection is useful to the vaccine industry and regulators by providing the ability to ensure lot-to-lot consistency of vaccine preparations. A new vaccine lot will be considered protective if it induces in vaccine recipients the level of a given immune function stipulated by the correlate of protection. The correlate of protection may be similarly used to demonstrate vaccine stability and determine the shelf life of a vaccine. For vaccines in which the correlate of protection involves measurement of serum antibody, it can provide a convenient means to determine the duration of protective immunity following vaccination. Many vaccines are now given in combination or are being considered for use in combination vaccines. In these instances, the simultaneous administration of several vaccines may unintentionally alter the immune response to a single component. A defined correlate of protection for each single vaccine component provides an objective measurement of the level of a particular immune response that must be achieved to ensure protective immunity. This information is critical for determining if the vaccine formulation must be adjusted to achieve protective immune levels by all vaccine components. For certain pathogens, the incidence of disease is very low, and outbreaks are unpredictable and geographically limited so that vaccine efficacy cannot be tested in clinical trials. This approach is also appropriate for the development of vaccines against bioterrorism agents for which there is no effective therapeutic treatment available. In these cases, identification of correlates or surrogates of protection during preclinical trials in relevant disease models in laboratory animals provides a basis for licensing a candidate vaccine. For this approach to work, the pathophysiology of the disease and the mechanism of interruption of the disease process by vaccines must be well understood. The vaccine effect must be demonstrated in one or more animal species in which the infection and disease process closely recapitulate the disease in humans, and the vaccine effect must be statistically linked with protection against end points that are relevant to human infection. Additionally, the pharmacodynamics of the vaccine must be known to allow identification of the correct vaccine dose and immunization schedule for humans. Under these circumstances, induction of the correlate or surrogate markers of protection in vaccine recipients would then be considered predictive of development of protection.

Mechanisms of vaccine-induced protection

Exotoxin-producing bacteria

Not surprisingly, the production of toxin-neutralizing antibodies correlates with protection against many bacterial exotoxins such as tetanus toxin and diphtheria toxin. Early studies of vaccine-mediated protection in laboratory animals led to the estimate of 0.01 IU/ml of serum neutralizing antibodies as the requirement to provide protection against disease caused by tetanus toxin. Although levels of protective antibodies determined in animal studies are not always indicative of protective requirements in humans, this dose was borne out in subsequent human studies. Today, the World Health Organization has established this titer

of neutralizing antibodies as the correlate of protection against tetanus toxin. The situation is somewhat less clear for vaccine-mediated protection against *B. pertussis*. In addition to the pertussis toxin, bacterial attachment molecules such as pertactin or fimbrial hemagglutinins are present in most pertussis vaccines and antibodies reactive with these proteins also contribute to and contribute to protection. This complicates the determination of protective effects due solely to neutralizing anti-pertussis toxin antibodies.

Yellow fever virus

Yellow fever virus is a member of the genus *Flavivirus* and is the causative agent of yellow fever. The virus is transmitted by the bite of infected mosquitoes and is responsible for approximately 200,000 infections in the tropical regions of the world. The 17D vaccine developed in the 1930s has been incredibly successful in preventing yellow fever and its mechanism of protection involves induction of neutralizing antibody. The induction of a serum neutralization index (SNI) of 0.7 neutralization units or a 50% plaque reduction neutralization text ($PRNT_{50}$) titer of 1 : 10 is considered indicative of protection. This level of antibody was derived from vaccine studies in nonhuman primates, which share many of the same disease manifestations with humans. Similar antibody-mediated mechanisms of protection have been identified for other flaviviruses including Japanese encephalitis virus, tick-borne encephalitis, and protection against challenge with homologous dengue virus serotypes. In all of these flavivirus examples, the presence of neutralizing antibody interrupts the viremia associated with viral infection.

Variola (Smallpox)

The World Health Organization proclaimed the eradication of smallpox in 1977, which ended the worldwide smallpox surveillance and immunization programs responsible for detecting and controlling smallpox outbreaks. With time, as the majority of the world's population was no longer immune to this pathogen, it was realized that smallpox could potentially be utilized as a weapon of bioterror. This realization resulted in renewed interest in vaccine production. During the mass vaccination campaigns of the smallpox eradication program, there were numerous reports of serious adverse events following administration of the smallpox vaccine, DryVAX, including death, vaccinial encephalitis, progressive vaccinia, and eczema vaccinatum. Given the high mortality rate associated with smallpox infection, the risk of developing these adverse events seemed acceptable. However, in the absence of natural smallpox infections, concerns over the risk of vaccination-related adverse events with the DryVAX vaccine led to the development of new and effective smallpox vaccines with more acceptable safety profiles. A hurdle to development of a new vaccine was that it was unknown what the correlates of immunity were for the DryVAX vaccine. Furthermore, since smallpox had been eradicated from nature, there was no way of determining what the correlates of protection were. In the original DryVAX immunizations, the development of a skin lesion at the site of scarification and vaccine application was indicative of successful vaccine "take." This surrogate of protection would not be useful for the new generation vaccines that were designed to be injected. It was, however, known that DryVAX immunization resulting in neutralizing antibody titers of 1:32 or greater protected vaccinees against disease. Vaccine-induced neutralizing antibody also protected laboratory animals against disease following challenge with related poxviruses. There is also strong evidence of a role for CD8$^+$ T cells in vaccine-mediated protection in animal models of poxvirus infection, leading to some question as to the identity of the correlates of immunity for the new smallpox vaccines. However, since variola virus no longer exists in nature, the true correlates of protection for the newly developed smallpox vaccines may remain an enigma.

Varicella zoster virus (chickenpox/zoster)

Varicella zoster virus (VZV) is a large double-stranded DNA virus in the *Herpesviridae* family and is the causative agent of chickenpox and herpes zoster. Although chickenpox is normally mild and the disease is of short duration in normal individuals, it may be more severe for very young infants, immune-compromised individuals, or pregnant women. VZV also establishes a lifelong latent infection in the dorsal root ganglia and is normally maintained in this state by virus-specific cell-mediated immunity. However, the virus may reactivate, particularly in persons with deficient cellular immune responses, resulting in a vesicular rash within a single dermatome. Herpes zoster may be painful and take several weeks to resolve. A further complication is the occasional development of postherpetic neural-

gia (PHN). PHN results in chronic pain and hypersensitivity of the skin to touch or temperature changes and may persist for several months. The live attenuated vaccine Varivax® prepared from the Oka Strain of VZV was approved for use in 1995 and is effective against chickenpox in young children and adults. Vaccine efficacy appears to be related to serum antibody titers although protection wanes more rapidly than can be explained by a drop in antibody titers, which suggests other mechanisms such as cell-mediated immunity may be critically involved in protection. The Zostavax® vaccine was approved in 2006 for protection against herpes zoster in individuals over 60 years of age. It provides a much higher virus dose than that provided by the Varivax vaccine given to children and young adults and is thought to boost the waning VZV-specific cell-mediated immunity of elderly individuals and thus maintain VZV latency. The live attenuated VZV vaccine has been shown to significantly reduce the incidence of herpes zoster. Additionally, the incidence and severity of PHN in vaccinees who developed zoster was significantly decreased compared to the placebo group. The duration of Zostavax-induced protection in this population is not currently known.

Rotavirus

Rotavirus is a member of the *Reoviridae* family and contains a segmented, double-stranded RNA genome. Group A rotavirus is a major cause of gastrointestinal disease in infants and young children and is responsible for an estimated 500,000 to 600,000 deaths per year worldwide. Live attenuated vaccines against rotavirus are highly protective against acute gastroenteritis, although the immune mechanisms responsible for protection are uncertain. Both antibody- and cell-mediated responses have been detected in animal models of rotavirus infection and following natural infection of humans, which are targeted against a variety of rotavirus proteins. Moreover, both neutralizing antibodies against the rotavirus outer layer proteins VP4 and VP7 and non-neutralizing antibody specific for VP6 has been shown to be protective in animal models; studies in humans find strong correlation between protection and high serum IgA antibody titers. Although rotavirus-specific T cells have been shown to play a role in virus clearance in animal models, and CD4$^+$ T cells can be detected in peripheral blood of humans following infection, there has been little study of the role of cell-mediated immunity in protection of humans. In humans immunized with live attenuated vaccines, protection seems to correlate with rotavirus-specific serum IgG and IgA levels although not necessarily with neutralizing activity.

Summary

- The innate immune system responds to conserved molecular patterns expressed by pathogens and with the production of immunologically potent compounds that activate and mobilize additional innate immune cells.

- The initial response by innate immune cells is important for activating and guiding the development of the adaptive immune response to the pathogen.

- The interaction of vaccines with the innate immune response is important for efficiently inducing an appropriate and durable adaptive immune response.

- The identification of specific types and levels of immune responses that correlate with protection allows for an objective measure of vaccine efficacy and can provide guidance for future vaccine improvement.

- A defined level of functional antibody serves as the correlate of protection for many licensed vaccines. However, as vaccines are developed against organisms with a complex structure or with complicated pathogenesis, it will be important to develop better methods of determining T-cell correlates of protection.

Further Reading

Amanna IJ and Slifka MK (2011). Contributions of humoral and cellular immunity to vaccine-induced protection in humans. Virology 411, 206–215.

Bonilla FA and Oettgen HC (2010). Adaptive immunity. Journal of Allergy and Clinical Immunology 125(2), S33–S40.

Borges O, Lebre F, Bento D, Borchard G, and Junginger HE (2010). Mucosal vaccines: recent progress in understanding the natural barriers. Pharmaceutical Research 27(2), 211–223.

Brandtzaeg P (2009). Mucosal immunity: induction, dissemination, and effector functions. Scandinavian Journal of Immunology 70, 505–515.

Plotkin SA (2010). Correlates of protection induced by vaccination. Clinical and Vaccine Immunology 17(7), 1055–1065.

Pulendran B (2004). Modulating vaccine responses with dendritic cells and Toll-like receptors. Immunological Reviews 199, 227–250.

Randall KL (2010). Generating humoral immune memory following infection or vaccination. Expert Review of Vaccines 9(9), 1083–1093.

Sallusto F, Lanzavecchia A, Araki K, and Ahmed R (2010). From vaccines to memory and back. Immunity 33, 451–463.

Vidor E (2010). Evaluation of the persistence of vaccine-induced protection with human vaccines. Journal of Comparative Pathology 142, S96–S101.

6 Adjuvants: making vaccines immunogenic

Gregg N. Milligan

Sealy Center for Vaccine Development, Department of Pediatrics, Department of Microbiology and Immunology, University of Texas Medical Branch, Galveston, TX, USA

Abbreviations

APC	Antigen-presenting cell	MyD88	Myeloid differentiation primary response protein 88
CpG	Cytosine-phosphate-guanosine		
CT	Cholera toxin	NAIP5	NOD-like receptor proteins neuronal apoptosis inhibitory protein 5
EMA	European Medicines Agency		
GM1	Monosialotetrahexosylganglioside	NLR	Nucleotide oligomerization domain receptor
HLP	Human papillomavirus		
IPAF	ICD protease activating factor	NOD	Nucleotide oligomerization domain
ISCOMS	Immune stimulating complexes	PAMPs	Pathogen-associated molecular patterns
LPS	Lipopolysaccharide		
LT	Heat labile enterotoxin of *E. coli*	PLG	Poly (lactide-co-glycoline)
MDP	Muramyl dipeptide	PRR	Pattern recognition receptor
MHC	Major histocompatibility complex	TLR	Toll-like receptor
MPL	Monophosphoryl lipid A	US FDA	US Food and Drug Administration

What is an adjuvant and why are they added to certain vaccines?

Adjuvant: Latin *adjuvare*, to help. A substance added to vaccines that increases the magnitude and/or duration of the immune response to the vaccine antigen. Adjuvants can also modulate the type of immune response elicited by the vaccine. Examples of licensed adjuvants currently used in approved vaccines in the USA or European Union include alum, oil in water emulsions such as MF59, and liposomes.

The adaptive immune system is capable of distinguishing "self" from "non-self" and reacts by producing antibodies or activated T lymphocytes specific for the foreign substance. Most infectious microorganisms and many crude preparations of their products can be recognized by the immune system as foreign and can elicit a vigorous immune response when injected into an individual. However, highly purified preparations of recombinant microbial proteins sometimes cannot, on their own, initiate the induction of the immune system or elicit a strong and protracted immune response. Under these circumstances, the addition of substances known as adjuvants is required to initiate and enhance the antigen-specific antibody and cell-mediated immune responses. Adjuvants are carefully formulated substances that improve the

Vaccinology: An Essential Guide, First Edition. Edited by Gregg N. Milligan and Alan D.T. Barrett.
© 2015 John Wiley & Sons, Ltd. Published 2015 by John Wiley & Sons, Ltd.

immunogenicity of a vaccine by increasing the potency or longevity of the immune response to the vaccine antigens. Normally, they do not become the target of the induced immune response but facilitate the initiation of an immune response to a coadministered antigen by either enhancing normal immune initiation processes or by changing the physical properties of the injected antigen so that it becomes more available to the immune system. Vaccine manufacturers utilize adjuvants to facilitate and enhance the immune response to their vaccine with the goal of inducing copious amounts of specific antibody and large populations of memory B and T lymphocytes. The list of currently approved adjuvants is very short (Table 6.1), and these compounds were developed based mainly on their ability to enhance the immune response (mostly antibody responses) with little understanding of how they worked. We now realize that vaccines

Table 6.1 Examples of Licensed and Developmental Adjuvants

Adjuvant	Classification	Description	Used in Vaccines Against
Licensed			
Alum	Aluminum salt	Aluminum-potassium sulfate	Diptheria, tetanus, pertussis, Hepatitis B, Human papilloma virus
		Aluminum-hydroxide Aluminum-phosphate	
MF59 (European Union)	Emulsion	Squalene in water	Influenza (Focetria® [pandemic influenza] and Fluad® [seasonal influenza])
Virosomes/liposomes (European Union)	Antigen delivery	Lipid vesicles	Hepatitis A, Influenza
AS03 (European Union)	Combination	Oil-in-water emulsion, α-tocopherol	Pandemrix® (pandemic influenza)
AS04 (European Union, US)	Combination	MPL, Alum	Hepatitis B (Fendrix® [EU only]), Human papilloma virus (Cervarix®)
In development			
MPL	Immunostimulant	TLR4 ligand	Visceral leishmaniasis, Hepatitis B
QS-21	Saponin	Quil A derivative	Breast cancer, prostate cancer, melanoma
PLG	Microparticle	polylactide-co-glycolide	HIV
Flagellin	Immunostimulant	TLR5 ligand	Influenza
Montanide	Emulsion	Water in oil	Malaria, cancer
ISCOMATRIX	Combination	Saponin, lipid mixture	Melanoma
AS01	Combination	MPL, liposomes, QS21	Malaria
AS02	Combination	MPL, oil-in-water emulsion, QS21	HIV, malaria, mycobacterium, tuberculosis
CPG 7909	Combination	CpG TLR9 ligand, Alum CpG TLR9 ligand, MF59	Malaria, hepatitis C virus

MPL, monophosphoryl lipid A; PLG, poly (lactide-co-glycoline); TLR, Toll-like receptor.

against some pathogens will require targeted initiation of specific immune response components, including specific populations of T lymphocytes, or will be delivered to mucosal sites, and will require adjuvants with different characteristics than currently approved adjuvants. Based on our current understanding of the role of the innate immunity in initiating adaptive immune responses, a number of candidate adjuvants with different properties and modes of action are currently under development.

Characteristics of a good adjuvant

There are a number of real and theoretical benefits provided by the utilization of adjuvants in vaccines. From a safety perspective, a vaccine should incorporate the least amount of antigen necessary to elicit a protective immune response. Addition of an effective adjuvant should decrease the amount of vaccine antigen required for development of protective immunity. Vaccine manufacturers obviously are also interested in minimizing the required antigen dose so as to control the cost of vaccine production and enable more doses of vaccine to be manufactured. This latter point may be particularly important in situations such as pandemics in which a limited vaccine antigen supply needs to be stretched to as many individuals as possible. Similarly, many vaccines require the administration of multiple doses in order to achieve sufficient levels of antibody or T lymphocytes necessary to protect against infection and disease. There are clear safety and economic benefits to reducing the number of times individuals must receive the vaccine, and the inclusion of effective adjuvants should be aimed at a reduction in the number of immunizations required for protection. Another approach to reducing the number of immunizations is to incorporate multiple antigens for different pathogens into a single vaccine. Unfortunately, some antigens cannot be combined easily due to competition to induce an immune response. Incorporation of adjuvants that are compatible with each vaccine antigen may potentially overcome the competition, resulting in vigorous responses to all vaccine antigens.

Increasing the immunogenicty of a vaccine with adjuvants also allows for immune responses to develop in individuals, such as the very young or elderly who have a limited capability to respond to immunization. Immune-compromised individuals cannot receive live attenuated vaccines. Therefore, effective adjuvants should augment vaccine responses to nonlive vaccines as a logical alternative approach to immune protection of these populations. It is important for immunization to result in the type of immune response required to prevent disease caused by a particular pathogen. Many of the vaccines we currently use work by eliciting protective antibody responses. However, for many pathogens, effective protection against disease will require a balanced immune response involving strong, vaccine-elicited T-cell responses, including both helper T-cell and cytotoxic T-lymphocyte populations in addition to antigen-specific antibody. It is also now clear that individuals with chronic infections have better outcomes if the T cells that respond to the pathogen express several effector functions; that is, the T-cell response is polyfunctional. Therefore, adjuvants may also be used according to their ability to guide the development of certain types of immunity or to develop T-cell populations with a broad range of effector functions. The use of adjuvants may be critical in instances of pandemic disease outbreak or intentional release of pathogens into population centers. The incorporation of adjuvants into pandemic vaccines would potentially decrease the time required for immunized individuals to develop protective immune responses. The shortened vaccine response time would likely be important for containment or control of disease spread.

Good candidate adjuvants should be developed using simple, inexpensive components that are readily obtained and in abundant supply. Moreover, adjuvants should be easy to produce such that that the physical and functional characteristics are consistently obtained without variability in product among production lots. The effective candidate should also be stable, preferably at ambient temperature, with a relatively long shelf life. However, once injected into humans, it should be easily biodegradable so that adjuvant components are not left long term at the injection site. Finally, it should be compatible with other adjuvants or immune potentiators so that further augmentation of the immune response or enhancement of antigen delivery might be achieved by combinations of these agents.

Safety

Reactogenicity: A toxic or pathogenic response to a vaccine component ranging from mild to severe in nature. Reactogenicity may also be immediate or long term. Examples of reactogenic events observed following vaccine administration include erythema, induration, swelling, or pain at the site of injection or systemic reactions such as fever, irritability, sleepiness, and malaise.

The goal of vaccines is to protect human and animal populations against disease, and the action of any component of the vaccine, including adjuvant, should be consistent with this goal. Because an overactivation of the immune system by adjuvant-containing vaccines may cause unintended damage to the tissues and organ systems of vaccine recipients, it is imperative that adjuvants are carefully formulated so that they are both effective and safe. Numerous candidate adjuvants have been shown to be efficacious in promoting vigorous immune responses but are not acceptable for use in humans. This is due mainly to safety concerns associated with potentially harmful responses elicited by the adjuvant that may be either short term or long term in nature. Short-term effects are due mainly to induction of significant inflammatory responses that result in acute reactogenicity or toxicity at the site of vaccine injection. These effects may include the development of chronic inflammation, abscesses, nodules, or ulcers at the injection site. Long-term effects are less easily observed or linked to a given adjuvant and include the potential for development of immune-mediated disorders, effects on pregnancy, and more theoretical concerns such as carcinogenesis or teratogenesis.

Many commonly used vaccines may cause short-term effects in some individuals, which are usually mild in nature and short in duration such as mild swelling, dull pain, or flu-like symptoms. Individuals who receive a vaccine are generally willing to tolerate some level of short-term discomfort to be protected against a particular disease. In fact, some level of reactogenicity associated with vaccine administration is usually unavoidable due to activation of the innate immune system. Important steps are taken to prevent or minimize these adverse effects and to determine the risk of development of adverse events compared to the benefit that inclusion of the adjuvant may provide. This risk-to-benefit ratio varies according to the different pathogens identified as vaccine targets and involves consideration of the incidence of infection and severity of disease. Individuals may be willing to tolerate more serious side effects if the risk of acquisition of a particular disease is great or if the disease is particularly severe or lethal.

Measures are taken during adjuvant development and production to reduce the reactogenicity of candidate adjuvants and monitor for adverse events. An important first step in this process is the careful formulation of the adjuvant and strict attention to quality control standards during initial manufacturing steps. Novel candidate adjuvants are considered new chemical entities and go through a series of preclinical toxicology studies both *in vitro* and in animals. This assessment includes single or repeat-dose toxicity studies in two animal species, and tests for genotoxicity including gene mutation, DNA damage, or chromosome aberrations, as well as tests for systemic hypersensitivity, injection site reactions, and pyrogenicity. The outcome of these studies may preclude further testing of some adjuvants identified as toxic and may identify safety concerns to be monitored in subsequent clinical studies for others. Adjuvants are not licensed as entities separate from candidate vaccines by regulatory authorities such as the US Food and Drug Administration (FDA) or the European Medicines Agency (EMA), and safety information is collected and evaluated as part of the preclinical evaluation and clinical trials for a given vaccine/adjuvant formulation. The complete vaccine including antigens, adjuvants, and any additives such as preservatives or excipients undergoes toxicology testing using the same formulation and dose as anticipated to be used in humans. The specifics of preclinical and clinical safety assessments will be covered in more detail in subsequent chapters (Chapters 11, 12, 15, 17). An example of safety monitoring of vaccines, including the use of adjuvants, is found in clinical testing of influenza vaccines either with or without incorporated adjuvants and in the H1N1 influenza pandemic of 2009–2010. The conventional, nonreplicating seasonal influenza vaccine administered in the USA does not contain adjuvant as it is not approved by the FDA. As a result, relatively large doses of antigen are required to induce protective antibody responses whereas influenza vaccines used in Europe contain adjuvants because they have been approved by the EMA. For some time, it has been argued that inclusion of an adjuvant into influenza vaccines would have several benefits, including the enhancement of the immune response to the vaccine in very young and elderly vaccine recipients, as well as reduction of the amount of antigen required per dose. This would obviously be beneficial in situations such as pandemic influenza outbreaks where the amount of antigen available could be "stretched" to protect many more individuals. Clinical trials were performed, primarily in Europe and China, to test the safety and immunogenicity of adjuvanted pandemic influenza vaccines in "at-risk" populations, including young children, pregnant women, immune-compromised populations, and in the elderly. In these studies, both local reactions such as tenderness, erythema, induration, swelling, pain or pruritis, and systemic reactions such as fever, irritability, sleepiness, diarrhea, vomiting, myalgia, and nasal discharge were carefully documented to establish the acceptability of these vaccines. Additionally, information was obtained to document the effects of these vaccines on the outcome of pregnancy in young women. As will be discussed in subsequent chapters (Chapters 15, 17), safety testing and monitoring of vaccine occurs not only in human clinical trials, but also throughout the vaccine approval and post-licensure stages. Currently, there is a great desire to develop integrated safety databases from data garnered during the testing and post-licensure monitoring processes that will be used to estimate the effectiveness and safety profile of the adjuvant for use in future vaccines. The end result of these efforts is to ensure the safety and acceptability of these products for use in vaccines developed for administration to humans.

Types of vaccine adjuvants

Adjuvants have been incorporated into vaccines for many years; however, until recently, we did not have a good understanding of how they worked. Much remains to be learned, but recent advances in our understanding of how the innate immune system detects the presence of different pathogens and how it responds to these stimuli have provided a good understanding of the basics of how a vigorous immune response is initiated. As will be discussed, many vaccinologists are currently using this information to develop adjuvants identical to or modifications of the pathogen-associated molecular patterns (PAMPs) responsible for "natural" stimulation of the innate immune response.

Pathogen-associated molecular patterns (PAMPs): Highly conserved, molecular structures or patterns preferentially expressed by viral, bacterial, or parasitic pathogens that are recognized by extracellular and intracellular receptors of the host, resulting in activation of innate immune responses. Examples of PAMPs include lipopolysaccharide, double-stranded RNA, flagellin, and unmethylated DNA oligonucleotides containing the CpG motif.

Pattern recognition receptors (PRRs): Host receptor molecules that recognize specific PAMPs. Signal cascades resulting from PAMP ligand binding to PRRs result in release of proinflammatory cytokines and induction of antimicrobial gene programs. Examples of PRRs include Toll-like receptors (TLRs), RIG-I, MDA-5, and C-type lectin receptors.

Other adjuvant strategies involve optimizing the physicochemical characteristics of vaccine antigens or developing novel methods to protect the vaccine antigen from degradation or to prolong antigen release. For these strategies, the adjuvant properties do not primarily rely on pathogen recognition receptor (PRR)-dependent stimulation of innate immune cells so much as on the physical nature of the antigenic particles presented or on the specific targeting of the antigen to specific cells or tissues of the immune system. While there are many different adjuvant strategies, it is useful to characterize candidate adjuvants as either antigen delivery vehicles or immunostimulatory agents.

Antigen delivery vehicles

Antigen delivery vehicles may be used to prolong antigen availability for efficient stimulation of B lymphocytes or to promote antigen uptake and internalization by innate immune cells for enhanced and targeted presentation to T lymphocytes. This can be accomplished in various ways, and different candidate adjuvants are currently under development that use different strategies to accomplish these aims. Antigen delivery adjuvants may act by multimerization of vaccine antigen or may incorporate the antigen into particles of an optimal size for efficient uptake by antigen scavenging cells. Because many vaccine antigens are easily degraded or metabolized, antigen delivery vehicles may protect the antigen, allowing for a protracted release of antigen. The specific targeting of vaccine antigen to specific tissues or cells may be accomplished by inclusion of ligands or antibodies specific for cell surface receptors. In some instances, the components of the delivery adjuvant particle may be formulated to allow delivery of antigen into the cytosol or endosomal compartments of antigen-presenting cells (APCs) for enhanced antigen presentation and delivery into the MHC class I antigen presentation pathway. Additionally, the addition of immunostimulatory agents to the adjuvant may allow induction of a proinflammatory reaction at the injection site, resulting in infiltration of innate immune cells including APCs. Thus, antigen delivery vehicles may be used in conjunction with distinct adjuvants that possess different functional properties and allow an additive or synergistic effect on vaccine immunogenicity.

Aluminum salt-based adjuvants

Aluminum salt adjuvants have a long history of safe and effective use in human vaccines, and at present these are the only universally approved adjuvants. In 1926, the successful and reproducible induction of vigorous antibody responses by injection of antigens precipitated with aluminum potassium sulfate (Alum) was reported. Subsequently, this approach was used in the production of vaccines against the toxins of *Clostridium diptheriae* and *C. tetani*. While the term "alum" is commonly used to describe any aluminum salt-based adjuvant, it specifically applies only to aluminum potassium sulfate. In the 1930s, the approach of adsorption of antigens onto aluminum hydroxide was developed, which resulted in a better-defined and standardized vaccine preparation, and large-scale production of alum-adsorbed vaccines began in the 1940s. Current aluminum salt adjuvants include aluminum hydroxide and aluminum phosphate to adsorb negatively charged and positively charged protein antigens, respectively. The adsorption process results in the formation of a lattice network in which vaccine antigen

is held in place by the aluminum salt. Each manufacturer has its own particular formulation of alum for inclusion in vaccines.

Although aluminum salt adjuvants have been used for decades in the USA, the mechanism responsible for the adjuvant activity has only recently begun to be elucidated. Early work on alum-precipitated vaccines found that antigen-containing alum precipitates could be detected for long periods in experimental animals vaccinated with alum-precipitated vaccines, but not in vaccines that lacked adjuvant. Moreover, emulsions of the precipitates from immune animals elicited a specific antibody response upon injection into nonimmune animals. Thus, the idea of an antigen depot and long-term release of antigen were believed responsible for the adjuvant activity of alum (Figure 6.1). More recently, it has been determined that proinflammatory cytokines and chemokines can be detected very soon after immunization with aluminum salt adjuvants and that neutrophils, myeloid dendritic cells, plasmacytoid dendritic cells, inflammatory monocytes, and eosinophils can be detected within 1 day of immunization at the injection site. Beyond recruiting these innate immune cells, aluminum salts have been shown to induce maturation of dendritic cell populations by upregulating MHC class II molecules, the co-stimulatory molecule CD86 and CD40 on the cell surface. This immunostimulatory activity was initially shown to occur independently of TLR signaling; subsequent studies have suggested that aluminum salts may result in the activation of the NLRP3 inflammasome. The exact mechanism of action by aluminum salt adjuvants remains uncertain, but these current studies certainly demonstrate a much more complicated and active role for aluminum salts in immune stimulation beyond merely serving as an antigen depot.

Immunization with aluminum salt-containing vaccines commonly results in a Th2-biased immune response with the production of high amounts of antibody of the IgG1 subclass (in mice). This bias has been shown to depend on the production of IL-4, which may stimulate differentiation of T cells toward Th2 responses and inhibit development of Th1 immune responses. Further, it has been determined that IL-4–producing eosinophils infiltrate the immunization site early after immunization and may serve as the source of IL-4 for eliciting the predominant Th2 immune response. The utilization of these adjuvants

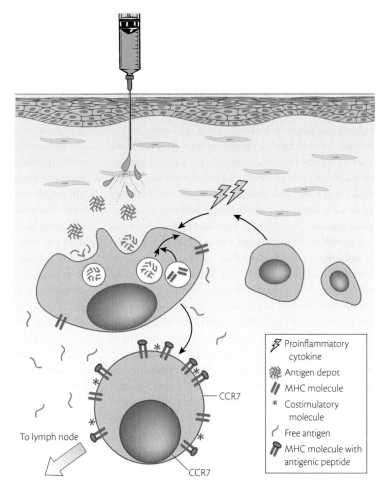

Figure 6.1 Local events following injection of vaccine formulated with an antigen delivery adjuvant. Antigen depots are deposited at the injection site and are maintained over time, resulting in a prolonged release of free antigen for activation of T and B lymphocytes in the lymph node. Inflammatory events from the injection result in local production of proinflammatory cytokines, which in turn attract tissue monocyte/macrophages or dendritic cells to the injection site. These cells take up and process antigen into antigenic peptides for association with MHC molecules and mature in the presence of the proinflammatory cytokines to express high levels of MHC molecules, co-stimulatory molecules, and the CCR7 molecule required for homing of the cells to the T-cell zone of the lymph node.

in vaccines also does not generally result in priming or cross-priming for vaccine antigen-specific CD8$^+$ T-cell responses.

The safety profile of aluminum salt-containing vaccines is very good, and there is no evidence that they are pyrogenic, carcinogenic, or teratogenic. Mild local reactions to the adjuvant have been reported. These include swelling, erythema, and induration at the site of injection, but in general these adjuvants are very well tolerated by humans. A limitation to the use of aluminum salt adjuvant-containing vaccines is that they cannot be frozen as the freeze–thaw process results in breakdown of the antigen lattice structures necessary for adjuvant activity.

Emulsions

Emulsions represent a type of commonly used adjuvant utilized in both human and veterinary vaccines that are usually prepared as either oil-in-water, or water-in-oil formulations. Early emulsions were water-in-oil formulations in which water droplets, stabilized by the addition of surfactants, were formed in a squalene or squalane oil base. Freund's incomplete adjuvant represents an early attempt at this type of adjuvant, and it was used to enhance antibody responses in human influenza vaccines. Its reactogenic properties and relative instability resulted in withdrawal of its use in human vaccines. More recent water-in-oil emulsions have proven less toxic. One current formulation,

Montanide 720, is currently being tested as a component in cancer vaccines.

Oil-in-water emulsions have generally proven to be less toxic and less reactogenic than their water-in-oil counterparts. The oil-in-water emulsion adjuvant MF59 is currently licensed in most of Europe and utilized as the adjuvant in influenza vaccines for humans. Squalene is utilized as the oil carrier in the presence of emulsifying agents such as Tween 80 and Span 85. Since squalene represents a natural precursor involved in cholesterol and steroid hormone syntheses, it is easily metabolized. This adjuvant platform approach is easily modifiable by the addition of immunomodulators to further potentiate the immune response. Recent testing has shown that use of MF59 in influenza vaccines resulted in higher antibody titers, required fewer doses and less antigen per dose, and increased the immunogenicity of the vaccine in elderly individuals. Importantly, these vaccines are safe and well tolerated. The mechanism of action for MF59 is not completely understood but is thought to involve enhanced uptake by APCs and the formation of long-term antigen release via a depot effect. Importantly, MF59 elicits a proinflammatory response characterized by the production and release of cytokines and recruitment of dendritic cells, monocytes, and granulocytes to the site of injection. Interestingly, microarray analysis revealed a more vigorous expression of cytokine genes, cytokine receptor genes, and genes involved in leukocyte migration and recruitment that was elicited following application of MF59 compared to either alum or cytosine-phosphate-guanosine (CpG) oligonucleotides. The mechanism responsible for the development of this response is currently unknown but may involve the direct stimulation of muscle fibers by MF59 in addition to effects on APC populations.

Liposomes

Liposomes are composed of lipid-bilayer membranes enclosing an aqueous-phase core. This approach is highly adaptable, and modifications to the vesicle size, lipid composition, and lipid-to-antigen protein ratio may be made to influence the adjuvanticity of the liposome. The entrapment of antigens into the aqueous core of liposomes generally occurs naturally during the production process but may be enhanced by conjugation of peptide or protein antigens to lipids for intercalation into the liposome membrane. The polar region of the membrane lipids generally confers a net electrical charge to the liposome surface and thus influences the adjuvant characteristics of the liposome. While some immunostimulation has been attributed to the liposome itself, its major function is to deliver the vaccine antigen to the immune system (Figure 6.2). This may be accomplished by providing an antigen-containing particle comparable in size to many pathogens for efficient uptake by APCs. The liposome composition may also be modified to enhance uptake by APCs. For example, it is thought that cationic liposomes may interact more efficiently with relatively negatively charged APC membranes. Alternatively, the incorporation of phosphatidylserine in the liposomal formulation may mimic the membrane of apoptotic cells expressing this lipid on their outer membranes and enhance uptake by APC. More specific targeting of liposomes to APCs may be accomplished by the incorporation of antibodies specific for APC membrane proteins such as IgG Fc receptors, mannose receptors, or MHC molecules. Lipid modifications may also result in delivery of antigen for enhanced processing. Utilization of pH-sensitive lipids in liposome formulations may allow destabilization of the liposomal membrane and release of antigen in the acid environment of endosomes. The liposome may also promote antigen presentation by preventing degradation of the vaccine antigen. Polymerization of liposomes by covalently cross-linking lipids may be utilized to resist enzymatic hydrolysis and may result in enhanced immunogenicity by extending the period of antigen release. Finally, incorporation of immunostimulatory adjuvants such as monophosphoryl lipid A (MPL), CpG oligonucleotides, or poly inosine:cytosine (poly I:C) in the liposome along with antigen may additionally enhance immunogenicity and increase the utility of liposome-mediated antigen delivery.

Several related approaches have been developed including archaeosomes, virosomes, and niosomes. Virosomes contain viral proteins in the bilayer membrane that enhance uptake by APCs or facilitate the delivery of antigen to intracellular compartments. Niosomes are also similar to liposomes but are composed of nonionic surfactants that confer membrane stability and thus a longer half-life to the particles. Archaeosomes contain glycerolipids of *Archaea* species, which also confer membrane stability. The utilization

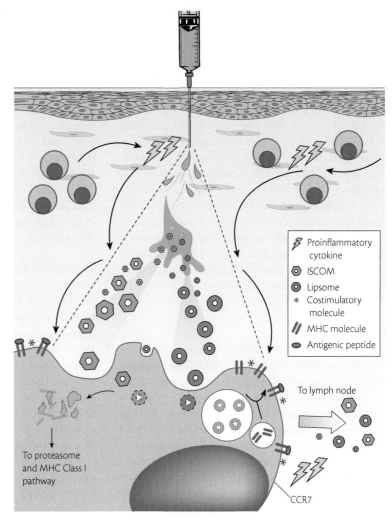

Figure 6.2 Local events following injection of antigen-loaded ISCOMs or liposomes. Inflammatory events following the injection result in recruitment of dendritic cells and monocyte/macrophages. Uptake of ISCOMs or liposomes may be accomplished through mechanisms such as phagocytosis, pinocytosis, or fusion with the plasma membrane such that the vehicles are delivered to endosomal or cytoplasmic compartments for degradation and presentation with cellular MHC proteins. Cell maturation events result in homing of the antigen presenting cell to T-cell zones in the lymph node. It is also possible that "free" liposomes or ISCOMs may reach the lymph node via the lymphatic system for activation of B lymphocytes or processing and presentation by lymphoid resident dendritic cells.

of archaeosomes as adjuvants has been shown to elicit strong antigen-specific antibody responses and to have the added benefit of promoting cross-priming of vaccine antigens, resulting in development of CD8[+] T-cell responses.

Microparticles/nanoparticles

Another approach to rendering antigens particulate has been to encapsulate them in biodegradable microcapsules. Utilization of encapsulation components with known rates of degradation would in theory result in prolonged and timed antigen release. The polymer poly (lactide-co-glycoline) (PLG), which has previously found use in biodegradable sutures, has

been tested for vaccine delivery and shown to be capable of eliciting strong antibody responses. Beyond the delayed-release benefits of this approach, the presence of a protective microcapsule may protect vaccine antigens from physical breakdown following the delivery process. For example, vaccines delivered by the oral route first must pass through the acid pH of the stomach followed by the mildly alkaline pH of the proximal end of the small intestine. This intestinal environment would also contain enzymes and surfactants of both host and normal flora origin. Thus, the presence of a temporal protective "coating" would aid in vaccine antigen protection and delivery to the site of uptake at mucosal immune inductive sites.

Microparticles may also be loaded with immunostimulatory agents or linked with molecules to target delivery of antigen to the microfold surface of intestinal immune inductive sites or for uptake by gut APCs.

A similar approach, taken on an even smaller scale, is the production of nanoparticles. Nanoparticles are usually of submicron size and are thought to provide advantages over microparticles by providing an increased surface area for the uptake of antigen. Additionally, the method of production may be simpler and more reproducible. While nanoparticles have also been shown to enhance the immunogenicity of delivered antigens in preclinical studies, there are still challenges in production and size stability during storage. Additionally, given the relatively high concentration of surfactants and excipients required in nanoparticle production, it will be essential to ensure that nanoparticle vaccines remain safe for human use.

Saponins

Saponins are a family of soluble triterpene glycosides isolated from plants. The most commonly used saponin in adjuvant formulations is Quil-A. This heterogeneous mixture of approximately 50 different saponins is obtained by extraction from the bark of the *Quillaja saponaria* tree. Although these compounds have good adjuvant activity, adverse events have been associated with their use in humans including development of granulomas and hemolysis. A purified fraction derived from Quil-A, QS-21, retains much of the adjuvanticity of the parental molecule yet is diminished in toxicity. QS-21 elicits proinflammatory cytokine release from innate immune cells although the mechanism responsible for this activity is unknown. QS-21 strongly associates with cell membranes and has been shown to facilitate entry of antigens to intracellular compartments. Thus, administration of antigens with QS-21 has been shown to elicit antigen-specific CD8$^+$ T-cell responses, strongly suggesting it enhances access of vaccine antigen to the class I MHC presentation pathway. QS-21 is also commonly used along with cholesterol and various phospholipids in the formulation of ISCOMS (immune stimulating complexes), a particulate adjuvant with a cage-like structure. Immunization with antigen incorporated into the physical structure of the adjuvant particle (ISCOMS) or with a derivative formulation in which antigen is mixed with the preformed adjuvant particle (ISCOMATRIX), has been shown to elicit a strong antibody response and extremely vigorous cell-mediated response. Perhaps due to the ability to deliver antigen directly into the cytosol and thus target efficient loading of antigenic peptides onto MHC class I molecules, ISCOMS are very efficient in priming for an antigen-specific CD8$^+$ T-cell response (Figure 6.2). Given the general inefficiency of most killed and subunit vaccines to elicit a vigorous antigen-specific CD8$^+$ T-cell response, the development of ISCOMS as a vaccine adjuvant may hold promise for eliciting this important T-cell subset in human populations that cannot receive live attenuated vaccines.

Immunostimulatory adjuvants

Many of the important cellular and molecular events involved in induction of adaptive immune responses have been identified from studies involving challenge of hosts with infectious organisms. We now know that innate immune cells such as monocytes and dendritic cells respond very quickly to the presence of pathogens and become activated via signaling through PRRs that recognize specific PAMPs. These signaling events result in cellular activation and the production and secretion of proinflammatory cytokines and chemokines that influence the activation, homing, and differentiation of other immune and somatic cells. PRR signaling also has a critical role in maturing resting, tissue-dwelling dendritic cells by increasing the expression of major histocompatibility complex and co-stimulatory molecules necessary for efficient presentation of antigen to naïve T lymphocytes. These PAMP-stimulated dendritic cells also express new chemokine receptors allowing them to respond to lymphoid tissue-produced chemokines and migrate from the site of activation to the regional lymph node. Once in the lymph node, these cells present the antigens collected at the site of infection to naïve T lymphocytes, thereby initiating the adaptive immune response (Figure 6.3). The types and quantities of cytokines produced by PAMP-stimulated innate immune cells also have a marked effect on the type and magnitude of B lymphocyte and CD4$^+$ T lymphocyte immune responses that develop. Additionally, secretion of some cytokines such as type I interferon

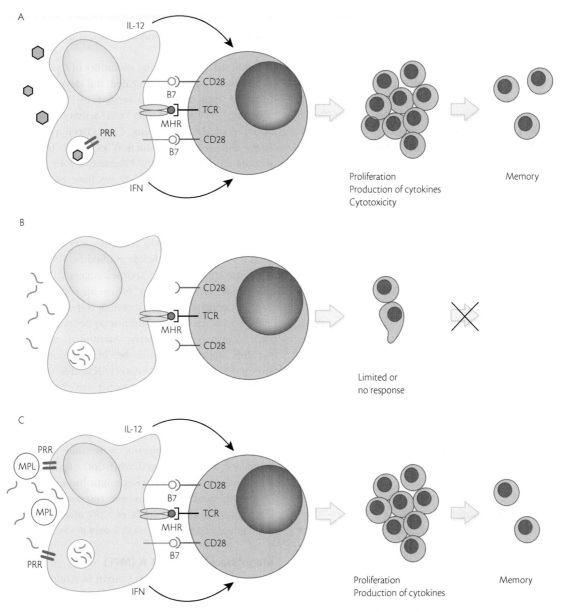

Figure 6.3 Immunogenicity of vaccine formulated with an immunostimulatory adjuvant. (A) Immunization with live attenuated vaccine results in maturation of dendritic cells and the production of co-stimulatory molecules (B7), proinflammatory cytokines, and type I IFNs. These cells provide all the antigen and co-stimulatory signals necessary to drive naïve T-cells to proliferate, produce cytokines and express cytotoxic activity and to differentiate into memory T cells. (B) Immunization with purified recombinant protein in the absence of any PAMP does not result in maturation of dendritic cells, and important co-stimulatory and cytokine signals are not provided so that the T-cell response is not maintained and T-cell memory is not induced. (C) Immunization of the same recombinant protein in the presence of an immunostimulatory adjuvant, in this case MPL, results in recognition of the adjuvant by cell-associated PRRs and subsequent maturation of dendritic cells. Again, appropriate cytokine and co-stimulatory signals are provided to drive proliferation of antigen-specific T cells with ultimate differentiation into memory T cells.

(IFN) enhance the ability of lymph node-resident dendritic cells to cross-present antigens to CD8$^+$ T lymphocytes. Thus, the stimulation of PRRs with specific microbial ligands (PAMPs) results in stimulation of the innate immune system and specifically the activation and maturation of dendritic cells. This is the critical step in immune stimulation by this very efficient process. Live attenuated vaccines that naturally contain PRR ligands are intrinsically adjuvanted, which is responsible, in part, for their effectiveness at eliciting vigorous immune responses. Additionally, the type of immunity elicited following stimulation of a particular PRR has been selected by evolution to be appropriate for the pathogen responsible for the stimulation. In this case, the live attenuated vaccine will elicit the type of immunity that will be effective against an encounter with the wild-type pathogen. Not surprisingly, an active area of adjuvant research is aimed at utilizing PRR ligands as adjuvants to increase the immunogenicity of subunit vaccines. A number of synthetic Toll-like receptor (TLR) agonists have been tested as adjuvants based on their ability to mimic the capacity of natural TLR-ligands to stimulate innate immune responses, including the maturation of dendritic cells and production of proinflammatory cytokines via activation of TLR-signaling pathways. Many of these agonists have been tested in preclinical experiments and some in clinical trials; they have great potential for use in enhancing the immunogenicity of candidate vaccines.

CpG oligodinucleotides

The study of the immunostimulatory properties of crude preparations of microbial products led to the discovery that bacterial and viral DNA were immunostimulatory and elicited an inflammatory response in vertebrate animals. It was soon determined that palindromic sequences including cytosine-phosphate-guanosine (CpG) motifs were particularly immunostimulatory and that the degree of methylation of cytosine in the CpG oligonucleotide (low in viral and bacterial DNA) was critical for this stimulatory effect. With the discovery of the TLR family of PRRs, it was soon recognized that TLR9 was responsible for sensing the stimulatory CpG oligonucleotides and for generating the signals required for activation of dendritic cells and production of proinflammatory cytokines. Species-specific motifs for humans, mice, chickens, cats, dogs,

horses, and pigs have been identified indicating the important role of surrounding nucleotides in the biological activity.

Initial studies examining the utility of CpG oligonucleotides as adjuvants revealed the development of immune responses characterized by the presence of strong Th1-like and CD8$^+$ CTL activity. This strong skewing of the developing CD4$^+$ T-cell response is likely due to the production of IL-12 from CpG stimulated dendritic cells. Likewise, strong antibody responses to a number of viruses have been elicited in animals by immunization with candidate vaccines that incorporate a CpG oligonucleotide adjuvant. In agreement with the nature of the T-cell response, the vaccine-elicited antibody response was made up of high levels of IgG2a subclass antibodies. The ability to stimulate strong T-cell responses suggests CpG oligonucleotide adjuvants may be useful components in vaccines designed to elicit immune responses in populations with inefficient immune systems such as the very young or the elderly. Additional applications for this approach would be in situations where strong T-cell responses are very desirable such as in therapeutic vaccines against hepatitis C virus, herpes simplex virus, human immunodeficiency virus (HIV), or cancer. CpG oligonucleotides have been used without obvious deleterious effects in preclinical studies in animals. Early concerns were that the strong T-cell responses generated with CpG oligonucleotide adjuvant-containing vaccines might increase the risk of development of autoimmune responses; however, the results of clinical trials of CpG oligonucleotide-adjuvanted vaccines suggest this may not be a concern.

Monophosphoryl lipid A (MPL)

Lipopolysaccharide (LPS) is known to strongly stimulate the innate immune system and has been shown in animal models to have strong adjuvant activity. These characteristics are dependent on signaling via TLR4 receptors in a MyD88-dependent fashion. Unfortunately, LPS is extremely toxic and not suitable for human use. It has been found that LPS can be made substantially less toxic through a series of acid–base hydrolysis steps to yield monophosphoryl lipid A (MPL). This compound contains the lipid A moiety of *Salmonella minnesota* LPS and possesses adjuvant activities by virtue of its ability to stimulate through the TLR4 receptor pathway. Interestingly, the signaling appears to be much less dependent on the MyD88 pathway than it is for the parental LPS. MPL has been administered to humans in vaccines as an adjuvant or as a component of allergy therapeutics. Its exceptional safety profile in humans has resulted in licensure in Europe and inclusion as an adjuvant for the hepatits B vaccine, Fendrix®.

TRL5 agonists: flagellin

Flagellin is a proteinaceous subunit of the flagellar structures found in many motile bacteria. Like other TLR agonists, flagellin has been shown to be highly stimulatory for both the innate and adaptive immune systems and has generated interest for development as an effective adjuvant. Flagellin is recognized not only at the cell surface by TLR5, but the cytoplasmic NOD-like receptor proteins neuronal apoptosis inhibitory protein 5 (NAIP5) and interleukin-1 beta-converting enzyme (ICE) protease activating factor (IPAF) have also been shown to detect the presence of flagellin. However, the relative contribution of each recognition pathway to the adjuvant activity of flagellin has not been fully determined. Flagellin adjuvants delivered either in association with vaccine antigens or physically linked as part of fusion protein have enhanced the development of both specific antibody and cell-mediated immune responses. Unlike TLR agonists such as CpG oligonucleotides that drive the developing cell-mediated response strongly toward IFN-γ production, flagellin-adjuvanted cellular immunity appears to be more heterogeneous with aspects of both Th1 and Th2 responses.

TLR3/RIG-I ligands

Both single- and double-stranded RNA molecules are capable of stimulating the innate immune system by virtue of their ability to be recognized by TLR3, RIG-I/MDA5 (double-stranded RNA), or TLR7 (single-stranded RNA). Poly I:C is a synthetic agonist for TLR3 and has potent adjuvant activities but it is unfortunately very toxic in humans, resulting in renal failure, coagulopathies, and hypersensitivity reactions. New dsRNA analogs have been produced such as poly [I]: poly [$C_{12}U$] that exhibit greatly diminished toxicity profiles yet retain the ability to stimulate production of proinflammatory cytokines and mature dendritic cells. TLR7 agonists such as Immiquimod and Resiquimod have also been shown to be highly stimulatory

for innate immune responses and have been licensed for use in antiviral therapies against HPV and against basal cell carcinoma. These synthetic agonists are highly immunostimulatory and have been shown to have adjuvant activity in laboratory animals. Given the excellent safety profile of these agents in humans, they may have possibilities as adjuvant candidates.

Muramyl dipeptide

Muramyl dipeptide (MDP) is a component of *Mycobacteria* cell walls and can be recognized by the NLR, NOD2. It also has been found to have profound adjuvant activities and was utilized as the active component of the complete Freund's adjuvant. Use of this adjuvant has been discontinued due to the extreme pyrogenic effects associated with its use. Less toxic analogs of MDP such as muramyl tripeptide phosphatidylethanolamine have been synthesized and are currently being tested for safety and efficacy.

Bacterial toxins

Bacterial toxins such as cholera toxin (CT) and the heat-labile enterotoxin of *Escherichia coli* (LT) have been shown to have very strong immunostimulatory activity. Also, since these toxins normally act at mucosal sites with high mucous content, there is much interest in development of these compounds as adjuvants for mucosal vaccines. These structurally related toxins exist as a complex of two subunits, an enzymatic A subunit, which possesses the adenosine diphosphate ribosyltransferase activity responsible for the toxin activity, and a B subunit made up of five B monomers, which binds to the GM1 ganglioside receptor found on nearly all host cell membranes. Preclinical studies revealed the potent adjuvant activity of CT and further demonstrated that the immunostimulatory effect depended primarily on the enzymatic activity. Mutations of single amino acids in the active site of the ADP ribosyltransferase of CT and LT were identified that significantly diminished enzymatic activity and thus the toxicity of these toxins, although much of the adjuvanticity of the complex was retained. The mechanism of action of CT and LT as adjuvants is thought to involve modulation of APC activity. Interestingly, both proinflammatory and anti-inflammatory effects have been reported following treatment with these molecules. Vigorous cell antigen-specific antibody responses are elicited using these adjuvants, with the majority of studies reporting a Th1-biased cell-mediated immune response.

Although CT and LT mutants with diminished toxicity hold much promise as adjuvants, hurdles still remain in their development. For example, these adjuvants have the capacity to bind to neurons and epithelial cells via the GM1 ganglioside receptor, which raises safety concerns and questions about the utility of their use in certain immunization schemes. One approach taken to overcome this hurdle is to abolish the promiscuous binding of the B subunit by the generation of gene fusion proteins in which the immunoglobulin binding D domains from *Staphylococcus aureus* is fused to the enzymatic A subunit of CT. Thus, further development and testing of genetically altered CT and LT may lead to adjuvants suitable for human use.

Combination adjuvants

The next generation of adjuvants is currently in various stages of clinical testing and takes advantage of recent developments in our understanding of the development of innate and adaptive immune responses, and the types of responses that will be effective against a given pathogen. Many of these are combinations of antigen delivery vehicles and immunostimulatory agents that have been carefully formulated to elicit enhanced antibody and cell-mediated immune responses. Many antigen-delivery adjuvants platforms such as liposomes, alum, or oil-in-water emulsions are amenable to incorporation of one or more immunostimulants to elicit specific, desired immune responses. Among the best-studied combination adjuvants are the antigen system (AS) adjuvants developed by Glaxo Smith Kline. ASO2 is a combination of oil-in-water emulsion, the TLR4 ligand MPL, and the saponin QS21. In this formulation, MPL provides signals required for enhanced antibody and cellular immune responses. QS21 also has marked effects for stimulation of T cell-mediated immunity and may help elicit $CD8^+$ T-cell responses. ASO3 combines α-tocopherol in an oil-in-water emulsion and has been used in pandemic influenza vaccines. ASO4 is a formulation composed of MPL and either aluminum hydroxide or aluminum phosphate, and combines the ability of MPL to drive Th1 type responses with the well-known adjuvanticity of aluminum salt-based adjuvants. AS03 and AS04 are currently licensed for use in vaccines in the European Union, and ASO4 has now been licensed for use in HPV vaccines in the USA. ASO1 is a three-component adjuvant containing MPL, QS21, and liposomes for antigen delivery. AS15 utilizes four components—CpG oligonucleotides, MPL, QS21, and liposomes—and is currently being utilized in immunotherapy. In each case, the effects of the adjuvant components on the developing immune response are additive and in some cases synergistic. This combination adjuvant approach holds great promise for optimizing antigen delivery and immunostimulation to elicit specific types of immune responses.

Adjuvants for veterinary vaccines

Adjuvants are also an important component of vaccines for veterinary use and, not surprisingly, share many of the same characteristics and requirements for acceptability as adjuvants for use in humans. Some of the adjuvants currently in development for humans are already available in veterinary vaccines (Table 6.2). However, the choice of which adjuvant to use is somewhat more complicated in animals due to the diversity of species to be vaccinated, the inability of some species to tolerate some commonly used adjuvants, and the less well-understood nature of the innate and adaptive systems of many companion and production animals.

As with humans, some element of mild reactogenicity to the vaccine is unavoidable and in most instances acceptable. However, there are differences in how well certain species tolerate specific adjuvant preparations. For example, bovines and poultry tolerate more reactogenic water-in-oil adjuvants, whereas less reactogenic oil-in-water adjuvants are appropriate for use with companion animals, horses, and pigs. Beyond the need to avoid adverse events that affect the general well-being of the animal, it is important to consider the effects of adjuvants on reproduction or growth rates, and whether they might create unacceptable blemishes on the coat or muscles of production animals. Severe adverse events that may occur at the site of injection include the development of inflammatory reactions, trauma, hemorrhage, or

Table 6.2 Utilization of Adjuvants in Vaccines for Veterinary Use

Species	Adjuvant	Used in Vaccines Against
Dogs	ISCOMATRIX	Parvovirus
	ISCOM	Rabies
Cats	ISCOM	Feline leukemia virus
Horse	ISCOM, Gene Gun	Influenza
	ISCOM, ISCOMATRIX	Equine herpes virus 2
Pig	Gene gun	Influenza
	PLG microsphere	*Escherichia coli*
	Liquid nanoparticles	Atrophic rhinitis/pleuropneumonia
Ruminants	ISCOMATRIX	Bovine virus diarrhea virus
	ISCOM	Bovine respiratory syncytial virus
Poultry	ISCOM	Influenza (H5N1)
	ISCOM	Newcastle disease virus
	Liposome	Infectious bursal disease viruses

ISCOM, immune stimulating complexes;
PLG, poly (lactide-co-glycoline).

granulomataous nodules. Postvaccination inflammatory responses have been associated with the rare development of fibrosarcomas, osteosarcomas, chondrosarcomas, rhabdomyosarcomas, and malignant fibrous histiocytomas in cats with similar events having been reported in dogs and ferrets.

Future challenges

Most of the human vaccines currently being utilized are effective due to the development of vigorous antigen-specific antibody responses. This type of immunity is sufficient for protection against many acute bacterial and viral pathogens. However, for some pathogens, protection will require vaccine-elicited T-cell responses and specifically, high numbers of memory T-cell responses capable of responding to exposure to a pathogen with a polyfunctional effector response. Vaccines against specific cancer antigens will likewise require the development of strong and appropriate T-cell responses. The challenge for candidate adjuvants is to drive the development of strong and appropriate T-cell responses, including CD8[+] T-cell responses. Novel approaches are needed to ensure that the elicited responses are balanced and provide protection without causing bystander tissue damage.

Infection with pathogenic microorganisms and inoculation with live attenuated vaccines often results in the development of memory B and T lymphocyte responses that last for years after antigen exposure. Unfortunately, for many types of nonlive vaccines, the antibody and T-cell responses that are elicited are not durable, which results in the need to periodically reimmunize to boost the immune response. An important goal for the vaccine industry remains the development of new vaccine strategies to elicit durable immune responses. An important challenge for adjuvant development is to achieve the goal of reducing the need to reimmunize, in a safe manner, thereby minimizing adverse effects of the vaccine.

Mucosal surfaces represent the largest body surface area that the immune system must defend. Since many of the most burdensome human pathogens infect at mucosal surfaces, it has been proposed that eliciting effective immune responses at the site of mucosal infection with vaccines may be the best approach to achieve protection. This approach would face many natural barriers such as the presence of mucous covering the mucosal epithelium, the presence of both host-derived and normal flora-derived enzymes capable of breaking down vaccine components, and the natural tolerogenic environment maintained at many mucosal surfaces. Additionally, new mechanisms must be developed to efficiently target vaccine antigens to mucosal immune inductive sites. Therefore, mucosal immunization approaches will require the development of novel vaccines and new adjuvants that will be amenable to mucosal delivery.

Summary

- The development of subunit vaccines containing highly purified and defined recombinant antigens requires the use of adjuvants to increase the immunogenicity of the vaccine and make possible the development of protective immunity.

- The addition of an adjuvant to a vaccine should reduce the amount of antigen, or the number of vaccinations required to elicit a protective immune response.

- Adjuvants should direct the development of an appropriate adaptive immune response in immunocompetent individuals and should elicit protective responses in populations with diminished capacities to respond to vaccine antigens.

- Adjuvants should be simple and inexpensive to manufacture and result in a stable product with consistent and well-defined properties.

- Adjuvants should be safe for use in human populations as well as companion and production animals.

- Candidate adjuvants currently under development fall into two major categories: (1) vaccine delivery vehicles and (2) immunostimulants.

- An understanding of the mechanisms of action of candidate adjuvants should allow development of novel combinations of adjuvants that can synergistically enhance vaccine immunogenicity resulting in immune responses "tailored" to protect against a specific pathogen.

Further reading

Chen W, Patel GB, Yan H, and Zhang J (2010). Recent advances in the development of novel mucosal adjuvants and antigen delivery systems. Human Vaccines 6(9), 706–714.

Coffman RL, Sher A, and Seder RA (2010). Vaccine adjuvants: putting innate immunity to work. Immunity 33, 492–503.

De Gregorio E, D'Oro U, and Wack A (2009). Immunology of TLR-independent vaccine adjuvants. Current Opinion in Immunology 21, 339–345.

Heegaard PMH, Dedieu L, Johnson N, Le Potier M-F, Mockey M, Mutinelli F, Vahlenkamp T, Vascellari M, and Sorensen NS (2010). Adjuvants and delivery systems in veterinary vaccinology: current state and future developments. Archives of Virology 156, 183–202.

Kwissa M, Kasturi SP, and Pulendran B (2007). The science of adjuvants. Expert Review of Vaccines 6(5), 673–684.

Lambrecht BN, Kool M, Willart MA, and Hammad H (2009). Mechanism of action of clinically approved adjuvants. Current Opinion in Immunology 21, 23–29.

Liang MT, Davies NM, Blanchfield JT, and Toth I (2006). Particulate systems as adjuvants and carriers for peptide and protein antigens. Current Drug Delivery 3, 379–388.

Lindblad EB (2004). Aluminium adjuvants—in retrospect and prospect. Vaccine 22, 3658–3668.

McKee AS, Munks MW, and Marrack P (2007). How do adjuvants work? Important considerations for new generation adjuvants. Immunity 27, 687–690.

O'Hagan DT and De Gregorio E (2009). The path to a successful vaccine adjuvant—"The long and winding road". Drug Discovery Today 14(11/12), 541–551.

7 Discovery and the basic science phase of vaccine development

Gavin C. Bowick

Department of Microbiology and Immunology, 301 University Boulevard, Galveston, TX, USA

Abbreviations

DIVA	Distinguish infected from vaccinated animals	TLR	Toll-like receptor
NA	Neuraminidase	VLP	Virus-like particle
NGS	Next-generation sequencing	VSV	Vesicular stomatitis virus

Basic science and translational research

Basic science is a general term that is used to describe a particular scientific paradigm: specifically studying a component of a complex system, often using "reductionist" methods, to further understanding into the role and function of that component. In the biological sciences, this may take the form of discovery of a previously uncharacterized gene and corresponding protein and knocking out expression of the novel protein from cells or animals to investigate the resulting phenotypic changes. Such changes can provide insight into the function of the protein and utilization of this information for drug or vaccine development.

Despite the incredible successes of many vaccines and campaigns to implement use of vaccines, the mechanisms by which vaccines induce protective immunity remain largely unknown. The majority of vaccines have been developed empirically, often following the maxim "identify, inactivate, inject." While vaccines produced using this approach have resulted in eradication or near eradication of diseases such as smallpox, rinderpest, and polio, this method does not build on the significant increases in our basic understanding of immunology, molecular biology, and the mechanisms of infectious disease. In the 21st century, regulators expect a detailed understanding of how a vaccine induces protective immunity and the mechanism of how it works before it can be licensed. Furthermore, with the increasing emphasis being placed on vaccine safety, utilizing the collected knowledge from basic science to rationally design the next generation of vaccines with enhanced immunogenicity and protection while eliminating potential adverse events, is becoming increasingly important.

Definition

Reductionism: The breaking down of complex systems into simpler subunits of constituent parts. An underlying philosophy of the contemporary scientific method, it allows complex biological systems to be studied "piece by piece." Modern "systems-biology" techniques (see text) are a good complement to this method, as they aim to describe biological systems in a more "holistic" fashion.

Vaccinology: An Essential Guide, First Edition. Edited by Gregg N. Milligan and Alan D.T. Barrett.
© 2015 John Wiley & Sons, Ltd. Published 2015 by John Wiley & Sons, Ltd.

The aim of this chapter is to link basic, fundamental bench research with aspects of the vaccine development process, many of which are described in detail in other chapters in this textbook. This chapter is not designed to describe a single, canonical route by which vaccines are designed *de novo* at the bench and moved into clinical practice, but rather to illustrate how developments and findings from many aspects of biology are contributing to the development of vaccinology, an overarching discipline that encompasses immunology, molecular and cell biology, computational biology, toxicology, virology and microbiology, neuroscience, oncology, materials sciences and chemistry, and many others. As an increasing number of scientific fields are becoming more multidisciplinary, vaccinology is becoming ever more dependent on developments in other areas of research as we move away from the "identify, inactivate, inject" paradigm.

The basic science techniques used for vaccine development are those used in every other biological discipline that can have an application to vaccine development. From tools such as high-throughput, whole-genome sequencing to the cell biology of signaling downstream of immunological pattern recognition receptors, the numerous advances in technology for basic science have facilitated the development of numerous and novel vaccine candidates. However, there remains a bottleneck in transitioning these bench advances to the clinical setting. In part, this is due to regulators expecting advanced scientific tools to be used for quality control of vaccines to improve their characteristics. For example, improved technology has enabled scientists to improve the level of detection of DNA from 1 nanogram (10^{-9} g) to 1 picogram (10^{-12} g) such that regulators now expect DNA contamination of vaccines to be less than 1 picogram. Translational science is a recent trend in research design, which aims to facilitate the transition of breakthroughs at the bench to the clinic.

Perhaps the advance that has most benefited vaccinology is the use of molecular biology techniques. These fundamental methods, developed in the 1970s, have driven the development of recombinant and subunit vaccines, allowing the production of vaccines for pathogens that cannot be grown for inactivation or attenuation by traditional methods. The first subunit recombinant vaccine was for hepatitis B, where hepatitis B surface antigen (HBsAg) was expressed in yeast and replaced hepatitis B particles that were purified from the plasma of infected individuals as the commercial vaccine.

Modern molecular biology came of age with the discovery of the first restriction enzyme *HindII* in 1970, for which Nathans, Arber, and Smith were awarded the Nobel Prize for Physiology or Medicine in 1978. The ability to cut DNA at specific points, and ligate in new sequences with complementary "sticky ends" has proven extraordinarily useful in virtually every area of biology. The subsequent field of recombinant DNA technology has made possible the creation of hybrid genomes or plasmids containing elements selected to confer particular phenotypic characteristics to genomes with regions "knocked out" or replaced with other sequences. The application of this technology can be used to investigate experimental systems, such as constructing a fusion between a protein of interest and a fluorescent protein, facilitating visualization in an experiment, to creating hybrid viruses as candidate vaccines. The application of these techniques to vaccine design is discussed in a subsequent section.

Mechanisms of disease and comparative pathogenesis

Understanding the basic molecular mechanisms that are responsible for a disease can play a critically important role in vaccine development. Most vaccines do not require the microorganism to be eliminated in order to be effective. In certain cases, it is possible to separate the disease from the organism, and develop vaccines against the mechanisms that drive the pathology.

A good example of this is the tetanus vaccine. This vaccine protects against the disease caused by *Clostridium tetani*, by raising an immune response, not against the bacterium, but against the toxin. Experiments in the 1880s demonstrated that *C. tetani* was the causative agent of tetanus and identified the toxin that the bacterium produced. Research continued and demonstrated that the toxin could be neutralized by antibodies and that passive immunization was effective in preventing disease. These findings led to the development of the tetanus toxoid (an inactive form of the toxin) vaccine by Descombey in 1924.

The example of development of the tetanus vaccine demonstrates how knowledge of the molecular basis of disease can lead to the development of a successful vaccine. Basic bench research into the bacterium provided the knowledge that allowed this vaccine to be developed. For this reason, experimental findings that can seem abstract or unrelated to an application can provide the building blocks for a vaccine, treatment, or product. This basic research into pathogenesis can be combined with modern molecular biology to develop or improve vaccines. For example, the pertussis toxoid vaccine has been redesigned using site-directed mutagenesis to produce a toxoid that is inactivated but that retains its ability to induce protective immunity.

Comparative pathogenesis refers to understanding the difference between a disease and non-disease state. There are two main variables in determining whether the outcome of a disease is severe or not. The first is the host. A population infected with a single pathogen will show the typical "iceberg" of disease (see Figure 7.1 for an example using West Nile virus). Many infected individuals will be asymptomatic; that is, they will seroconvert without ever presenting with clinical symptoms or having been aware that they were infected. A smaller number will show a mild

clinical disease, and a smaller number still will present with a severe or fatal outcome. The relative proportions of these disease manifestations vary from disease to disease, and it is often difficult to determine accurate numbers, as those who were infected but who did not show any clinical symptoms are unlikely to seek medical attention. The changes in outcome to infection are likely driven primarily by host genetics, although other lifestyle and socioeconomic factors can also be involved.

The other major determinant of outcome is at the level of the pathogen. Closely related virus and bacterial species, or different strains or variants of the same virus or bacterium, may give rise to strikingly different courses of disease, from a completely asymptomatic disease to a severe or lethal infection. Again, this is driven by genetics, with sequence differences in the pathogen genome leading to alterations in protein structure and function.

Multi-segment viruses

Some viruses, including the influenza virus and rotavirus have genomes made up from multiple genome segments (8 and 10–11, respectively). This genome structure lends itself to manipulation. By infecting cells with multiple virus strains simultaneously, *reassortant* viruses can be generated, containing genome segments from different strains. This approach is ideally suited to disease-causing viruses for which nonpathogenic species or strains exist, or strains with different hosts can be reassorted. For example, reassortment has been used to develop licensed (cold-adapted) live attenuated influenza and human–bovine reassortant rotavirus vaccines. In the case of vaccines against Lassa fever, a candidate vaccine was produced by creating a reassortant virus between Lassa virus and Mopeia virus. This virus, which is made up of the glycoprotein and nucleoprotein from Lassa virus, and the Z protein and polymerase from Mopeia virus, was shown to protect against disease following Lassa virus challenge in guinea pigs and a nonhuman primate model.

A key factor in the ability to produce vaccine candidates by reassorting the viral genome segments is the genetic location(s) of the determinants of pathogenesis. Let us consider a hypothetical family of viruses with two-segment genomes. One segment encodes the surface proteins, which are the "targets"

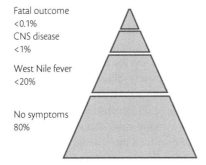

West Nile virus Disease

Fatal outcome
<0.1%
CNS disease
<1%

West Nile fever
<20%

No symptoms
80%

Figure 7.1 The "iceberg" of infection.

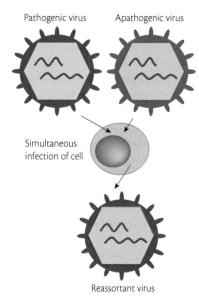

Figure 7.2 Virus reassortment.

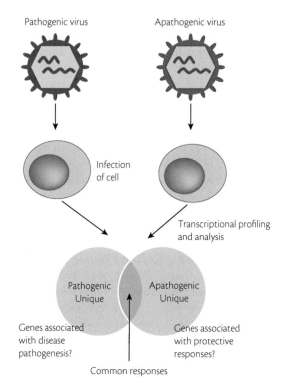

Figure 7.3 Comparative pathogenesis by expression profiling.

of a protective immune response, the other segment encodes the additional proteins the virus needs to replicate. If there are two viruses in this family, one that causes disease and one that is pathogenic, and it is known that a protein encoded on the non-envelope segment leads to disease, a reassortant virus that encodes the surface protein(s) segment of the virulent virus and the second segment from the apathogenic virus may be a suitable vaccine candidate (see Figure 7.2). However, if the envelope protein itself, or other proteins encoded on that segment, contribute to disease, the resulting reassortant may still be pathogenic and not suitable for direct use as a vaccine candidate. In these cases, knowledge of the molecular basis of disease mechanisms may, in the future, allow these viruses to be further attenuated by rational site-directed mutagenesis to ablate these key "disease-causing" functions of specific proteins.

Overlapping areas of research

Beyond the originally intended rationale for conducting a given experiment, basic bench science also contributes to the global collection of data, which ultimately might be used for a number of related downstream applications. For instance, comparing the effects of infection with a pathogenic and an attenuated virus or bacteria pair provides a wealth of infor-

mation that can potentially advance a number of areas of research. Consider the case of an mRNA expression profile experiment in which the cellular responses to a pathogenic strain of a virus or bacterium (*P*) are compared to those seen following infection with an attenuated (or apathogenic) strain (*A*) or to mock infection (see Figure 7.3). Those responses that are common between *P* and *A* may be those that are a general response to a viral infection or infection with a virus or bacterium of that family. The responses unique to *P* may illuminate the molecular mechanisms of pathogenesis, may suggest targets for novel therapeutics that aim to suppress these events, or could be used to develop patterns of signature biomarkers to develop new diagnostics or prognostics. The responses unique to *A* may reveal which genes are required to develop a protective immune response and which new vaccine candidates may need to activate. They could also feed into the biomarker development pathway, revealing signatures of gene expression that correlate with a mild or subclinical infection.

Definition

Biomarker: A portmanteau of "biological marker," biomarkers are "signatures" that can be used to determine a particular biological state, disease, response, etc. Biomarkers can include metabolites, pathogen nucleic acids or proteins, host proteins etc. For example, elevated levels of prostate-specific antigen (PSA) in the serum can be used as a biomarker for prostate cancer; levels of enzymes such as aspartate aminotransferase (AST) and alanine transaminase (ALT) are biomarkers of liver damage.

Molecular biology and recombinant vaccines

As described above in the section on basic science and translational research, the continuing development and use of molecular biology techniques have enabled the assembly of hybrid genomes, incorporating specific regions from specific organisms. Over the past several years, a large number of candidate vaccines have been developed and undergone nonclinical testing in animal models. The majority of these, however, do not advance into clinical trials for a variety of reasons. One particular strategy that continues to be explored is that of expressing a gene (or genes) from a pathogen, into the genome of a virus or bacterium that does not cause disease. A common strategy is to replace a surface expressed protein of a nonpathogenic vector virus or bacterium (e.g., poxviruses such as vaccinia or canarypox, or bacteria such as listeria) with the candidate vaccine antigen (usually a surface expressed protein from the target pathogen), thereby exposing the host to a live, multiplying virus or bacterium, which is likely to induce stronger, longer-lasting immune responses with fewer boosters than if the target vaccine antigen were produced as a subunit vaccine that will not multiply in the host. In the veterinary field, canarypox and other pox vectors have been used to successfully express many viral and bacterial antigens as commercial vaccines. In humans, the first recombinant vectored vaccine has recently been licensed for Japanese encephalitis in Australia and Thailand where the live yellow fever 17D vaccine virus was used as a vector to express the membrane and envelope protein genes of Japanese encephalitis virus.

In the field of vaccines against biodefense agents and emerging viruses, vesicular stomatitis virus (VSV) has proved a useful starting point for the development of recombinant vaccines against Marburg, Ebola, and Lassa viruses. By replacing the VSV glycoproteins with those from the target virus, protective immunity has been demonstrated in nonhuman primate studies. The use of VSV as a backbone to carry the target viral glycoprotein has proven successful, largely due to the fact that an immune response to the glycoprotein alone appears to offer sufficient protection against the challenge virus. It would also appear that the actively replicating VSV induces the correct humoral versus cell-mediated immune response required for protection.

While live recombinant viruses efficiently induce protective immunity, the fact that they are actively replicating may limit their potential use in "special" populations, such as pregnant women or immunocompromised individuals, due to the potential of adverse events. While this may not be relevant in the case of vaccines against viruses such as Ebola or Marburg, where routine vaccination is unlikely to be performed, it may limit this strategy for vaccines that would be administered routinely to large populations.

An alternative strategy is the virus-like particle (VLP), another development of modern molecular biology tools. Basic research into the function and biology of specific viral proteins led to the observation that expression of certain viral structural proteins in cells resulted in the spontaneous assembly of structures that resembled viral particles, despite lacking the complete complement of viral structural proteins or viral genomes. These particles contain the viral proteins in the same conformation in which they would be presented in the complete, infectious virus particle, which may not be the case when viral proteins are administered as subunit vaccines. Cloning of the required virus proteins into expression plasmids allows for production in a number of cellular systems, such as yeast or baculovirus (an insect virus) expression systems, which allows for high levels of particle production. This approach has been used to great effect to develop human papillomavirus vaccines based on VLPs expressed in yeast and baculoviruses that have been licensed in the past 7 years.

Molecular biology can also play additional important roles in vaccine development. In the case of a number of veterinary vaccines, serology is often used to determine whether or not an animal has been infected with a particular agent. This was critically important in the outbreaks of foot-and-mouth disease in the UK in the 2000s. A potential problem with vaccination in these cases is the inability to differentiate between an animal that is seropositive due to infection with the wild-type virus or bacterium and an animal that has been vaccinated. This problem is mediated by the fact that a good vaccine will lead to production of antibodies against the same immunodominant epitopes as the antibodies induced following infection with the virulent pathogen. This inability to distinguish vaccinated from infected animals (DIVA) confounds efforts to monitor livestock populations for disease outbreaks and has significant implications for animal health, as well as major economic implications.

A major goal of veterinary vaccination, at least for regions where the pathogen is not endemic, is to develop "marker vaccines," which allow vaccinated animals to be DIVA. One strategy that has been employed is to engineer viruses that contain heterologous proteins from other viral strains. A vaccine developed against avian influenza uses the hemagglutinin (HA) protein from the virus against which protection is to be raised, but has been engineered to contain the neuraminidase (NA) of a different viral strain, allowing the discrimination of vaccinated and infected birds. Other strategies have generated recombinant vaccines, for example, where the NA protein is modified to include an immunodominant peptide from the murine hepatitis virus S2 glycoprotein. A serological test

against this epitope will be negative in the case of infected birds.

Therapeutic vaccines and vaccines against noninfectious agents

Prophylactic immunization to prevent acute infectious diseases (i.e., when vaccines are administered in order to prevent disease in individuals who are not infected with the pathogen nor have the disease) is not the only area in which vaccination can play an important role in controlling or preventing disease. Chronic infectious and noninfectious diseases, such as hepatitis C, Parkinson's disease, and arthritis, or diseases such as cancer, can also be targeted with novel vaccination strategies. This chapter will discuss how basic bench science and clinical research can be applied to the development of vaccines for these conditions.

As with vaccines for infectious diseases, the first step is to sufficiently understand the mechanisms of the disease process in order to identify targets for vaccination. In the case of vaccines against noninfectious diseases, this can be a more complicated process because the proteins involved are host-derived, raising potential problems due to the effects of immune tolerance, or the risk of raising autoimmunity, or off-target effects. The identification of specific forms/conformation of proteins that are associated with disease is an important step in the development of vaccines to these conditions, and these findings come from investigations into the molecular pathology of the disease process.

A significant emerging field is that of vaccines against cancer, either as prophylactic (i.e., prevent disease) vaccines, or therapeutic vaccination (i.e., give the vaccines after the individual has the infection or disease) as potential treatments following a cancer diagnosis. Given the self-derived nature of the tumor cells, identifying specific antigens for vaccination is more challenging than for infectious agents. Historically, the terms *tumor-specific antigen* and *tumor-associated antigen* have been used to classify these antigens. Tumor-specific antigens are expressed only by the transformed tumor cells, such as a mutated form of a protein (e.g., the p53 tumor suppressor, a protein that is mutated in over 50% of human cancers). Tumor-associated antigens are not specific to the tumor. They

---

Definitions

Active vaccination: The use of an antigen—such as a viral protein or bacterial toxoid—to induce the development of a protective immune response.

Passive vaccination: The transfer of preexisting antibodies produced in one individual to another.

Prophylactic vaccination: The administration of a vaccine as a preventative measure before exposure to a pathogen or development of a disease.

Therapeutic vaccination: The administration of a vaccine against a preexisting disease as a treatment strategy.

may show aberrant or ectopic expression in the tumor cells, but they are normally expressed in other cells or tissues; overexpression of the epidermal growth factor receptor family member ErbB2 is an example of a tumor-associated antigen.

Cancer is a multistep process dependent on the cells acquiring a range of mutations that facilitate a constitutive ability to proliferate, resist antiproliferative signals, and disarm cellular pathways, which trigger apoptosis in response to unrestricted movement through the cell cycle and induce vascular formation. Each one of these mutations could potentially lead to a tumor-specific or tumor-associated antigen. Many of these mutations may be patient, tumor, or cell specific. However, if basic research into the molecular basis of the cancer pathology can define common tumor-specific or tumor-associated antigens, could these be targeted with anticancer vaccines? The discovery of naturally produced cytotoxic T cells that are specific to cancer antigens, such as a mutated cyclin-dependent kinase 4 in melanoma, suggests that it is possible to raise an immune response to mutated host proteins.

Research is beginning to identify antigens that may be targeted to either prevent progression to cancer from earlier stage disease, or serve as therapeutic targets following progression to cancer. The antigen MUC1 has been shown to be overexpressed and hypoglycosylated in colonic adenomatous polyps. The use of MUC1 peptide as a vaccine has been shown to flatten polyps in a mouse model system. Naturally produced MUC1 antibodies in patients with adenocarcinomas have been associated with increased survival, again supporting the hypothesis that immune priming with vaccines can be an effective cancer treatment or preventative strategy. Currently, there are a number of therapeutic vaccines based on monoclonal antibodies that recognize cancer antigens. This situation is termed *passive immunization*, where the monoclonal antibodies are "humanized" so that the human immune system does not recognize them as foreign, and they are given as a drug regimen with multiple doses over a period of time depending on the half-life of the antibody.

While the accumulation of mutations of cancer cells allows for the cancer cell antigens to become sufficiently different from the "self" antigens to allow specific immune targeting, the continued ability of the cancer cells to mutate allows for "escape mutants" to evolve. As an effective immune response would lead to killing of the transformed cells that displayed the appropriate mutated protein, there is a large evolutionary pressure selecting for cells that do not display this form of the mutated form and therefore escape immune-mediated killing.

Proliferating cancer cells may also escape the immune response by producing their own immunomodulators, secreting cytokines to modulate the immune system and reducing its effectiveness. The cytokine transforming growth factor β (TGF-β) is produced by a variety of solid tumors and is a potent immunosuppressant; TGF-β can inhibit the maturation of dendritic cells and the proliferation of T cells. Additionally, TGF-β can lead to an increase in the production of regulatory T cells (Tregs), providing a further mechanism for inhibiting immune-mediated killing.

Vaccination against self-derived antigens is not limited to cancer. Alzheimer's disease is a progressive neurodegenerative disease in which neurofibrillary tangles form inside nerve bodies and amyloid beta (Aβ) plaques are deposited extracellularly. It is believed that hyperphosphorylated forms of the protein tau mediate the formation of these tangles or directly cause pathology through the formation of tau oligomers. This being the case, would it be possible to vaccinate against these forms of the tau protein or Aβ plaques to raise an immune response that may protect against Alzheimer's and other *Tauopathies*? Passive immunization using antibodies against Aβ has shown positive results, suggesting that immune-mediated control of these diseases may be possible.

A further example of the use of targeting host proteins is the case of experimental vaccines against rheumatoid arthritis. This disease is characterized by chronic inflammation mediated in part by the proinflammatory cytokine tumor necrosis factor-α (TNF-α). Experimental DNA vaccines, which encode the TNF-α gene under the control of a viral promoter, suggest that immunizing against a host-produced immune mediator can be effective in treating autoimmune diseases. This type of treatment strategy has potential pros and cons compared to treating with anti-TNF-α antibodies or soluble receptors. While the half-life of these proteins is short compared to the immunological memory produced by vaccination, could the short half-life be advantageous? What are the long-term effects of raising antibodies against an important immune regulator? As laboratory studies continue to define the basic immune mechanisms that underlie both the disease and the response, we will be better placed to answer these questions.

Definition

DNA vaccine: A vaccine that is administered in the form of a DNA molecule that contains the gene encoding for the antigen under the control of appropriate promoter and regulatory sequences to allow the transcription and subsequent translation by the host cell after vaccine administration. The DNA molecule can be engineered to encode protein adjuvants such as cytokines and chemokines. The first licensed DNA vaccine is an equine vaccine against West Nile virus; there are currently no DNA vaccines licensed for human use.

Immunology of protection and adjuvants

As we continue to move forward with the rational design of novel vaccines, as opposed to attempting to attenuate live pathogens by serial passage, understanding the role of the various immune effectors in controlling the infection becomes increasingly relevant. In particular, the relative balance of cell-mediated immunity versus humoral mechanisms, such as anti-bodies, can be critically important in determining protection.

With the emergence of DNA vaccines, new strategies for enhancing immune responses are gaining importance. Additionally, with the potential difficulties of certain live vaccines due to concerns regarding adverse events, adjuvants may become more important in order to induce long-lasting immunity with the minimum number of doses. DNA vaccination offers a unique advantage given the form of the vaccine. Because the vaccine comprises a DNA molecule that contains the coding sequence for the antigen under the control of an appropriate promoter, it is possible to include the coding sequences for other proteins or peptides in the same vaccine. This allows for the inclusion of cytokines and chemokines in the vaccine, which can be expressed from the site of vaccination. The inclusion of cytokines and chemokines is designed to recruit appropriate immune cells to the site of vaccination and drive the development of a particular type of immune response. Table 7.1 shows a list of soluble factors currently being studied for this purpose.

The increase of knowledge in the underlying immunological mechanisms of protection also plays a role in the development of adjuvants. Adjuvants are additional molecules or compounds added to a vaccine in order to improve immunogenicity. Adjuvants are described in detail in Chapter 6 but will be discussed

Table 7.1 Potential Roles of Cytokine and Chemokine Adjuvants

Cytokine/Chemokine	Function	Potential Uses
CCL27	Recruitment of T cells to the skin	Adjuvant for DNA vaccination
CCL28	Chemoattractant of lymphocytes to a number of tissues including the mucosa	Adjuvant for DNA vaccination
IL-1α	Inflammatory cytokine, contributes to febrile response	Mucosal immunity to HIV
IL-12	Differentiation of naïve T cells	DNA vaccine/vaccinia virus prime-boost; HIV
IL-15	Proliferation of NK cells; production of cytotoxic granule proteins	Adjuvant for DNA vaccination
IL-18	Produced by macrophages, induced cell-mediated immunity; stimulates release of interferon-γ by NK cells and T cells	Mucosal immunity to HIV
GM-CSF (granulocyte macrophage colony stimulating factor)	Production of monocytes, neutrophils, eosinophils and basophils	Multiple myeloma

here in the context of novel adjuvant discovery and design from the perspective of basic research. Of interest to this chapter is to understand how and why novel adjuvants function, and which adjuvants may be most effective or appropriate to complement a particular vaccine. Studies using the live attenuated yellow fever vaccine, 17D, are delineating the initial interaction events of the host with the vaccine that are required to generate protective immune responses. These studies have shown that the activation of multiple upstream pathways, driven by Toll-like pattern recognition receptors leads to the strong, lasting protection induced by this vaccine.

When adjuvants go wrong

A good example of the need to understand the major immune mechanisms for viral control is provided by *Ectromelia virus*, the etiological agent of mousepox. The protective response to ectromelia is mediated predominantly by the T_H1-type cytotoxic response, which express predominantly interleukin (IL)-2 and interferon (IFN)-γ. The antibody-mediated response, based around B-cell maturation and expansion, is mediated by T_H2-type T cells that produce IL-4. These responses involve positive feedback on themselves, while negatively regulating the other, pushing the immune response toward being mediated predominantly by either cytotoxic T cells or antibody. To investigate the response, a recombinant ectomelia virus was engineered containing the gene for murine IL-4. It might be hypothesized that this virus would stimulate the production of high levels of antibody, leading to an effective immune response. However, this recombinant virus gave rise to a lethal infection in mice that were genetically resistant to wild-type mousepox. The IL-4 produced during the infection suppressed the production of natural killer cells and cytotoxic T cells, as well as inhibiting the production of interferon-gamma, key mediators of the protective response to infection with the wild-type virus.

Using high-throughput methods to characterize host gene expression changes following vaccination, correlated with functional immune responses, and analyzed computationally, the data illustrate that the response to a vaccine is complex, involving myriad cellular pathways and transcriptional responses, and they highlight the importance of studying multiple aspects of host responses in a "global" context and applying emerging "systems biology" approaches (discussed below). These findings are leading to the development of adjuvants that stimulate these upstream pathways and that aim to generate a similar level of protection to a live attenuated virus using a safer subunit vaccine. Indeed, an influenza vaccine study provided strong evidence of the power of this strategy, using nanoparticles to deliver an influenza virus subunit antigen along with ligands for the pattern recognition receptors TLR4 and TLR7. By stimulating these receptors and downstream pathways, the immune response showed strong evidence of persisting, despite the use of a subunit antigen.

The finding that engineering the mousepox virus to encode the B-cell growth factor IL-4 increases virulence illustrates the importance of having an understanding of the appropriate immune effector mechanisms required to protect against the infection. Given the multiple attenuating mutations that contribute to the lack of virulence of live vaccines, this type of situation is unlikely to arise in a vaccine candidate. However, it does illustrate that a vaccine will be most effective if it can induce the appropriate immune effector functions. A vaccine may be shown to produce very high levels of neutralizing antibodies, but if cellular immunity is the key effector of protection, then the vaccine may not be very effective.

High-throughput methods and systems biology

The scientific method that we traditionally think of is *reductionist*, where we reduce the complexity of a system and study its components in isolation, attempting to reduce the number of variables involved. For example, many studies that characterize the effect of viral infection on a specific cellular function use a cell line and infect at a high multiplicity of infection to ensure that the majority of cells are infected in order to minimize the averaging effects due to uninfected bystander cells. However, *in vivo* the infected cell will likely be interacting with other cell types; many will be uninfected, and the cells will be communicating to each other via surface protein expression and cytokine production. Additionally, if the host is responding by initiating a fever response, the cell might be at temperatures of 38 °C or 39 °C, rather than the 37 °C at which cells are traditionally incubated in culture. All of these additional variables could alter the effect of infection on the function that was under study. However, considering, and controlling for, the multiple variables at play in this system can be experimentally complicated.

Definition

Systems biology: A term describing an emerging paradigm that aims to characterize biological mechanisms as part of an integrated "system" of interactions. This field differs from more traditional basic science approaches, which aim to apply reductionist approaches by using methods that allow a more holistic view of the biological system. Systems biology approaches typically involve high-throughput "-omics" experiments such as cDNA microarrays and proteomics.

Systems biology attempts to investigate biological processes at a more holistic level, defining how these multiple parameters are integrated and characterizing the functional consequences. Systems biology-type experiments often utilize high-throughput methods, often exploiting what are called the "-omics" technologies; a description of some of these is given in Table 7.2. Transcriptomic microarrays are the most widely used of these tools, given their comparative affordability, and the fact that gene expression of virtually every gene can be easily quantified. This contrasts with proteomics, traditionally performed using two-dimensional electrophoresis, which requires protein "spots" to be stained on the gel, "picked," and the amino acid sequence determined by mass spectrometry. This is technically more challenging to perform, as well as more expensive, due to the fact that spot sequencing is relatively low throughput

Table 7.2 Overview of "-Omics" Technologies

"-Ome"	Description	Technologies
Genome	The complete genetic sequence of an organism	High-throughput sequencing, SNP chips
Transcriptome	The collection of mRNAs expressed at a particular time in a particular cell or group of cells	cDNA microarrays, high-throughput sequencing
Proteome -phospho-proteome -sumoylome	The complement of expressed proteins. Subfields of this often look at post-translational modifications such as phosphorylation or sumoylation	Two-dimensional electrophoresis, liquid chromatography, mass spectrometry
Metabolome/metabonome	The collection of small-molecule metabolites in a given system	Mass spectrometry methods coupled to chromatography such as liquid or gas phase
Lipidome	The lipid complement of a system	Gas-phase mass spectrometry
Glycome	The entire complement of sugars	Mass spectrometry
Interactome	The complete complement of molecular interactions in a system	Yeast 2-hybrid screening, computational interaction prediction
Immunome	The complete set of antigens targeted by the immune system in a given pathophysiological condition	Serological proteome analysis (SERPA)
Peptidome	The complement of small peptides/protein fragments of a system	Mass spectrometry
Kinome	The collection of kinases in a system (proteins that phosphorylate other proteins)	Phosphorylation screening, peptide substrate chips

compared to the data produced by transcriptomic microarrays. While proteomics has its limitations, microarrays are limited in that they may not detect differences in splicing variants, suffer from a limited dynamic range (a "compression" of the range of expression values over which they are reliably quantitative), and do not show whether the mRNA is translated into protein.

Despite their limitations, however, transcriptomic microarrays have perhaps been the single most useful tool in bringing about the "-omics" revolution. Their combination of high throughput (in terms of data points per sample as opposed to number of samples) and relative affordability have allowed significant advances in our understanding of the host responses to challenge. By comparing the mRNA transcriptional profile of unchallenged cells to that seen following virus infection, for example, it is possible to determine the global cellular response to that particular stimulus in an unbiased way.

Before the advent of these high-throughput methods, the effects of a particular stimulus were investigated in the context of a suspected altered output. For example, if a particular stimulus was suspected to alter the expression of a particular protein, cells would be stimulated, cell extracts prepared and then assayed for protein expression using a method such as western blotting. While consistent with the basis of hypothesis-driven research, this type of approach is limited in that it is unlikely to identify effects on cellular systems that are as yet uncharacterized with respect to that specific stimulus, or with which the particular researcher is not familiar. Even with the advent of microarray technology, the large datasets produced by these types of analyses were often overwhelming, producing more data than could be analyzed, validated, and placed into a functional context. Analyses were often limited to genes that exhibited the highest-fold changes, or genes that were already known to be involved in the response to the particular challenge.

Recent advances in bioinformatic and computational tools have allowed these high-throughput datasets to be used to a greater potential. As results from basic biochemistry and cell biology continue to define the fundamental interactions that define cell function, these findings can be curated into databases, which can be interrogated with gene expression data in order to place findings into a functional context and allow the development of additional hypotheses for further testing. A number of commercial and academic or open-access software tools and databases are available to facilitate these types of analysis; these are summarized in Table 7.3. By overlaying expression data over known networks of interaction, it is possible to go beyond simply looking at genes that show the highest level of differential expression and look for regulatory networks or functional systems that show clustering of expression changes, potentially indicating an involvement or role for this group of genes in controlling the response to stimulation or challenge.

High-throughput gene expression data can also be used to infer upstream events that led to the observed pattern of gene expression, rather than limiting further analyses to "gene x was upregulated, what is the role of gene x in disease?" By turning the question around and asking, "gene x is upregulated, *what events led to the upregulation of gene x?*" hypotheses can be generated that can lead to defining the proteins and pathways responsible for controlling a particular response. High-throughput gene expression data, combined with complete genome sequencing and well as fundamental biochemical findings, provide a useful platform to begin to answer these questions. With the knowledge that a particular gene shows increased or decreased expression and setting this against the background of the complete sequence of that gene and its upstream regulatory sequences, the transcription factor binding sites responsible for control of expression of that particular gene can be inferred. When looked at in the context of the complete transcriptome and genome, it is possible to compute a statistical likelihood that particular transcription factors are responsible for controlling the majority of the transcriptional response. For example, if the complete transcriptome of an organism contains 30,000 genes, of which 5% contain the binding site for a particular transcription factor, but that binding site is seen in 90% of gene promoters because of the transcripts differentially expressed following stimulation, it is likely that this transcription factor is centrally important in regulating cellular responses to that stimulus.

These types of approaches have significant implications in vaccinology. By using high-throughput profiling to identify the responses produced by historically successful vaccines, it is possible to begin to

Table 7.3 Commonly Used Bioinformatics/Systems Biology Analysis Software Applications and Databases

Application/Database	Description
Cytoscape	Open source application for the visualization of complex pathways and datasets. The open source nature of the application has led to numerous developers contributing additional "plug-ins" to perform specific functions.
Ingenuity Pathways Analysis	A commercial software application, which acts as the front end to construct networks following interrogation of a database of functional interactions and processes curated from the scientific literature.
KEGG (Kyoto Encyclopedia of Genes and Genomes)	The pathway database integrates information on molecular interactions and functional metabolic and signaling pathways.
Gene Set Enrichment Analysis	GSEA is an application developed by the Broad Institute. The application analyzes gene expression data and identifies sets of genes that show differential expression and are involved in similar functions, or are similarly regulated or located in similar chromosomal regions.
PSCAN	PSCAN is a Web-based tool that looks for statistical overrepresentation of transcription factor binding sites in the promoters of differentially expressed genes following RNA expression analysis.
PathVisio	PathVisio is a Web-based application that allows the graphical visualization of datasets and interaction data.
REACTOME	REACTOME is an open-access curated database of biological signaling pathways.

define the types of response that lead to the development of a protective response. By identifying the key transcription factors that are implicated in the development of this expression profile, the so-called master regulators, it may be possible to tailor future vaccines to activate the appropriate upstream pathways that lead to activation of these transcription factors and lead to the development of a protective immune response. This represents a further area of overlap between systems biology/vaccinology and adjuvant design.

Additionally, as other studies in other areas of research continue to contribute to the knowledge base, the association of particular patterns of gene expression with other responses, such as adverse events or other off-target effects, may be able to be predicted by analyzing the gene expression profile. In the case of the development of a number of vaccine/adjuvant candidates using modern molecular approaches, systems biology may provide a means of selecting the most promising candidates for continued investigation prior to clinical trials.

Definitions

In vivo: Experiments performed in living organisms
In vitro: Literally *in glass*; describes the use of techniques such as cell culture as an experimental system
In silico: The use of computer modeling, simulation, and prediction

Bioinformatics and reverse vaccinology

Bioinformatics is the mathematical and computational study of biology and can range from performing statistical analysis and interpreting the results of a transcriptomic microarray experiment, to developing tools to model cellular signaling pathways *in silico*. Bioinformatics has grown considerably in the past two decades, and computational approaches can now play a lead role in the vaccine development process.

A number of algorithms are available that can predict immunodominant epitopes of a pathogen on the basis of primary sequence data alone. In tandem with the development of DNA and peptide vaccines,

this represents a powerful strategy to generate a number of candidates for *in vitro* and *in vivo* testing. Additionally, by serving to triage the vast number of potential epitopes of a pathogen, this approach can drastically reduce the time and cost involved in moving through this stage of the process compared to manually testing every pathogen component for immunogenicity using traditional "wet lab" methods.

Reverse vaccinology has been made possible by the advances in high-throughput methods such as whole genome sequencing and proteomics. A conventional approach to vaccinology might involve purifying a selection of candidate antigens and investigating their ability to induce protective immunity (see Figure 7.4). This approach is limited in a number of ways including its time-consuming, low-throughput nature and the

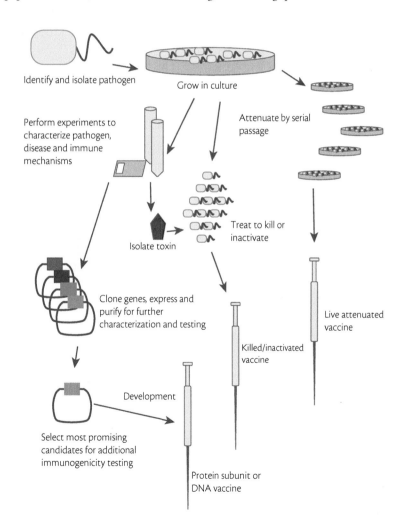

Figure 7.4 The classical vaccine development pathway.

fact that it is likely to only be able to test proteins expressed by the organism in culture, whereas the proteome expressed by the organism during infection of a host could be significantly different. With reverse vaccinology, the complete genome sequence can be searched for likely candidates for immunization, using computational algorithms to determine which proteins should be selected for further testing on the basis of motifs for protein location, or predicted T-cell epitopes (see Figure 7.5). While this approach has its own limitations, such as only considering proteins as antigens, it opens up the complete genome/proteome to vaccine candidate development.

Reverse vaccinology was employed in the development of the group B meningococcus vaccine. Effective purified polysaccharide vaccines against *Neisseria meningitidis* are available for the A, C, Y, and W135 serogroups of the bacterium. However, the surface carbohydrates of the group B organisms share cross-reactive antigens with host carbohydrates and so were unsuitable for a group B vaccine. The complete genome sequence of *N. meningitidis* was analyzed using computer programs, which looked for genes that coded for proteins predicted to be expressed on the surface of the bacterium. After this initial screen, candidate open reading frames (ORFs) were assayed for their conservation across serogroups. Recombinant proteins were then expressed from the set of filtered ORFs and used in mouse vaccination studies. From an initial 570 ORFs identified by the first computational analysis, 28 proteins were found to lead to a bactericidal antibody response. This list of candidate proteins can then be further filtered on the basis of bactericidal performance using multiple assays and a predicted lack of phase variation—an immune evasion strategy characterized by mutation rates at specific sites that

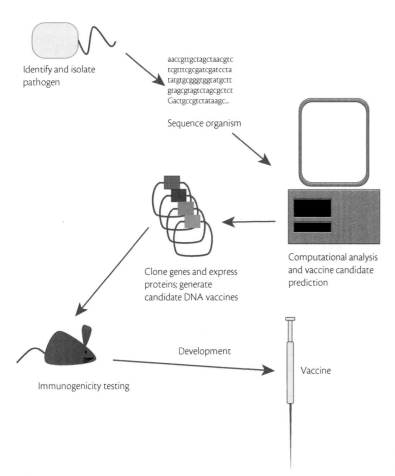

Identify and isolate pathogen

aaccgttgctagctaacgtc
tcgtttcgcgatcgatccta
tatgtgcgggtggtatgctt
gtagcgtagtctagcgctct
Gactgccgtctataagc...

Sequence organism

Computational analysis and vaccine candidate prediction

Clone genes and express proteins; generate candidate DNA vaccines

Immunogenicity testing

Development

Vaccine

Figure 7.5 The reverse vaccinology pathway.

are higher than would normally occur. This has resulted in two candidate group B meningococcal vaccines, each consisting of up to five immunogens.

The reverse vaccinology paradigm is ideally poised to take advantage of technological developments such as next-generation sequencing (NGS), or deep sequencing, which allows the sequences of variants in a population to be analyzed. As NGS is more widely used and whole genome sequencing becomes ever more affordable, we will likely see an explosion in the numbers of whole genome sequences available for analysis, not only for representative strains of a pathogen, but for a whole spectrum of strains that show differing levels of virulence, ability to replicate under different conditions, etc.

Additional roles for basic science in vaccine development

Iterative cycle of vaccine development

As discussed in the section on comparative pathogenesis, the ability to compare cellular responses to pathogenic and avirulent strains can provide clues into which host responses are associated with disease, and which can lead to the development of a protective immune response and control of the pathogen. In the case of live attenuated vaccines, the development of the vaccine strain represents a tool to feedback into the vaccine development pathway.

Vaccine delivery

The development of a promising vaccine candidate and an appropriate adjuvant that is predicted to elicit the correct immune responses is not the end of the process: The vaccine must be administered to the vaccinee (or delivered) in an effective way that facilitates the development of the most effective immune response. The mechanism of delivery must be considered in the context of the type of vaccine, with a DNA vaccine requiring a different method of delivery from an attenuated virus vaccine to produce the best immune response. This field integrates research and technologies from diverse fields such as molecular biology and materials science to mechanical engineering. An additional aspect to consider with respect to the clinical administration of vaccines is that of the use of prophylactic antipyretic drugs to control the fever response following vaccination. While this is com-

monly used to reduce excessive febrile responses following vaccination, some studies suggest that this could reduce the magnitude of the immune response to some vaccines. Continued basic research is required to understand the effects of these drugs to ensure maximum vaccine effectiveness.

Virosomes and VLPs are non-replicating "empty shells" of viruses, in which the viral proteins required for particle assembly are used to drive formation of a particle that does not include viral nucleic acid or other viral proteins. In addition to being used as viral vaccines, these particles can also be used to deliver other antigens. Viral, bacterial, and tumor-associated antigens and peptides, as well as nucleic acids, have been delivered using virosomes, and the nature of the delivery system can allow presentation via the MHC-I or MHC-II pathways. These particles can also have an intrinsic adjuvant effect. Additional applications of basic science have led to technologies such as the gene gun for delivering DNA vaccines, as well as tools that include various types of nanoparticles, cell-permeable peptides, ultrasound techniques, cationic polymers, and laser light alteration of cell membrane permeability, that can be used to deliver antigens and adjuvants.

Definitions

Virosome: Hollow particles with lipid-bilayer membranes that contain influenza virus proteins, which allow them to fuse with cells.

Virus-like particle (VLP): Noninfectious particles derived from viruses, which contain the virus proteins but no genetic material. These particles morphologically resemble the virus from which they are derived, as they contain the virus structural proteins and those required for assembly and budding.

Nanoparticle: Small particles (1–10,000 nm), which, for vaccine purposes, can be coated with or conjugated to antigens or adjuvants.

Toward personalized vaccinology

Currently, vaccines are not 100% effective across all populations. As has been described previously, genetic differences of the host can lead to different responses to a vaccine, in the same way that they can produce the characteristic "iceberg" of infection following infection with the virulent pathogen. Would vaccination be more effective if more than one vaccine for a particular disease was available and the most appropriate vaccine used for a specific individual or population? With technologies such as next-generation high-throughput sequencing becoming more affordable and driving the proliferation of genome-wide association studies, our ability to associate phenotype with genotype will continue to improve and may eventually lead to accurate predictions of diseases and responses to specific treatments. In vaccinology, it would be advantageous to know if a person is likely to produce a strong immune response following one dose of a vaccine, whether they are likely to require several doses, or if there is an increased likelihood of an adverse event. Also, the quantity of vaccine in a dose may vary according to the vaccinee. As these types of studies become more widely performed, in the future it may become possible to design vaccines—from a stock of "on the shelf" components—for specific individuals based on their genetic code, perhaps selecting a particular combination of antigens based on MHC haplotype, and combining these with a "cocktail" of adjuvants, perhaps based on polymorphisms in Toll-like receptor or immune signaling genes.

Definition

Genome-wide association study (GWAS): The use of genome characterization to study the association of particular mutations with disease incidence. Typical studies have used microarray technology to analyze hundreds of thousands of single-nucleotide polymorphisms (SNP chips) and look for correlation with disease, such as the incidence of a particular cancer.

Conclusions

Vaccines are perhaps medical science's most significant achievement, having saved hundreds of millions of lives since the time of Jenner. In their more recent history, the increased profile of vaccine-associated adverse events has led to questions about the balance between vaccine safety and vaccine efficacy. This shift in society's view—which assumes all vaccines are 100% effective but questions their safety—has necessitated changes in how we consider the design and

development of new vaccines. In this chapter, we have explored the numerous ways in which basic science is involved in the vaccine development pipeline. From seemingly the most fundamental discovery of the tools for molecular biology, to novel computational methods, basic science has enabled the development of many vaccines as we begin to move away from the conventional empirically derived vaccine.

There are numerous other areas in which basic science contributes to vaccinology, which have not been discussed in this chapter. The techniques of the laboratory bench are also applied to vaccine testing and characterization at various stages of the vaccine development process, from assaying the levels of antibody production using enzyme-linked immunosorbant assays (ELISAs) or techniques such as viral plaque reduction to define the magnitude of B-cell responses, to investigating the host responses following vaccination, to defining signatures for vaccine efficacy, or defining the molecular mechanisms underlying any adverse events. In the future, techniques familiar to many bench scientists may become commonplace in the clinic, as physicians perform a genetic or metabolic test to see to which vaccine or adjuvant formulation a patient may best respond.

In summary, the majority of vaccines licensed for use in humans are based on techniques developed several decades ago. While the vast majority of scientific research is performed to further our understanding of the fundamental "nuts and bolts" of biology, this work has been slow to impact vaccinology, and many experimental and regulatory bottlenecks complicate the transition of basic discoveries into novel treatments. The research paradigm "translational medicine" serves to bridge the basic and clinical disciplines, identifying laboratory advances that could be brought into the clinic, and assessing clinical need to drive appropriate basic research. The modern field of vaccinology is complex and interdisciplinary, encompassing disciplines such as immunology, virology and microbiology, molecular biology, materials science, and public health and social policy. While there may not be one linear, defined pathway through which a vaccine can be designed from the first principles of basic science, the fundamental knowledge gained across many fields at the bench has allowed the next generation of vaccines to move beyond the methods used by the vaccinologists of the 19th century.

Summary

- Basic science and a knowledge of the molecular basis of disease has been instrumental in the development of many historical vaccines such as the tetanus vaccine.

- The techniques of basic science are becoming increasingly important in the development of novel, rationally designed viruses.

- Basic molecular biology studies, which uncover novel mechanisms of phenomena such as host restriction, can lead to new strategies for vaccine development.

- An understanding of the immunological basis for protection can lead to the design of novel adjuvants.

- Translational medicine is emerging as a paradigm to link fundamental bench science with clinical development.

- Large basic research projects, such as the human HapMap project, may provide useful tools as we move towards personalized medicine and vaccinology.

- Continued research in virology is leading to new methods of vaccine delivery, such as virosomes and recombinant viruses, in addition to new viral vaccine candidates.

Further reading

Bachmann MF and Jennings GT (2010). Vaccine delivery: a matter of size, geometry, kinetics and molecular patterns. Nature Reviews. Immunology 10, 787–796.

Beatty GL and Vonderheide RH (2008). Telomerase as a universal tumor antigen for cancer vaccines. Expert Reviews of Vaccines 7, 881–887.

Flower DR, Macdonald IK, Ramakrishnan K, Davies MN, and Doytchinova IA (2010). Computer aided selection of candidate vaccine antigens. Immunome Research 6 Suppl 2, S1.

Jones SM, Feldmann H, Ströher U, Geisbert JB, Fernando L, Grolla A, Klenk HD, Sullivan NJ, Volchkov VE, Fritz EA, Daddario KM, Hensley LE, Jahrling PB, and Gesibert TW (2005). Live attenuated recombinant vaccine protects nonhuman primates against Ebola and Marburg viruses. Nature Medicine 11, 786–790.

Kasturi SP, Skountzou I, Albrecht RA, Koutsonanos D, Hua T, Nakaya HI, Ravindran R, Stewart S, Alam M, Kwissa M, Villinger F, Murthy N, Steel J, Jacob J, Hogan RJ, Garcia-Sastre A, Compans R, and Pulendran B (2011). Programming the magnitude and persistence of antibody responses with innate immunity. Nature 470, 537–547.

Kennedy RB and Poland GA (2011). The top five "game changers" in vaccinology: toward rational and directed vaccine development. Omics: A Journal of Integrative Biology 15, 533–537.

Kim DY, Atasheva S, Foy NJ, Wang E, Frolova EI, Weaver S, and Frolov I (2011). Design of chimeric alphaviruses with a programmed, attenuated, cell type-restricted phenotype. Journal of Virology 85, 4363–4376.

Kutzler MA, Kraynyak KA, Nagle SJ, Parkinson RM, Zharikova D, Chattergoon M, Maguire H, Muthumani K, Ugen K, and Weiner DB (2010). Plasmids encoding the mucosal chemokines CCL27 and CCL28 are effective adjuvants in eliciting antigen-specific immunity in vivo. Gene Therapy 17, 72–82.

Lambert PH and Laurent PE (2008). Intradermal vaccine delivery: will new delivery systems transform vaccine administration? Vaccine 26, 3197–3208.

Li S, Nakaya HI, Kazmin DA, Oh JZ, Pulendran B (2013). Systems biological approaches to measure and understand vaccine immunity in humans. Seminars in Immunology 25, 209–218.

Li S, Rouphael N, Duraisingham S, Romero-Steiner S, Presnell S, Davis C, Schmidt DS, Johnson SE, Milton A, Rajam G, e S, Carlone GM, Quinn C, Chaussabel D, Palucka AK, Mulligan MJ, Ahmed R, Stephens DS, e HI, e B (2014). Molecular signatures of antibody responses derived from a systems biology study of five human vaccines. Nature Immunology 15, 195–204.

Lukashevich IS, Patterson J, Carrion R, Moshkoff D, Ticer A, Zapata J, Brasky K, Geiger R, Hubbard GB, Bryant J, and Salvato MS (2005). A live attenuated vaccine for Lassa fever made by reassortment of Lassa and Mopeia viruses. Journal of Virology 79, 13934–13942.

Poland GA, Ovsyannikova IG, Jacobson RM, and Smith DI (2007). Heterogeneity in vaccine immune response: the role of immunogenetics and the emerging field of vaccinomics. Clinical Pharmacological and Therapeutics 82, 653–664.

Pulendran B, Li S, and Nakaya HI (2010). Systems vaccinology. Immunity 33, 516–529. Pulendran B, Oh JZ, Nakaya HI, Ravindran R, Kazmin DA (2013). Immunity to viruses: learning from successful human vaccines. Immunol Rev 255, 243–255.

Querec TD, Akondy RS, Lee EK, Cao W, Teuwen D, Pirani A, Gernert K, Deng J, Marzolf B, Kennedy K, Wu H, Bennouna S, Oluoch H, Miller J, Vencio RZ, Mulligan M, Aderem A, Ahmed R, and Pulendran B (2009). Systems biology approach predicts immunogenicity of the yellow fever vaccine in humans. Nature Immunology 10, 116–125.

Rappuoli R (2000). Reverse vaccinology. Current Opinion in Microbiology 3, 445–450.

Rappuoli R, Black S, and Lambert PH (2011). Vaccine discovery and translation of new vaccine technology. Lancet 378, 360–368.

Seib KL, Dougan G, and Rappuoli R (2009). The key role of genomics in modern vaccine and drug design for emerging infectious diseases. PLoS Genetics 5, e1000612.

Söllner J, Heinzel A, Summer G, Fechete R, Stipkovits L, Szathmary S, and Mayer B (2010). Concept and application of a computational vaccinology workflow. Immunome Research 3 Suppl 2, S7.

Uttenthal A, Parida S, Rasmussen TB, Paton DJ, Haas B, and Dundon WG (2010). Strategies for differentiating infection in vaccinated animals (DIVA) for foot-and-mouth disease, classical swine fever and avian influenza. Expert Reviews of Vaccines 9, 73–87.

Vergati M, Intrivici C, Huen NY, Schlom J, and Tsang KY (2010). Strategies for cancer vaccine development. Journal of Biomedicine and Biotechnology 2010, 596432.

Vivona S, Gardy JL, Ramachandran S, Brinkman FSL, Raghava GPS, Flower DR, and Filippini F (2008). Computer-aided biotechnology: from immuno-informatics to reverse vaccinology. Trends in Microbiology 26, 190–200.

Weiner LM, Surana R, and Murray J (2010). Vaccine prevention of cancer: can endogenous antigens be targeted? Cancer Prevention Research 3, 410–415.

8 Microbial-based and material-based vaccine delivery systems

Alfredo G. Torres, Jai S. Rudra, and Gregg N. Milligan

Sealy Center for Vaccine Development, University of Texas Medical Branch, Galveston TX, USA

Abbreviations

Ag85	An antigenic protein of Mycobacterium tuberculosis currently being tested for inclusion in tuberculosis vaccines.	F protein	Fusion protein
		G protein	Guanine nucleotide-binding proteins
		Gag protein	Group specific-antigen proteins that form the capsid of retroviridae
AIDA-I	Adhesin involved in diffuse adherence		
APCs	Antigen-presenting cells	H5, H7 proteins	Influenza hemagglutinin proteins
BCG	Bacillus Calmette–Guérin	Hsp	Heat shock protein
BG	Bacterial ghost	ICAM-1	Intercellular adhesion molecule 1
BoHc/A	Subunit fragment of *Clostridium botulinum* type-A neurotoxin	IFN	Interferon
		IgA	Immunoglobulin A
B7-1	T-cell co-stimulatory molecule	IgG	Immunoglobulin G
cCHP	Cationic cholesteryl-group-bearing pullulan	Inp	Ice-nucleation protein
		kb	Kilo base
cDNA	Complimentary DNA	LFA-3	Lymphocyte function-associated antigen 3
CFP10	Culture filtrate protein 10kDa of *M. tuberculosis*	LipL	Lipoproteins of *Leptospira interrogans*
CpGs	Cytosine-phosphate-guanosine motif		
		LPS	Lipopolysaccharide
CTA	Cholera toxin A subunit	LT	Labile toxin
CTB	Cholera toxin B subunit	MAP	Multiple antigenic peptide
CTL	Cytotoxic T lymphocyte	MHC	Major histocompatability complex
DAMPs	Damage-associated molecular patterns	mRNA	Messenger RNA
		Nef	A retroviridae protein that influences virion replication *in vivo*
DCs	Dendritic cells		
dmCT	Double-mutant cholera toxin	NF-κB	Nuclear factor κB
DNA	Deoxyribonucleic acid	NLRs	Nod-like receptors
E Genes	Envelope genes	NSs	A nonstructural protein encoded by the bunyavirus, Rift Valley Fever virus
ESAT6	Early secretory antigenic target protein 6 of Mycobacterium tuberculosis		
		Omp	Outer membrane protein

(*Continued*)

Vaccinology: An Essential Guide, First Edition. Edited by Gregg N. Milligan and Alan D.T. Barrett.
© 2015 John Wiley & Sons, Ltd. Published 2015 by John Wiley & Sons, Ltd.

PAL	Peptidoglycan-associated lipoprotein	tat	A transactivator of transcription protein
PAMPs	Pathogen-associated molecular patterns	TB	Tuberculosis
		Th	T helper cells
PEG	Poly(ethylene-glycol)	Th1	Type 1 T helper cell
PLGA	Poly(lactic-co-glycolic acid)	TLR	Toll-like receptor
pol	A retroviridae protein required for virus replication	V proteins	Virus-coded proteins
		vif	A retroviridae protein that enhances infectivity of virus
prM Genes	Premembrane genes		
PRRs	Pattern recognition receptors	VirG	A virulence factor of *Shigella* sp. that plays a role in spread of the bacterium
rBCG	Recombinant BCG		
RD1	Region of difference of Mycobacterium tuberculosis		
		VLPs	Virus-like particles
rev	The retroviridae protein that is responsible for export of viral RNAs from the nucleus	Vpr	A retroviridae protein that influences cell cycle
		Vpu	A retroviridae membrane protein that enhances virus production
RLRs	RIG-I-like receptors		
RNA	Ribonucleic acid		

Virus vectors as vaccine platforms

Viruses have evolved efficient mechanisms for binding to and delivering their genome into host cells, utilizing host metabolic pathways for the production of new viral nucleic acids and viral proteins, assembling viral proteins into infectious virions, and disseminating newly formed virions to new target cells. These activities result in the production of large amounts of viral proteins and nucleic acids as well as the stimulation of host pattern recognition receptors by virus-encoded molecules. As a result, infection with most viral pathogens results in the induction of innate immunity and ultimately the activation of vigorous humoral and cell-mediated responses. Vaccinologists have long taken advantage of live attenuated (weakened) virus or bacteria as vaccines to elicit strong immune responses against the homologous wild-type (virulent) pathogens. Advances in molecular genetics have made it possible to specifically alter many diverse types of viruses so as to attenuate their natural pathogenicity and to express a foreign protein or proteins of interest for the purpose of inducing an immune response to that protein.

There are several advantages in the use of virus vectors as vaccines: (1) Insertion of one or more relevant genes into a virus vector results in focusing the immune response on important vaccine antigens so as

> **Advantages of using virus vectors as vaccines**
>
> - Insertion of one or more relevant genes into a virus vector results in focusing the immune response on important vaccine antigens.
> - Virus infection results in expression of high levels of both structural and nonstructural proteins on a particle of appropriate size for recognition by immune cells.
> - Most viruses induce high levels of innate immunity; this immunity provides an intrinsic adjuvant effect and results in a larger and more durable adaptive immune response with efficient development of humoral and cell-mediated memory responses.
> - The use of viruses as vectors makes possible the delivery of antigen to induce a full array of adaptive immune responses.
> - Take advantage of the cellular or tissue tropism of the virus used as vector for effective delivery of antigen.
> - Many virus genomes are simple and relatively easy to manipulate by molecular genetics techniques.

to interfere with infection or enhance clearance of the targeted pathogen. It also represents an opportunity to immunize against cross-reactive epitopes shared among different pathogen serotypes and provide protection against closely related pathogens. (2) Virus infection results in expression of high levels of structural proteins on a particle of appropriate size for recognition by immune cells. Further, proteins incorporated into the virion structure efficiently induce an immune response due to effective concentration and presentation of appropriately folded and modified proteins by the virus particle. (3) Most viruses induce high levels of innate immunity following recognition of virion components by host pattern recognition receptors. This immunity provides an intrinsic adjuvant effect and results in a larger and more durable adaptive immune response with efficient development of humoral and cell-mediated memory responses. Additionally, through incompletely understood mechanisms, the specific nature of the innate immune response results in development of specific types of effector mechanisms by adaptive immune cells. (4) The use of viruses as vectors makes possible the delivery of antigen to induce a full array of adaptive immune responses. For example, beyond inducing vigorous antibody responses, live vectors can deliver antigen into the major histocompatability complex (MHC) class I antigen-presentation pathway and provide efficient generation of cytotoxic T lymphocytes against important pathogen epitopes. Additionally, virus vectors can deliver antigen to induce different types of $CD4^+$ T cell responses, favoring overall development of either humoral or cell-mediated responses to vaccine antigen. (5) It is possible to take advantage of the cellular or tissue tropism of the virus used as vector for effective delivery of antigen. Virus vectors can deliver genes for selected pathogen proteins to specific cells (for example, alphavirus delivery of vaccine genes to dendritic cells) or tissues (for example, adenovirus delivery of vaccine genes to mucosal surfaces). Finally, many virus genomes are simple and relatively easy to manipulate by molecular genetics techniques, including RNA virus genomes that can now be engineered by reverse genetics. Genes of interest can be inserted into specific sites, deletion of virus structural protein genes allows the replication of virus vectors but not the production of infectious virion progeny (termed *single-cycle viruses*), and virus-encoded

immune evasion genes can be deleted to attenuate the vector. Additionally, the molecules binding host cell receptors can be altered or switched for those of related viruses to allow multiple rounds of vaccine boosting in the presence of vigorous immune responses against the initial vaccine.

There are, however, potential difficulties with the use of vaccine vectors. Perhaps the most common difficulty encountered results from preexisting immunity in the immunized individual against the viral vector. If a commonly encountered virus is used as vector, the vaccine recipient may already have been naturally exposed to the pathogen and have mounted a vigorous response to vector-specific antigens. The end result is that it may be difficult or impossible to induce an immune response to the inserted gene of the vector in the face of the individual's immune response to and rapid removal of the vector. For example, adenovirus vectors may not be as efficacious in individuals who have been previously infected with adenovirus. Additionally, the immune response from the priming immunization using a given vector may preclude reuse of the same vector for boosting immunization. However, not all virus vectors are inhibited by previous immunization with the virus and/or vector, including measles and yellow fever vaccine viruses. For those vectors that are negatively affected by a previous antiviral immunity, the use of different serotypes of the original vector (e.g., adenovirus) or related but antigenically distinct viruses (avipox and orthopox vectors) as boosting vectors can avoid this problem. Constraints on the size or type of gene insert that can be used in some virus vectors may limit the utility of the vector. Additionally, the quantity of antigen produced may vary among different types of virus vectors or vary as a result of the relative persistence of the virus vector in the immunized individual such that relatively low levels of the target protein are available to the host immune system.

The characteristics of a good vaccine vector include assurance that vector DNA does not integrate into the host genome. Many of the most-utilized DNA virus vectors replicate in the cytoplasm and avoid this issue. For DNA virus vectors that replicate in the nucleus, it is important to ensure that the viral DNA does not become incorporated into the host genome. It is also important to ensure that the virus vector is stably attenuated in such a manner that it cannot revert to wild type (virulent) through mutation or recombination events. Importantly, it must be easy to produce and purify large quantities of the vector in a cost-efficient manner. Based on these characteristics, a number of different types of virus vectors have been constructed from both RNA and DNA viruses. The utility of a given vector is largely a reflection of the physical properties of the vector, its infectious and replicative properties, and how it interacts with the host immune system.

DNA viruses

Poxviruses

Poxviruses are in the family *Poxviridae*, and the most common poxvirus vaccine vectors are derived from the genera *Orthopoxvirus* and *Avipoxvirus*. These viruses have very large double-stranded DNA genomes ranging in size from 150 to 350 kb. The orthopoxviruses include the human pathogen smallpox virus as well as a number of viruses that infect a wide variety of animal species and a wide range of cell types including dendritic cells. The value of these viruses as vectors lies in part in the stability of the genome due to a very low mutation rate and that the entire replication cycle takes place in the cytoplasm, which makes incorporation into the host genome unlikely. Additionally, mul-

tiple vaccine genes may be inserted into the vector without affecting replication.

Vaccinia virus, which was widely used as the vaccine against smallpox, was first utilized as a vaccine vector in experimental animal models and resulted in high levels of vaccine protein expression and induction of both antibody and cell-mediated immune responses. Vaccinia virus vectors first found use in the veterinary setting as a rabies virus vaccine encoding the G protein of rabies virus (Raboral VR-G). This vaccine was incorporated into edible bait, spread in the wild, and achieved remarkable success in control of rabies. Use of this vaccine resulted in the elimination of rabies from red foxes in Western European countries, control of rabies outbreaks in coyote populations in Texas (USA) and of raccoon rabies in the eastern USA. Although most individuals have not been naturally exposed to poxviruses, preexisting immunity in individuals vaccinated with vaccinia virus against smallpox may limit its use as a vaccine vector. More importantly, the original (wild-type) vaccinia virus is reactogenic and should not be used in immunocompromised individuals and individuals with certain skin conditions.

Two attenuated vaccinia virus variants have been produced to increase vaccine safety: modified vaccinia virus Ankara strain (MVA) and NYVAC. MVA was attenuated by 570 serial passages in chick embryo

Virus abbreviations

AAV	Adeno-associated viruses	RVFV	Rift Valley Fever virus
CAEV	Caprine arthritis encephalitis virus	SAD B19	A live attenuated rabies virus vaccine
CMV	Cytomegalovirus	SARS	Severe acute respiratory syndrome
DENV	Dengue virus		
FIV	Feline immunodeficiency virus	SFV	Semliki Forest virus
HIV	Human immunodeficiency virus	SINV	Sindbis virus
HSV	Herpes simplex virus	SIV	Simian immunodeficiency virus
JEV	Japanese encephalitis virus	TROVAC-AIV-H5	A fowlpox virus expressing the avian influenza H5 hemagglutinin gene
MVA	Modified vaccinia virus (Ankara strain)		
NDV	Newcastle disease virus	VEEV	Venezuelan equine encephalitis virus
NYVAC	A highly attenuated vaccinia virus strain derived from the Copenhagen vaccine strain	VSV	Vesicular stomatitis virus
		WNV	West Nile virus
RV	Rabies virus	YFV	Yellow fever virus

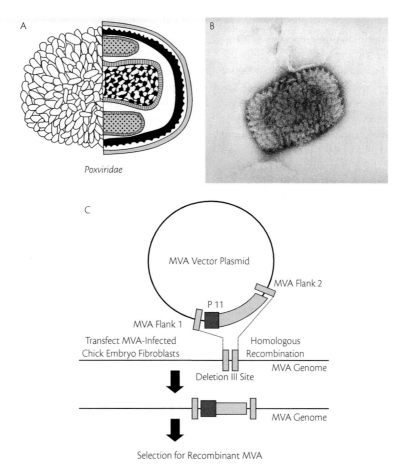

Figure 8.1 (A) Stylized depiction of poxvirus structure (from http://www.utmb.edu/virusimages/ with permission of Frederick Murphy, University of Texas Medical Branch [UTMB], Galveston, Texas). (B) A smallpox virion visualized by negative stain electron microscopy. Magnification about ×150,000. Micrograph from Frederick Murphy, UTMB, Galveston, Texas. (C) Plasmids encoding a vaccinia virus promoter and vaccine gene flanked by regions homologous to the insertion region of MVA genome are transfected into MVA-infected chick embryo fibroblasts. The promoter and vaccine gene are inserted into the MVA genome by homologous recombination. Recombinant MVA virions expressing the protein of interest are selected and plaque purified.

fibroblasts, resulting in loss of approximately 15% of the virus genome. This virus is very attenuated with a good safety profile in humans and has been used in clinical trials of malaria and HIV vaccines (Figure 8.1). NYVAC is a plaque isolate of the Copenhagen strain of vaccinia virus, which was attenuated by deletion of 18 open reading frames of genes encoding virulence proteins. NYVAC also has a good safety profile in humans and has been used as a vector for a candidate malaria vaccine.

As mentioned previously, potential difficulties with the use of poxvirus vectors arise from the presence of preexisting immune responses. This problem can arise most often in cases where the same poxvirus vector is used to prime and boost the recipient but can be circumvented by the use of poxvirus vectors engineered from alternative poxviruses that infect other species. In particular, the avipoxviruses that naturally infect bird species have been utilized as vectors for use in vaccine regimens in conjunction with other poxvirus vectors. It is generally thought that avipoxviruses do not productively infect mammalian cells so that the virus will not spread within the mammalian vaccine recipient. Fowlpox and canarypox vectors do not

131

generate vigorous antivector antibody responses, making these vectors useful in prime/boost immunization regimens. Further, current evidence suggests the immunity elicited by human orthopox vectors will not interfere with a subsequent avipox-based vaccine boost. This regimen has been utilized in the clinical trial of a prostate cancer vaccine in which vaccinia virus encoding a prostate cancer-specific antigen and human B7-1, ICAM-1, and LFA-3 proteins was used for priming followed by a fowlpox (avipox) vector with the same gene inserts as a boost. An alternative approach to circumventing preexisting immunity is found in the development of a prime/boost regimen in which individuals are primed with a DNA vaccine encoding the gene of interest and then boosted by a poxvirus vector encoding the same antigen. The boosting effect of this type of regimen is greater than that elicited by delivery of virus vector followed by DNA boost. Although the reason for this phenomenon is not completely clear, the lack of inflammation during priming with DNA vaccines may result in preferential differentiation of responding T cells into memory T cells.

Beyond the successful development and implementation of the poxvirus-vectored rabies vaccine, orthopox and avipox vectors are also being developed for use in veterinary vaccines. For example, a canarypox vector has been utilized as a platform technology for use in veterinary vaccines against canine distemper virus, feline leukemia virus, West Nile virus, and equine influenza virus, and other infectious agents (see Chapter 10 for more examples). An avipox virus has been engineered to express the H5 and H7 proteins of avian influenza virus (TROVAC™-AIV-H5) and has been used to vaccinate chickens against avian influenza virus. Similar vaccine strategies utilizing myxoma virus vectors to express genes for feline calicivirus, and rabbit hemorrhagic disease virus and capripox virus vectors to express antigens from *peste des petit ruminants* virus and bluetongue virus are currently under development.

Adenovirus

Adenoviruses belong in the family *Adenoviridae*, genus *Mastadenovirus*, carry a double-stranded DNA genome, and are the causative agents of upper respiratory infections in humans. Adenoviruses are generally species specific, and many serotypes of adenovirus

exist that infect humans (e.g., adenovirus serotype 5 is commonly used as a vaccine vector). The virus attaches to host cell receptor proteins via the knob domain of the capsid fiber protein. Manipulation of this protein by exchange with other adenovirus serotype fiber proteins or by construction of chimeric fibers results in alteration of the target cells for the adenovirus vector. Adenovirus E1 proteins play an essential role in viral replication, and deletion of the E1 region results in loss of replication competency, thereby increasing the safety of the vector. The E3 gene is nonessential and can also be deleted to increase the cloning capacity of the vector. Replication competent adenovirus vectors can encode a 3–4 kb insert while replication defective adenoviruses deleted of the E1 or E1 and E3 genes can carry up to a 7–8 kb insert (Figure 8.2). Recently, helper-dependent or "gutless" adenoviruses have been developed, in which nearly all viral genes have been deleted, and they are capable of expressing large amounts of foreign genetic material with very little development of anti-adenovirus immunity. Many humans have been naturally infected with adenoviruses, and many military recruits have been immunized with a live enteric adenovirus vaccine. Therefore, a substantial proportion of the human population has developed specific immune responses to adenovirus that can interfere with successful immunization with adenovirus vectors. Fortunately, the problem of preexisting immunity can be overcome by use of adenovirus vectors derived from serotypes that infrequently cause human infection (e.g., adenovirus serotype 35), with vectors expressing genetically altered surface proteins, or with chimpanzee adenovirus-derived vectors as vaccines to deliver boosting immunizations.

A number of candidate human vaccines utilizing adenovirus vectors have been developed and tested in clinical trials, including a cancer vaccine and prime/boost regimens for vaccines against malaria, HIV, SARS, and Ebola. Adenovirus vectors have also been tested in a number of veterinary vaccines including rabies virus and foot-and-mouth virus vaccines.

Adeno-associated viruses

Adeno-associated viruses (AAV) are single-stranded DNA viruses of the family *Parvoviridae*, genus *Dependovirus*. These viruses require coinfection with a helper virus such as adenovirus or herpesvirus for productive

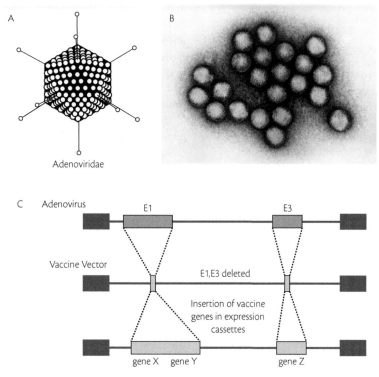

Figure 8.2 (A) Stylized depiction of adenovirus structure (from http://www.utmb.edu/virusimages/ with permission of Frederick Murphy, UTMB). (B) Colorized transmission electron micrograph of adenovirus. Micrograph from Dr. G. William Gary, Jr., Center for Disease Control and Prevention. (C) Genes encoding vaccine antigens can be inserted into expression cassettes located at the sites of adenovirus gene deletion. A first-generation replication defective adenovirus vector with deletions of E1 and E3 genes is shown.

replication. In the absence of a helper virus, AAV becomes latent without production of progeny virions. AAV binds to heparin sulfate proteoglycans, fibroblast growth factor receptor, or the integrin $\alpha_v\beta_5$ on the host cell surface and is internalized by endocytosis. A number of AAV serotypes are known. Although some can infect humans, no known human diseases are associated with AAV infection. This virus generally induces only weak immunity although this response is sufficient to complicate a boosting vaccination. As discussed for other viruses, the use of alternative AAV serotypes as vectors or inclusion of AAV vectors in a prime/boost regimen can overcome this barrier. Due to the prolonged expression of AAV genes and weak immune response to AAV proteins, this virus is being studied extensively as a gene delivery vector in gene therapy studies. However, there is also interest in AAV-derived vectors as vaccine delivery vectors due to the ability of the vector to accommodate up to 5 kb of

gene insert if all virus genes are deleted. AAV vectors are produced in packaging cell lines that provide all AAV genes and helper virus functions. AAV has been tested as a vector for SIV and HIV, CMV, and HSV vaccines.

RNA viruses

Alphavirus vectors

These viruses are arthropod-borne, single-stranded positive-sense RNA viruses in the family *Togaviridae*, genus *Alphavirus*. Alphaviruses replicate in the cell cytoplasm and are highly cytolytic. Several alphaviruses can infect humans, causing a range of illnesses ranging from rash and fever to lethal encephalitis. Three alphaviruses have been most often utilized as vaccine vectors: Sindbis virus (SINV), Venezuelan equine encephalitis virus (VEEV), and Semliki Forest

133

Packaging cell lines

Some viral vectors have been engineered by deletion of the genes encoding the proteins necessary for packaging the replicated viral genome into a new virion, thereby preventing further rounds of infection by the viral vector. In order to produce a virus vector capable of only a single round of infection, the missing packaging protein functions must be provided in such a way that the genes encoding the packaging proteins and the transgene vector sequence are present in the same cell but are physically kept separate. This is usually accomplished by transfection of plasmids containing vaccine vector genes into mammalian cells that have been stably transfected with plasmids encoding the packaging genes (constitutive production of the packaging proteins). Alternatively, mammalian cells can be cotransfected with plasmids encoding the transgene vector sequence and separate plasmids encoding the packaging genes. The packaging genes and vector sequence genes are engineered to prevent recombination and formation of a "wild-type" infectious particle. The packaging proteins (but not the genes) are therefore provided in *trans* to the developing vector particle, and a particle capable of only a single round of infection is produced.

virus (SFV). Alphaviruses are particularly useful as vaccine vectors because they have a broad host range, and there is no risk of the RNA genome of the vector being incorporated into the host genome. These viruses target dendritic cells for infection, relatively high levels of encoded proteins can be expressed, and there is very little natural exposure of humans to these viruses, which results in a very low incidence of pre-existing immunity to alphavirus vectors. Another important characteristic that enhances the vaccine potential of these viruses lies in the fact that alphaviruses elicit a very strong innate immune response that intrinsically adjuvants the adaptive immune response to the alphavirus vector itself or for recombinant proteins administered simultaneously with the vector. A 26S subgenomic RNA controlled by a viral subgenomic promoter amplifies viral structural genes, which results in very high level expression of the encoded proteins. Vaccine transgenes that are inserted here in place of viral structural protein genes are amplified, and high levels of vaccine antigen are expressed as a result. To further enhance vaccine protein processing

and expression, the vaccine gene can be inserted in-frame with an alphavirus enhancer element encoded in the first 34 residues of the capsid gene. A foot-and-mouth disease virus 2a protease element may be inserted between the capsid gene enhancer and the vaccine gene to remove the truncated capsid protein from the vaccine protein.

Three main types of alphavirus vectors have been developed for use as vaccine vectors: virus-like particles, layered DNA–RNA vectors, and replication competent alphavirus vectors (Figure 8.3). Virus-like particles are vectors in which the vaccine transgene replaces the alphavirus structural proteins. This type of vector can undergo only one round of replication and must be produced in "packaging cell lines" transfected with plasmids encoding envelope and capsid genes that have been deleted of packaging signal so they cannot be incorporated into the vector genome. Layered DNA–RNA vectors consist of a vaccine gene-containing alphavirus replicon encoded by cDNA driven by the CMV promoter. Vector RNA including the transgene of interest is transcribed from the DNA. Although there is usually a low efficiency of vaccine cDNA transfection, the vaccination results in high vaccine protein production, and the use of cDNA immunization circumvents any preexisting immunity during vaccination. Replication competent alphavirus vectors contain both the vaccine transgene and virus structural genes. In this scheme, two subgenomic RNAs are produced: one for the transgene and one for the structural proteins, which have been mutated to attenuate the vector. Given the ability of alphaviruses to cause disease in humans, there is obviously concern over the potential for reversion of vector to wild-type virus. These concerns have been addressed through the use of highly attenuated strains for vector development and by genetically engineering the vector to prevent recombination events. Recently alphaviruses that infect only mosquitoes have been discovered and described. Since this newly discovered virus does not infect vertebrate cells, it offers further opportunities for development of novel alphavirus vaccine vectors.

Experimental vaccines utilizing alphavirus vectors expressing the HIV Gag protein gene by SINV, or VEEV VLPs; expressing Japanese encephalitis virus genes by replicating SINV virus vector; expression of mumps and rubella genes by SFV VLPs; expression of Ebola, Norwalk, or Marburg genes inserted into VEEV VLPs;

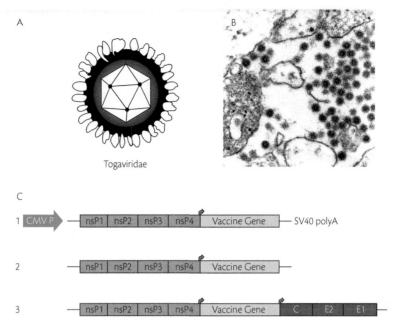

Figure 8.3 (A) Stylized depiction of alphavirus structure (from http://www.utmb.edu/virusimages/ with permission of Frederick Murphy, UTMB). (B) Ultra-thin section of a Vero cell culture infected with Eastern equine encephalitis virus (24-hr infection) (from http://www.utmb.edu/virusimages/ with permission of Frederick Murphy). Magnification approximately ×70,000. Micrograph from F.A. Murphy, UTMB, Galveston, Texas. (C) Vector construction of three types of alphavirus vectors. The small green arrow indicates the site of the subgenomic promoter. (1) Layered DNA–RNA vector. (2) Virus-like particle vector. (3) Replication competent alphavirus vector.

and hantavirus and malaria genes expressed by SINV DNA/RNA vaccines have been tested preclinically. Tumor vaccines against melanoma (SINV DNA–RNA), glioma (SINV VLP, SFV VLP), prostate cancer (VEEV VLPs), and breast cancer (VEEV VLPs) have also been tested. Alphavirus vectors have also been tested in veterinary vaccines against pseudorabies and classical swine fever (SINV DNA–RNA), *Brucella abortus* (VEEV VLP), and bovine viral diarrhea (SFV VLPs).

Newcastle disease virus (NDV)

NDV is a negative-sense, single-stranded RNA virus in the family *Paramyxoviridae*, genus *Avulavirus*. NDV infects and causes disease in all species of birds ranging in outcomes from asymptomatic to fatal. NDV has a genome of approximately 15 kb encoding six structural genes, including a nucleocapsid protein, a phosphoprotein, a polymerase, a matrix protein, a hemagglutinin–neuraminidase protein involved in attachment of the virus to its cellular receptor, and a fusion (F) protein, which mediates entry into the cell by fusion of the viral envelope with the host cell membrane. The genome contains a 3′ leader and a 5′ trailer that are necessary for transcription and virus replication. Two important properties of NDV affect its use as a vector. First, the viral polymerase attaches to the viral genome and reads through the open reading frames sequentially but because the polymerase is prone to become detached from the viral RNA template, early gene sequences are transcribed preferentially. Therefore, foreign gene sequences inserted near the 3′ end are transcribed with higher frequency. Second, the tropism of NDV for infection of different cell types is regulated to a large extent by the number of basic amino acids encoded in the F protein cleavage site. The addition of an F protein cleavage site that contains several basic amino acids can be cleaved by many different cellular proteases, whereas cleavage sites that contain few basic residues are cleaved preferentially by proteases found in respiratory tract cells. Thus, the pathogenicity and the cellular tropism of the vector can be engineered by control of basic amino acids at this important protein cleavage site. The use of NDV as a vector is limited in that it cannot accommodate large foreign genes or multiple genes. To enhance the ability of NDV to serve as a vector, a NDV vector with a bisegmented genome has been engineered and shown to be capable of expressing large proteins encoded on each genome segment.

The NDV vector system holds potential for use in humans. Because NDV is not a natural pathogen of humans, potential recipients do not have preexisting immunity against the virus, an important attribute for potential vaccine vectors. Importantly, NDV has been shown to be safe in humans. NDV vectors carrying genes for severe acute respiratory syndrome virus (SARS-CoV), respiratory syncytial virus, and parainfluenza virus type 3 have undergone preclinical testing. Additionally, NDV vectors encoding granulocyte/macrophage colony stimulating vector, interleukin 3, and interferon gamma have undergone preclinical tests as cancer vaccines.

Because NDV is a natural pathogen for bird species, it has found use as a vector for veterinary use, particular in the poultry industry. Most notably, hemagglutinin genes from high pathogenic avian influenza virus have been inserted into NDV vectors for the immunization of chickens. Similarly, a NDV vector expressing the VP2 protein of infectious bursal disease virus has been constructed to protect chickens against acquisition of this immunosuppressive agent.

Other related viruses are also being investigated as vectors including bovine parainfluenza virus 3 (genus *Respovirus*) and simian parainfluenza virus 5 (genus *Rubulavirus*).

Measles virus

Measles virus is an enveloped virus containing a single-stranded RNA genome also of the family *Paramyxoviridae*, genus *Morbillivirus*, and is the causative agent of measles in humans. The virus binds to receptors on host cells via hemagglutinin and fusion proteins and can efficiently infect dendritic cells. It has been proposed as a vaccine vector due to its intrinsic stability and excellent safety record as a live attenuated vaccine. Measles virus can accommodate two to three gene inserts for simultaneous delivery of multiple vaccine antigens. Since this vaccine has been proven safe in children, it has been suggested as a useful delivery vehicle for pediatric vaccines, including

potential vaccination against HIV, and many candidate recombinant vaccines are in preclinical development, including a dengue virus vaccine. Although many people have been vaccinated with measles vaccines, the preexisting immunity does not prevent boost effect upon subsequent immunizations.

Vesicular stomatitis virus and rabies virus

The family *Rhabdoviridae* includes nonsegmented RNA viruses with negative-sense genomes such as vesicular stomatitis virus (VSV, genus *Vesiculovirus*) and rabies virus (RV, genus *Lyssavirus*). VSV is an arthropod-borne virus that causes severe disease of livestock characterized by vesicular lesions very similar to that of foot-and-mouth disease. Infections of humans are predominantly asymptomatic or result in a mild, flu-like illness, although encephalitis has been reported. Infection with VSV begins with the viral spike glycoproteins binding to an unknown cell surface receptor. The virus is then internalized by endocytosis and replication takes place in the cytoplasm followed by cytopathic release of progeny virions. The genome of VSV is 11 kb and can accommodate gene inserts of up to 4.5 kb. A useful characteristic of VSV is that it can encode vaccine glycoproteins for expression on the virion surface. The highly repetitive protein structure of the VSV particle results in induction of vigorous humoral and cell-mediated immune responses to these surface-exposed proteins.

RV is the causative agent of rabies and results in lethal infection in humans if not treated prior to virus invasion of the central nervous system. However, RV vectors can be effectively attenuated to maintain immunogenicity while decreasing pathogenicity. For example, the RV vaccine is derived from the SAD B19 strain, which has extremely limited ability to invade the central nervous system. Large vaccine transgenes can also be inserted stably into RV with mid to high expression of vaccine antigen, resulting in induction of strong adaptive immune responses. Because of the low incidence of VSV and RV infection of humans, preexisting immunity to both rhabdoviruses occurs at low levels in the human population so priming with these vaccine vectors is not considered problematic. However, neutralizing antibody to these rhabdoviruses is very effectively induced and will prevent boosting effects if the same vector is utilized. As discussed for other virus vectors, alternating the serotype of the VSV vector used for boosting immunization can overcome this obstacle. Alternatively, for RV vectors, the ectodomain of the RV glycoprotein can be replaced with VSV glycoprotein in the boosting vaccine. Preclinical studies of rhabdovirus-based vector vaccines for hepatitis C, HIV, and SIV, and preclinical studies of VSV-vector vaccines for H5N1 avian flu, Ebola and Marburg, *Yersinia pestis*, hepatitis C viruses have been reported.

Flaviviruses

Flaviviruses are arthropod-borne viruses with a single-stranded, positive-sense RNA genome. The family *Flaviviridae*, genus *Flavivirus* includes many important human pathogens including yellow fever virus (YFV), dengue virus (DENV), Japanese encephalitis virus (JEV), and West Nile virus (WNV). In the 1930s, a YFV vaccine was developed by serial passage of YFV, resulting in the live attenuated YFV 17D vaccine. This vaccine has a long history of success in preventing yellow fever disease in humans and elicits immunity in approximately 95% of recipients within days of vaccination. The vaccine also has an excellent safety record with only rare accounts of serious adverse events resulting from YFV 17D immunization. Recently, this successful vaccine has been utilized as a vaccine platform using an infectious clone of the 17D vaccine virus for the expression of important immunogenic proteins of other flaviviruses. The most successful approach has been to construct chimeric flaviviuses where the premembrane (prM) and envelope (E) genes of a flavivirus of interest are exchanged for those same genes from the YFV 17D vaccine. This approach was taken in development of ChimeriVax™ technology. Chimeric virus vaccine candidates have been prepared that express the nonstructural and capsid proteins from YFV 17D and the prM and E proteins from JEV, WNV, or DENV. A ChimeriVax-based vaccine for JEV (ChimeriVax-JE) has successfully undergone phase I, II, and III testing. It has been found to be safe and highly immunogenic in humans and has been licensed in Australia and Thailand. An identical approach has been utilized to develop a ChimeriVax-based vaccine for dengue virus although the development process is more complicated (Figure 8.4). Because there are four serotypes of dengue virus (DENV-1 to DENV-4), each of which can cause disease ranging from dengue fever to dengue shock syndrome,

a candidate vaccine must be able to protect against all four serotypes. Although promising preclinical and clinical phase I and II trial results were obtained with a tetravalent ChimeriVax-DENV vaccine containing chimeric viruses representing all four dengue serotypes, this vaccine recently gave inconclusive immunogenicity data in a phase IIb clinical trial, but phase III trials are proceeding. Additional candidate dengue vaccines are being clinically evaluated using chimeric viruses based on attenuated DENV-2 or DENV-4 backbones.

Insertion of non-flavivirus foreign genes into flavivirus vectors is theoretically possible. However, there are insert size constraints, and the inserted gene must be placed either behind an internal ribosome entry site or at specific sites within the flavivirus genome for expression. Some success with this approach has been reported from studies in which short stretches of nucleotides encoding epitopes recognized by malaria-specific cytotoxic T lymphocytes were successfully incorporated into a 17D vector. This vaccine construct was also shown to decrease parasite burden in a malaria challenge study. Similar constructs have been made for Lassa virus and tumor antigens and are in preclinical development.

Lentiviruses

Viruses of the family *Retroviridae*, genus *Lentivirus*, contain a diploid RNA genome that is converted to double-stranded DNA by reverse transcriptase before being integrated into the host cell genome. Lentiviruses express the structural genes gag, pol, and env as well as the tat, rev, vif, vpr, nef, and vpu genes that control viral replication and infection. Clinically, the most important member of the lentiviruses is the human immunodeficiency virus type 1 (HIV-1) although other viruses are important animal and veterinary pathogens, including simian immunodeficiency virus (SIV), feline immunodeficiency virus (FIV), and caprine arthritis encephalitis virus (CAEV). The consideration of lentiviruses as vectors derives from their ability to stably encode large vaccine gene inserts, to infect both dividing and nondividing cells due to the action of the lentiviral preintegration complex, development of low levels of antivector immunity, and long-term expression of vaccine proteins due to integration of genome into host cell chromosomes. However, this last characteristic also

137

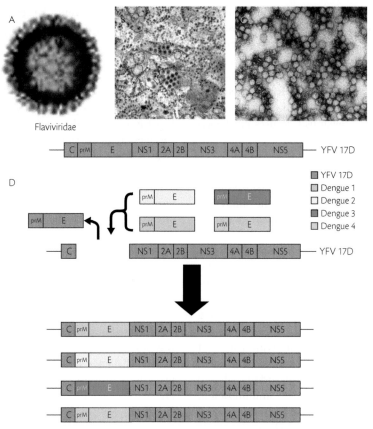

Figure 8.4 (A) Stylized depiction of flavivirus structure (from http://www.utmb.edu/virusimages/ with permission of Frederick Murphy, UTMB, Galveston, Texas). (B) Transmission electron micrograph of dengue virus. Photo taken by Fredrick Murphy and provided by Frederick Murphy and Cynthia Goldsmith, Center for Disease Control and Prevention. (C) Electron micrograph of yellow fever virus (×234,000). Electron micrograph from Erskine Palmer, Center for Disease Control and Prevention. (C) Construction of the ChimeriVax dengue vaccine. The genes for the premembrane (prM) and envelope (E) proteins of yellow fever virus are deleted and replaced with the prM and E genes from dengue1, dengue 2, dengue 3, or dengue 4. Precise amounts of each vaccine virus must be mixed to provide protective immunity against all four dengue serotypes.

presents a potential safety issue to be addressed before widespread use as a vaccine vector. Lentivirus-based vaccines have been shown to effectively induce strong cell-mediated responses including the induction of vaccine gene-specific cytotoxic T lymphocytes.

Most lentivirus vectors are derived from HIV-1 but significant progress has also been made using vectors derived from SIV and FIV. Current lentivirus vectors are termed third-generation self-inactivating lentivirus vectors that lack the nonessential HIV-1 genes vif, vpr, nef, and vpu. The vector has been rendered "self-inactivating" by deletion in the 3' long terminal repeat that abolishes the 5' long terminal repeat promoter

activity and reduces the risk of vector mobilization. Other changes to the vector, including codon optimization of the gag-pol gene, changes in the long terminal repeat region, addition of a rev-responsive element to the vector, addition of a polypurine tract to the pol gene, and replacement of the lentivirus env glycoprotein with the vesicular stomatitis virus glycoprotein gene result in optimization of the production and uptake of the vector. Recently an integration-deficient lentivirus vector system has been developed that minimizes integration of the vector into the genome by mutations in the integrase protein in the lentivirus particle.

Immunization with lentivirus vectors represents a relatively new field, although a number of vaccines have been constructed against infectious agents including HIV and hepatitis B. Lentivirus-based vaccines encoding genes for melanoma, hepatoma, or prostate cancer proteins are also in development. Vigorous cell-mediated immune responses, including development of antigen-specific cytotoxic T-lymphocyte responses, resulted from vaccination with these lentivirus vaccines.

Other vaccine vectors

A number of other viruses have characteristics amenable to encoding and expressing vaccine antigens and are currently being developed as vaccine vectors. For example, bunyaviruses contain a genome comprising three RNA segments and include the important human and veterinary pathogen, Rift Valley Fever virus (RVFV). Genetically engineered strains of RVFV deleted of the NSs gene, which functions as an interferon (IFN) antagonist, are attenuated and can accept insertion of a foreign gene. Since bunyaviruses infect many species and many cell types, work is being done to develop attenuated RVFV strains as safe, attenuated vaccine vectors. Coronaviruses, which include viruses responsible for the common cold, have a large positive-sense RNA genome that could theoretically accommodate large gene inserts. They are also natural pathogens of mucosal surfaces and might be useful for delivery of vaccine antigen to respiratory or intestinal mucosa. Importantly, from a safety perspective, many nonpathogenic strains are available for vector development.

Hepatitis B virus vectors in the form of virus-like particles are currently being developed and tested as vaccines. Although the utility of this type of vector may be limited due to its ability to accept only a relatively small vaccine gene insert, immunization with these particles has been shown to generate strong cytotoxic T lymphocyte responses. Picornaviruses are a group of viruses containing a positive-stranded RNA genome and include the human pathogen, poliovirus. Because the virus spreads via the oral mucosal surface during natural infection, it may be useful as a vector for mucosal vaccine delivery. A potential limitation of this approach is that many individuals worldwide have been immunized with the poliovirus vaccine, and the resulting neutralizing antibody response may interfere with widespread utility of this type of vector. Although much work remains to be done to ensure the safety, efficacy, and affordability and reproducibility production of viral vectors for the delivery of vaccine antigens, the wide range of vector options and potential for development of strong, durable immune responses make this an attractive approach for future vaccine development.

Bacterial vectors as vaccine platforms

Most studies on bacterial vectors as vaccines are either in the discovery or preclinical development phase. Few constructs have proceeded to clinical trials, and only a couple, including a *Salmonella* vaccine and an anthrax vaccine, have been licensed for human use. Nonetheless, there are a number of promising bacterial systems. To develop protective immune responses against mucosal bacterial pathogens, the delivery route for vaccination is important. Therefore, novel antigen delivery systems are under development that show great potential as effective and safe mucosal vaccines against various pathogens. Highly developed systems such as bacterial cell surface displays (for example, autotransporters and fusion proteins), together with the traditional use of bacterial surface-exposed proteins, have brought additional capabilities for the carriers to expose foreign molecules on the cell surface. Bacterial peptide display (consisting of the genetic fusion of a peptide of interest to a surface-expressed protein to allow its presentation at the bacterial surface) has successfully competed with other epitope mapping techniques (including several processes of identifying the immunoreactive epitopes in the target antigens) and proven useful in identification of the entire set of pathogen antigens targeted by the immune system. In addition, the development of novel delivery systems has significantly advanced by using intracellular pathogens for genetic immunization. Delivery of DNA vaccine plasmid and even translation-competent mRNA directly to the cytosol of the antigen-presenting cells can be efficiently achieved by self-destructing live bacterial carriers. Bacterial ghost (BG) delivery systems (BGs are cell envelopes derived from Gram-negative bacteria) have become popular for heterologous antigen presentation and also have been tested for DNA vaccination. Yet another technique, the use of protein secretion systems, has opened new horizons of using "inverted pathogenicity" for vaccine purposes. The purpose of this section is to introduce several recent approaches to induce mucosal immunity with vaccines, with an emphasis on new bacteria-based delivery systems.

> The "inverted pathogenicity" concept refers to the use of virulence mechanisms for prevention or therapy of disease. Specifically, this approach exploits the microbial toxins, other virulence factors, and the cellular mechanisms normally exploited by the pathogen for preventive or therapeutic purposes.

Bacterial cell surface display systems

Surface display of protein structures has two main applications in vaccine development. First, the use of cell surface-exposed heterologous antigens has always been considered beneficial for efficient exposure of expressed antigens to the immune system, resulting in induction of a vigorous antigen-specific immune response. Second, live vaccines can be loaded simultaneously with different antigens or their specific immune epitopes and receptor-specific ligands for specific vaccine-targeting, or co-displayed with adhesin proteins that may increase the efficiency of the immune response to the vaccine antigen. In general, attenuated pathogens or nonpathogenic commensal bacteria are used as candidate live vaccine carriers (e.g., *Vibrio* and *Salmonella* attenuated strains or lactic acid bacteria). The display of different colonization factors (fimbriae, flagella, or other adhesins) on the surface of nonpathogens could be particularly advantageous for mucosal immunization, since these vaccine vehicles do not normally invade the host, and, therefore, the co-display of adhesins can increase colonization of mucosal epithelium, leading to better stimulation of the local immune response.

Gram-negative display systems

Gram-negative as well as Gram-positive bacteria have been used as vaccine vectors to present foreign molecules on their surface. The initial vector systems employed outer membrane proteins (Omps) as carriers for the display of heterologous peptides or proteins to be displayed. Because integral outer membrane proteins possess membrane-spanning regions containing surface exposed loops, the major task was to identify the "permissive" sites within these loops that could tolerate insertions without the loss of biological functions. The limitations of this approach were both the size and nature of the foreign antigen (passenger domain) used to modify the carrier protein. Some examples of carrier outer membrane proteins that were used to display the passenger amino acid sequence of different sizes include the outer membrane proteins OmpA, OprF, LamB, OmpS, and PhoE. Most of these carrier proteins have been expressed in enteric bacteria and successfully used to elicit a strong immune response to the foreign passenger protein, following delivery as a live vaccine (Figure 8.5).

Another example of an outer membrane protein employed in bacterial display systems is the invasin of *Yersinia pseudotuberculosis*. This approach has been proposed to be effective for the selection of anti-adhesion agents for use in anti-adhesion therapy (preventing the interaction between the bacteria and the target host cell, therefore reducing the ability to cause pathology) against bacterial diseases. A recent example

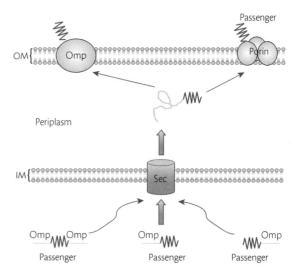

Figure 8.5 Examples of carrier outer membrane proteins (Omp or Porin) used to display the passenger amino acid sequence of a foreign antigen.

of this application is *Lactobacillus plantarum*, a bacterium that has been proposed as a potential delivery vehicle for mucosal vaccines. Because the inherent immunogenicity of vaccine antigens by themselves is in many cases insufficient to elicit an efficient immune response, the proinflammatory properties of *L. plantarum* were evaluated by expressing a long or short version of the extracellular domain of invasin from the human pathogen *Y. pseudotuberculosis*. All the constructs mediated surface display of invasin and several of the engineered strains were potent activators of NF-κB. The study demonstrated that the proinflammatory *L. plantarum* strains represent promising mucosal delivery vehicles for vaccine antigens.

In addition to outer membrane proteins, surface-exposed lipoproteins have been tested as bacterial display systems. Examples include the plasmid-encoded lipoprotein TraT involved in conjugation, the peptidoglycan-associated lipoprotein (PAL) from *E. coli*, and the ice-nucleation protein Inp of *Pseudomonas syringae*, which have been tested as anchor sequence display systems. A recent successful application of this strategy includes expression of LipL32 and LipL21, which are the conserved outer membrane lipoproteins of *Leptospira interrogans* and are considered vaccine candidates. Two predicted B- and T-cell combined epitopes of LipL21 and four of LipL32 were expressed in a phage display system, and these epitopes were recognized by CD4(+) T lymphocytes that were polarized toward a Th1 phenotype. Further data indicated that epitopes that have both B- and T-cell immune reactivities are critical for designing an effective vaccine for leptospirosis.

Autotransporter proteins have also been employed for surface display. These proteins are characterized by a single polypeptide chain that is able to provide all functions necessary to translocate a "passenger domain" across the Gram-negative cell envelope and to display this domain in a stable manner on the bacterial surface. The natural passenger domains of several autotransporter proteins have been replaced by heterologous proteins or protein domains, resulting in display of these determinants on the cell surface of Gram-negative bacteria. Autotransporter proteins that have been used for display of heterologous antigens include the IgA1 protease from *Neisseria gonorrhoeae*, VirG of *Shigella*, and *E. coli* adhesin involved in diffuse adherence (AIDA-I). An example of the use of

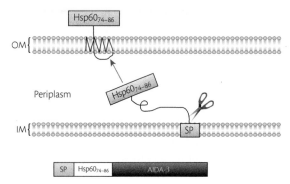

Figure 8.6 The AIDA-I autotransporter protein used in vaccine design to display the *Y. enterocolitica* heat shock protein Hsp60 (Hsp6074-86).

autotransporter proteins in vaccine design is the translational fusion between the MHC class II-restricted epitope of the *Y. enterocolitica* heat shock protein Hsp60 ($Hsp60_{74-86}$) and the autotransporter domain of the *E. coli* AIDA-I. This construct was expressed in a *Salmonella enterica* serovar Typhimurium vaccine strain and resulted in surface localization of the $Hsp60_{74-86}$ epitope. Colonization studies in mice vaccinated with *Salmonella* expressing $Hsp60_{74-86}$ AIDA-I fusion proteins demonstrated that the bacterial vector displayed a high genetic stability *in vivo*. Furthermore, a pronounced T-cell response against *Yersinia* $Hsp60_{74-86}$ was induced in mice following vaccination with the *Salmonella* vector vaccine (Figure 8.6).

Gram-positive display systems

A major advantage of Gram-positive microorganisms for surface display applications is the fact that these cells possess a single outer membrane with common mechanisms for surface anchoring of surface-expressed proteins. The display systems of Gram-positive bacteria have been classified into three groups: cell wall-bound, cell membrane-anchored, and cell surface-associated proteins. Examples of the first group include protein A of *Staphylococcus aureus*, the M6 protein of *Streptococcus pyogenes*, the surface protein antigen P1 from *S. mutans*, and the cell wall-bound proteinase PrtP of *L. lactis*. Representatives of the second group include the lipoprotein DppE of *Bacillus subtilis*, the autolysin modifier protein CwbA of *B. subtilis*, and *M. tuberculosis* lipoprotein Mtb19. The third group consists of proteins such as the beta-D-fructosyltransferase Ffts of *S. salivarius*, and the S-layer proteins EA1 and Sap of *Bacillus anthracis*. New efforts in bacterial display in combinatorial protein engineering have focused on a recently developed system for display using the Gram-positive bacteria *Staphylococcus carnosus*. This system has been successfully used to select binding proteins from large combinatorial libraries displayed on the surface of this bacterium. For example, the staphylococcal-displayed library can be subjected to flow-cytometric sorting and then selection for binding to human factors, such as TNF-α. The cell surface display of cloned peptides on *S. carnosus* has been extensively used for determination of antibody-binding epitopes using an antigen-focused, library-based approaches.

Novel tuberculosis vaccines

Tuberculosis (TB) is a potentially fatal contagious disease that mainly infects the lungs and is caused by the tubercle bacillus, *Mycobacterium tuberculosis*. The Bacillus Calmette–Guérin (BCG) vaccine is a century old and the only available vaccine against tuberculosis. The vaccine is prepared from a strain of the live attenuated bovine tuberculosis bacillus, *Mycobacterium bovis*. BCG is the most widely administered vaccine in the world, and although it is currently an officially recommended vaccine in more than 180 countries, excluding the USA, the efficacy of BCG as a vaccine against tuberculosis remains controversial. BCG provides significant protection against severe forms of TB, i.e., the disseminating and meningeal forms. However, the protective efficacy of BCG against pulmonary TB (which represents the transmissible form of this disease) in adults is inconsistent and incomplete, and despite the relative efficacy of BCG in infants, a major question that remains unanswered is why BCG fails to prevent pulmonary TB in adolescents. Because BCG is clearly insufficient for worldwide TB control, there is a strong need to develop a vaccine that can either boost BCG's initial priming and protective effects or replace it as a more effective vaccine. The current approaches being investigated include the construction of either improved recombinant BCG (rBCG) or the genetic attenuation of *M. tuberculosis*. Two major rBCG approaches have been explored: one includes introducing immunodominant *M. tuberculosis*-specific

antigens that are absent in BCG (such as the RD1 locus-encoding antigens ESAT6 and CFP10) or by overexpressing BCG antigens such as cognates of the Ag85 complex that are only expressed in distinct phases of infection. A second approach to improving BCG is by introducing genetic modifications to enhance or facilitate cross-priming and to inhibit its ability to neutralize phagosomal maturation, which are key processes associated with *M. tuberculosis* survival and persistence.

In the case of *M. tuberculosis* attenuation, the approaches currently investigated include the deletion of essential metabolic genes to create auxotrophic mutants or the inactivation of major virulence genes. Recent studies exemplifying this approach include the engineering of *M. microti* to express *M. tuberculosis* RD1antigens, or the use of a *M. smegmatis* attenuated strain complemented by the transfer of the *M. tuberculosis* esx-3 locus. Both vaccine candidates result in improved protection against experimental tuberculosis.

Despite progress with these approaches, an important area of investigation to create better TB vaccines is the development of subunit vaccines. Subunit vaccines against TB are mostly based on recombinant proteins admixed with proper adjuvants, or the use of attenuated viral vectors. Although subunit vaccines theoretically could be used as priming vaccines, the current consensus is that the subunit vaccine could be used as a boosting vaccine to be administered after BCG or rBCG vaccination, producing strong, long-lived immune responses that will persist to levels high enough to protect susceptible individuals against TB disease.

Novel delivery systems

Bacterial ghost system

The bacterial ghost (BG) platform technology is an innovative system for vaccine, drug, or therapeutic agent delivery, and for applications in biotechnology. BGs are cell envelopes derived from Gram-negative bacteria that are devoid of all cytoplasmic content but have a preserved cellular morphology including all cell surface structures. The original approach to produce a BG of Gram-negative bacteria included the controlled non-denaturing method of lysis by the PhiX174 bacteriophage protein E. The resulting BG is generally free from nucleic acids, ribosomes, and other intracellular components; however, outer and inner membranes largely remain intact. In contrast to heat, irradiation, or chemical inactivation of pathogens for vaccine purposes, BG preserves its native antigenic structure, and the membrane-associated lipopolysaccharide (LPS) and peptidoglycan retain their immunostimulatory activity. BGs exhibit intrinsic adjuvant properties and trigger an enhanced humoral and cellular immune response to the target antigen. Multiple antigens of the native BG envelope and recombinant protein or DNA antigens can be combined in a single type of BG. Antigens can be presented on the inner or outer membrane of the BG as well as in the periplasm that is sealed during BG formation.

The BG system has been utilized for presentation of envelope and/or heterologous antigens of many medically important bacterial agents such as *V. cholerae*, pathogenic *E. coli*, *Salmonella* spp., *Actinobacillus pleuropneumoniae*, *Francisella tularensis*, *Brucella melitensis*, and *Bordetella bronchiseptica*. BGs have also been successfully tested as a platform technology for DNA delivery following the loading of lyophilized BG in the DNA-containing buffer or by developing a procedure for the targeted immobilization of plasmid DNA in the cytoplasmic membrane of the carrier (Figure 8.7).

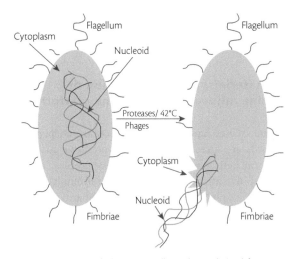

Figure 8.7 Bacterial ghosts are cell envelopes derived from Gram-negative bacteria devoid of all cytoplasmic content but preserving immunogenic cell surface structures.

> **DNA vaccines** are composed of bacterial plasmids encoding antigens under the control of strong eukaryotic promoters. Typically, DNA vaccines are injected intramuscularly or intradermally in their naked form and induce antigen-specific humoral and cellular immune responses.

Genetic vaccination

Genetic vaccination is a technology that has emerged in recent years and represents one of the most notable tools under development in the field of vaccinology. In general, DNA vaccines are composed of bacterial plasmids encoding antigens under the control of strong eukaryotic promoters. Typically, DNA vaccines are injected intramuscularly or intradermally in their naked form and induce antigen-specific humoral and cellular immune responses. However, delivery of DNA vaccine plasmids into mammalian cells by intracellular bacteria (bactofection) might allow more specific targeting of a variety of host cells, including professional antigen-presenting cells (APCs) and is amenable for mucosal administration. In most cases, bacteria used as DNA vaccine carriers are attenuated pathogens that can be classified into three categories: extracellular pathogens (some strains of *E. coli*, *Yersinia* spp.); intraphagosomal pathogens (*Salmonella* spp.); and intracytosolic pathogens (*Shigella* spp., *L. monocytogenes*). For example, *Y. enterocolitica* is an extracellular enteropathogen that multiplies in abdominal lymphoid tissue. Normally, the pathogen is resistant to phagocytosis due to the presence of a virulence plasmid-encoding type III secretion system. Nevertheless, a virulence plasmid-cured variant (the lack of the plasmid eliminates the major virulence factors blocking Yersinia phagocytosis) could be phagocytosed by APCs, thus providing a basis for the DNA vaccine delivery. *Salmonella* cells can promote their own uptake into phagocytes and avoid the killing mechanism of phagocytes following internalization. Virulent strains will multiply in the phagosomal compartment. However, attenuated live vaccine carriers of *Salmonella* die there, resulting in release of the DNA vaccine vectors into the phagosome and consecutively from the phagosome via phagosomal leakage into the cytosol. Upon invasion of APCs, *Shigella* spp., unlike *Salmonella* spp., can rapidly escape from endocytic vacuoles to the cytosol of the mammalian cell. Therefore, attenuated vaccine carriers, which are lysed in the cytosol, can deliver the plasmids directly to this intracellular compartment. *L. monocytogenes*, the only Gram-positive carrier for bacterial DNA vaccine, can multiply within the cytosol and disseminate through tissue by intercellular spread. Like the *Shigella*-based vaccine delivery platform, *Listeria* carriers deliver DNA vaccine to the cytosol of a broad spectrum of host cell types. Further, inactivation of *L. monocytogenes* genes involved in invasion led to a reduced ability of the *L. monocytogenes*-based carrier to deliver DNA vaccine. Moreover, most of the bacterial carriers for DNA vaccination are designed to lyse when bacteria enter the host cell. The impaired cell wall synthesis (*Shigella*, *Salmonella*, invasive *E. coli* carriers) and production of a phage lysin (*Listeria*) are the common ways to achieve specific autolysis of the bacteria into the cytosol compartment.

Definitions

Extracellular pathogens: Pathogenic bacteria able to attach to or colonize host cells, eliciting their virulence properties without invading the target cell.
Intraphagosomal pathogens: Pathogenic bacteria that invade the host cell and that have evolved a number of mechanisms to be able to survive phagocytosis.
Intracytosolic pathogens: Pathogenic bacteria that enter host cells entrapped in a membrane-bound compartment from which it is able to escape, reaching the cytosol and surviving intracellularly.

One of the major limiting factors in using bacterial carriers for DNA vaccination is the import of plasmid DNA from the cytosol into the nucleus where the expression takes place. The nuclear membrane represents a significant barrier for efficient gene transfer. Recently, a self-destructing *L. monocytogenes* carrier was used to release translation-competent messenger RNA (mRNA) directly into the cytosol of epithelial cells, macrophages, and human dendritic cells. The transfer of functional mRNA into mammalian cells using a bacterial carrier represents a totally novel delivery system for vaccine development.

Plant vectors

MucoRice

A rice-based oral vaccine (MucoRice) has been receiving global attention as a new form of cold chain-free vaccine, because it is stable at room temperature for a prolonged period. Further, the benefits associated with the use of rice-based vaccine include its delivery route (powder form versus using edible intact plants). This mucosal delivery system is derived from initial work done expressing *Streptococcus mutants* protein antigens on tobacco leaves and the development of edible plant-based vaccines expressing diverse antigens. Initial generation of the oral vaccine included rice-expressing cholera toxin B (CTB) subunit, which effectively induces enterotoxin-neutralizing immunity. A third generation of this rice-based vaccine, MucoRice, has been developed, which expresses a nontoxic double-mutant cholera toxin (dmCT) containing the CTA and CTB toxin subunits. Oral administration of MucoRice-dmCT induced CTB-specific, but not CTA-specific, serum IgG and mucosal IgA antibodies, generating protective immunity against cholera toxin without inducing rice protein-specific antibody responses. Further, results showed that oral MucoRice-CTB can effectively induce CT-specific, neutralizing, serum IgG Ab responses in nonhuman primates, and inducing CTB-specific SIgA-mediated longstanding protection against *V. cholerae*-induced diarrhea or LT-enterotoxigenic *E. coli*-induced diarrhea. MucoRice has the potential to be used as a safe multicomponent vaccine expression system.

Biomaterials: a new generation of vaccine adjuvants and vaccine platforms

Vaccines based on recombinant protein and peptide subunits are increasingly being favored due to their chemical definition and better safety profiles. Compared to live attenuated vaccines that multiply in the vaccinee, "killed" vaccines or recombinant antigens are poorly immunogenic and require coadministration with substances called *adjuvants* to elicit robust immune responses. Most currently used adjuvants are chemically heterogeneous mixtures of plant- or pathogen-derived products, formulations of mineral

Definition

Biomaterials: Materials that are derived from natural sources or chemically synthesized in the laboratory for interaction with biological systems. Biomaterials, owing to their diverse physicochemical and biological properties, can be designed for the following: (1) development of vaccines that can be tailored for sustained antigen release, (2) delivery to specific cell types, and (3) activation of innate immunity.

salts, or emulsions, which suffer from poor definition and have some associated toxicity and reactivity (see Chapter 6 for information on adjuvants). Also, the heterogeneous chemical composition of most adjuvants makes their exact mechanism of action unclear. Even after 80 years of extensive use, the exact mechanism of action for clinically approved adjuvants, such as alum, is still not completely understood. In the past decade, a number of small molecule adjuvants have been developed for potent activation of antigen-presenting cells to elicit robust immune responses; however, none of them have been licensed for clinical use. Therefore, there is an urgent clinical need for vaccine adjuvants that are chemically defined in composition, maximally immunogenic, and minimally reactogenic.

Biomaterials offer an attractive platform for the development of vaccines with excellent chemical homogeneity and the ability to probe and modulate the immune system. The generation of protective immunity after vaccination is dependent on various factors among which antigen availability, delivery of the vaccine to antigen-presenting cells, and activation of innate immunity are the key factors. The versatility in the design and engineering of materials offers a distinct advantage, where the immunobiology of the disease can be mimicked for the optimal induction of effector B- and T-cell responses and immunological memory. A few examples of biomaterials-based vaccination strategies investigated to date include sustained antigen release, targeting of vaccines to dendritic cells, cell-based immunotherapies, polarizing immune responses through cytokine release, and activation of innate immunity. The flexibility in designing and engineering biomaterials on a molecular scale has led to

their application as adjuvants not only for vaccines against infectious diseases but also in immunotherapies for cancer and autoimmune diseases. This section will briefly discuss the application of a few popular biomaterials-based strategies in vaccine development, including aspects such as antigen encapsulation, targeted delivery, and activation of innate immunity. For a detailed understanding of the breadth and scope of the field please refer to the reviews at the end of the chapter.

Strategies for antigen encapsulation and presentation

Vaccine antigens comprise a wide variety of molecules including but not limited to peptides, proteins, DNA, whole cells, and bacterial or viral vectors. In immunotherapies (i.e., therapeutic immunization) for cancer, tumor lysates are often employed as antigens. The choice of an appropriate biomaterial for antigen encapsulation will depend on multiple aspects of the vaccine: the nature of the antigen, the intended rate of release, and the type of immune response desired. A number of natural and synthetic biomaterials have been investigated for antigen encapsulation. The most successful and popular biomaterial for antigen encapsulation has been the biodegradable polymer poly (lactic-co-glycolic acid) (PLGA), which is a clinically approved polymer and is used extensively in the manufacturing of surgical sutures. Antigen-loaded PLGA microparticles (μM [10^{-6} m] in diameter) and nanoparticles (nM [10^{-9} m] in diameter) have shown enhanced vaccination efficiency for a variety of infectious diseases and cancer. It was initially assumed that PLGA enhanced immune responses through sustained release of the antigen similar to the depot effect of alum. However, recent studies have shown that the polymer has immunomodulatory properties, which leads to the maturation of dendritic cells and macrophages. Additionally, a variety of Toll-like receptor (TLR) ligands have also been coencapsulated along with antigens into PLGA matrices for programming the adaptive immune response. Other polymer systems investigated for antigen encapsulation include block copolymers and charged polyelectrolytes. Stimulus-responsive polymers such as the pH-sensitive poly (beta-aminoester), acid degradable polyketals, and polyanhydrides have been developed for the dual purpose of encapsulation and releasing the antigen into the acidic endosomal compartment after uptake by dendritic cells. Antigen encapsulation strategies based on liposomes and micelles have also been investigated for the induction of antibody and cytotoxic T-cell (CTL) responses and delivering DNA to cells. A liposome is a vesicle composed of lipid monomers with a hydrophilic head and a hydrophobic tail, which are oriented such that the hydrophobic head groups are inside the bilayer. The aqueous core of the liposome allows for encapsulation of hydrophilic molecules such as peptides, proteins, and DNA, including TLR agonists such as CpGs. Another highly versatile strategy called *layer-by-layer assembly* uses a sacrificial core template onto which antigens are adsorbed and then coated with several bilayers of polymers. The polymers used have opposite charges at neutral pH, which allows for the deposition of a thin polymer layer over another. Finally, the core templates are dissolved, yielding hollow capsules loaded with antigens. The capsules protect the antigen from premature degradation before being taken by antigen-presenting cells. The capsule surface can be further functionalized with chemical moieties for attaching TLR ligands, antibodies, or other cues for enhanced uptake by dendritic cells and targeted delivery.

A second system of antigen delivery involves multivalent presentation of antigens on material surfaces rather than encapsulation. A multiple antigenic peptide (MAP) display system was developed to improve the poor immunogenicity of subunit peptide vaccines for infectious diseases like malaria and influenza and cancer. In a MAP system, multiple copies of antigenic peptides are simultaneously bound to the α- and ε-amino groups of a nonimmunogenic lysine-based dendritic scaffold. These MAPs promote high avidity and enhanced molecular recognition by immune cells, thereby inducing strong immune responses. Recently, fibrous biomaterials based on short self-assembling peptides have been recognized as powerful immune adjuvants. Their activity is dependent on the physical conjugation of the antigen to the self-assembling domain, which allows multivalent presentation of the antigen and enhanced immunogenicity. The multivalent presentation of antigens on simple self-assembling peptide scaffolds represents an attractive platform for vaccine systems and provides opportunities for further improvements for the delivery of whole protein antigens. Although the mechanism of adjuvant action still remains to be determined, the synthetic nature and chemical definition of self-assembling peptides makes them attractive as immune adjuvants. Other strategies based on multivalent antigen presentation include virus-like particles (VLPs) based on self-assembled synthetic or naturally derived protein capsids, which are highly effective at mimicking natural viruses and inducing powerful immune responses without a potential for infectivity. This approach was used to develop the human papillomavirus vaccine, via expression of VLPs in yeast or insect cells, that was licensed in the mid-2000s.

A few naturally derived biomaterials have also been proposed and tested for vaccine development. Chitosan, a modified natural polysaccharide derived from chitin, a major component of crustacean and insect exoskeleton, is a natural-based cationic polymer. Owing to its high positive charge, chitosan and its variants have been investigated for the encapsulation and delivery of negatively charged antigens such as DNA and viral vectors. Such a strategy causes dendritic cells that take up the DNA or the vector to produce antigen over an extended period of time. Alginate, a heteropolysaccharide derived from seaweed, is another biomaterial which has been investigated for its adjuvant effects via activation of the innate immune system. Alginate hydrogels, containing autologous dendritic cells loaded with antigens, have been shown to be effective carriers for dendritic cell-based vaccines. Taken together, biomaterials, whether natural or synthetic, are attractive for encapsulation of a wide variety of vaccine antigens.

Strategies for antigen delivery

Other aspects of the vaccine such as the delivery route and the tissue or cell type to which the vaccine needs to be delivered are important determinants of vaccine efficacy and will need to be considered for the generation of long-term memory. A number of design strategies have been applied for targeted antigen delivery using biomaterials. Depending on their physicochemical properties, biomaterials can deliver antigens

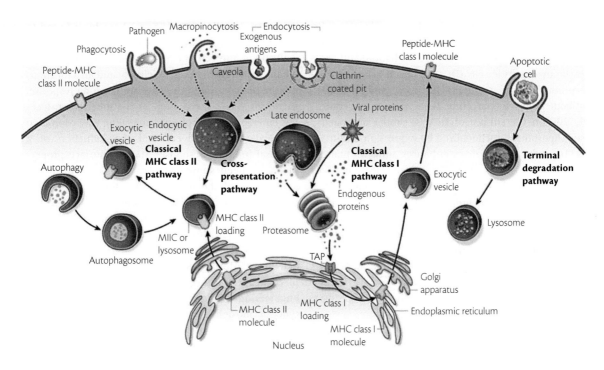

Figure 8.8 A simplified view of antigen presentation by dendritic cells. Left, exogenous particles, proteins or pathogens can be taken into the cell through various pathways, including phagocytosis (for particles >1 μm), macropinocytosis (<1 μm), and endocytosis from caveolae (~60 nm) or clathrin-coated pits (~120 nm). Exogenous antigens are then processed in endocytic vesicles (phagosomes, endosomes, lysosomes and/or endolysosomes; dashed arrows represent multiple vesicular steps). Processed antigen (peptide) is subsequently loaded onto MHC class II molecules (which have been assembled in the endoplasmic reticulum, transported through the Golgi apparatus and targeted to endocytic compartments) in a lysosome or MHC class II compartment (MIIC). The peptide–MHC class II complexes then move through exocytic vesicles to the cell surface, where antigen presentation occurs. MHC class II loading of endogenous antigen provided by autophagy can also occur, particularly when the cell is under stress. Right, antigen can be loaded onto MHC class I molecules through two main pathways. In the classical pathway, endogenous or viral proteins in the cytosol are processed through the proteasome, transported into the endoplasmic reticulum through the molecule TAP (transporter associated with antigen processing), loaded onto MHC class I molecules, and then transported through the Golgi apparatus and exocytic vesicles to the cell surface for presentation. In addition, exogenous antigens that have been phagocytosed, macropinocytosed, or endocytosed can be cross-presented on MHC class I molecules by some subsets of the dendritic cell. In this pathway, antigen either may be loaded in endocytic compartments (not shown) or may escape endosomes and arrive in the cytosol, where it is processed through the proteasome as usual, loaded onto MHC class I molecules and transported to the surface. Finally, terminal degradation pathways can occur (for example, when apoptotic cells are internalized). Reprinted by permission from Macmillan Publishers Ltd: Hubbell JA, Thomas SN, Swartz MA (2009). Materials engineering for immunomodulation. Nature, 462:449–460.

through diverse mechanisms and will be processed differently by the immune system (Figure 8.8). For example, particulate biomaterials like PLGA and polystyrene have been shown to cause phagosomal acidification leading to activation of the inflammasome pathway, similar to alum. Cationic polymers like chitosan can affect tight junctions between epithelial cells and open them transiently to allow an increased paracellular transport of molecules.

Definition

Paracellular transport: The transfer of small molecules across the epithelial barrier by passing through the intercellular space between the cells.

Thus, depending on the antigen delivery needs, the choice of biomaterials will differ. In addition to relying on intrinsic material properties, functionalization of biomaterials with molecules focused on immune recognition, has also been investigated. Enhanced antigen uptake by dendritic cells (DCs) has been achieved by decorating PLGA nanoparticles with anti-DEC205 antibodies and by targeting the endocytic receptor DEC205 on the surface of DCs. A similar approach using liposomes functionalized by expression of anti-CD11c antibody derivatives enhances antigen uptake by CD11c+ DCs. For controlled antigen release in the cytosol after uptake by DCs, acid-degradable materials, based on poly (beta-aminoester), polyketals, and acetylated dextran have been developed. Another simple strategy that has been extensively investigated is the use of antigens encapsulated in or conjugated to biomaterials that are stabilized by disulfide linkages. After uptake, these biomaterials degrade rapidly in the reductive intracellular environment, thereby releasing the antigen.

After antigen uptake, DCs migrate to the secondary lymphoid organs (where the adaptive immune responses are mainly induced) and present the antigens to cognate T cells. Therefore, developing vaccines for delivery to the lymph nodes via lymphatic drainage represents an attractive strategy for the induction of a faster immune response. Targeted antigen delivery to the lymph node has been achieved via simple control of vaccine particle size. Antigen-conjugated, polypropylene sulfide nanoparticles of smaller diameter (approximately 25 nm) have been shown to effectively enter the lymphatic system and concentrate in the lymph nodes, compared to larger nanoparticles (approximately 100 nm).

Definition

Nanoparticle: A particle with dimensions less than or equal to 100 nanometers (100 × 10⁻⁹ meters).

Studies have shown that smaller nanoparticles enter the lymph node via the subcapsular sinus where they are taken up not only by the resident lymphoid DCs, but also macrophages and B cells, thus targeting a broader population of immune cells. Also, in a liposome-based antigen delivery strategy, large diameter liposomes (greater than 225 nm) have been found to induce a Th1-type response whereas small diameter liposomes (smaller than 155 nm) have been found to preferentially induce a Th2-type response. Therefore, controlling the vaccine particle size is an effective means for targeted antigen delivery and also for modulating the polarity of the adaptive immune response. In recent years, vaccination at the mucosal surfaces has emerged as a simple and appealing way compared to needle-based delivery and the induction of a mucosal immune response. Material surface properties have been shown to play a major role in the penetration of the mucosa. The clinically approved hydrophilic polymer poly (ethylene-glycol) (PEG) has been used for surface functionalization of PLGA and polystyrene particles for enhanced mucosal penetration. Thus, the strength of biomaterials as a vaccine delivery platform lies in their inherent and diverse physicochemical properties. Additionally, the ease of engineering existing biomaterials for tissue and cell-type specific delivery of antigens makes them a powerful tool for the development of next generation vaccines.

Nanogels

The application of a relatively new type of nanoparticles (lipobeads), a liposome–hydrogel encapsulating antigen, has shown significant potential as a novel vaccine and immunotherapy delivery system. An appropriate assemblage of spherical hydrogel particles and liposomes combines the properties of both classes of materials and may find a variety of applications, including the development of nanometer-sized (less than 100 nm) bioadhesive polymer hydrogel systems. The nanometer-sized hydrogel (*nanogel*) consists of a cationic type of cholesteryl-group-bearing pullulan (cCHP) forming self-assembly associated polymers as physically cross-linked nanogels in water. However, CHP nanogels can capture proteins inside and form a hydrated nanogel polymer network (nanomatrix), without aggregation, maintaining the native form of the trapped protein. For example, a nontoxic subunit fragment of *Clostridium botulinum* type-A neurotoxin (BoHc/A) can be cross-linked to cCHP nanogel (cCHP-BoHc/A) and administered intranasally, which results in continuous adherence to the nasal epithelium and is demonstrated to be effectively taken up by mucosal dendritic cells after its release from the cCHP nanogel. This application indicates that cCHP nanogel can be used as an alternative universal protein-based antigen-delivery vehicle for adjuvant-free intranasal vaccination.

Strategies for activating innate immunity

It is now well known that most adjuvants act through the stimulation of the innate immune system, which further regulates the adaptive response. This primitive line of defense has evolved to recognize conserved signals called *damage-associated molecular patterns* (DAMPs, associated with tissue damage and inflammation) or *pathogen-associated molecular patterns* (PAMPs, molecules expressed by pathogens of their outer surface). Antigen-presenting cells (such as DCs) express pattern recognition receptors (PRRs) that recognize DAMPs and PAMPs, which subsequently lead to their maturation and expression of co-stimulatory molecules along with antigen processing and presentation. The most studied PRRs are the TLRs. A total of 11 different TLRs have been identified in humans and are found on the surface of DCs and macrophages and in their intracellular compartments. Depending on the TLRs, triggered DCs secrete different cytokine profiles, which in turn control the strength and polarity of the adaptive immune response. Thus, the use of TLR agonists as adjuvants has become one of the most exciting areas of vaccine development at the present time. Other promising potential adjuvants, which include ligands or agonists for alternative families of PRRs such as Nod-like receptors (NLRs) and RIG-I-like receptors (RLRs), are currently under investigation.

In recent years, polymeric biomaterials like PLGA, alginate, and chitosan have been shown to activate TLRs by mimicking PAMPs. DCs and macrophages exposed to biomaterials in culture have shown to upregulate maturation markers; however, the exact mechanism of action is not yet clear. Although the development of novel materials that are strong intrinsic activators of innate immunity is still an emerging field, biomaterials have been used to coencapsulate TLR agonists, along with recombinant antigens, for the induction of robust protective immunity with considerable success. Different strategies have been pursued to evoke synergistic responses while combining antigen loading and delivery with the stimulatory properties of TLR agonists. This has been achieved by either simple mixing and coencapsulation of the

antigen and TLR ligand in a single construct, or encapsulation of the antigen and TLR agonists in separate constructs delivered together, or by physically linking the TLR agonist to the antigen via chemical modifications prior to encapsulation. Activation of TLR3, TLR7, and TLR 9 using a nanoparticle-based delivery system has been shown to induce strong CD4 and CD8 effector T-cell responses. Strong antibody responses have been reported for delivery systems incorporating TLR5 and NALP3 (a member of the NLR family of receptors) agonists. These studies have also observed that combining certain TLR agonists along with antigens also steered the immune responses to a Th1 type. Therefore, it is possible that by incorporating the desired TLR ligand, or a combination of TLR ligands one can modulate the immune response to induce a Th2- or Th17-type depending on the disease target. Recently, a novel approach for the activation of the immune complement using surface-functionalized polypropylene sulfide nanoparticles has also been reported. Nanoparticles with hydroxylated surfaces were shown to result in strong activation of DCs, initiation of the complement cascade. and to elicit robust humoral and cellular responses when compared to nanoparticles with methoxylated surfaces. Synthetic peptide adjuvants based on short self-assembling peptides have also been shown to activate innate immunity. The humoral responses associated with one self-assembling peptide, Q11, have been shown to be myeloid differentiation primary response protein 88 (MyD88)-dependent. It is not yet known if all self-assembling peptides can activate the innate immune system as most of these novel classes of materials are still in their early stages of development.

Conclusions and future directions for biomaterials

Engineered biomaterials have clearly demonstrated success as antigen encapsulation and delivery platforms to enhance the immune response to antigens for a wide variety of diseases. Some biomaterials can also act as immune adjuvants through activation of innate immunity. The ability to engineer materials for antigen encapsulation, targeted delivery, sustained release, and activation of innate immunity present multiple avenues for the development of preventive and therapeutic vaccination strategies. The design and development of immunotherapeutic biomaterials is an emerging field that lies at the intersection of medicine, biology, chemistry, and engineering. We are also are currently limited by our knowledge and understanding of immunobiology, as interactions between immune cells is still a developing area. Open questions with respect to practical aspects of large-scale vaccine production, storage requirements, and booster regimens still need to be addressed. Therefore, as our knowledge of immunobiology and immune activation grows, we can rationally design new biomaterials-based platforms that will form the basis for the next generation of vaccines.

and the use of live attenuated bacteria as delivery system for plasmid DNA has emerged as a promising alternative to overcome many potential pitfalls.

- Natural and synthetic biomaterials with a variety of physicochemical and biological properties are an attractive platform for vaccine development.

- Microparticles and nanoparticles, liposomes, virus-like particles, self-assembling peptides, block copolymers, and polysaccharides have been investigated as platforms and adjuvants for materials-based vaccines.

- The ability to engineer biomaterials for antigen encapsulation, targeted delivery to specific cells and tissues, and activation of innate immunity provides multiple avenues for the development of next generation vaccines.

Summary

- The ease of manipulation of virus genomes by molecular genetics techniques and the efficiency of viruses in infecting host cells and expressing high levels of protein from encoded genes makes them useful as vaccine vectors.

- Following recognition by pattern recognition receptors, most virus vectors induce high levels of innate immunity that provide an intrinsic adjuvant effect and result in a larger, more polyfunctional, and durable adaptive immune response.

- The safety of vaccine vectors can be enhanced by creation of replication defective vectors, modification of the vector genome to prevent recombination, or insertion into the host chromosome and deletion of virus-encoded immune evasion genes to attenuate the vector.

- The molecules binding host cell receptors can be altered or switched for those of related viruses to allow multiple rounds of vaccine boosting in the presence of vigorous immune responses against the initial vaccine.

- The display of protein or peptide antigens with a distinct function at the surface of the Gram-negative or Gram-positive bacterial cell has an increasing impact in many areas of vaccine development.

- Besides many other immunostimulatory components, the bacterial ghost (BG) system is as a potent vaccine delivery system with intrinsic adjuvant properties.

- DNA vaccination represents one of the most notable tools under development in the field of vaccinology,

Further reading

Ali OA and Mooney DJ (2011). Immunologically active biomaterials for cancer therapy. Current Topics in Microbiology and Immunology 344, 279–297.

Atkins GJ, Fleeton MN, and Sheahan BJ (2008). Therapeutic and prophylactic applications of alphavirus vectors. Expert Reviews in Molecular Medicine 10(33), 1–18.

Brun A, Albina E, Barret T, Chapman DAG, Czub M, Dixon LK, Keil GM, Klonjkowski B, Le Potier MF, Libeau G, Ortego J, Richardson J, and Takamatsu HH (2008). Antigen delivery systems for veterinary vaccine development. Viral-vector based delivery systems. Vaccine 26, 6508–6528.

Curtiss R 3rd, Xin W, Li Y, Kong W, Wanda SY, Gunn B, and Wang S (2010). New technologies in using recombinant attenuated Salmonella vaccine vectors. Critical Reviews in Immunology 30, 255–270.

Demento SL, Siefert AL, Bandyopadhyay A, Sharp FA, and Fahmy TM (2011). Pathogen-associated molecular patterns on biomaterials: a paradigm for engineering new vaccines. Trends in Biotechnology 29, 294–306.

Dietrich G, Spreng S, Favre D, Viret JF, and Guzman CA (2003). Live attenuated bacteria as vectors to deliver plasmid DNA vaccines. Current Opinion in Molecular Therapeutics 5, 10–19.

Fujkuyama Y, Tokuhara D, Kataoka K, Gilbert RS, McGhee JR, Yuki Y, Kiyono H, and Fujihashi K (2012). Novel vaccine development strategies for inducing mucosal immunity. Expert Review of Vaccines 11, 367–379.

Hubbell JA, Thomas SN, and Swartz MA (2009). Materials engineering for immunomodulation. Nature 462, 449–460.

Jones KS (2008). Biomaterials as vaccine adjuvants. Biotechnology Progress 24, 807–814.

Langemann T, Koller VJ, Muhammad A, Kudela P, Mayr UB, and Lubitz W (2010). The Bacterial Ghost platform system: production and applications. Bioengineered Bugs 1, 326–336.

Liniger M, Zuniga A, and Naim HY (2007). Use of viral vectors for the development of vaccines. Expert Review of Vaccines 6, 255–266.

Liu MA (2010). Immunologic basis of vaccine vectors. Immunity 33, 504–515.

Löfblom J (2011). Bacterial display in combinatorial protein engineering. Biotechnology Journal 6, 1115–1129.

Ofek I, Hasty DL, and Sharon N (2003). Anti-adhesion therapy of bacterial diseases: prospects and problems. FEMS Immunology and Medical Microbiology 38, 181–191.

Ottenhoff TH and Kaufmann SH (2012). Vaccines against tuberculosis: where are we and where do we need to go? PLoS Pathogens 8, e1002607.

Rollier CS, Reyes-Sandoval A, Cottingham MG, Ewer K, and Hill AVS (2011). Viral vectors as vaccine platforms: deployment in sight. Current Opinion in Immunology 23, 377–382.

Swartz MA, Hirosue S, and Hubbell JA (2012). Engineering approaches to immunotherapy. Science Translational Medicine 4, 148rv9.

Walsh SR and Dolin R (2011). Vaccinia viruses: vaccines against smallpox and vectors against infectious diseases and tumors. Expert Review of Vaccines 10(8), 1221–1240.

9 Licensed vaccines for humans

Alan D.T. Barrett

Departments of Pathology and Microbiology & Immunology, Director, Sealy Center for Vaccine Development, University of Texas Medical Branch, Galveston, TX, USA

Abbreviations

APC	Antigen-presenting cells		IPV	Inactivated polio vaccine
att	Attenuated		LF	Lethal factor
AVA	Anthrax vaccine adsorbed		MenB	*Neisseria meningitidis* serotype B
AVP	Anthrax vaccine precipitated		MVS	Master vaccine strain
BEI	Binary ethylene-imine		NA	Neuraminidase
BPL	Beta-propiolactone		NAD	Neisserial adhesin A
ca	Cold adapted		NHBA	Neisseria heparin binding antigen
CVJE	ChimeriVax-Japanese encephalitis		OMPC	Outer membrane protein
DTP	Diphtheria, tetanus, and pertussis		OMV	Outer membrane vesicles
E	Envelope		OPV	Oral polio vaccine
EF	Edema factor		ORF	Open reading frame
fHBP	Factor H binding protein		PA	Protective antigen
GM-CSF	Granulocyte-macrophage colony-stimulating factor		PAP	Prostatic acid phosphatase
			PBMC	Peripheral blood mononuclear cells
HA	Hemagglutinin		prM	Premembrane
HBsAg	Hepatitis B surface antigen		PRP	Polyribosyl-ribitol-phosphate
HEV	Hepatitis E virus		SC	Subcutaneous
Hib	*Haemophilus influenzae* type b		ts	Temperature sensitive
HPV	Human papillomavirus		VAPP	Vaccine-associated paralytic poliomyelitis
ID	Intradermal			
IM	Intramuscular		VLP	Virus-like particle
IN	Intranasal		YFV	Yellow fever virus

Introduction

This chapter provides information on each type of vaccine that has been developed and licensed for use in humans. The description of the vaccines is not exhaustive but provides information on those that have been used in different countries. It should be noted that the exact formulation, immunization dosing regimen, and recommendations will vary depending on decisions made by national regulatory authorities and national ministries of health. Chapter 10 describes veterinary vaccines. Note that there are many more vaccines for animals than humans due in part to the need to demonstrate long-term safety in

Vaccinology: An Essential Guide, First Edition. Edited by Gregg N. Milligan and Alan D.T. Barrett.
© 2015 John Wiley & Sons, Ltd. Published 2015 by John Wiley & Sons, Ltd.

humans prior to licensure and that the requirements for licensure in humans are continually being increased by regulatory authorities because of advances in science.

Immunization strategies

Immunization

The terms *immunization* and *vaccination* are often used interchangeably and refer to the process where the host immune system is exposed to molecules that are foreign to the host (termed *nonself*). The nonself molecule is considered an immunogen if it stimulates an immune response. Active immunization is where the immunogen stimulates the immune system to produce antibodies and/or T cells. Traditionally active immunization is induced by live or inactivated vaccines (see Table 9.1 for a definition) but in the past 50 years major advances have been made in subunit vaccines. (Table 9.2 shows examples of diseases where we have successful vaccines today). The immune system remembers the foreign agent due to the host memory immune response, which involves stimulation of memory B and T cells (an adaptive immune response), such that when the immune system is subsequently exposed to the foreign agent it can rapidly develop a protective immune response against the foreign agent. This normally consists of induction of antibodies and T-cell responses and is described in detail in Chapter 5.

Immunization

- Prophylactic or therapeutic
- Active or passive

Immunization is normally associated with the process where the host induces a memory immune response prior to seeing the foreign agent by administration of an immunogen. This is termed *prophylactic immunization*. Such immunization is normally given to healthy people who can "trigger" or "induce" a good immune response, but in recent years immunization is now also targeted at those who have an impaired immune system due to either very young (individuals who do not have a mature functioning immune

Table 9.1 Definitions of Different Types of Vaccines

- **Live attenuated vaccines**: An organism whose virulence for humans is reduced by adaptation to a different host; can be cells or different animal. Gives protective immunity after one or a few doses.
- **Inactivated vaccines**: Chemically or heat-inactivated organisms that induce protective immunity after multiple immunizations.
- **Toxoid vaccines**: Toxins produced by bacteria that have been inactivated (e.g., formalin) to avoid toxic effects while producing a protective immune response.
- **Polysaccharide vaccines**: Purified sugar molecules taken from the surface of selected bacteria that can stimulate the immune system to generate antibodies.
- **Conjugate vaccines** (also termed *polysaccharide–protein conjugate vaccines* or *glycoconjugate vaccines*): Second-generation polysaccharide vaccines that enhance the immunogenicity of capsular polysaccharides by conjugation (chemical linking) of the polysaccharide to protein carriers.
- **Recombinant vaccines**: Specific immunogens, usually surface proteins from viruses that are often expressed as virus-like particles, shown to stimulate the major components of the antimicrobe immune response.
- **DNA vaccines**: Naked DNA encoding one or a few genes with no proteins. None have been licensed for humans but a few have been licensed for veterinary use.
- **Single-round infectious particle vaccines**: These lack a complete genome and so only go through one round of replication and hence cannot produce infectious particles. Currently in clinical development.

system) or old age (due to immunosenescence), immunocompromised (the lack of a completely functioning immune system), or immunosuppressed (the immune system is incapacitated due to a drug treatment regimen, e.g., transplant patients).

Therapeutic immunization refers to immunization of individuals who already have the clinical condition for which the vaccine is to be used. The objective is to eliminate, manage, or reduce the clinical condition. For example, many individuals are infected with varicella virus when they are children and may get the disease chickenpox. Once infected with the varicella virus, the virus remains dormant in dorsal root ganglia and may reactivate later in life to cause shingles (also known as *zoster*). Administration of the varicella

Table 9.2 Examples of Licensed Vaccines

Live attenuated vaccines	Viruses: Adenovirus types 4 and 7 (US military only), chickenpox/zoster, hepatitis A (China only), influenza, Japanese encephalitis, measles, mumps, polio, rotavirus, rubella, smallpox and yellow fever Bacteria: *Mycobacterium bovis* BCG (tuberculosis) and *Salmonella typhi* (typhoid)
Inactivated vaccines	Viruses: Hepatitis A, influenza, Japanese encephalitis, poliovirus, rabies, and tick-borne encephalitis Bacteria: *Salmonella typhi* (typhoid) and *Vibrio cholerae* (cholera)
Toxoid vaccines	*Bordetella pertussis* (pertussis), *Clostridium tetani* (tetanus), and *Corynebacterium diphtheriae* (diphtheria)
Recombinant viral vaccines	Hepatitis B, hepatitis E (China only), human papillomavirus, and influenza
Polysaccharide vaccines	*Streptococcus pneumonia* (pneumonia), *Neisseria meningitides* (meningitis), and *Salmonella enteroritica* serovar typhi (typhoid)
Conjugate vaccines	*Corynebacterium diphtheriae* (diphtheria), *Haemophilus influenzae* type b (Hib), *Neisseria meningitidis* (meningitis), and *Streptococcus pneumoniae* (pneumonia)

vaccine to those over the age of 50 can help prevent or lessen episodes of shingles.

Prophylactic immunization

Active immunization
- To stimulate an immune response following administration of an "immunogen"

Passive immunization
- To provide short-term protection against infection or clinical condition
  - Antibodies – monoclonal or polyclonal
  - For example, CytoGam® licensed for prophylaxis against Cytomegalovirus after transplantation
- Hypersensitivity – also known as "serum sickness"

Table 9.3 Examples of Immunoglobulins Available for Passive Immunization

Clostridium botulinum (botulinum; antitoxin)
Cytomegalovirus
Corynebacterium diphtheriae (diphtheria antitoxin)
Hepatitis A
Hepatitis B
Rabies
Respiratory syncytial virus[a]
Respiratory syncytial virus (monoclonal antibody)[a]
Clostridium tetani (tetanus antitoxin)
Vaccinia
Varicella zoster

[a]Both a monoclonal antibody and an immunoglobulin are available for respiratory syncytial virus

Passive immunization

There are many diseases for which no active vaccines are available. In this situation, passive immunization is sometimes used to provide short-term protection against infection or a particular clinical condition. This is where presynthesized elements of the immune system are transferred to a person so that the body does not need to produce these elements itself. Passive immunization most often involves the administration of antibodies, either polyclonal or monoclonal, by the intravenous or intramuscular routes. This method of immunization begins to work very quickly (within 48 hours), but it is short-lived (no more than 3–6 months), because the antibodies are naturally broken down by the liver, and if there are no B cells to produce more antibodies, they will disappear. Table 9.3 provides examples of immunoglobulins available. Most are polyclonal and derived from people who have antibodies to the particular microbe. Monoclonal antibodies are now being used for passive immunization. The first one licensed was a monoclonal antibody against respiratory syncytial virus.

Currently, there are clinical trials for immunotherapy where autologous peripheral blood mononuclear cells are activated against a particular antigen. The section on personalized vaccines provides information on the first licensed immunotherapy for prostate cancer.

In addition to artificial passive immunization described above, the body also undertakes natural passive immunization when antibodies are transferred from mother to fetus by crossing the placenta during pregnancy to protect the fetus before and shortly after birth.

Active immunization

Active immunization refers to the induction of an immune response following administration of an "immunogen." A vaccine immunogen takes different forms from live attenuated, to inactivated, to subunit vaccines (see Table 9.1 for definitions of different vaccine types). Each type of vaccine induces differential stimulation of antibody and cellular immune responses. These are summarized in Figure 9.1.

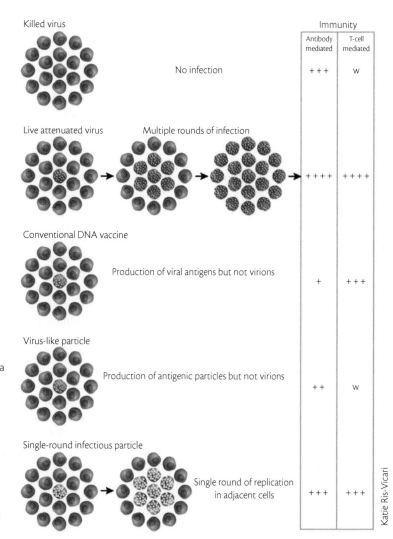

Figure 9.1 Comparison of the mechanisms associated with different vaccination strategies. Whereas immunization with killed virus elicits mainly antibody-mediated immunity and delivery of conventional DNA vaccines confers primarily cell-mediated immunity, a "split-genome" DNA construct generates single-round infectious particles that generate both humoral and cell-mediated protection almost as potent as the response to a live attenuated virus. Single-round infectious particles eliminate concerns about the safety of infection with live attenuated viruses w, weak response. (From Barrett, AD [2008]. Flavivirus DNA vaccine with a kick. Nature Biotechnology 26, 525–526.)

155

Live attenuated (or weakened) vaccines are based on organisms whose virulence for the natural host is reduced by adaptation to a different host. This can be due to passage in cells (e.g., *Mycobacterium bovis* Bacillus Calmette–Guérin [BCG] in potato medium) or in an animal species that is not normally a host for the organism (e.g., yellow fever 17D vaccine in embryonated chicken eggs). A live attenuated vaccine can give protective immunity after one or few doses due to stimulation of both B- (antibody) and T-cell responses. In comparison, inactivated (or killed) vaccines, often chemically (e.g., formalin, beta-propiolactone [BPL], binary ethylene-imine [BEI]), or heat-inactivated, induce protective immunity after multiple immunizations and induce an antibody response with a weak T cell response. Consequently, live attenuated vaccines are often considered to be better immunogens than inactivated vaccines. However, the major question for all live attenuated vaccines is their safety. Do they have any residual virulence? Since there are examples of incomplete attenuation of live vaccines, inactivated vaccines are often considered to be safer than live vaccines as there is very little risk of residual virulence if the activation process is undertaken correctly. In addition to the vaccine immunogen, other components in a vaccine formulation (termed *excipients*) may raise questions over safety, including chemicals used to stabilize a vaccine. Overall, all vaccines must maximize both long-term immunogenicity and safety to give a licensed product that is approved for use in humans.

Maternal immunization

Maternal immunization describes immunization during pregnancy to protect pregnant women and fetuses or infants. In recent years this has become a very active area for immunizations due to the significant opportunities to protect both the mother and fetus. In addition, administration of nonlive vaccines during pregnancy provides passive protection to the baby via transfer of vaccine-induced immunoglobulin across the placenta. Clearly, live vaccines are contraindicated for pregnant women due to the potential risk of reversion to virulence, but studies with a number on nonlive vaccines have shown that immunization is as effective in pregnant women as women who are not pregnant. Currently, there are recommendations for using only a few vaccines in pregnant women,

including inactivated influenza (not the live influenza vaccine), pertussis, diphtheria, and tetanus. Maternal and neonatal tetanus is worthy of specific mention. This disease particularly affects those in the poorest countries, and the tetanus toxoid vaccine is extremely effective. As such, the World Health Organization has a program to eliminate neonatal tetanus.

In addition, following birth, postpartum women can receive all vaccines recommended by the national authorities that were not administered during pregnancy (e.g., live vaccines).

Cocooning (maternal and family/household vaccination)

Most vaccines cannot be given to newborns, and the immune system of infants younger than 6 months of age is not mature or developed enough to produce antibodies against many infectious diseases. Thus, cocooning (also known as the *Cocoon Strategy*) is a vaccination strategy that aims to protect newborn infants by administering vaccines to mothers, family members, and any individuals who could come into regular contact with the newborn infant. Thus a vaccination ring, or cocoon, is established around the newborn infant where the vaccinated individuals are both protected from getting the infectious disease and passing it to the infant. The best-known example of this strategy is to protect newborn infants from becoming infected with *Bordetella pertussis* (whooping cough) by administering the combination tetanus, diphtheria, and acellular pertussis (Tdap) booster vaccine to mothers, family members, and any individuals who could come into regular contact with the newborn infant. The same strategy can also be used for influenza.

Ring immunization

Ring immunization is the identification, immunization, and quarantine of all contacts of cases and the contacts of contacts. This regimen was successfully used to enable the elimination and ultimately the eradication of smallpox.

Booster immunizations

The ideal vaccine should give lifelong protection after one dose. Only a few vaccines achieve this goal (e.g., yellow fever). Other vaccines need booster doses to maintain protective immunity. This may take the form of a series of doses to give the initial protective immune response, and/or it may take the form of a booster dose after a certain period of time to maintain protective immunity (e.g., rabies).

Cell culture used to prepare vaccines

Bacteria multiply in liquid or solid media whereas viruses multiply inside cells. Very few cell culture substrates have been approved to prepare virus vaccines because of the need to ensure the cells are free from contamination that may potentially be administered with the vaccine, and thereby leading to a clinical condition. This includes components of some nonhuman cell types that may have the potential to lead to reactogenicity if they are included in vaccine formulations. Examples of cell substrates approved to prepare virus vaccines include WI-38 human diploid (cells with a finite life span and passaged in tissue culture) lung fibroblasts, MRC-5 human fetal diploid fibroblasts, primary chick embryo fibroblasts, embryonated chicken eggs, primary hamster kidney cells, Madin–Darby canine kidney, and African green monkey kidney Vero cells. Specific virus vaccines are only approved to be produced in particular cell types shown to be free of adventitious agents (see Table 9.4).

Vaccine excipients

These are the substances that are included with the vaccine immunogen in a dose of vaccine. They often include the adjuvant (for nonlive vaccines), preservatives, stabilizers, and possibly trace materials from the process used to manufacture the vaccine. Such trace materials include the medium used to grow a bacterial vaccine or cell components for viral vaccines (e.g., egg proteins from vaccines produced in eggs), and the chemical used to inactivate a killed vaccine. Note that the manufacturing process involves steps to remove the materials described above such that only trace amounts are found in the final product. National regulatory authorities set limits on the quantity of nucleic acid (DNA and RNA) and protein that can be included in a vaccine.

Hypersensitivity

Hypersensitivity refers to the rare occasions where reactogenicity is produced by the normal immune system. For active immunization this is due to sensitivity to one of the vaccine components. The best known example is reactogenicity to vaccines produced in chicken eggs or chicken cells because of sensitivity to egg proteins. For passive immunization, reactogenicity can be to those particular immunoglobulins that are derived from a nonhuman origin, e.g., some antitoxin antibodies.

Route of administration

Induction of protective immunity requires that the vaccine protect against natural infection. The route of natural infection and target tissue/organ varies for different infectious diseases. The major routes for the digestive, respiratory, nervous, or liver systems are respiratory, fecal–oral, and skin lesions, and tropism. Consequently, the route of administration of the vaccine is important as it must induce an immune response after administration that will protect from disease, and hopefully infection by the microbe via its normal route of entry. Vaccines tend to be given either by the oral (e.g., live polio, adenovirus and rotavirus, BCG, plus inactivated cholera and live/polysaccharide typhoid), respiratory (intranasal: live influenza), or parenteral (most vaccines, e.g., diphtheria, measles, killed influenza, killed polio, etc.) routes. For the oral and respiratory routes of administration, the goal is to mimic the natural route of infection and induce a mucosal immune response. Currently, the measles vaccine is given by the subcutaneous (SC) route but an aerosol-based measles vaccine is undergoing clinical evaluation since the disease is spread by aerosol. For the parenteral route, vaccines are given by the intramuscular (IM), SC, and intradermal (ID) (sometimes referred to as *transdermal immunization*) routes. Smallpox vaccine is unique in that it is given by scarification. There is much interest in using ID administration as it results in stimulation of dendritic cells, which are often the first line of defense and stimulate both the innate and adaptive immune responses. However, ID administration requires a skilled vaccinator to avoid SC or IM administration (i.e., the depth of the needle). To overcome this problem, a number of devices have been developed that ensure the needle goes to the correct depth in the skin for ID administration. Although the costs of the devices are decreasing, they are often more expensive than the vaccine that they administer, and this has limited the use of these devices. Table 9.4 shows the route of administration of commonly used vaccines.

Table 9.4 Number of Doses and Route of Administration for Commonly Used Vaccines

Vaccine Type	Infectious Agent	Production	Route of Administration	Primary Immunization Regimen
Live virus	Adenovirus types 4 and 7	WI-38 human-diploid fibroblast cell culture	Oral	One dose
	Chickenpox/ herpes zoster (shingles)	MRC-5 cells	Prevention of chickenpox: SC Prevention of herpes zoster (shingles) in individuals 50 years of age and older: SC	One dose
	Influenza	Allantoic fluid of embryonated chicken eggs	IN	One dose
	Japanese encephalitis	Primary hamster kidney cell culture (SA14-14-2) and African green monkey (Vero) cells (Chimerivax-Japanese encephalitis)	SC	One dose
	Measles	Chick embryo cell culture	SC	One dose
	Mumps	Chick embryo cell culture	SC	One dose
	Polio	African green monkey (Vero) or primary monkey kidney cells	Oral	Three doses
	Rotavirus	African Green monkey kidney (Vero) cells	Oral	Two or three doses, depending on particular vaccine
	Rubella	WI-38 human diploid lung fibroblasts or MRC-5	SC	One dose
	Smallpox	African Green monkey kidney (Vero) cells	Percutaneous (scarification) using 15 jabs of a bifurcated needle	One dose
	Yellow fever	Embryonated chicken eggs	SC	One dose
Live bacterium	*Mycobacterium bovis* BCG (tuberculosis)	NA	Pericutaneous	One dose
	Salmonella typhi (typhoid)	NA	Oral	Four doses
Inactivated virus	Hepatitis A	MRC-5 human diploid cells	IM	Two doses

Table 9.4 (*Continued*)

Vaccine Type	Infectious Agent	Production	Route of Administration	Primary Immunization Regimen
	Hepatitis E	*E. coli*	IM	Three doses
	Influenza	Allantoic fluid of embryonated chicken eggs, or Madin–Darby canine kidney (MDCK) cells	IM	One dose
	Japanese encephalitis	African Green monkey kidney (Vero) cells	IM	Two doses
	Polio	African Green monkey kidney (Vero) cells	IM or SC	Three doses
	Rabies	MRC-5 human diploid cells, or primary chick embryo fibroblasts	IM	Preexposure: two or four doses, depending on the vaccine Postexposure: Four or five doses. Some patients receive human rabies immune globulin (HRIG), 20–30 IU per kg body weight, or equine rabies immune globulin (ERIG), 40 IU per kg body weight, at the time of the first dose
	Tick-borne encephalitis	Chick embryo fibroblast cells	IM	Two (travelers) or three (endemic areas) doses
	Vibrio cholera (cholera)	NA	Oral	Two doses
	Salmonella typhi (typhoid)	Cell surface Vi polysaccharide extracted from *Salmonella typhi* Ty2 strain	IM	One dose
Acellular bacterium	*Bacillus anthracis* (anthrax)	NA	IM or SC	Three or four doses
	Bordetella pertussis	IM	IM	Three doses
Toxoid bacterium	*Corynebacterium diphtheriae* (diphtheria)	NA	IM	Three doses
	Clostridium tetani (tetanus)	NA	IM	Three doses

(*Continued*)

Table 9.4 (*Continued*)

Vaccine Type	Infectious Agent	Production	Route of Administration	Primary Immunization Regimen
Polysaccharide bacterium	*Neisseria meningitidis* (A, C, W135, and Y)	NA	IM	Three doses
	Streptococcus pneumoniae	NA	IM	Three doses
	Salmonella enterica serovar Typhi (typhoid)	Cell surface Vi polysaccharide extracted from *Salmonella enterica* serovar Typhi, S typhi Ty2 strain	IM	One dose
Conjugate bacterium	*Haemophilus influenzae* type b (Hib)	NA	IM	Three dose
	Neisseria meningitidis (A, C, W135, and Y)	NA	IM	Two doses
	Streptococcus pneumoniae	NA	IM	Three doses
Subunit virus	Hepatitis B	*adw* subtype of hepatitis B surface antigen (HBsAg) produced in yeast cells	IM	Three doses
	Hepatitis E	*E. coli*	IM	Three doses
	HPV types 16 and 18	L1 proteins are produced in separate bioreactors using the recombinant baculovirus expressed L1 protein in *Trichoplusia ni* insect cells	IM	Three doses
	HPV types 6, 11, 16, and 18	L1 proteins are produced by separate fermentations in recombinant *Saccharomyces cerevisiae* and self-assembled into VLPs	IM	Three doses
	Influenza	Purified HA proteins produced in a continuous insect cell line (*expres*SF+®) that is derived from Sf9 cells of the fall armyworm, *Spodoptera frugiperda*	IM	One dose
	Neisseria meningitidis (B)	*E. coli*	IM	Two or three doses

IM, intramuscular; IN, intranasal; NA, not applicable, SC: subcutaneous.

Dosing regimen

The number of doses of a vaccine required to induce an initial protective immune response varies according to a number of factors, including live or inactivated/subunit vaccine, the quantity of vaccine in a dose, route of administration, and whether or not an adjuvant is used. Live vaccines often require only one dose while inactivated/subunit vaccines may need 2–6 doses depending on the number and quality of the immunogen(s) incorporated in the vaccine. Table 9.4 shows the number of doses needed to give a protective immune response for commonly used vaccines.

Mucosal-based vaccines

In addition to the infectious disease vaccines delivered by the oral and respiratory routes described above (see Table 9.4), there are noninfectious disease vaccines licensed in Europe that stimulate mucosal immunity. Anti-allergy vaccines have been licensed in Scandinavia and France for birch pollen, cat allergen, Timothy grass, and for grass pollen and dust mites in Russia. These are the first anti-allergy vaccines to be marketed and it is likely that other anti-allergen vaccines will be licensed in the future.

Specific vaccine types

Table 9.5 shows the characteristics of the ideal vaccine. Not surprisingly, a vaccine that is safe with no reactogenicity protects 100% of vaccinees against the disease after one dose for their entire life is a very tough goal. Nonetheless, there are approximately 30 diseases that are controlled by 40–50 vaccines. A

Table 9.5 Characteristics of an Ideal Vaccine

- Protective immune response: Gives life-long immunity
- Dosing regimen: One dose induces protective immunity
- Safety: No side effects
- Stability: Retains biological activity for a long time at different temperatures
- Ease of administration: Can be coadministered with other vaccines at one visit
- Manufacture: Can be easily scaled-up and at low cost

Table 9.6 Different Types of Vaccines

- Live attenuated vaccines
- Inactivated vaccines
- Toxoid vaccines
- Polysaccharide vaccines
- Conjugate vaccines
- Recombinant vaccines

number of strategies (see Table 9.6) have been utilized to develop specific vaccines based in part on the disease caused by the microbe. The sections below describe the different types of vaccines that have been developed and provide examples of common infectious diseases.

Live attenuated vaccines

These vaccines consist of weakened viruses or bacteria that multiply in the host and stimulate strong cellular and antibody responses similar to those induced by the natural disease. They are organisms whose virulence for humans was reduced by adaptation to a different host, which can be cells (viruses), media (bacteria), or different animal models. They usually give protective immunity after one or a few doses. Examples include BCG, cholera, polio, rotavirus, and typhoid (oral), influenza (intranasal), measles, mumps, rubella, smallpox, varicella, and yellow fever. A live hepatitis A vaccine is available in China only. It should be noted that in most situations the wild-type infectious agent will stimulate the immune system to induce lifelong immunity against the specific infectious disease while live vaccines stimulate long-term immunity that may be lifelong (e.g., yellow fever) or not (e.g., measles). Thus, for some live vaccines, booster doses are needed to maintain protective immunity years after the initial immunization, while other vaccines require two doses to provide an initial protective immune response (e.g., rotavirus).

Despite the advantages of live attenuated vaccines, there are some downsides. All organisms are naturally mutating, and the organisms used in live attenuated vaccines are no different. The remote possibility exists that an attenuated organism in the vaccine could revert to a virulent form and cause disease. This is a very rare event as live vaccine organisms have been attenuated by adapting to a nonhuman host. Nonetheless, continued testing of live vaccines for genetic stability and safety testing, including animals, is important for all live vaccines. Also, not everyone can safely receive live attenuated vaccines. For their own protection, individuals who are immunocompromised or immunosuppressed should not normally be given live vaccines. Recommendations on who should and who should not receive a live vaccine are vaccine specific and depend on many criteria. Table 9.7 shows typical considerations when deciding who should receive a live vaccine.

Another limitation is that live attenuated vaccines usually need to be refrigerated to stay potent, and excipients are added to maintain stability. A live vaccine may not be the best choice if the vaccine needs to be shipped overseas and stored by health care workers in developing countries where the ambient temperature is high and there is a lack of widespread refrigeration.

Table 9.7 Conditions That May Affect Whether or Not to Receive a Live Vaccine

(Note that any decision will be vaccine-specific such that a decision to not give a particular live vaccine may not preclude an individual from receiving a different live vaccine.)

Immunosuppression
- Acquired immunodeficiency syndrome or other symptomatic manifestations of human immunodeficiency virus (HIV) infection. (Note, asymptomatic individuals may be able to receive a vaccine).
- Leukemia, lymphoma, thymic disease, generalized malignancy.
- Individuals whose immunologic responses are suppressed by drug therapy, e.g., corticosteroids (often considered with respect to greater than the standard dose of topical or inhaled steroids), alkylating drugs, or antimetabolites.
- Radiation therapy.
- Individuals who have had transplantation and may be immunosuppressed.
- Individuals receiving tumor necrosis factor (TNF)-α inhibitors, and interleukin (IL)-1 blockers and monoclonal antibodies targeting immune cells.
- Individuals who have received systemic corticosteroids for 14 days or more; it may be advisable to delay vaccination until at least 1 month after completing the course.

Hypersensitivity
- Allergy to vaccine components.
- Serious hypersensitivity reactions (e.g., anaphylaxis) after a previous vaccine administration.
- Reaction to eggs or chicken proteins if the live vaccine is produced in eggs or chick embryo cell culture.
- Reaction to antibiotics that may be in a vaccine dose, e.g., kanamycin and/or erythromycin.
- Chronic disease such as asthma or other breathing disorder, diabetes, kidney disease, or blood cell disorder such as anemia.
- History of seizures.

Age
- Infants or the elderly may be excluded due to weakened immune responses.

Current severe febrile illness and/or a compromised general health state
- Immunization may be delayed until the individual has recovered.

Pregnancy
- Normally live vaccines are not given to pregnant women, unless under epidemiological emergency circumstances, following express recommendations from the health authorities.
- Some vaccines can cause abnormal effects on the fetus.

Traditionally, live attenuated vaccines have proven easy to generate for certain viruses, particularly viruses with RNA genomes due to the higher mutation frequency of their RNA-dependent RNA polymerase compared to viruses with DNA genomes and their DNA-dependent DNA polymerase (e.g., herpesviruses), which have very low mutation frequencies. Virus-based vaccines often contain 10^5 or less infectious units of virus per dose of vaccine. Live attenuated vaccines are more difficult to generate for bacteria than viruses. Bacteria have thousands of genes, which are all DNA, and thus are much harder to manipulate to generate a stable live attenuated phenotype. The live attenuated typhoid vaccine, *Salmonella typhi* Ty21a strain, was generated by chemical mutagenesis of parental virulent strain of *Salmonella typhi* Ty21. This vaccine is licensed in some countries, but not the USA, and is given orally using gelatin capsules, which are coated with an organic solution to render them resistant to dissolution in stomach acid. Each enteric-coated capsule of the vaccine contains about $2–7 \times 10^9$ colony-forming units of bacteria. Live bacterial vaccines typically contain more than 10^9 colony-forming units per dose of vaccine.

Virus reassortment

The development of cell culture to grow organisms was critical for approaches that gave rise to live attenuated vaccines. Subsequently, cell culture was used for reassortment of gene segments for those viruses that had their genome divided between multiple segments rather than containing the entire genetic information in one piece of RNA. The genome of influenza virus has 8 segments of single-stranded RNA while that of rotavirus has 11 segments of double-stranded RNA. Genetic reassortment takes place when a single cell is infected with more than one virus (see Figure 9.2). The gene segments from different viruses can segregate independently and the new "reassortant" viruses produced from that cell can contain genes from either parent resulting in multiple strains that are different from the initial ones.

Live attenuated virus vaccines for strains of type A and type B influenza were developed by serial passage in chick embryo fibroblasts at 25 °C until they became "cold adapted" (ca). Briefly, they multiply efficiently at 25 °C, a temperature that does not allow replication of many wild-type influenza viruses, and conversely they are temperature sensitive (ts) (i.e., they are limited in replication at 37 °C or above, the temperature of humans and at which many wild-type influenza viruses multiply efficiently). Further, they have an attenuated (att) phenotype when tested in humans and in animal models, such as the ferret model of human influenza infection. At least five genetic loci in three different internal gene segments contribute to the ts and att phenotypes of the type A influenza master vaccine strain (MVS) while at least three genetic loci in two different internal gene segments contribute to both the ts and att properties; for the type B influenza master strain, five genetic loci in three gene segments control the ca property. Thus, the combined ca, ts, and att phenotypes are multigenic, and the chance of reversion to virulence is very low and has not been seen in vaccinees.

Influenza vaccine: low or high dose, one dose or two, adjuvant or no adjuvant?

More manufacturers produce influenza vaccine than any other vaccine, in part because people need to be immunized each year and the wide age range for the vaccine. The goal is to immunize children, adults and senior citizens. As such, the vaccine is being tailored to each population.

The routine inactivated vaccine for adults given by the intramuscular route is trivalent or quadrivalent and consists of 15 μg of each virus HA component (i.e., 3×15 μg or 4×15 μg) given as a one dose vaccine. A vaccine given by the intradermal route has also been developed and this contains less HA per dose (3×9 μg). Senior citizens often have an immune system that is not as effective as that in younger adults below the age of 65, because of immunosenesence. Consequently, a single, high-dose vaccine (3×60 μg) has been developed for persons aged 65 years and older that gives a superior immune response to the routine adult vaccine. The recently licensed recombinant HA vaccine produced in insect cells contains more HA than the inactivated vaccines (3×45 μg). Some influenza vaccines are adjuvanted (e.g., alum, MF59, or virosomes) while others have no adjuvant. Finally, young children are given two doses of the routine inactivated vaccine.

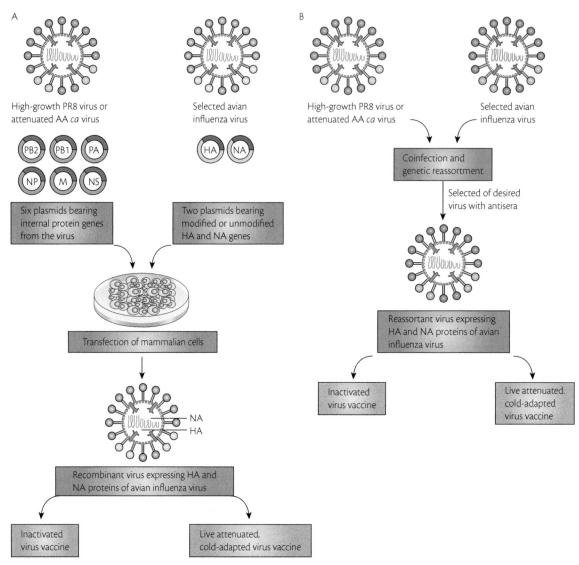

Figure 9.2 The eight-plasmid reverse-genetics system. Generation of recombinant vaccines for pandemic influenza. (a) Six plasmids encoding the internal proteins of the high-growth influenza A/Puerto Rico/8/34 (PR8) donor virus or the attenuated, cold-adapted (ca) H2N2 A/Ann Arbor/6/60 (AA) donor virus are cotransfected with two plasmids encoding the avian influenza virus haemagglutinin (HA; modified to remove virulence motifs, if necessary) and neuraminidase (NA) glycoproteins into qualified mammalian cells and the recombinant virus is then isolated. Recombinant viruses containing internal protein genes from the PR8 virus are used to prepare inactivated influenza virus vaccines. Recombinant viruses containing internal protein genes from the attenuated, cold-adapted AA virus are used to prepare live attenuated influenza virus vaccines. (b) The generation of pandemic influenza vaccine viruses by classical reassortment. The reassortant viruses derive six internal protein genes from the vaccine donor virus and the HA and NA genes from the circulating avian influenza virus. The reassortant virus is selected using antisera specific for the HA and NA glycoproteins of the donor virus. M, matrix protein; NP, nucleoprotein; NS, nonstructural protein; PA, polymerase acidic protein; PB, polymerase basic protein. (From Subbarao K and Joseph T [2007]. Scientific barriers to developing vaccines against avian influenza viruses. Nature Reviews Immunology 7, 267–278.)

Vaccine strains are prepared by the reassortment of gene segments from an MVS and a putative epidemic strain (see Figure 9.2). The six internal gene segments responsible for ca, ts, and att phenotypes are derived from an MVS, and the two segments that encode the two major immunogens of the virus, hemagglutinin (HA) and neuraminidase (NA), are from the putative epidemic strain such that the vaccine induces a protective immune response against the epidemic strain. A major concern for generation of reassortants is that such viruses must multiply well to give high yields of virus that can be grown at manufacturing scale. Most prototype MVS seed viruses are provided to the manufacturers by government agencies, which generate high-yielding strains through the "classical" reassortment process (described above) with a high-yielding laboratory strain, A/PR/8/34 (designations such as A/PR/8/34 are the nomenclature used for influenza virus; this indicates that the virus was type A, isolated from specimen number 8 obtained from a patient in Puerto Rico in 1934). In addition, reverse genetics is being applied to influenza vaccines. The eight segments of the influenza virus genome of the MVS and epidemic strain are copied in to complementary DNA versions such that reassortants can be made to order based on the six internal genes from the MVS and two (HA and NA) from the epidemic strain that are used to infect cells so that the cells have only the eight segments needed for the candidate reassortant vaccine virus (see Figure 9.2). Currently, most influenza vaccines are trivalent and consist of three viruses: two type A virus strains and one type B virus strain; however, new quadrivalent vaccines have just been licensed that include two type A strains and two type B strains.

Rotavirus vaccines to prevent rotavirus gastroenteritis in infants and children were also developed by reassortment but two concurrent, yet independent, approaches were used to develop the vaccine. Rotateq™ is a pentavalent human/bovine reassortant vaccine (i.e., it contains five strains) based on bovine strain WC3 as the parent strain with three viruses having the VP7 gene from human G1, G2 or G3 serotypes, one virus containing a VP4 gene substitution with a human P[8] serotype, and the fifth virus containing a human G4 VP7. It is given as a three-dose course. By comparison, Rotarix™ is a monovalent, non-reassortant, human virus based on the attenuated human strain 89-12, which was an isolate obtained from an infant with gastroenteritis in Cincinnati, USA, and attenuated by cell culture adaptation; it is given as a two-dose course. Note that Rotarix prevents disease by G1, G3, G4, and G9, while Rotateq prevents disease caused by serotypes G1, G2, G3, G4, and G9.

Definition

Adjuvant: Latin *adjuvare*, to help. A substance added to vaccines that increases the magnitude and/or duration of the immune response to the vaccine antigen. Adjuvants can also modulate the type of immune response elicited by the vaccine. Examples of licensed adjuvants currently used in approved vaccines in the USA or European Union include alum, oil-in-water emulsions such as MF59, and liposomes.

Inactivated vaccines

These contain whole-cell killed bacteria or viruses and require several doses, with the first dose to "prime" the immune system and then "boost" the immune response with one or more doses to provide protection. Nearly all inactivated vaccines contain an adjuvant to enhance the immune response induced by the vaccine. The adjuvant is needed because the inactivated vaccine cannot multiply in the host and continually stimulate the immune response. As would be expected, live vaccines induce superior immune responses to inactivated vaccines as they multiply in the host. Inactivated vaccines tend to induce antibodies and weak cellular immune responses.

Correspondingly, inactivated vaccines induce protective immunity for relatively short periods of time (e.g., 1–5 years) compared to live vaccines (10 years or more), and more booster doses are needed to maintain a protective immune response. The length of time between prime and boost(ers) is vaccine specific and depends on many criteria, including the age of the vaccinee, the amount of vaccine in a dose, and the adjuvant used in the vaccine. The need for booster immunization may be a drawback in areas where people do not have routine access to immunizations and cannot receive booster doses in a timely manner. Inactivated vaccines are produced by killing the disease-causing organism with chemicals (e.g., formalin, BPL, BEI), heat, or radiation. As such, inactivated vaccines are more stable and safer than live vaccines.

165

Furthermore, inactivated vaccines usually do not require refrigeration, and they can be easily stored and transported in a freeze-dried form, which makes them more accessible to people in developing countries. However, the costs to produce inactivated vaccines are often higher than those to produce live vaccines. Examples of inactivated viral vaccines include hepatitis A, influenza, Japanese encephalitis, polio, rabies, and tick-borne encephalitis.

Only a few vaccines have multiple uses

Most vaccines are developed as one vaccine for one species for one disease/condition. Rabies vaccine is an exception. The rabies vaccine is used for humans as a prophylactic preexposure vaccine as well as a therapeutic postexposure vaccine. Not only is the rabies vaccine given to humans, but it is also used to immunize many animal species, including dogs, foxes, raccoons, etc.

The Cutter incident

There are very few examples of where inactivated vaccines have been inadequately inactivated. One of the most cited examples is the "Cutter Incident." In 1955, Jonas Salk developed a formalin-inactivated poliovirus vaccine. The vaccine was manufactured by five companies, including Cutter Laboratories in Berkeley, California. Cutter Laboratories was licensed to manufacture vaccine on April 12, 1955, and despite the lots of vaccine that passed safety tests, some lots contained live wild-type polio virus. Cutter Laboratories withdrew its vaccine from the market on April 27, 1955, after reports of vaccine-associated polio disease. Very regrettably, 200,000 people were inadvertently injected with live wild-type polio virus. Seventy thousand became ill, 200 were permanently paralyzed, and 10 died. A subsequent investigation showed that there were no problems with the production method; rather, the problem was due to the inactivation process where it proved difficult to completely inactivate all virus in a particular lot. This incident demonstrates the very important role played by regulatory authorities in ensuring adequate quality control and assurance in producing vaccines.

The disease cholera is caused by a toxin secreted by serogroups O1 and O139 of the bacterium *Vibrio cholerae* and is prevented by an inactivated cholera vaccine.

There are two variants of this oral vaccine currently in use, termed WC-rBS and BivWC. WC-rBS is a monovalent inactivated vaccine containing killed whole cells of *V. cholerae* serogroup O1 plus additional recombinant nontoxic B subunit-binding portion of the cholera toxin (cholera toxin B subunit; CTB). BivWC is a bivalent inactivated vaccine containing killed whole cells of *V. cholerae* serogroups O1 and O139. The vaccine acts by inducing mucosal immunity against both the bacterial components and CTB. The antibacterial intestinal antibodies prevent the bacteria from attaching to the intestinal wall and bacterial colonization. The antitoxin intestinal IgA antibodies prevent the cholera toxin from binding to the intestinal mucosal surface and prevent the toxin-mediated diarrheal symptoms.

Bacterial subunit vaccines

Every component of a vaccine has to be evaluated for immunogenicity and safety before a vaccine is licensed. Whole-cell bacteria vaccines contain many components that are not involved in inducing a protective immune response and may increase reactogenicity of the vaccine. As such, "component" vaccines offer opportunities to focus the immune response induced by the vaccine and decrease reactogenicity.

Acellular pertussis

The disease whooping cough is caused by *Bordetella pertussis*. Bacterial virulence factors include pertussis toxin (PT), filamentous hemagglutinin (FHA), 69kDa outer-membrane protein (also known as pertactin; PRN), fimbriae (FIM) type 2 and type 3, adenylate cyclase toxin (ACT), tracheal cytotoxin (TCT), lipooligosaccharide, and *B. pertussis* endotoxin.

The original pertussis vaccine was a whole cell-inactivated vaccine (wP), which was inactivated by a combination of heat and formalin. It had good immunogenicity but was associated with reactogenicity, including minor local and systemic side effects in many vaccinated infants. Thus, a second generation acellular vaccine (aP) was developed in the 1980s that used selected antigens of *B. pertussis* to induce immunity, with manufacturers using different components and inactivated methods (chemically or genetically detoxified PT, FHA, PRN, FIM-2, and FIM-3 antigens) in different concentrations, with variable adsorption methods, and different adjuvants. Furthermore, the aP immunogens are derived from different strains of *B. pertussis* and different purification methods. No correlates of protection have been established for pertussis vaccines, and it is conceivable that the mechanism of protective immunity differs among the various aP vaccine formulations. The aP vaccine is considered safer than wP vaccine because it uses fewer antigens than the wP, and this is consistent with the reported 90% reduction in side effects compared to wP. However, the aP is more expensive, and evidence suggests that it may not be as immunogenic as wP.

Toxoid vaccines

Some bacteria secrete toxins and toxoid vaccines (i.e., detoxified toxins) have been developed. These vaccines are used when a bacterial toxin is the main cause of illness. These contain toxins produced by bacteria that have been inactivated (e.g., formalin) to avoid toxic effects while producing a protective immune response. When the immune system receives a vaccine containing a toxoid, it induces antibodies that recognize the natural toxin, lock on to, and block the toxin. Vaccines against diphtheria (caused by *Corynebacterium diphtheriae*) and tetanus (caused by *Clostridium tetani*) are examples of toxoid vaccines.

Since the 1970s, the development of techniques in genetic engineering and recombinant DNA has made it possible to produce safer and more effective vaccines. In particular, toxoids have been genetically modified to decrease side effects.

Note that tetanus is a unique disease because individuals who recover from tetanus disease still need to be immunized against tetanus, as immunity is not acquired after tetanus. Thus, in comparison to most other infectious diseases, so-called natural immunity to tetanus does not occur.

Currently, a combined diphtheria, pertussis, and tetanus (DPT) vaccine is used in children and adults, and these vaccines are not identical. For adults, the combination booster vaccination is termed "Tdap" (tetanus, diphtheria, acellular pertussis) and is given as one dose whereas the childhood vaccine is called "DTaP" (diphtheria, tetanus, acellular pertussis) and given in a three-dose regimen, with the major difference that the adult version contains smaller amounts of the diphtheria and pertussis components; this is indicated in the name by the use of lowercase "d" and

"p" for the adult vaccine. The lowercase "a" in each vaccine indicates that the pertussis component is acellular.

Polysaccharide vaccines

The polysaccharide vaccines contain purified sugar molecules taken from the surface of bacteria that can stimulate the immune system to generate antibodies. Examples include meningococci, pneumococci, and typhoid.

Many Gram-positive bacteria are surrounded by a polysaccharide capsule, which contains the important antigens recognized by antibodies that mediate protective immunity (in this case type-specific antibodies that enhance opsonization, phagocytosis, and killing of bacteria by leukocytes and other phagocytic cells) and other antigens that determine the virulence of these bacteria. While polysaccharide vaccines are easy to generate, they induce only short-term protective immunity for a few years (as seen with inactivated vaccines). The immune response is slow with antibody levels rising slowly, and there is a lack of a memory immune response due to lack of induction of a T-cell response (what is termed a *T-cell independent response*). Thus, when an individual is subsequently exposed to the wild-type bacteria, the immune response is slow to develop and this is somewhat similar to the situation when the individual is naïve to the antigens. Furthermore, these vaccines are not effective in infants and young children (under 18 months of age) and frequent booster vaccinations are avoided because of evidence of immune tolerance where there is a poorer immune response to each successive dose of vaccine. Finally, there is evidence that the vaccine may not prevent bacterial colonization due to lack of mucosal immunity, e.g., of the nasopharynx by meningococci (*Neisseria meningitidis*). Thus, while the vaccine may provide protection to the individual immunized, the vaccinee may still pass the bacteria to other individuals, and so the vaccine will not contribute to herd immunity. Consequently, polysaccharide vaccines are not ideal for national vaccination programs but are excellent vaccines for travelers who need short-term protective immunity.

The first polysaccharide vaccine was for pneumonia caused by *Streptococcus pneumoniae*, which has 92 known serotypes. The first pneumococcal vaccine was derived from a capsular polysaccharide and developed in the

1940s with a 14-valent version produced in the 1970s. The polysaccharide antigens were used to induce serotype-specific antibodies that enhanced opsonization, phagocytosis, and killing of pneumococci by phagocytic cells. The latest version of this vaccine developed in the 1980s contains a mixture of polysaccharide components for 23 serotypes (1, 2, 3, 4, 5, 6B, 7F, 8, 9N, 9V, 10A, 11A, 12F, 14, 15B, 17F, 18C, 19F, 19A, 20, 22F, 23F, and 33F).

Neisseria meningitidis has 13 clinically significant serogroups, which are classified according to the antigenic structure of their polysaccharide capsule. Six serogroups—A, B, C, W-135, X, and Y—are responsible for nearly all cases of clinical disease, and serogroups A, C, W-135, and Y are represented in the polysaccharide vaccine. The first meningococcal vaccine was approved in the 1970s, and only one is still in use today because conjugate vaccines have been developed (see below). A major reason for its continued use is that it is the only vaccine licensed for use in those over 55; the conjugate vaccines are only approved for use up to age 55. As with the pneuomcoccal polysaccharide vaccine, immunity is short-lived at 3 years or less in children aged under 5 because it does not generate memory T cells, and boosters result in a reduced antibody response. There is no serogroup B polysaccharide vaccine because the capsular polysaccharide on the type B bacterium is too similar to human neural antigens to be a useful target for a vaccine but a type B vaccine has been developed using reverse vaccinology (see below).

The Vi capsular polysaccharide vaccine is one of two typhoid vaccines (the other is a live vaccine) and is made from the purified Vi capsular polysaccharide from *Salmonella enterica* serovar Typhi, S typhi Ty2 strain. The Vi capsular polysaccharide vaccine is licensed for use from age 2 years and older, and boosters are required every 3 years.

Haemophilus influenzae type b (Hib) causes meningitis (an infection of the covering of the brain and spinal cord), pneumonia (lung infection), epiglottitis (a severe throat infection), and other serious infections. The first Hib vaccine licensed was a purified polysaccharide vaccine, which was developed in the 1980s. As with the other polysaccharide-based vaccines, the immune response to the vaccine was found to be age-dependent, with the major target population, children under 18 months of age, not producing antibodies in response

to the vaccine. Consequently, the polysaccharide vaccine was withdrawn in the late 1980s.

Conjugate vaccines

Polysaccharide–protein conjugate vaccines (also termed *glycoconjugate vaccines*) are improvements on polysaccharide vaccines and are based on different technologies. They can be considered as second-generation polysaccharide vaccines that enhance the immunogenicity of capsular polysaccharides. Specifically, the major advantage of conjugate vaccines is that they offer improved long-term protection compared to polysaccharide vaccines. Improved immunogenicity is due to the polysaccharides being weak T-independent antigens (i.e., a T-cell independent response) and its conjugation to protein carriers provides T-cell help to enhance immunogenicity (i.e., it is a T-cell dependent response). The first conjugate vaccine was the pneumococcal 7-valent vaccine, which consists of the individual oligosaccharides conjugated to a carrier protein consisting of purified *Corynebacterium diphtheriae* CRM197 protein (CRM197 is a nontoxic variant of diphtheria toxin isolated from cultures of *C. diphtheriae* strain C7 [β197]) that was licensed in 2000. This was subsequently replaced by a 13-valent vaccine, which is licensed for the prevention of pneumonia and invasive disease caused by *S. pneumoniae* serotypes 1, 3, 4, 5, 6A, 6B, 7F, 9V, 14, 18C, 19A, 19F, and 23F in persons 50 years of age or older. This vaccine is also licensed for the prevention of invasive disease caused by *S. pneumoniae* serotypes 1, 3, 4, 5, 6A, 6B, 7F, 9V, 14, 18C, 19A, 19F, and 23F for use in children 6 weeks through 17 years of age, and the prevention of otitis media caused by *S. pneumoniae* serotypes 4, 6B, 9V, 14, 18C, 19F, and 23F for use in children 6 weeks through 5 years of age. Thus, one vaccine may be licensed for multiple uses based on the ages of vaccinees and the diseases that it is used to prevent. In addition to the 13-valent vaccine, a 10-valent vaccine has also been developed that utilizes the protein D from nonspecific *H. influenzae* as the main carrier protein. Note that while the conjugate vaccine is more efficacious than the polysaccharide vaccine it protects against many fewer serotypes of disease than the 23-valent polysaccharide vaccine.

In the case of meningococcal disease, conjugate vaccines were first licensed in the mid-2000s. The four serotype (A, C, W-135, and Y) polysaccharides are produced by bacterial fermentation, treated with formaldehyde, and purified. The individual oligosaccharides are conjugated to purified *C. diphtheriae* CRM197 protein by hydrolysis, sizing, and reductive amination, followed by covalent linking to the CRM197 protein to form the four glycoconjugates in the vaccine product. There are four versions of the conjugate vaccine produced by different manufacturers and with specific vaccines licensed in different countries around the world. The conjugate vaccine is approved for ages from 9 months to 55 years; the polysaccharide vaccine is the only one approved for those over 55 years of age. The conjugation results in enhanced duration of protection, increased immunity with booster vaccinations, and effective herd immunity, all of which were limitations of the polysaccharide vaccine.

In Europe and North America, the 4-valent vaccine is used due to the distribution of meningococcal serotypes, whereas in sub-Saharan Africa serogroup A is responsible for the vast majority of meningococcal disease. Thus, a tetanus toxoid conjugated serotype A specific vaccine, known as MenAfriVac, has been developed and used to successfully control much of the serotype A meningococcal disease in this region.

The limitations of the *Hib* polysaccharide vaccine led to the production of the Hib conjugate vaccine based on conjugation of *Hib* polysaccharide to one of three protein carriers that varied by producer (inactivated tetanus toxoid, mutant diphtheria protein, or outer membrane protein complex [OMPC] of the B11 strain of *Neisseria meningitidis* serogroup B). The polysaccharide is the capsular polysaccharide polyribosyl-ribitol-phosphate (PRP), high molecular weight polymer prepared from the *Hib* strain that is heat inactivated and purified prior to conjugation. As with other conjugate vaccines, protective immunity was greatly enhanced in young children compared to the polysaccharide vaccine. Note that the Hib vaccine is produced by different producers. The strain of Hib used to prepare PRP differs by manufacturer as does the protein carrier. Hib vaccine is not effective against non-type B *H. influenzae*. However, non-type B disease is rare in comparison to pre-vaccine *H. influenzae* disease.

Viral subunit vaccines

Viral subunit vaccines consist of specific immunogens, usually surface proteins from viruses that are shown to stimulate the major components of the antiviral immune response. One of the major benefits of recombinant vaccines is that they only contain the essential immunogens and not all the other molecules that make up the organism, thus the potential of reactogenicity to the vaccine is correspondingly lower. Such vaccines are considered to be very safe since they do not contain any genetic material from the microbe and better immunogens than inactivated vaccines.

All of the licensed recombinant vaccines are based on one or more proteins but a number of candidate vaccines in development involve only epitopes (the specific parts of the protein antigen that antibodies or T cells recognize and bind to).

Definition

Virus-like particles (or VLPs) are virus particles that lack part or the entire virus genome and one or more virus proteins. VLPs mimic the structural organization and conformation of wild-type virus particles such that they contain the protein immunogens needed to induce an immune response. Further, most VLPs self-assemble, which makes them very amenable for use as vaccines because they can be produced in a variety of cell culture systems, including mammalian cell lines, insect cell lines, yeast, and plant cells. Because they lack the virus genome they are non-infectious and cannot multiply in cells to produce more virus particles. Thus they are considered safe and economical vaccines, although multiple doses are normally needed to generate a protective immune response.

Virus-like particles

Virus-like particles (or VLPs) are virus particles that lack part or the entire virus genome and one or more virus proteins. VLPs mimic the structural organization and conformation of wild-type virus particles such that they contain the protein immunogens needed to induce an immune response. Further, most VLPs self-assemble, which makes them very amenable for use as vaccines because they can be produced in a variety of cell culture systems, including mammalian cell lines, insect cell lines, yeast and plant cells. Because they lack the virus genome, they are non-infectious and cannot multiply in cells to produce more virus particles. Thus, they are considered safe and economical vaccines, although multiple doses are normally needed to generate a protective immune response.

Advantages of recombinant DNA-derived vaccines

- Consist of specific immunogens, usually surface proteins from viruses or bacteria that are shown to stimulate the major components of the antimicrobe immune response
- Better immunogens than inactivated vaccines
- Considered to be very safe since they do not contain any genetic material from the microbe
- Less reactogenic than live or inactivated vaccines
- Do not contain genetic material of microbe
- Superior characterization compared to live and inactivated vaccines

Recombinant hepatitis B vaccine

Recombinant DNA technology has been critical in advances made for subunit vaccines. The first licensed recombinant subunit vaccine was developed for hepatitis B virus, a virus with a double-stranded DNA genome, by insertion of the hepatitis B surface antigen (HBsAg) gene into yeast (*Saccharomyces cerevisiae*). The yeast was then grown at large scale to express HBsAg in cells, released from yeast cells by cell disruption, and purified as VLPs for use in the vaccine, which is administered with an adjuvant. The subunit vaccine replaced an inactivated vaccine that was derived by collection, inactivation, and purification of hepatitis B virus from the plasma of chronically infected carriers of the virus. The vaccine produced in yeast has been shown to be comparable to the plasma-derived vaccine in terms of animal potency (mouse, monkey, and chimpanzee) and protective efficacy (chimpanzee and human). Clearly, the subunit vaccine was a major advance compared to the inactivated vaccine.

Influenza vaccines: an example of where multiple technologies are used by different producers to make a vaccine

Influenza is an acute respiratory disease that is caused by a virus whose genome is divided into eight segments. The major immunogens are the hemagglutinin (HA) and the neuraminidase (NA). There are three major types of influenza virus termed *types A, B*, and *C*, each of which are genetically and serologically different viruses. Most disease is associated with type A, some disease by type B, and little disease is associated with type C. Type A influenza consists of multiple subtypes that are distinguished by the HA (H1–18) and NA (N1–11). Thus, in theory there can be 198 combinations of HA and NA on influenza type A viruses. Not all influenza A subtypes infect humans, but a significant number do (e.g., H1N1, H1N2, and H3N2). In addition, influenza type B consists of two major groups, types 2A and 2B. It is necessary to produce influenza vaccines each year due to the variability in the influenza virus immunogens and limited (termed *antigenic drift*, e.g., H1N1 and H1N2) or lack (termed *antigenic shift*, e.g., H1N1 and H3N2) of cross-protective immunity between particular subtypes. From a global perspective, more manufacturers produce influenza vaccine than any other vaccine, in part because people need to be immunized each year. Vaccines are produced using five different technologies. Technologies 2–4 are trivalent and contain three influenza viruses (two type A and one type B). Technology 1 was a trivalent vaccine but has now transitioned to a quadrivalent vaccine consisting of two type A and two type B influenza strains. Technology 5 is also a quadrivalent vaccine.

1. Live attenuated reassortant (natural or reverse genetics) given by the intranasal route.
2. Inactivated whole virus given by the intramuscular route.
3. Split virus particles that are prepared from inactivated virus particles disrupted with detergents. These vaccines have been shown to induce fewer side effects and were found to be as immunogenic as whole virus vaccine, and are given by the intramuscular route. This is sometimes referred to as a subunit (purified surface antigen) influenza virus vaccine.
4. Recombinant baculovirus expressed hemagglutinin given by the intramuscular route.
5. Inactivated quadrivalent vaccine containing two type A and two type B influenza viruses given by the intramuscular route.

Recombinant human papillomavirus vaccine

Human papillomavirus (HPV), the cause of cervical carcinoma, is also a virus that has a double-stranded DNA genome. A subunit HPV vaccine (officially termed *recombinant HPV-like particle vaccine*) has been licensed based on expression of the L1 protein, the major capsid protein, that forms VLPs. Two recombinant HPV vaccines have been produced, one produced in *Saccharomyces cerevisiae* as described above for HBsAg vaccine above and the other in insect cells. The latter vaccine contains recombinant L1 protein and is produced in bioreactors using a recombinant baculovirus expression vector system in *Trichoplusia ni* insect cells. The L1 protein is not secreted from cells but rather accumulates in the cytoplasm of the cells, and L1 protein is released by cell disruption and subsequently purified. Assembly of the L1 proteins into VLPs occurs at the end of the purification process. The purified, non-infectious VLPs are then adsorbed onto the adjuvant.

Recombinant hepatitis E vaccine

Hepatitis E virus (HEV) is a calicivirus, which is a non-enveloped virus with a single-stranded RNA virus genome where open reading frame 2 (ORF2) encodes the one capsid protein of the virus particle. Expression of amino acids 368-606 of ORF2, which contains HEV neutralizing epitopes, in *E. coli* generates proteins that assemble as homodimers, and then as VLPs. This *E. coli* expressed VLP was licensed as a vaccine in China in 2011, marketed in 2012, and is the first human vaccine to be licensed based on expression of a recombinant protein in *E. coli*. The vaccine has a three-dose regimen (0, 1, and 6 months).

Recombinant influenza vaccine

Most recently a baculovirus-insect cell expression has been used to develop a subunit influenza vaccine. Briefly, recombinant influenza HA protein is expressed in a continuous insect cell line (*expres*SF+®) that is derived from Sf9 cells of the fall armyworm, *Spodoptera frugiperda* using a baculovirus vector (*Autographa californica* nuclear polyhedrosis virus). HA protein is purified from the cell culture medium. There is no adjuvant with this subunit influenza vaccine.

DNA vaccines

DNA vaccines are considered "third-generation vaccines" and take immunization to a new technological level. These vaccines dispense with all components of the both the microbe and subunit proteins, and consist only of the portion of the microbe's genetic material that encodes the protective immunogens. Thus, the vaccine lacks all the genes necessary to make the microbe but can make the immunogens associated with protective immunity. Devices have been designed that enable the DNA to be taken up directly into cells by either generating a brief electric stimulation (termed *electroporation*) to induce temporary holes (or pores) in the membranes of cells to allow the DNA to directly enter cells, or by high-pressure gas to shoot microscopic gold particles (nanoparticles) coated with DNA directly into cells, or by traditional needles that enable intradermal immunization such that the DNA is seen by antigen-presenting cells in the skin.

Even if a vaccine is licensed, it is not always successful

Rotashield™

Two live rotavirus vaccines are currently licensed: Rotateq™ and Rotarix™ and have proved to be safe and highly effective. However, Rotashield™ was the first live rotavirus vaccine developed and was a trivalent reassortant vaccine based on a simian virus, RRV, backbone. It was extensively evaluated in clinical trials prior to licensure in 1998. However, less than 1 year post licensure, 15 cases of intussusception (a form of intestinal blockage caused when a segment of the bowel prolapses into a more distal segment of the intestine) were reported 3 to 14 days after the first dose of the three-dose regimen. Investigations by the US Advisory Committee on Immunization Practices led to the conclusion that an association existed between administration of the vaccine and development of intussusception. The risk of intussusception was age related and increased substantially in children older than 3 months of age, such that it was recommended that subsequent rotavirus vaccines be given to infants younger than 3 months old. It should be noted that the exact mechanism of the association of the Rotashield™ vaccine and intussusception has not been determined.

LYMErix™

Lyme disease is a tick-borne disease caused by *Borrelia burgdorferi*. The clinical manifestations of early stage disease in humans are generally nonspecific. However, long-term infection can lead to serious dermatological, arthritic, cardiac, and neurological conditions that can cause significant morbidity. LYMErix™ is a vaccine

(Continued)

based on recombinant outer surface protein A (OspA) of *B. burgdorferi* expressed in *E. coli* and adsorbed to alum adjuvant. It was licensed in 1998 as a two 30-µg dose regimen, administered 1 month apart, with a booster vaccination at 12 months. Within a year of its introduction, LYMErix™ was being anecdotally associated with development of arthritis. The putative association between the vaccine and these adverse events was well publicized. While concerns, whether real or perceived, continued to increase, post-licensure phase IV studies of LYMErix™ safety were undertaken by the manufacturer, and the data did not demonstrate an association between vaccination and development of arthritis. Further, the US Vaccine Adverse Event Reporting System (VAERS) analyzed data obtained between December 1998 and July 2000. They found that there were 1.4 million doses distributed and 905 adverse events reported, of which 102 were coded as forms of arthritis and 12 as facial paralysis, both of which had been hypothesized to be sequelae of Lyme disease. There was no apparent temporal association between the development of arthritis and vaccine administration, although reports of arthritis were more often reported after the second and third immunizations. Significantly, the reported rate of both arthritis and facial paralysis was below what was expected as background in the population. The conclusion of the VAERS study was that there were no unexpected or unusual patterns of adverse events associated with LYMErix™ vaccination. Consequently, in 2001, a US Food and Drug Administration panel found no reason to remove the vaccine from the market or modify its labeling. Continued media coverage of the putative vaccine-associated adverse events led to decreased acceptance of the LYMErix™ vaccine and sales continued to decline. LYMErix™ vaccine was withdrawn from the market in 2002 due to poor sales.

Once inside the cells, the DNA encoding the immunogen is transcribed to make a messenger RNA that is translated on ribosomes to generate the protein immunogen. The cells secrete the immunogen and/or display it on their surfaces. Thus, the body's own cells manufacture the vaccine that stimulates the immune system to induce protective immunity. In theory, the DNA vaccine will induce a strong antibody response to the immunogen secreted by cells and a strong cellular response against the immunogens displayed on cell surfaces. Economically, DNA vaccines are relatively easy and inexpensive to design and produce.

While the technology is straightforward, no DNA vaccine has been approved for humans as candidate DNA vaccines have been found to have reduced efficacy in higher animal species, and immunity is predominantly T-cell mediated with weak antibody responses. However, recent clinical trials with genetically modified candidate DNA vaccines suggest that they have significant improvements in induction of neutralizing antibody and T-cell responses. Nonetheless, two DNA vaccines have been approved for animals: West Nile and canine melanoma. The former has been in clinical trials in humans with safety and immunogenicity demonstrated. However, no efficacy trials have been undertaken. The latter vaccine utilizes a DNA copy of the human tyrosinase gene (found in melanomas) and is administered via a transdermal device, which delivers the vaccine without the use of a needle. It has been shown to extend survival of dogs with stage II or stage III oral canine melanoma. This was the first approved, therapeutic vaccine for the treatment of cancer, in either animals or humans.

Reverse genetics

Recent years have seen much emphasis of vaccine research based on molecular studies. One technology that had great promise for vaccine development is so-called reverse genetics. This is the situation when the genome of a virus with a messenger RNA genome is converted into a complementary DNA (cDNA) where the whole genome is in one cDNA molecule. Transcription of the cDNA will result in an RNA molecule that is equivalent to the RNA genome of the virus. Although there are not techniques to genetically manipulate RNA, there are many approaches for genetic manipulation of cDNA. Consequently, it is possible to genetically manipulate the cDNA molecule of the virus genome and incorporate mutations that can be rescued when the cDNA is transcribed into RNA. Clearly, these techniques, collectively known as "reverse genetics," can be used to genetically manipulate genomes of RNA viruses to develop candidate vaccines. To date, only one example has progressed to a licensed vaccine. ChimeriVax-Japanese encephalitis (CVJE) utilizes technology to genetically manipulate the genome of the licensed live attenuated yellow fever 17D vaccine virus (see Figure 9.3). Note, only

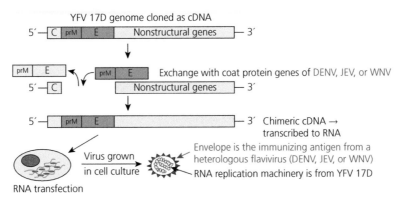

YFV 17D genome cloned as cDNA

Exchange with coat protein genes of DENV, JEV, or WNV

Chimeric cDNA → transcribed to RNA

Virus grown in cell culture

Envelope is the immunizing antigen from a heterologous flavivirus (DENV, JEV, or WNV)

RNA replication machinery is from YFV 17D

RNA transfection

Figure 9.3 Construction of ChimeriVax-based vaccines. Chimeric flaviviruses vaccines are constructed by replacing the genes coding for premembrane (prM) and envelope (E) proteins from yellow fever virus (YFV) 17D-204 vaccine with those of heterologous flaviviruses (dengue [DENV], Japanese encephalitis virus [JEV] or West Nile virus [WNV]). After DNA cloning, RNA is transcribed and transfected into Vero cells to obtain chimeric viruses possessing the YFV 17D replication machinery and the external coat of the relevant heterologous flavivirus.

CVJE is licensed; other ChimeriVax vaccines are in clinical development. Yellow fever virus (YFV) is a flavivirus, which has a genome that is one single-stranded, positive-sense RNA molecule approximately 11,000 nucleotides in length. YFV has three structural proteins termed *capsid* (which surrounds the RNA genome), *membrane* (which is synthesized as a precursor called *premembrane* [prM]) and *envelope* (which is the major surface glycoprotein of flaviviruses) (E). The prM and E genes of YFV were "swapped" for those of the live attenuated Japanese encephalitis virus (another flavivirus) vaccine strain SA14-14-2 to generate the chimeric vaccine virus called CVJE. It was licensed in Thailand and Australia in 2010 as a one-dose vaccine given by the subcutaneous route. In addition to being the first recombinant-derived live vaccine virus, it is a chimera between two different viruses, and as such it is the first genetically manipulated organism as a live vaccine and was subject to a number of careful evaluations as a genetically manipulated organism. The CVJE vaccine is produced in monkey kidney Vero cells and so it is the first live vaccine produced on a continuous cell line and given by injection. All other human vaccines produced in Vero cells are inactivated except for live polio vaccine, which is given by the oral route.

Reverse vaccinology

Reverse vaccinology refers to the approach of developing a vaccine based on the genomic content of an organism. The genome of the organism is sequenced, the open reading frames (ORFs) are identified, and the proteins potentially expressed by each ORF are analyzed to identify putative surface expressed proteins. Each putative surface protein is expressed as a recombinant protein, and the proteins are used to immunize animals (usually mice). Properties of mouse antisera are then examined to identify those proteins putatively associated with surface proteins on the organism and antibodies associated with protective immunity. This approach has been used to develop two candidate *N. meningitidis* serotype B (MenB) vaccines because vaccines against serotype B meningococcal disease have proved difficult to produce. This is in part due to the capsular polysaccharide cross-reacting with host components and that MenB consists of three major antigenic variants. Unfortunately, the three variants do not induce cross-protective immunity to each other. Therefore, antigens representative of the different major variants need to be included in the vaccine. Interestingly, although the same approach was used to develop the two vaccine candidates, they did not identify the same immunogens, which indicates a vaccine may be developed using more than one approach and with different immunogens. One of the meningococcal B vaccines, 4CMenB (see Figure 9.4 for its derivation), has been licensed in Europe and the other is in phase III clinical trials. The 4CMenB vaccine contains factor H binding protein (fHBP), a member of the regulators of complement activation

Determination of genomic sequence of *Neisseria meningitis* type B genome

↓

Identify Open Reading Frames (ORFs) and genes therein predicted to encode surface exposed proteins and conserved between strains (n ~600)

↓

Express candidate surface exposed protein ORFs/genes in *E. coli* (n=350)

↓

Purify proteins and immunize mice (n=91)

↓

Evaluate mouse antisera to see if potential protein is surface exposed and antibacterial activity (bactericidal and opsonophagocytosis) (n=28)

↓

Test positive mouse antisera for antibacterial activity against a range of *N. meningitis* variants/serogroups

↓

Prioritize mouse antisera based on broadness of variant/serogroup cross-reactivity (n=5)

↓

Identify candidate immunogens for inclusion in vaccine (n=4)

Figure 9.4 Development of a *Neisseria meningitidis* type B candidate vaccine by reverse vaccinology.

family and a complement binding protein from variant #1; Neisserial adhesin A (NadA); Neisseria heparin binding antigen (NHBA); and outer membrane vesicles (OMV) from *Neisseria meningitidis* group B strain NZ98/254 measured as amount of total protein containing the PorA P1.4. Note, all but OMV are produced as proteins expressed in *E. coli*. The other MenB vaccine is bivalent with two fHBPs, one representative of each of two of the major antigenic variants of MenB.

Combination vaccines

The above sections demonstrate that a number of vaccines have been developed, in particular for childhood diseases. It is clear that if an individual wants to receive all of the vaccines they will have many injections on multiple visits to their health care provider. It is well-known that getting individuals to undertake multiple visits to complete an immunization course is difficult, and it would be better for the vaccinee and vaccine policy groups if multiple vaccines could be given in one visit. Giving multiple vaccines at one visit

is known as *coadministration*. Table 9.8 shows examples of vaccines that are often used together. Note, recommendations for combinations vary by country and are based on many considerations taken by health officials and regulatory authorities. One of the most widely coadministered vaccines is Hib. This can be given with DTP, DTaP, oral poliovirus, MMR, hepatitis B, and occasionally inactivated poliovirus vaccine.

Clearly, mixing vaccines must be done with care so that the immunogenicity and safety of each component is not compromised. The general rule is that live vaccines should either be given simultaneously or not be given within 28 days of each other to prevent potential interference in induction of immune responses, whereas inactivated and subunit vaccines can often be given at the same time as there are no multiplying components in the vaccines. If multiple vaccines are going to be given at the same visit they can either be mixed in one dose or given as single vaccines at different anatomical sites, e.g., one immunization in each arm, depending on the particular formulation of the vaccines are available (see Table 9.8).

Table 9.8 Examples of Multiple Vaccines Given on the Same Day

DPT	Diphtheria + pertussis + tetanus
DT (or TD)	Diphtheria + tetanus
DTP	Diphtheria + tetanus + inactivated poliovirus (Netherlands and France only)
DTwP	Diphtheria + whole-cell pertussis + tetanus
DTap	Diphtheria + acellular pertussis + tetanus
DTaP + HBV + IPV	Diphtheria + acellular pertussis + tetanus + hepatitis B (recombinant) + inactivated poliovirus
dT + IPV	Diphtheria + tetanus+ inactivated poliovirus
DTaP + IPV	Diphtheria + acellular pertussis + tetanus + inactivated poliovirus
DTaP + IPV + Hib	Diphtheria + acellular pertussis + tetanus + inactivated poliovirus + *Haemophilus b* conjugate
DPT + IPV + Hib +HBV	Diphtheria + acellular pertussis + tetanus + inactivated poliovirus + *Haemophilus b* conjugate + hepatitis B (recombinant)
Hib + HBV	*Haemophilus b* conjugate (meningococcal protein conjugate) and hepatitis B (recombinant)
HAV + HBV	Inactivated hepatitis A + hepatitis B (recombinant)
HAV + typhoid	Inactivated hepatitis A + Vi polysaccharide
Men C + Hib	*Neisseria meningitidis* serogroup C capsular polysaccharide antigens + *Haemophilus influenzae* type b
Men CY + Hib	*Neisseria meningitidis* serogroup C and Y capsular polysaccharide antigens and Haemophilus b
Tdap	Adult low dose diphtheria + adult low dose acellular pertussis + tetanus
MMR	Measles + mumps + rubella
MMRV	Measles + mumps + rubella + varicella
MMRV + Hib	Measles + mumps + rubella + varicella + Haemophilus b Conjugate vaccine (Meningococcal Protein Conjugate)
MR	Mumps + rubella

Definitions of vaccines administered together

Coadministration: Vaccines administered within 4 weeks of each other. This can be giving multiple vaccines at one visit, either vaccines mixed in one dose or given as single vaccines at different anatomical sites.
Combined: Vaccines administered on the same day at the same location (mixed prior to injection).
Concomitant: Vaccines administered at the same day but in different anatomical sites (e.g., left and right arms).
Simultaneous: Same as concomitant.

Both live and inactivated vaccines

For some diseases there are both live and inactivated vaccines available (cholera: live and polysaccharide; Japanese encephalitis: live and inactivated; polio: live and inactivated; and typhoid: live and polysaccharide). This raises the important question: Why have different vaccines been developed for one disease? The answer is complicated and differs by vaccine. For example, different manufacturers distribute vaccines in different countries and so it may relate to approval processes by national regulatory authorities. Market size may also play a role, as a particular manufacturer may decide it is not economical to go through the national approval process to get licensure. Alternatively, cost and availability of the vaccine and how the immunization regimen would be integrated into the national immunization policy (i.e., does the dosing schedule complement visits to health care providers for other vaccines) may be a consideration for national ministries of health. Furthermore, some vaccines may not be used because the disease is not found in the particular country. Thus, the market may be for travelers' vaccines and that may or may not be economical.

In addition to the above, two major considerations are comparable for the immunogenicity of vaccines, the dosing regimen and need for booster doses, and the potential side effects of live attenuated vaccines and utilization of inactivated vaccines that normally have a superior safety profile but may be less immunogenic. The best example of the above relates to polio vaccine. Poliovirus consists of three serotypes that do not induce cross-protective immunity; therefore, polio vaccine needs to be trivalent. The live attenuated oral polio vaccine (OPV) is very efficacious and has superior immunogenicity to the inactivated polio vaccine (IPV). However, the first dose of OPV can give rise to a condition known as *vaccine-associated paralytic poliomyelitis* (VAPP). The incidence of VAPP is estimated to be 4 cases per million birth cohort per year in countries using OPV and is only seen in primary vaccinees. Although VAPP is very rare, it is a major concern for OPV. Thus, the OPV has been used in mass and routine vaccination campaigns to get a high level of protection and herd immunity. This has been successfully undertaken in the Americas and Europe to the extent that the OPV vaccine has now been replaced by the IPV since it is safer, will eliminate VAPP, and the major vaccination requirement is to vaccinate the birth cohort rather than continue to immunize the entire population.

Unfortunately, OPV campaigns have proved difficult in a very few countries (e.g., Nigeria, Pakistan, and Afghanistan), and it has proved very difficult to eliminate wild-type poliovirus in these countries. However, there is considerable evidence that wild-type poliovirus serotype 2 has been eradicated as there has been no isolation of this virus since 1999. Consequently, there are now plans to modify the polio vaccine from trivalent to bivalent. The poliovirus eradication efforts are described in detail in Chapter 3.

Vaccines for special populations

Vaccines for biodefense and biothreat agents

Throughout the ages there have been examples of humans utilizing infectious agents as biological weapons. While these attempts have been in limited geographic areas and populations, there is always the potential that some very pathogenic infectious agents can be used as a biological weapon on either a small or large scale. Due to this potential, a number of vaccines have been developed for infectious agents with the greatest risk of causing mass morbidity or casualties, be it to military and/or civilian populations. The objective is that these vaccines will not be administered; rather, their availability will persuade those thinking of developing biological weapons not to do so. The two major vaccines in this area are smallpox and anthrax.

In addition to vaccines for biothreat agents, this category sometime includes use of vaccines for geographic areas where a biothreat agent causes natural endemic disease, e.g., plague in areas where *Yersinia pestis* is transmitted by the bite of a flea.

The smallpox vaccine was one of the first-ever vaccines developed and consists of a live attenuated vaccine based on the vaccinia strain. It was widely used over several hundred years, and a concerted vaccination program resulted in the eradication of the disease smallpox in the 1970s (see Chapter 3). Consequently, smallpox vaccination ceased, and manufacturers no longer produce the vaccine. In the early 2000s, the lack of vaccination led to concern about smallpox being used as a biological weapon. The US government undertook development of a new smallpox vaccine that would be stockpiled. This was based on a plaque purification cloning from Dryvax® (calf lymph vaccine, New York City Board of Health Strain) and propagated in African green monkey Vero cells. The vaccine is not routinely used.

The disease anthrax is caused by the three-protein exotoxin secreted by virulent strains of *Bacillus anthracis*. Anthrax toxin is composed of a cell-binding protein, known as protective antigen (PA), and two enzyme components, called edema factor (EF) and lethal factor (LF). A number of anthrax vaccines have been licensed. There are two acellular vaccines. In the USA, the "Anthrax Vaccine Adsorbed (AVA)" vaccine has been stockpiled and is produced from cell-free filtrates of microaerophilic cultures of an avirulent, nonencapsulated strain of *B. anthracis* known as V770-NP1-R. The final product, prepared from the sterile filtrate culture fluid, contains proteins, including the PA protein (but all three toxin components [LF, EF, and PA] are present in the product), released during the bacterial growth phase and contains no dead or live bacteria. The primary vaccination regimen consists of three subcutaneous doses at 0, 2, and 4 weeks, and three booster vaccinations at 6, 12, and 18 months, and annual single dose boosters to maintain protective immunity. In Britain, the Anthrax Vaccine Precipitated (AVP) vaccine is used based on a sterile filtrate of an alum adjuvant precipitated anthrax antigen from the Sterne strain. The vaccine is given by the intramuscular route with a primary course regimen of four doses at 0, 3, and 6 weeks, followed by a 6-month dose, which is followed by a single booster dose given once a year.

Live attenuated, unencapsulated spore vaccines have been developed and used in Russia and China and can be given by aerosol, scarification, or subcutaneous routes.

The disease known as "plague" is caused by *Yersinia pestis*. Clinically, different forms of plague are recognized, including bubonic (due to infection by fleas) and pneumonic (due to infection by aerosol). Early plague vaccines consisted of heat-killed *Y. pestis*, which conferred protection against bubonic plague but induced reactogenicity, including high fever in the majority of vaccinees. A formalin-killed whole-cell vaccine was developed in the mid-20th century in the USA and used to protect military personnel, but it also caused reactogenicity, did not induce protection against pneumonic plague, and was discontinued in 1999. Live attenuated plague vaccines were developed in the early 20th century using the EV strain and its derivatives, and were used in mass vaccination campaigns in Madagascar in the 1930s. Unfortunately, this vaccine was associated with side effects, including residual virulence. The live attenuated EV76 and EV88 strains are still in use in Russia and Central Asian countries. However, no vaccine confers long-term protection against bubonic plague nor is there a vaccine that protects against pneumonic plague.

In addition, live brucellosis (caused by *Brucella* spp.) and tularemia (caused by *Francisella tularensis*) vaccines are available in Russia.

Q fever is a bacterial disease with acute and chronic stages caused by *Coxiella burnetii*. The bacterium is highly infectious for humans. A whole-cell, inactivated vaccine is available in Australia that is given by the intradermal route. A single dose of vaccine provides protective immunity for many years and booster vaccination is not generally required.

Travelers' vaccines

We live in an era where air travel enables an individual to get to any destination in the world within 24 hours. Thus, a particular disease may not be found in the country of residence of a traveler but may be found in the destination country. Accordingly, the traveler will want to be immunized against vaccine-preventable diseases that are found in the destination country, and some countries have immunization requirements for travelers who enter that country. Such vaccines are considered to be "traveler" vaccines for the country of residence. Travel medicine clinics are found in many developed countries that provide immunizations for travelers for a fee because a particular vaccine may not be part of the country of residence's national immunization policy since that disease is not found in the traveler's home country. Similarly, many vaccine manufacturers have travel vaccine divisions that specialize in marketing these specialized vaccines, which are often marketed at a profit as the traveler is only looking for short-term protection while in the destination country. The best example of a travel vaccine is the yellow fever vaccine. Yellow fever disease is found in tropical areas of sub-Saharan Africa and South America and is the only vaccine required for visitors in the International Health Regulations (IHR). Surprisingly, there is no other vaccine requirement to those countries in the IHR. For more details on travelers' vaccines, see Chapter 16.

Noninfectious disease vaccines

Noninfectious disease vaccines are sometimes termed *noncommunicable disease vaccines*.

There are anti-allergy vaccines that have been licensed in Scandinavia and France for birch pollen, cat allergen, and Timothy grass, and for grass pollen and dust mites in Russia. These are the first anti-allergy vaccines to be marketed, and it is likely that other anti-allergen vaccines will be licensed in the future.

In addition, there are cancer vaccines for liver cancer and cervical carcinoma that utilize hepatitis B and HPV vaccines, respectively. Interestingly, these two vaccines are marketed as noncommunicable disease vaccines, even though both diseases are caused by viruses.

Other considerations

Vaccines in the 20th and 21st centuries

The 20th century was an era when there was a dramatic increase in the number of vaccines available (see Plotkin and Plotkin [2011] in the Further Reading section). This was in part due to the development of vaccines to protect children from life-threatening infectious diseases. At the start of the 20th century childhood mortality due to infectious diseases was a major public health problem, and scientists responded with the generation of a large number of vaccines (currently 40 to 50) that have resulted in the control of many major infectious diseases (see Table 9.9), including poliomyelitis, diphtheria, measles, rubella, pertussis, smallpox, and others. The US Centers for Disease Control and Prevention ranked vaccines number 1 in the top 10 public health achievements of the 20th century. To date, the only organism eradicated is smallpox, but many of the childhood diseases are caused by organisms that infect humans only (see Table 9.10), such that vaccination can theoretically eradiate a number of these diseases, including measles and polio (see Chapter 3).

In the 21st century, the focus is shifting to enabling adults to live longer. The World Health Organization has published two very important statistics. First, the number of senior citizens worldwide will double by 2025. Second, many major diseases in adults are chronic in nature, and by 2020, chronic diseases are predicted to be the leading cause of disability worldwide. Consequently, managing or preventing chronic illnesses at the early stages may greatly reduce disease burden. Accordingly, we are seeing many of the childhood disease vaccines being reformulated for adults and/or senior citizens. Examples are DTP, influenza, meningococcal and pneumococcal, Hib and varicella vaccines, which have either reduced quantities of vaccine in a dose for booster doses in adults or larger quantities of vaccine per dose for senior citizens due to immunosenescence in the elderly.

Why are there no generic vaccines?

Vaccines are complex biological preparations that contain not only the vaccine but other components (vaccine excipients) to maintain the vaccine potency.

Table 9.9 Impact of Childhood Vaccines in the USA in the 20th Century

Disease	Pre-Vaccine Morbidity	1998 Morbidity
Smallpox	48,164	0
Diphtheria	175,885	1
Pertussis	147,271	7,405
Tetanus	1,314	41
Polio (paralytic)	16,316	1
Measles	503,282	100
Mumps	152,209	666
Rubella	47,745	364
Congenital rubella	823	7
H. influenzae type b	20,000	61

Table 9.10 Infectious Diseases That Can Be Eradicated...We Have Vaccines

- Smallpox (eradicated 1977)
- Polio (continuing attempts to complete eradication campaign [termed *endgame*])
- Measles (proposed for eradication vaccination campaign)
- Mumps
- Rubella
- Chickenpox
- Hepatitis A
- Hepatitis B

The stability of the vaccine over time and at different temperatures becomes an important consideration. Thus, a live vaccine must retain viability from the time it is prepared to the time it is administered to the vaccinee, and it must retain viability when stored for long periods of time. For nonliving vaccines, immunogens must retain the correct conformation that induces a protective immune response. In many situations, the goal of a vaccine is to have a shelf-life of 3 years and be able to withstand low and high temperatures between manufacture and administration of the vaccine. Further, vaccines use multiple technologies (see the section on vaccine types) that require expensive dedicated manufacturing facilities to meet regulatory requirements. Therefore, unlike drugs, "copying" a vaccine is very difficult; that is why there have been no generic vaccines to date.

Personalized vaccines

The first of a new generation of personalized therapeutic vaccines has been recently licensed for prostate cancer. Such therapeutic vaccines are used after the patient shows a clinical disease and utilizes the host immune response for the benefit of the patient. As such, the vaccine/immunotherapy is individual specific; hence the term *personalized vaccine*. It has also been termed *active immunotherapy* and a *new class* of drugs. Briefly, it is an autologous cellular immunotherapy for the treatment of asymptomatic or minimally symptomatic metastatic castrate resistant (hormone refractory) prostate cancer.

The patient's peripheral blood mononuclear cells (PBMCs) are obtained via leukapheresis. These autologous PBMCs, including antigen-presenting cells (APCs), are activated by culturing with recombinant human PAP-GM-CSF (prostatic acid phosphatase [PAP], an antigen expressed in prostate cancer tissue, that is linked to granulocyte-macrophage colony-stimulating factor [GM-CSF], to stimulate the immune cells). Subsequently, approximately 3 days later, at least 50 million autologous $CD54^+$ cells that have been activated with PAP-GM-CSF are infused back into the patient. $CD54^+$ (also known as ICAM-1) is a cell surface molecule that plays a role in the immunologic interactions between APCs and T cells and is considered a marker of immune cell activation.

The precise mechanism of action is unknown, but this autologous cellular immunotherapy is designed to induce an immune response targeted against PAP, an antigen that is expressed in most prostate cancers. Clinical trials have shown that this immunotherapy extends the life of prostate cancer patients but does not cure the patient of the cancer.

Summary

- Early vaccines consisted of live attenuated or chemically/heat-inactivated vaccines.

- The 20th century saw the development of many vaccines to prevent childhood infectious diseases. This included not only new live attenuated and inactivated vaccines but also second-generation vaccines that utilized subunits of the microbe, such as polysaccharide and conjugate vaccines.

- The last quarter of the 20th century saw the development of recombinant DNA technology to enable genetic manipulation of viral and bacterial genes to generate the first recombinant subunit vaccines. Such vaccines have improved safety but may or may not have improved immunogenicity.

- The start of the 21st century has seen great advances made in structural biology and genomics that have led to the development of vaccines using reverse genetics and reverse vaccinology.

- Vaccine development has moved from childhood infectious diseases to infectious diseases affecting adults and senior citizens.

- Vaccines have recently been developed for noncommunicable diseases such as allergies and cancer.

Further reading

European Center for Disease Control and Prevention. http://www.ecdc.europa.eu/en/activities/diseaseprogrammes/vpd/Pages/index.aspx

European Medicines Agency. http://www.ema.europa.eu/ema/index.jsp?curl=pages/regulation/general/general_content_000407.jsp&mid=WC0b01ac058002958b

Immunize Australia Program. http://www.immunise.health.gov.au/

New Zealand Ministry of Health. http://www.health.govt.nz/our-work/preventative-health-wellness/immunisation

Plotkin SA and Plotkin SP (2011). The development of vaccines: how the past led to the future. Nature Reviews. Microbiology 9, 889–893.

Public Health Agency of Canada. http://www.phac-aspc.gc.ca/im/index-eng.php

United Kingdom National Health Service. http://www.nhs.uk/Conditions/vaccinations/Pages/vaccination-schedule-age-checklist.aspx

United States Centers for Disease Control and Prevention. http://www.cdc.gov/vaccines/default.htm

World Health Organization. http://www.who.int/immunization/en/

10 Veterinary vaccines

A. Paige Adams
Kansas State University, Olathe, KS, USA

Abbreviations

AABP	American Association of Bovine Practitioners	COBTA	Council on Biologic and Therapeutic Agents
AAEP	American Association of Equine Practitioners	CVB	Center for Veterinary Biologics
AAHA	American Animal Hospital Association	DIVA	Differentiating infected from vaccinated animals
AASRP	American Association of Small Ruminant Practitioners	DTH	Delayed type hypersensitivity
		FAO	Food and Agriculture Organization
APHIS	Animal and Plant Health Inspection Service	PGL	Poly(lactide-co-glycolide)
		PGLA	Poly(lactic-co-glycolic acid)
AVMA	American Veterinary Medical Association	USDA	US Department of Agriculture
CDC	US Centers for Disease Control and Prevention	WHO	World Health Organization

Vaccine selection for companion and food-producing animals

Given the wide range of animal species and the large number of vaccine products available on the market for veterinarians, decisions concerning vaccine selection and administration protocols have become complicated. Factors affecting these decisions include the following: (1) ongoing changes in the understanding of the immune system and its response in different animal species, (2) changes in either local or regional population susceptibilities to various diseases, (3) increased animal appraisal and related liabilities, (4) longer animal life expectancies due to an improved quality of care, (5) improved medical record keeping, which allows for better tracking of the effects of vaccine use and administration, (6) discoveries of new understanding of infectious diseases and pathogenesis, (7) improved understanding of the biologic regulatory licensing and labeling process by veterinarians, and (8) the heightened awareness of potential risks to human health associated with vaccine use and administration

Vaccinology: An Essential Guide, First Edition. Edited by Gregg N. Milligan and Alan D.T. Barrett.

in animals. Moreover, the American Veterinary Medical Association (AVMA) Council on Biologic and Therapeutic Agents (COBTA) has recognized that there is insufficient data available to scientifically determine a single best vaccination protocol regimen for application to *all* animals globally. Therefore, COBTA recommends a more customized approach to vaccination as the safest and most effective method to medically address the increasing diversity of animal patients presented for immunization.

Factors in selecting vaccine targets

(1) Ongoing changes in the understanding of the immune system and its response in different animal species

(2) Changes in either local or regional population susceptibilities to various diseases

(3) Increased animal appraisal and related liabilities

(4) Longer animal life expectancies due to an improved quality of care

(5) Improved medical record keeping, which allows for better tracking of the effects of vaccine use and administration

(6) Discoveries of new understanding of infectious diseases and pathogenesis

(7) Improved understanding of the biologic regulatory licensing and labeling process by veterinarians

(8) Increased awareness of potential risks to human health associated with vaccine use and administration in egg- and milk-producing animals

To simplify the task of selecting appropriate vaccines for companion and food-producing animals, vaccines can be generally categorized as either "core" or "noncore." Core vaccines are those that protect animals from diseases that are endemic to a region, protect the human public from diseases that can be transmitted from animals, are required by law, protect against highly virulent or infectious diseases, and/or clearly demonstrate efficacy and safety with a high level of patient benefit/low level of risk to justify their use in the majority of patients. Noncore vaccines are

intended for a minority of animals and are targeted for diseases that are of limited risk in the region, protect against diseases that present less severe threats to infected patients, have a benefit/risk ratio that is too low to justify the use of the veterinary product in all circumstances, and/or lack adequate scientific information to allow regulators to fully evaluate the safety and/or efficacy of the product. Vaccination schedules are also categorized based on other factors, including age or immune maturity of the animal and general living conditions (indoor versus outdoor, single versus multiple animal ownership, etc.). The AVMA and several AVMA-recognized associations have published recommended vaccination schedules for core and noncore vaccines on their respective web-sites, including the American Association of Feline Practitioners (AAFP), American Animal Hospital Association (AAHA), American Association of Equine Practitioners (AAEP), American Association of Bovine Practitioners (AABP), and American Association of Small Ruminant Practitioners (AASRP).

Factors affecting the cost-effectiveness of a vaccine

(1) Vaccine cost (including labor)

(2) Incidence of the disease

(3) Average treatment and production cost of the disease

(4) Vaccine efficacy

When considering the use of a vaccine in food-producing animals, there are economic factors that must be carefully considered. Often, veterinarians and animal producers overseeing the care of food animals will perform a cost-benefit ratio analysis of a vaccine before adding it to an existing preventive health care program. Fundamentally, vaccines decrease the incidence and severity of a disease, and thus decrease the associated treatment costs and production losses if the animal were to become exposed to the pathogen. However, the cost-effectiveness of a vaccine is actually dependent on at least four factors when considering its use for a large group of animals: (1) vaccine cost (including labor), (2) incidence of the disease, (3) average treatment and production cost of the disease, and (4) vaccine efficacy. As predicted, some of these factors can be highly variable, and therefore accurate information is required in order to make an informed decision. There are some published studies that describe the cost-benefit analysis of either vaccines or vaccination schemes for certain diseases. For herd health management, there are also health cost-benefit calculators that are available online that, after user input, calculate the cost-benefit of vaccination as well as the marginal rate of return.

Definitions

Companion animal: Domesticated or domestic-bred animals whose physical, emotional, and social needs can be readily met as companions in the home, or in close daily relationships with humans; the more usual word is "pet."

Food-producing animal: Animals used in the production food for humans, including animals that produce meat, eggs, and milk.

Status of veterinary vaccines for infectious and noninfectious diseases in companion and food-producing animals

The primary focus of this chapter is veterinary vaccines for infectious diseases; however, vaccines are also available for animals for noninfectious diseases and fertility/production control. Noninfectious disease vaccines have been primarily developed for allergies and cancers in both companion and food-producing animals, and to control wildlife populations or alter reproductive functions. For the latter, vaccines are targeted against either gamete antigens or specific reproductive hormones, which affect the function of the hypothalamic–pituitary–gonadal axis.

As discussed in detail below, there are various forms and formulations for veterinary vaccines against viruses, bacteria, parasites, and fungi, and there are variable degrees of immune protection that are generated from these vaccines that must be factored in when selecting them for a vaccination program.

Definitions

First-generation vaccine: Whole-organism vaccines that are either live and weakened or killed forms.
Second-generation vaccine: Subunit vaccines, consisting of defined protein antigens or recombinant protein components.
Third-generation vaccine: Typically DNA vaccines, which are often composed of a small, circular piece of bacterial DNA (called a plasmid), genetically engineered to produce one or two specific proteins (antigens) from a pathogen after being transfected into host cells via direct injection, or injection with electroporation or gene gun.

Viruses

Table 10.1 shows a partial list of viruses that are of global importance in veterinary medicine that affect companion (dogs, cats, horses) and food-producing (cattle, sheep, pigs, poultry) animals. Depending on their composition, vaccines are generally categorized as "first-generation," "second-generation," or "third-generation" vaccines. For viruses, first-generation vaccines include conventional live and inactivated (killed) vaccines, which have been used for decades in routine vaccination protocols. These vaccines account for more than 2,000 US Department of Agriculture (USDA) licensed vaccines for use in animals and are available for both companion and food-producing animals. The majority of licensed first-generation vaccines are inactivated, but nearly 25% of them are live attenuated formulations.

Live attenuated virus vaccines

Most live vaccines have been selected for attenuation by either obtaining live organisms from nontarget hosts or passaging wild-type viruses in cell culture or chicken embryos (eggs). Attenuation of live viruses has also been achieved by the selection of mutations in the viral genome by passaging in a host or cell type that the virus does not normally replicate. There is adaptation to the new host, and the virus no longer causes disease in the normal host. Live attenuated viruses usually replicate in the target cells of the wild-type virus, causing a mild infection and inducing robust cellular and humoral immune responses. Live attenuated viruses also have the potential to revert to

Table 10.1 Partial Listing of Viruses That Are of Global Importance in Veterinary Medicine, Listed by Target Animal[a]

Dogs	Rabies virus Canine distemper virus (CDV) Canine adenovirus (hepatitis; CAV-2) Canine parvovirus Canine parainfluenza virus Canine coronavirus	Cattle	Rabies virus Bovine respiratory disease complex (BRDC) Foot-and-mouth disease virus (FMDV) Rinderpest virus (cattle plague) Lumpy skin disease Vesicular stomatitis virus (VSV)
Cats	Rabies virus Feline panleukopenia virus (FPV; feline distemper) Feline viral rhinotracheitis (FHV-1; feline influenza) Feline parvovirus Feline calicivirus (FCV) Feline leukemia virus (FeLV) Feline immunodeficiency virus (FIV; feline AIDS)	Pigs	Classical swine fever Foot-and-mouth disease virus (FMDV) Porcine reproductive and respiratory syndrome (PRRS) African swine fever Swine influenza Porcine circovirus-2 Parvovirus
		Sheep	Bluetongue virus (BTV; multiple serotypes) Foot-and-mouth disease virus (FMDV) Capri poxviruses Avian influenza virus
Horses	Herpes viruses (EHV) Equine influenza virus (EIV) West Nile virus (WNV) Eastern equine encephalitis virus (EEEV) Venezuelan equine encephalitis virus (VEEV) Western equine encephalitis virus (WEEV) African horse sickness Equine arteritis virus (EAV) Equine infectious anemia virus (EIAV)	Poultry	Paramyxoviruses (including Newcastle disease) Marek's disease virus (MDV) Infectious laryngotracheitis virus Duck herpes virus (DHV-1) Avian infectious bronchitis virus (IBV) Infectious bursal disease virus (IBDV) Chicken anemia virus (CAV)

[a]Vaccines are available for most of the viruses listed, but with variable efficacy and availability; some vaccines are also important for preventing zoonotic transmission of these viruses (e.g., rabies virus, VEEV).

a pathogenic phenotype and can sometimes be the source of an outbreak. However, they have also been crucial in the successful control and prevention of many important viral diseases. For example, a live attenuated vaccine (the so-called Plowright vaccine [for Walter Plowright, the inventor of the vaccine]) was primarily responsible for the recent global eradication of the rinderpest virus (RPV). In 2011, rinderpest was recognized as the second disease in history to be completely eliminated from the world, following smallpox, which was the first.

Inactivated or killed virus vaccines

For inactivated (killed) vaccines, viral inactivation is achieved with the use of either heat or chemicals (e.g., formaldehyde, thiomersal, ethylene oxide, and β-propriolactone). When compared to live attenuated vaccines, inactivated vaccines are more stable and pose less risk for reversion to virulence. However, they are also less protective, because they are unable to multiply in the vaccinee, infect target cells, and activate cytotoxic T-cell responses. For this reason, the use of adjuvants and multiple doses are usually required to induce a sufficient level of immunity.

Rationally designed virus vaccines

Conventional vaccines are available and effective for many viral diseases of livestock; however, some countries do not allow these vaccines to be used in routine vaccination programs due to the inability to serologically distinguish vaccine from wild-type strains. This would result in the loss of the country's disease-free status and their ability to compete in international trade. A good example of this problem is foot-and-mouth disease (FMD), which affects cloven-hoofed animals (e.g., cattle, sheep, pigs, goats). Although conventional vaccines are available for FMD and have been shown to be effective in controlling the disease, they are not used in FMD-free countries, and often a slaughter policy is used instead to control the spread of infection in the event of an outbreak. "Marker vaccines" are becoming favorable for use in disease-free countries, which would provide a method for differentiating infected from vaccinated animals (DIVA), and importantly, contribute to the efforts in disease control and eradication. By selectively deleting gene(s) in a marker vaccine, this approach provides a way to distinguish between the antibody responses to the vaccine strain with that of the wild-type strain such that there would be no antibodies generated against the deleted gene(s) of the vaccine strain. DIVA vaccines and their companion diagnostics tests are either available or in the development process for several important infectious diseases, including FMD, Rift Valley fever, infectious bovine rhinotracheitis (IBR), pseudorabies, and classical swine fever (CSF).

Subunit vaccines are considered to be second-generation vaccines, and a large number of them are in the veterinary market today. Subunit vaccines are noninfectious and composed of either purified or recombinant viral antigens that are capable of stimulating an immune response. Unfortunately, these vaccines generally induce poor protective immunity, usually requiring multiple doses and/or the addition of strong adjuvants to induce immunity.

Other rationally designed vaccines include those in which specific mutations or deletions have been introduced into the viral genome, producing a stably attenuated live vaccine; these vaccines can also be inactivated using conventional methods. In addition, engineered from at least two different viral genomes, chimeric viruses have been used successfully as vaccines. Chimeric vaccines for porcine circovirus type 2 (PCV2), avian influenza virus, and West Nile virus (WNV) have been licensed for use in animals. Live viral vectored vaccines are also widely used in animals and are primarily based on poxviruses, including vaccinia virus, fowlpox virus, and canarypox virus. Poxviruses are used as vectors for the expression of viral proteins in mammalian cells, which result in the induction of a protective immune response. The canarypox virus system ALVAC has been used exten-

sively as a platform for several veterinary vaccines, and the oral recombinant vaccinia-rabies vaccine has been extremely successful in controlling rabies in Europe (foxes) and the USA (coyotes, raccoons, and foxes).

DNA vaccines are considered third-generation vaccines that offer many advantages over live vaccines when it comes to safety and stability; however, these vaccines have not been particularly effective due to poor immunogenicity. DNA vaccines have become particularly useful for fish viruses, including infectious hematopoietic necrosis (IHN) virus in salmon, and a DNA vaccine for WNV has been licensed for use in horses. Table 10.2 lists second- and third-generation licensed and commercialized veterinary viral vaccines that are available for different animal species.

Table 10.2 Second- and Third-Generation Licensed/Commercialized Veterinary Viral Vaccines, Listed by Target Animal

Target Animal	Target Pathogen(s)
Pigs	Porcine circovirus virus, type 2 Pseudorabies virus Classical swine fever virus
Cattle	Bovine herpesvirus, type 1
Horses	Equine influenza virus West Nile virus
Poultry	Marek's disease virus Herpes turkey virus Infectious bursal disease virus Newcastle disease virus Avian influenza virus (H5N1)
Cats	Rabies virus Feline leukemia virus
Wildlife, canines	Rabies virus
Dogs	Canine parvovirus Canine coronavirus Canine distemper virus
Fur animals	Canine distemper virus
Salmon	Infectious hematopoietic necrosis virus

Adapted from Meeusen et al. (2007).

Bacteria

Similar to viral vaccines, a large number of live attenuated and inactivated bacterial vaccines have been used for decades to vaccinate animals against bacterial diseases. In most cases, the basis for attenuation has not been determined for these vaccines as they were derived and licensed prior to the development of molecular biology and genetic manipulation techniques. The method for conventional attenuation of live bacteria is similar to that used for viruses, in which bacteria are passaged in media or cells to acquire attenuating mutations and/or adapted to a new host, in which they no longer cause disease in the usual host. Inactivated vaccines usually consist of bacterins (i.e., formalin-inactivated bacterial cultures) or more well-defined subunit antigens that have been formulated in an oil or aluminum hydroxide adjuvant. With the advances of new technologies, there has been a concerted effort to develop more molecularly defined vaccines for bacteria. Several bacterial vaccines have been engineered with specific mutations or deletions of previously characterized genes to attenuate the bacteria. For example, a gene-deleted vaccine has recently been developed for strangles, a highly infectious respiratory disease in horses and caused by the bacterium *Streptococcus equi* subspecies *equi*. Based the partial deletion of the *aroA* gene, this live attenuated vaccine provides protection following submucosal administration. Table 10.3 lists recently commercialized veterinary bacterial vaccines that are available for different animal species.

There has been particular interest in vaccine development against zoonotic bacteria, including *Salmonella* and *Campylobacter* in poultry, brucellosis in cattle and small ruminants, *Streptococcus suis* in swine, and *Escherichia coli* (*E. coli*) in cattle. Vaccines against food-borne bacteria have been an area of increasing interest due to their potential impact in preventing human disease worldwide. Periodic, but often explosive, outbreaks of *E. coli* infections in humans due to contaminated produce and meat products can result in serious health consequences. A notable *E. coli* outbreak occurred in May and June 2011 in northern Germany, in which a strain of *E. coli* O104:H4 caused serious food-borne illness, including hemolytic uremic syndrome (HUS) and death. The outbreak involved cases in at least 15 other countries, including the USA, and

Table 10.3 Recently Commercialized Veterinary Bacterial Vaccines, Listed by Target Animal

Target Animal	Target Pathogen(s)
Pigs	*Actinobacillus pleuropneumoniae*
	Lawsonia intracellularis
Cattle	*Brucella abortus*
Sheep	*Chlamydophila abortus*
Horses	*Streptococcus equi*
Poultry	*Mycoplasma synoviae*
	Mycoplasma gallisepticum
	Bordetella avium
	Salmonella
Dogs	*Porphyromonas gulae*
	Porphyromonas denticanis
	Porphyromonas salivosa
Fish	*Yersinia ruckeri*
	Aeromonas salmonicida
	Vibrio anguillarum

Adapted from Meeusen et al. (2007).

there were economic losses associated with restrictions on the importation of European Union (EU) produce by other countries. By the end of the outbreak, the World Health Organization (WHO) reported that there were at least 908 HUS cases, 3167 cases of enterohemorrhagic *E. coli* (EHEC) infection, and 50 deaths associated with the outbreak.

According to the Centers of Disease Control and Prevention (CDC), more than 63,000 Americans acquire food-borne pathogens every year after consuming contaminated foods such as ground beef or raw vegetables. Of those, approximately 2138 individuals will require hospitalization, and 20 will die from the infection. In 2009, a vaccine against bacterial proteins involved in seeking and binding iron (which are important for sustaining *E. coli* growth) was made available to the USA under a conditional license from the USDA to reduce shedding of *E. coli* O157:H7 from cattle. Based on the field trials, it was determined that this vaccine was able to effectively reduce the number of cattle testing positive for the bacteria, and in the cattle that did test positive, the concentration of bacteria in the fecal samples was significantly reduced when compared to the cattle receiving placebos. As of 2012, there were two promising vaccines for *E. coli* O157:H7 that were awaiting approval by the Center for Veterinary Biologics (CVB) at the USDA Animal and Plant Health Inspection Service (USDA-APHIS) for conventional licenses.

Parasites

Currently, drugs that treat economically important parasites might be considered sufficient for most purposes, especially since they are commercially available, safe, cheap, and effective against a broad spectrum of parasites. However, drug resistance and residue problems are becoming significant challenges, both of which are exacerbated by increased prophylactic use of drugs. Therefore, the threat of resistance to these antiparasitic drugs has become a major motivator for the development of parasite vaccines. Indeed, for some protozoal diseases, there are no effective chemotherapeutics available, and the only control method is vaccination. This includes vaccines that prevent abortion in cattle and sheep due to the protozoans *Neospora caninum* and *Toxoplasma gondii*, respectively.

in humans or animals, the development of vaccines for parasites can be extremely challenging due to several factors, most of which are primarily due to the antigenic complexity of parasites during the different stages of their life cycle within an animal. Other factors that have contributed to the slow development of vaccines include (1) for some parasites, the lack of vaccine effectiveness at the site of infection, (2) the immune effector mechanisms that are not clearly defined, (3) variation in the host immune response to different parasites and to different parasite stages, (4) difficulty screening potential vaccine antigens, (5) vaccines with a narrow spectrum of protection, which are often restricted to a strain, and (6) in certain situations, lack of economic incentive by manufacturers. There are only a few veterinary vaccines that have been investigated for helminths and ectoparasites; however, a large number of protozoal vaccines have been available for many decades and are primarily based on live attenuated organisms. Several killed or subunit vaccines have recently been developed and are commercially available, and it is speculated that more vaccines will become available as our understanding of parasite genes lead to the identification of antigens that are immunologically relevant. Table 10.4

Factors that have contributed to the slow development of parasite vaccines

1. For some parasites, the lack of vaccine effectiveness at the site of infection
2. Immune effector mechanisms that are not clearly defined
3. Variation in the host immune response to different parasites and to different parasite stages
4. Difficulty screening potential vaccine antigens
5. Vaccines with a narrow spectrum of protection, which are often restricted to a strain
6. In certain situations, lack of economic incentive by manufacturers

---

Recent technological advances have increased knowledge and understanding of parasites; however, commercially available vaccines that are based on this information have yet to be exploited. Whether for use

Table 10.4 Veterinary Protozoal Vaccines, Listed by Target Animal

Target Animal	Target Pathogen(s)
Cattle	*Theileria parva*
	Theileria annulata
	Theileria hirci
	Babesia bovis
	Babesia bigemina
	Neospora caninum
Sheep	*Toxoplasma gondii*
Horses	*Sarcocystis neurona*
Poultry	*Eimeria* spp.
	Eimeria tenella
	Eimeria maxima
Dogs	*Giardia duodenalis*
	Babesia canis
	Leishmania donovani

Adapted from Meeusen et al. (2007).

lists commercially available veterinary protozoal vaccines that are available for different animal species.

Fungi

Similar to vaccines for parasites, veterinary vaccines for fungi are also a challenge to develop, and a better understanding of the immune response to these infections is needed in order to develop effective vaccines. However, there are several useful fungal vaccines that are available in veterinary medicine. Equines and other mammals (including dogs) infected with *Pythium insidiosum* develop a debilitating cutaneous, subcutaneous, or systemic disease. Two vaccines have been useful for both the prevention (prophylactic vaccination before clinical disease) and treatment (therapeutic vaccination after the start of clinical disease) of horses infected with *P. insidiosum*. One of these vaccines is composed of sonicated hyphal antigens, whereas the other vaccine is prepared from culture filtrate antigens. Although the specific immunogens from each preparation have not yet been identified, work is ongoing to identify the specific constituents of these extracts that are responsible for eliciting protective immunity.

Dermatophytosis (or ringworm) is another important fungal infection that affects the hair and superficial keratinized cell layers of the skin of both animals and humans. Several species of the genera *Microsporum*, *Trichophyton*, and *Epidermophyton* can cause clinical infections in animals, and dermatophytosis is a zoonotic disease. Some of the dermatophyte species can infect a variety of hosts, but there is a certain degree of host specificity. The disease spreads easily from one animal to another by direct contact or indirectly via environmental contamination or fomites. In some countries, ringworm in cattle and fur-bearing animals is a notifiable disease, and to limit the spread of disease, certain control measures are often imposed on affected herds, which includes restricting the sale of affected animals, access to grazing pastures, and participation in livestock shows.

In some countries, mass vaccination programs have been used to successfully control and eradicate dermatophytosis in cattle and fur-bearing animals, which has also significantly decreased the number of human cases due to zoonotic transmission. Current vaccines are largely first-generation vaccines; of these, the most effective and widely used vaccines for this disease are live attenuated vaccines, which stimulate a cell-mediated immune response and confer long-lasting immunity against subsequent exposure to the fungus. There are several commercially available live attenuated vaccines for use in different countries for cattle, horses, and fur-bearing animals, which can be used for either prophylactic or therapeutic administration.

Inactivated dermatophyte vaccines are also available for use in cattle, horses, dogs, and cats in some countries; however, the scientific literature supporting the efficacy of these vaccines (especially for companion animals) has been rather limited. Despite attempts to prepare subunit vaccines based on virulence factors (including keratinases) and heat shock proteins (hsp) derived from different dermatophyte species, these second-generation vaccines have been limited in their success. When assessing the efficacy and safety of vaccine candidates in a target animal species, a delayed type hypersensitivity (DTH) skin test is often used to assess the cell-mediated immune response, a key factor in developing protective immunity to this fungal disease. There is also clear evidence that candidate antigens must be able to stimulate strong T helper 1 cell responses in order to confer protection against dermatophyte infections. Therefore, future research will need to focus on the identification of major T-cell epitopes that specifically elicit a DTH reaction.

Status of vaccines for aquaculture

Aquaculture is the fastest growing sector of agriculture in the world, and today it accounts for almost 50% of the world's supply of fish for human consumption. Fish is also a vital source of protein for people around

---

Definition

Aquaculture: The cultivation of aquatic organisms, such as fish, shellfish, and even plants, for human consumption. Aquaculture can range from land-based to open-ocean production and involve either marine or freshwater species.

---

the world, and in 2000, the Food and Agriculture Organization (FAO) of the United Nations estimated that about 1 billion people worldwide rely on fish as their primary source of animal protein. In North America and Europe, fish supply less than 10% of the total animal protein consumed, but in Africa, Asia, and China, fish supply at least 17%, 26%, and 22%, respectively, of total animal protein consumed. Fish also have substantial social and economic importance. In 2000, the FAO estimated the value of fish traded internationally to be $51 billion per annum with over 36 million people employed directly through fishing and aquaculture. With the growing human population, consumption of food fish is increasing, having risen from 40 million tons in 1970 to 86 million tons in 1998; in 2008, it reached 115 million tons.

With such a rapidly growing industry providing a significant portion of the world's food fish, it is important that losses of any kind are minimized. Thus, infectious diseases can be particularly devastating to this industry, and effective prophylactic and therapeutic regimens are vital. Vaccination against fish pathogens is playing an ever-increasing role in large-scale commercial fish farming and has been a key reason for the success of salmon and trout cultivation. In addition, commercial vaccines have reduced the use of antibiotics, and they are becoming more available for other types of farmed fish, including channel catfish, European seabass and sea bream, Japanese amberjack and yellowtail, and tilapia and Atlantic cod. Proper fish management with good hygiene and limited stress are also important in the prophylaxis of infectious diseases and a necessity for the optimal effect of vaccines.

Fish can be immunized by (1) injection, usually intraperitoneally (or intramuscularly, if administering a DNA vaccine), (2) immersion, typically by dipping fish in a diluted vaccine solution, or (3) oral administration of the vaccine. Several factors must be addressed when considering these routes of administration for a particular vaccine, including antigen delivery, level of protection, side effects, practicality, and cost-benefit ratio. Only the injection and immersion methods are used at the industrial level, and in the commercial production of salmonids, both procedures are well-established practices.

The mechanisms involved in antigen uptake and presentation to the host's immune system after immersion and oral vaccination are poorly understood. However, it is clear that the mucosal immune system plays a central part in immune protection since the first encounter with a pathogen occurs through the mucosal surface. For oral vaccination, research has focused on protecting the antigens from digestion and decomposition during passage through the stomach and anterior portion of the hindgut, with the ultimate goal of antigen absorption and stimulation of the immunocompetent tissues in the posterior hindgut. Encapsulation of antigens in alginate microcapsules has been one approach to improve antigen delivery in the gut. Other approaches for oral vaccine delivery include the use of transformed microalgae, nanoparticles or microparticles composed of either natural or synthetic polymers, chitosan microparticles, poly(lactide-co-glycolide) (PGL) or poly(lactic-co-glycolic acid) (PGLA) particles, and biofilms.

There are several empirically developed vaccines based on inactivated bacterial pathogens that are currently on the market, which have proven to be efficacious in fish with relatively few side effects. In contrast, there are fewer vaccines that are commercially available for viruses, and no parasite vaccines exist.

Bacterial infections of fish caused by Gram-negative bacteria, including *Vibrio*, *Aeromonas*, and *Yersinia* species, have been effectively controlled by vaccination with inactivated vaccines. In particular, furunculosis, caused by the bacterium *Aeromonas salmonicida* subspecies *salmonicida*, is one of the most serious bacterial diseases of wild and farmed salmonids in the world. The disease is named after the raised liquefactive muscle lesions (furuncles), which sometimes occur in chronically infected fish, whereas acute infection usually results in fatal septicemia. At first, furunculosis was regarded as a disease occurring exclusively in salmonids; however, during the past decade, several cases of *A. salmonicida* infections have been reported in non-salmonids. With furunculosis, the success of vaccination has been largely due to the use of injectable vaccines that contain adjuvants. Interestingly, the first scientific publication concerning a fish vaccine was reported in 1942 by Duff, which was based on the effective use of an inactivated vaccine for *A. salmonicida*. Vaccines against several other important bacterial infections have been studied and found to be technically feasible. In particular, immunoprophylaxis against fish pasteurellosis and streptococcosis (lactococcosis) has been the focus of more recent studies.

Most commercially available virus vaccines for aquaculture are based on either inactivated viruses or recombinant subunit antigens, and when administered by either injection or immersion, they have been shown to elicit protective immunity. However, sometimes the level of protection by this formulation can be too low for commercial use, which has been observed for some viral diseases, including IHN (as previously mentioned), viral hemorrhagic septicemia (VHS), spring viremia of carp (SVC), and channel catfish virus disease (CCVD). In contrast, vaccines against infectious pancreatic necrosis (IPN) and grass carp hemorrhagic disease (GCHD) have proven to be successful in commercial fish farming when administered by injection. Red sea bream iridoviral disease (RSIVD) is a relatively recent threat to Japanese marine aquaculture, but a formalin-killed vaccine against RSIVD is commercially available and effective in protecting fish against disease. Live attenuated vaccines have been tested with good results; however, there are concerns about the safety of these vaccines that have hindered their use as commercial vaccines due to their potential to revert to virulence.

There are no commercially available vaccines against parasitic diseases in fish, and parasitic diseases, such as amoebic gill disease, white spot disease, whirling disease, and proliferative kidney disease (PKD), can create severe problems in fish farming. However, based on previous studies of the immune response to some of these parasites, one of the candidate diseases for immunoprophylaxis is cryptobiosis. Rainbow trout (*Oncorhynchus mykiss*) vaccinated with a live attenuated strain of *Cryptobia salmositica* were protected when challenged with this pathogenic hemoflagellate. Salmon lice (*Lepeophtheirus salmonis*) infections in the Northern hemisphere can be the source of major epizootics in both farmed and wild salmon. As a result, a number of studies are underway to examine various antigens of this ectoparasite as potential vaccine targets, particularly those antigens associated with the gastrointestinal tract and reproductive endocrine pathways.

Advanced technology has stimulated the development of new fish vaccines, including DNA vaccines, that demonstrate considerable efficacy, but in order for these vaccines to become commercially available, vaccine production must be economical, and all safety and environmental concerns must be carefully addressed. Although there is a considerable amount of research devoted to the development of fish vaccines by manufacturers, there is limited information about these vaccines in scientific publications. Currently, carps, barbels, and other members of the cyprinid family dominate fish aquaculture and account for 46% of the total value of cultivated fish in the world. Conversely, salmonids account for 16% of the total value of cultivated fish, and they have been the primary focus of scientific literature and vaccine development in the aquaculture industry. Therefore, future research efforts in vaccine development should continue to expand to include other species of farmed fish and the diseases that affect them.

Future challenges

Overall, veterinary vaccines improve animal health and productivity. And in most cases, they are more cost-effective than treating sick animals; however, they can also make a significant impact on human health in terms of reducing the exposure to zoonotic pathogens as well as potentially harmful veterinary pharmaceuticals. With new technological advances in vaccine development, the veterinary vaccine market is forecast to grow exponentially, and this growth will be stimulated even further as recognized pathogens become resistant to drug therapies and new pathogens are discovered. As the population of the world continues to expand, the demand for nutrient sources, including protein from food-producing animals, will increase. This situation will require the continuous development of vaccines that are not only effective in preventing infectious disease but which must also be economical for animal producers. This will be a formidable task as the global population is predicted to reach between 7.5 and 10 billion by 2050. The development of future veterinary vaccines for both companion and food-producing animals depends in part on the discovery of new technologies that achieve selective induction of effective immune responses. To make an impact on animal health, collaborative efforts between researchers, manufacturers, and government regulatory agencies will be critically important for the successful of development and marketing of veterinary vaccines in the future.

Summary

- As new vaccines become available on the market, veterinarians caring for companion and food-producing animals must carefully consider several different factors before selecting them for routine use.

- Most veterinary vaccines on the market are derived and produced by conventional attenuation and/or inactivation processes; however, a large number of genetically engineered and subunit vaccines have been and will continue to be developed and marketed to improve safety and efficacy against a wide range of infectious diseases.

- When it comes to veterinary vaccines that are based on scientific advances and new technology, commercialization of these vaccines for viruses and bacteria far outweigh those of parasites and fungi; however, with the discovery of new antigen targets for parasites and fungi, subunit vaccines are currently being investigated for their ability to provide protective immunity.

- With the global demand of fish for human consumption, the aquaculture industry relies heavily on the success of their vaccination programs to prevent infectious diseases and the economic losses associated with an outbreak.

Further reading

Blanco JL and Garcia ME (2008). Immune response to fungal infections. Veterinary Immunology and Immunopathology 125, 47–70.

Gudding R, Lillehaug A, and Evensen O (1999). Recent developments in fish vaccinology. Veterinary Immunology and Immunopathology 72, 203–212.

Lund A and DeBoer DJ (2008). Immunoprophylaxis of dermatophytosis in animals. Mycopathologia 166, 407–424.

Meeusen ENT, Walker J, Peters A, Pastoret P-P, and Jungersen G (2007). Current status of veterinary vaccines. Clinical Microbiology Reviews 20, 489–510.

Patel JR and Heldens JGM (2009). Immunoprophylaxis against important virus diseases of horses, farm animals, and birds. Vaccine 27, 1797–1810.

Sommerset I, Krossoy B, Biering E, and Frost P (2005). Vaccines for fish in aquaculture. Expert Review of Vaccines 4, 89–101.

Tollis M (2006). Standardization or tailorization of veterinary vaccines: A conscious endeavor against infectious diseases of animals. Annali Dell'istituto Superiore Di Sanita 42, 446–449.

Vercruysse J, Knox DP, Schetters TPM, and Willadsen P (2004). Veterinary parasitic vaccines: pitfalls and future directions. Trends in Parasitology 20, 488–492.

11 Development of vaccines for microbial diseases

Dennis W. Trent and David W.C. Beasley

Sealy Center for Vaccine Development, University of Texas Medical Branch, Galveston, TX, USA

Abbreviations

AFC	Antibody-forming cells	HIV	Human immunodeficiency virus
ATCC	American Type Culture Collection	IND	Investigational new drug
BLA	Biologics License Application	MCB	Master cell bank
CBER	Center for Biologics Evaluation and Research	MHC	Major histocompatibility complex
		NDA	New drug application
CDC	US Centers for Disease Control and Prevention	NIBSC	National Institute for Biological Standards and Control
CEF	Chick embryo fibroblast	OECD	Organization for Economic
CFR	Code of Federal Regulations		Cooperation and Development
ECACC	European Collection of Cell Cultures	QA	Quality assurance
		QC	Quality control
ELISA	Enzyme-linked immunosorbent assay	SOP	Standard operating procedure
		TFF	Transgential flow filtration
FD&C	FDA and Cosmetic Act	US FDA	US Food and Drug Administration
GCP	Good clinical practice	VSD	Vaccine safety datalink
GLP	Good laboratory practice	WCB	Working cell bank
GMP (or cGMP)	Good manufacturing practice	WHO	World Health Organization

Introduction

Vaccines provide an effective means to prevent and control transmission of serious infections in the human population for the good of public health. In the USA and Western Europe, the incidence of the most vaccine-preventable human diseases has declined 95–99% as compared the pre-vaccine era. In addition to immunization and protection of the individual, the rate that diseases are transmitted between individuals in the community is affected when a significant pro-portion of the population is vaccinated (see Chapters 3 and 18). The contribution of vaccines to preventing epidemics of once common childhood infections has been dramatic. Epidemics of human smallpox virus have been eradicated, while the incidence of other infectious disease has been significantly reduced (polio, measles, mumps, rubella) as a result of vaccination.

It is critical that new vaccines are developed to prevent diseases caused by infectious agents that anti-genically change (e.g., influenza and HIV) and for

Vaccinology: An Essential Guide, First Edition. Edited by Gregg N. Milligan and Alan D.T. Barrett.
© 2015 John Wiley & Sons, Ltd. Published 2015 by John Wiley & Sons, Ltd.

Table 11.1 Key Considerations for Vaccine Development

Consideration	General Comments
Antigen identification	Conserved virulence factors, B/T cell epitopes depending on pathogen
Development of production methods	Product dependent—manufacture requirements specific; intact organism, purified subunit, cell-culture systems, bio-fermentation
Relevant CD4+ Th target	Th1 versus Th2 versus Th17 epitopes depending on pathogen
Needed for/CD8+ T cells	Intracellular pathogens specific need
Specific memory subset needed	Central memory (Tcm) versus peripheral memory (Ptem)
Avoidance of excessive Treg	Treg inhibit effecter T-cell development for long-term memory
Adjuvant selection	Alum salts enhance Ab responses; Toll-like receptor agonists, oil/water enhance T cells
Vaccine delivery method	B- versus T-cell responses; ideally mimic natural pathogen invasion strategy
Vaccination schedule	Mucosal versus systemic vaccination depending on biology of the pathogen and nature of vaccine
Immunological biomarkers of immunity	Molecular signature associated with optimal immune response; antibodies versus cell-mediated immunity
Phase I to III clinical trials	Optimization of dosing schedule and potency; safety first, then immunogenicity and correlates of protective immune efficacy

newly emerging diseases. Diseases for which effective vaccines have not been developed can emerge from isolated ecosystems (e.g., zoonotic bacteria and viruses that make the "jump" from animals to humans [e.g., SARS {severe acute respiratory syndrome} and Nipah/ Hendra viruses]) and may rapidly spread in an immunologically naive population. In spite of an extensive research and development effort, over the past 30 years few new human and animal vaccines have been licensed. Recent developments in molecular biology, genetics, immunology, pathology, and vaccinology (see Chapter 7) have opened avenues for development of new vaccines that are safer, highly immunogenic, and prime anamnestic immune responses that limit infection and prevent clinical disease (Table 11.1).

Principles of vaccine design

The research and development process to create new vaccines requires an interdisciplinary scientific effort involving principles of molecular biology, immunol- ogy, microbiology, biochemistry, epidemiology, clinical vaccinology, bioinformatics, and regulatory affairs

---

Definition

Regulatory affairs define every interaction that a company has with a regulatory authority, be that authority national, state or provincial, or local. They involve every internal department or individual that might need something from, or need to provide something to, a regulatory authority. This interaction continues for the entire life cycle of the product, from conception to marketing and every type of interaction between the company and the authorities, over all times, and for all products.

It is essential to remember the broad possibilities of experiences when dealing with regulatory affairs colleagues as their expectations and perspective can be very broad and not specific or with unique perspective and sometimes with narrow views of the field.

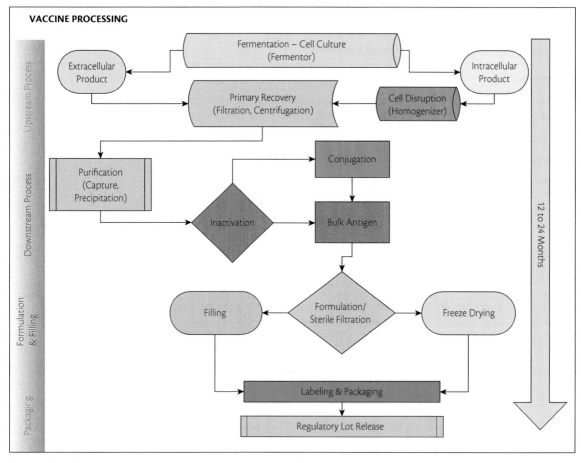

Figure 11.1 Generalized outline indicating the major steps involved in the vaccine research and development pathway.

(Figure 11.1). This process requires a significant financial investment and may require as long as 10 to 18 years to develop, manufacture, and obtain regulatory approval to conduct clinical trials and license for use vaccine in the population at risk. Clinical studies to demonstrate safety, potency, and efficacy in humans are conducted with approval of national regulatory authorities who license vaccines for use in the intended population at risk (see Chapters 12 and 15).

This chapter will describe key components in the design and development of vaccines with insight into strategies to create and produce experimental vaccines to be tested for immunogenicity, efficacy, and safety in animal models. This process requires research sup-

ported by the sciences of chemistry, physics, physiology, immunology, microbiology, clinical medicine, and public health. Creation of new vaccines requires much of the work to be done in a regulated environment to ensure that purity, efficacy, and safety information is appropriate and accurate. It is critical that vaccine development programs communicate with regulatory authorities early in the process to share and receive information critical to the process. Once the nonclinical studies are completed, an investigational new drug (IND) application containing laboratory study results of the vaccine candidate is submitted to the regulatory authorities to request permission to conduct studies in humans (Figure 11.2).

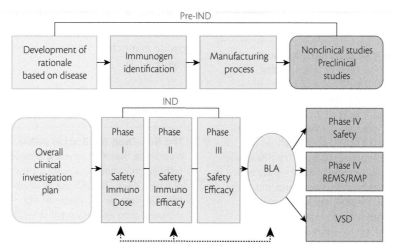

Figure 11.2 Outline of the sequence of events involved in identification of vaccine antigens, manufacture of the vaccine, and overall clinical investigation plan through licensure of the vaccine with regulatory authorities.

Regulatory terminology

Potency: Specific ability or capacity of the product, as indicated by appropriate laboratory tests or from adequately controlled clinical data obtained through administration of the product in the manner intended, to give a given result. Potency is defined as the ability of the product to perform as claimed and is usually associated with some measurable effect and/or correlate with some quantitative laboratory finding.

Purity: Relative freedom from extraneous matter, regardless of whether it is harmful to the recipient or deleterious to the product. Usually, the concepts of purity and safety coincide; purity most often relates to freedom from such materials such as pyrogens, adventitious agents, and chemicals used in manufacture of the product.

Safety: Relative freedom from harmful effect to people affected directly or indirectly by a product when prudently administered, taking in to characterization the character of the product in relation to the condition of the recipient. Thus, safety is relative and cannot be ensured in an absolute sense.

Vaccine efficacy (VE): The percentage reduction in disease incidence attributable to vaccination, calculated by means of the following formula equation: VE% = (U − V)/U × 100 where U = incidence in unvaccinated people and V = incidence in vaccinated people.

Product development pathway

Development of a new vaccine begins with the concept that immunization can prevent or modify a clinical disease of known etiology (Figure 11.2). For example, of the approximately 30 vaccines licensed for human immunization in the USA, 12 are pediatric vaccines developed in response to a medical need to prevent these infectious diseases in children. Public demand for safe and effective vaccines continues to be strong. Therefore, research and development to create new vaccines for infections such as malaria, HIV/AIDS, dengue, respiratory syncytial virus, herpes simplex, and hepatitis C are in progress. The challenges involved are scientifically complex, expensive, require specialized facilities, and are demanding due to the need to meet rigorous government regulatory requirements. A significant hurdle in translating basic science advances into vaccines is correlating efficacy in animal models when human efficacy studies are not appropriate or possible to undertake (Figure 11.2; see Chapter 12). For a vaccine with wide utility, the manufacture of tens of millions of doses per year is required. The goal is that each and every dose is equivalent, safe, and effective. The regulatory burden is the level of proof and documentation necessary to provide guarantees that this broad goal is achieved for every vaccine lot.

The quest to prevent infectious disease requires more than understanding the antigenic structure of the infectious agent and definition of protective epitopes on structural and nonstructural proteins (Figure 11.1, Table 11.1; see Chapters 4, 5, and 7). How the antigens will be presented and the type of vaccine that will be developed must be determined whether an inactivated organism, subunits/recombinant protein, or attenuated organism. In addition, how the vaccine will be produced is essential to the development plan: fermentation, cell culture, genetic engineering, recombinant DNA, or a combination of methods. During and after the experimental vaccine has been prepared testing must be done to certify the vaccine is pure, safe, efficacious, potent, and stable.

The central issue related to technology is the evolution and translation of a procedure used to make vaccines in a basic research laboratory into a process that can be scaled up to operate in a manufacturing environment to make tens of millions of doses per year. There are many academic and governmental research laboratories and fledgling biotechnology companies with the ability to innovate and generate interesting new vaccine product candidates, which is the first step in the vaccine development process. However, this stage is just the beginning of a cycle of intense activity that requires great skill, sophisticated facilities, determination, and much patience, and, accordingly, a long period of time. Development of information to demonstrate efficacy and safety of a vaccine to enable application for licensure with submission of a new drug application (NDA) to regulatory authorities may require as much as $900 million and 18 years of work (Figure 11.1).

Identification of vaccine protective antigens

The first task in vaccine development is identification and characterization of the antigen to be the immunological target for the protective immune response (Table 11.1). To be effective, the vaccine antigen must induce a primary immune response and significant immune anamnestic response upon second exposure of the host. The immune response should be directed against highly conserved antigens expressed by all or most subtypes of a particular pathogen that will minimize the chance of the pathogen immunological escape. Targeting virulence factors essential for multiplication of the pathogen is critical so that immunological neutralization will render the pathogen innocuous. If protective epitopes are located in hypervariable regions of the protective antigen, it is likely mutations will accumulate in response to the vaccine enabling immunological escape and spread of mutants for which the vaccine will not be protective. Vaccine development and design is based on laboratory studies using immunological methods to identify key antigens, selection of a method for antigen presentation, optimization of a method(s) for production of the antigen, and development of tests to measure desired immunological responses to critical epitopes on the vaccine antigen.

Immunological definitions

Immunogenicity: The ability of an antigen to stimulate B- and/or T-cell mediated immune responses in the challenged host, resulting in the production of antibodies and/or T cells that react specifically with the stimulating antigen.

Immunoglobulins: A group of glycoproteins present in the serum and tissue fluids of all mammals. Some are present on the surface of B cells, where they act as receptors for specific antigens. Others (antibodies) are present in blood or lymph. Contact between B cells and antigen is needed to cause the B cells to develop into antibody-forming cells (AFCs), also called plasma cells, which secrete large amounts of antibody. Five distinct classes of immunoglobulin molecules are recognized in higher animals, namely IgG, IgA, IgM, IgD, and IgE. They differ in size charge, amino acid composition, and carbohydrate content.

Anamnestic response: The immune response that follows a second or subsequent encounter of the immunocompetent cells of the immune system with a particular common antigen. The response to the antigen occurs soon after stimulation, the antibody immune response can be primarily IgG, and the antibody titers resulting from the repeated stimulation are usually higher.

Selecting antigens with conserved epitopes that stimulate a protective immune response is essential in identification of antigens that will be the immunological vaccine target. To effectively simulate immunological protection against an extracellular pathogen, linear as well as conformational peptides, polysaccharides, glycopeptides, and glycolipid epitopes expressed on the surface of the pathogen may be ideal targets for stimulation of protective immunity. High-affinity antibody responses can prevent pathogen infection and/or opsonize the pathogen for uptake and killing by phagocytes. The induction of optimal antibody responses normally requires help from CD4+ helper T cells.

Conversely, to stimulate immunity that provides protection against an intracellular pathogen, conventional αβ T cells reactive with short peptide epitopes presented by major histocompatibility complex (MHC) class I and II proteins on the surface of an infected cell are critical for protective immunity. T cells, unlike antibodies, recognize infected cells expressing short pathogen-specified peptides presented by MHC surface molecules. The activated T cell can inhibit intracellular pathogen growth by a variety of mechanisms which include (i) activation of cytokines that have microbiocidal activity, (ii) induction of cellular apoptosis, or (iii) release of cytolytic granules containing enzymes that can kill the infected cells.

Vaccine antigens contain potent epitopes immediately recognized by the host immune system and stimulate an immediate immune response that will inactivate the pathogen early in the infection. On the other hand, immunodominant epitopes may prevent a broad protective immune response essential to facilitate immunologically mediated immune clearance of the pathogen. Therefore, effective vaccines must contain antigens whose neutralizing epitopes are potent and genetically stable. Genetically unstable pathogens that have highly mutable and unstable immunodominant epitopes can facilitate immune escape of the pathogen and enable long-term survival of the pathogen in the host and frustrate a protective immune response by vaccination. Failure to develop effective vaccines against HIV is a classic example of this phenomenon.

Antibody responses to vaccine antigens are elicited by the exposure of B cells in the lymph nodes to freely diffusing vaccine antigens and/or antigens in association with macrophages and dendritic cells (DCs). Protein antigens activate both B and T cells, resulting in the initiation of B-cell differentiation in organs in which antigen-specific B cells can proliferate and differentiate into antibody-secreting plasma memory B cells. Polysaccharide antigens that fail to activate T cells do not trigger DCs and therefore elicit weaker and shorter antibody responses, and no immune memory.

Definition

Pivotal study: During the licensure of a vaccine, the initial clinical studies (phase I) are focused on safety and initial investigation of dose required to stimulate an appropriate immune response. Phase II studies focus on dose and immunization schedule in addition to acquisition of additional safety information. Phase III clinical studies are pivotal, in that the efficacy, safety, dose, and schedule of the immunization are established in earlier studies are used to vaccinate a large population a risk to show that the vaccine can prevent the disease as intended and that all other features of the immunization are satisfactory to be proposed in the Biologics License Application (BLA).

Vaccine development pathway

Vaccine development involves taking an antigen or vaccine identified in research studies as stimulating a protective immune response and developing that into a vaccine drug product that is antigenically stable, immunologically potent in humans or animals (as appropriate), and a safe human immunogen. The antigen or vaccine can be manufactured on a commercial scale and be approved by regulatory authority such as the FDA, European Medicines Agency (EMA), Therapeutic Goods Administration, etc., for human clinical trials. This process involves development of systems for production, purification, potency titration, confirmation of replication properties, chemical characterization, and that it is stable, immunogenic, efficacious, and safe (Figure 11.3). During this process, research programs are transformed from a basic investigation to determine the character of the immune response and confirm protective immunity (the so-called discovery phase) to work in a commercial regulated environment where studies are conducted according to principles of good laboratory practice (GLP) and good manufacturing practice (cGMP) (as part of the so-called nonclinical phase). In this environment, assays and processes are validated and records of experimental work reviewed by quality assurance (QA) with quality control (QC) management of materials and processes. Production is expanded from tissue culture flasks (25–150 mL) to 1000-L continuously stirred fermenters. Vaccines used in early phase I clinical trials to demonstrate safety must be manufactured according to

Process definitions

Good laboratory practice (GLP): GLP regulations govern laboratory facilities, personnel, equipment, and operations. Compliance with GLPs requires procedures and documentation of training, study schedules, processes, and status reports, which are submitted to facility management and included in the final study report to the FDA.

Quality assurance (QA): A QA program is a defined system, and the quality assurance unit (QAU) is the personnel who are independent of the study conduct that execute the program, which is essential to ensure test facility management of compliance with the principles of good laboratory practices.

Quality assurance unit (QAU): The role of the QAU is critical in establishing and maintaining GLP compliance. The QAU, as defined by GLPs, must be independent of the study conducted, which is a common element of a quality organization. Key responsibilities of the QAU are to maintain a master schedule of all studies conducted at the testing facility, maintain copies of protocols, conduct inspections of studies at intervals adequate to assure integrity of the study, submit written reports to management and study directors and assess and document deviations from protocols and standard operating procedures (SOPs).

Quality control (QC): The processes employed to ensure a certain level of quality of a product or service. Essentially, QC involves examination of the product, service, or process for certain minimal levels of quality. Quality control involves evaluating a product, activity, process, or service. In contrast, QA ensures a product or service is manufactured, implemented, created, or produced in the right way. QC is concerned with the product, while QA is process oriented.

protocols and processes used to manufacture the commercial product according to cGMPs. Vaccines used in phase III clinical trials are manufactured by fully developed processes as commercial products and comply with all requirements for licensure.

The vaccine development and manufacturing processes are divided into two broad categories of work that are referred to as upstream and downstream processes (Figure 11.3). The upstream process begins with selection and characterization of the organism (virus, bacteria, yeast, fungi or *Rickettsia*) or purified molecule that contains the vaccine antigens to be produced. The

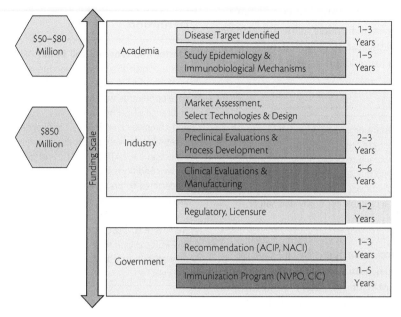

Figure 11.3 Generalized process model for production, purification, and formulation of vaccines in culture initiated by fermentation, purification, characterization, formulation, and regulatory release.

next step is selection and characterization of systems for production of vaccine antigens, which will depend upon the biology of the organism to be cultured (Figure 11.3). Viruses can be cultured and harvested from embryonated chicken eggs, tissues of animals and *in vitro* cultures of cells. Bacteria and yeast are typically grown by fermentation in a selective broth. *Rickettsia* are usually grown in embryonated chicken eggs.

Upstream processes

Selection and characterization of the vaccine antigen

It is essential the virus, bacterium, yeast, *Rickettsia*, or fungi that contains the vaccine antigen is well characterized and all critical testing of the organism documented. The source of the cell cultures, embryonated eggs, media reagents, and all components needed for propagation of the vaccine antigen must also be documented (Figure 11.3). If the antigen is a microorganism, the source of the organism must be documented together with validated testing information to establish identity, antigenic subtype of the organism (if appropriate), passage history, genetic information, nucleotide sequence of the genome (if appropriate),

freedom from adventitious agents, cell-culture systems and/or bacteriological media used to propagate the organism, virulence for experimental animal hosts, and so on. It is critical that master and working seeds of the microorganism to be used as the antigen and/or cultures used for production of the vaccine are acceptable to the regulatory authorities and that all testing to determine identity and purity are documented and carried out in accordance with the GLP regulations.

An ideal source for well-characterized microorganisms suitable for vaccine development is the American Type Culture Collection (ATCC) or the European Collection of Cell Cultures (ECACC), which maintain and make available for commercial vaccine development many strains of cell culture, bacteria, yeast, fungi, viruses, *Rickettsia*, and *Chlamydia* that are appropriate for preparation of master and working seeds. Microorganisms suitable for development of vaccines and information about animal disease models may also be obtained from collections held agencies such as the US Centers for Disease Control and Prevention (CDC), and US National Institutes of Health and the UK National Institute for Biological Standards and Control (NIBSC). If the microorganism that is the vaccine candidate or used to produce the vaccine cannot be obtained from a registered source with appropriate credentials, the investigator is obligated to conduct sufficient testing to ensure identity, purity, and safety.

Definition

Adventitious agents are organisms found in unexpected places that are out of the usual or normal place. During the manufacture of biologics, the products are tested for adventitious agents, microorganisms, and other materials, which are not expected to be in the product and are not acceptable for purity and safety standards.

Propagation of vaccine antigens in cell culture

Cell cultures for propagation of vaccines must be certified by the FDA, EMA, or regulatory authorities in countries where the vaccine will be prepared and used (Figure 11.3). For example, human diploid embryonic lung cells (MRC-5 and WI-38 cells) are suitable and have been used for the production of attenuated rubella, varicella, and hepatitis A human vaccines. African green monkey kidney (Vero 10-87) cells have been used to produce live attenuated and inactivated human vaccines. Certified Vero10-87 cells are maintained by the ATCC and ECCAC, and can be obtained with approval of the regulatory authorities, including the FDA. Vero cells are used for the production of inactivated polio virus vaccine, live attenuated measles virus, live attenuated chimeric yellow fever 17D–Japanese encephalitis virus, and experimental live attenuated dengue and Japanese encephalitis virus vaccines. It is essential that certified samples of designated cell cultures received from validated collections be managed properly if they are to be used to produce vaccines. Master cell banks (MCB) of the cells should be prepared and these cells tested to ensure genetic lineage and freedom from adventitious agents (bacteria, mycoplasma, yeast, and fungi). Cells from the MCB are expanded by limited passage to produce a working cell bank (WCB) that is expanded to provide cell cultures for production of vaccines. Vero cells used for production of vaccine can be passed a limited number of times (approximately passage 147) in this process. Therefore, each production lot of vaccine is usually produced in cells expanded from the WCB for production of a single vaccine lot.

Definition

Master and working cell banks: Well-defined cultured cells in which the biologic/vaccine is to be produced are established to in order to provide research and development as well as manufacture of the product assurance of purity, consistency, reproducibility, security, and compliance with GLP. Cells validated to be acceptable for vaccine production are from a validated collection (i.e., ATCC, NIBSC) and grown in medium and under conditions that freedom from contamination can be certified to prepare the MCB. These cultures will be expanded, from which the WCB will be ultimately prepared. Cells in the MCB will be extensively tested for sterility, retroviruses, adventitious agents, and by qPCR/qRT-PCR (reverse transcriptase) for agents that the cells may contain but do not produce cytopathic effects in the cells.

Primary cultures of chicken embryo cells are used for preparation of measles and mumps vaccines and embryonated chicken eggs are used for production of both live attenuated and inactivated subunit influenza and yellow fever virus vaccines. The chicken embryo fibroblast cell cultures and embryonated chicken eggs used for production of vaccines are obtained from chick flocks that are certified to be free from infectious agents and maintained as isolated flocks by the manufacturer for this specific purpose.

Downstream processes

Purification of the vaccine antigen

The strategy for production, purification, and characterization of vaccine in a crude harvest to enable formulation of the final, highly purified vaccine drug product requires multiple steps by which the vaccine antigen is separated from the substrate in which it has been produced. An outline of this generalized process for a vaccine produced in cell culture is presented in Figure 11.3. The process begins with harvest of the crude vaccine substance followed by purification using physical and chemical methods that do not inactivate the antigen or destroy protective antigenic epitopes while facilitating separation of the vaccine antigen from undesirable host proteins, nucleic acids, carbohydrates, and lipids. Each vaccine is unique, and therefore the processes for production and purification

Table 11.2 Quality Control Testing of a Viral Vaccine Product from Harvest to Filled Drug Product

Virus harvest		Virus bulk	Bulk drug substance	Release of bulk drug substance	Filled drug product
Biosafety tests	In-process tests	Release tests	Identity tests	Identity tests	Identity tests
Sterility	Potency	Potency	Potency	Potency	Potency
Mycoplasma	Identity	Identity	Residual DNA with sizing	pH	pH
Adventitious viruses	Residual host cell protein	Residual host cell protein	Residual host cell protein	Appearance	Appearance
Retroviruses	Endotoxin		Bioburden	Endotoxin	Endotoxin
			Endotoxin	Sterility	Sterility
					General safety

to produce the bulk drug product are significantly different.

To ensure purity, potency, and identity of the product during the manufacturing process, QC testing of the vaccine is done at each critical step (Table 11.2). This process begins with the virus harvest and continues at each step: (1) bulk drug substance, (2) bulk drug product, (3) filled drug product, and (4) finished drug product. The QC tests are done to determine biosafety, and confirm product purity and characteristics during the in-process purification of the product. Specific testing will vary according to product; however, the tests indicated are typical and essential for production of both experimental and clinical lots of vaccine.

Definition

Good manufacturing practices (cGMPs) are regulations that govern the manufacture of human and veterinary drugs, biologics, and medical devices to ensure the identity, strength of purity, and quality of the finished product. The cGMPs are based on fundamental principles of quality assurance: (i) quality, safety, and effectiveness must be designed and built into the product; (ii) quality cannot be inspected or tested into the product; (iii) each step of the manufacturing process must be controlled to maximize the likelihood that the product will meet acceptable criteria.

Testing of vaccine potency and immunogenicity

During vaccine development systems are established to measure vaccine potency and immunogenicity in animal models as well as humans (Table 11.3). Testing vaccine potency is essential to ensure that critical antigenic characteristics of the vaccine are retained and the vaccine antigen potency is maintained during growth and purification. If the vaccine is highly purified and free from contaminating materials, potency may be expressed in terms of micrograms or milligrams of protein or carbohydrate polysaccharide, i.e., hepatitis B HBsAg, tetanus toxin, diptheria toxin, streptococcal polysaccharides. Live attenuated yellow fever, influenza, and polio vaccine potency is usually expressed as infectious plaque-forming units or tissue culture infectious doses. Examples of vaccine potency tests include hemagglutination of erythrocytes, infectivity for animals and cell culture, immunochemical tests such as the enzyme-linked immunosorbent assay (ELISA) and micrograms of polysaccharide. Table 11.3 provides examples of different types of vaccines are presented with the potency of the final product and the tests used to determine their immunogenicity in animal models and humans. The potency of inactivated influenza virus vaccine that contains HA and NA from two influenza A strains and one influenza B strain is determined by radial immunodiffusion. The potency of live attenuated influenza vaccine is determined by plaque-forming units. Hepatitis B vaccine is

Table 11.3 Vaccine Potency Assays with Recommended Human Vaccine Dose

Vaccine	Vaccine Antigen	Vaccine Antigen Potency Test	Vaccine Potency per Dose	Test for Vaccine Immunogenicity
Influenza	Virus HA and NA antigens	Radioimmunoassay	15 µgm of each of the three HA antigens	Hemagglutination inhibition antibody and neutralization
Influenza	Attenuated virus	Tissue culture infectious doses	10^6–10^7 tissue culture infectious doses	Hemagglutination inhibition antibody and neutralization
Measles	Attenuated virus	Plaque-forming units	10^3 tissue culture infectious doses	Virus neutralizing antibody
Hepatatis A	Inactivated virus	ELISA	ELISA immunoadsorbent units (ELU), variable	ELISA milli-International Units per ml (mIU/ml)
Hepatitis B	HBsAg surface protein	ELISA	3–40 µg HBsAg	ELISA anti-HBs >10 mIU/ml
Tetanus	Tetanus toxoid	ELISA	40 IU	Toxin neutralization test in mice of ELISA
Meningococcus	Capsular polysaccharide	Microgram	50 µg per dose of each component polysaccharide	Serum bactericidal assay
Streptococci	Capsular polysaccharide	Microgram	1–10 µg per dose of each component polysaccharide	Enzyme immune assay (EIA) for IgA, IgM, and IgG
Polio	Inactivated virus	ELISA—D antigen units	Type 1 = 40; Type 2 = 8; Type 3 = 32 Units	Virus neutralizing antibody
Diptheria	Toxoid	ELISA	1500 international flocculating units	Vero cell neutralization or ELISA
Yellow fever	Attenuated virus	Tissue culture infectious doses	$\geq 10^4$ plaque-forming units	Virus neutralizing antibody

prepared from yeast cells transformed with HBsAg and is a highly purified antigen measured in micrograms. Inactivated poliovirus vaccine is measured in terms of D protein antigen in an ELISA, whereas potency of the live polio virus is measured in cell-culture plaque-forming units.

The examples provided in Table 11.3 are typical of those developed for the specific product during early stages of vaccine development. Each test has a defined accuracy and reproducibility that can be validated. It is essential that tests to measure the immune response to the vaccine are also developed and reproducible. These assays measure effectiveness of the vaccine to stimulate the host immune response and establish immune correlates of vaccine efficacy in terms of antibody and/or immune cells. For many vaccines the neutralizing titer of serum antibody to the vaccine is expressed as the dilution of serum that will neutralize 50% (or some other percentage) of the virus/bacterium added to a specific dilution of serum (NT_{50}). The measure of influenza virus immunity following immunization is measured in terms of the serum dilution that will prevent virus hemagglutination (hemagglutination inhibition; HAI).

Examples of vaccine development and production

Selected models of vaccine production and downstream purification process are presented in limited detail in Table 11.3 as examples for production and

Correlates of protection: Assessing the relationship between immunogenicity and prevention of disease has relied upon comparisons of aggregate measures such as comparisons of vaccine efficacy and geometric mean titers of antibodies. An alternate possibility is to combine information about incidence of disease and antibody concentrations in different subgroups of the study population. Correlates of protection can also be determined on the individual by determining the level of antibodies from longitudinal follow-up data on individuals who contacted the infection in spite of vaccination.

Serologic correlates: Several parameters of the immune antibody response to vaccination must be considered: (1) specificity of the antibody being tested for antigenic variants of the infecting organism, (2) quantitative assessment of the immune response may not be adequate and qualitative characteristics of antibodies should be considered, and (3) induction of immune memory must be considered because anamnestic responses may occur after a weak primary response.

Seroprotection: Animal and clinical data support functional antibody as the basis for protection against disease, but IgG antibody concentration has conventionally been the principal immunologic parameter for non-inferiority comparisons to establish protection from disease. However, antibody affinity maturation may contribute to protection, but its role is usually not established. Immunologic memory may be useful for evaluation of seroprotection stimulated by new vaccine types. Establishing a threshold IgG antibody level that would exceed the anticipated minimum level of protection is a more conservative estimate of short-term protection and easier to define.

testing of different types of vaccines. During the process of vaccine development, assays for vaccine potency are developed and validated to ensure accuracy, sensitivity, and reproducibility for manufacture of the finished drug product. The information provided in Table 11.4 has been extracted from the manufacturers package inserts when provided. The inactivated influenza vaccine is formulated to contain 15 μgm of a specific hemagglutinin antigen from two type A and one type B influenza strains. Live attenuated vaccines for influenza, measles, and yellow fever are formulated to contain a specified infectious titer as determined by plaque assay or tissue culture infectious dose. Inacti-

vated polio vaccines, hepatitis B, hepatitis A, diphtheria, and tetanus are expressed in terms of antigenic ELISA units.

Development of vaccine antigens for immunization to prevent disease against specific infectious pathogens requires production of antigens from a wide variety of organisms by different processes. The early stages of vaccine development define the upstream technologies for production of the vaccine bulk, requiring the development of tests to monitor the host cells, the master and working seeds, and growth of the virus or bacterial antigen. Examples of vaccine production provide insight into the processes involved and the analytical testing required to ensure vaccine potency, purity, and stability of the final finished drug product.

Recombinant protein (hepatitis B)

The hepatitis B virus (HBV) surface protein consists of a mixture of large and small HBsAg proteins in both glycosylated non-glycosylated forms. During virus replication the HBsAg protein is encoded and expressed only by the HBsAg. The licensed recombinant hepatitis B vaccine consists of a 226-amino acid S gene product (HBsAg) that is expressed in yeast and purified by physical separation techniques including chromatography and filtration. Recombinant *S. cerevisiae* cells expressing the HBsAg are grown in stirred tank fermenters. The growth medium consists of yeast extract, soy peptone, dextrose, and mineral salts. At the end of fermentation, intracellular HBsAg antigen is harvested by lysing the yeast cells. The HBsAg particles assembled by hydrophobic interaction are purified by size-exclusion chromatography. The purified HBsAg protein spontaneously assembles into 22-nm particles, representing the same antigen as is present in the blood of HBV-infected persons, which is highly immunogenic and stimulates protective antibodies. This was the first human vaccine based on recombinant DNA technology.

Bacterial polysaccharide (*Streptococcus pneumoniae*)

Capsular polysaccharide is the most important virulence factor of *Streptococcus pneumoniae*, but not the only one. Pneumococcal virulence depends in part on several serotype specific characteristics. The different pneumococcal serotypes vary in virulence depending on their ability to activate the alternative complement pathway, to deposit and degrade the complement

Table 11.4 Examples of Vaccine Manufacturing Processes (Source: Vaccine package insert)

Disease	Trade Name	Production System	Vaccine Purification	Final Product
Measles, mumps, rubella, and varicella	ProQuad (live attenuated)	Measles—chick embryo cell culture; mumps—chick embryo cell culture; rubella—WI-38 human diploid cells Varicella—MRC-5 human diploid cells.	Not disclosed	Lyophilized
Pneumococcal and diptheria	Prevnar	*Streptococcus pneumonia* serotypes 4,6B, 9V, 14,18C, 19F, and 23R grown in soy peptone broth. *C. diphtheria* grown in broth containing casamino acids and yeast extract.	Polysaccharides purified by precipitation, ultrafiltration & chromatography	Aluminum hydroxide suspension
Meningococcal and diptheria	Menactra	Menigococcal strains cultured on Muller Hinton agar and Watsobn Schrep media. Diphtheria grown on modified Muller medium.	Polysaccharides centrifugation, precipitation, extraction and filtration. Diptheria purified by precipitation and filtration.	Sodium phosphate buffered isotonic sodium chloride.
Polio	IPOL (live attenuated)	Type 1, 2 and 3 viruses grown individually in Vero cells	Clarified and concentrated	Medium -199
Influenza	Fluzone (inactivated HA subunits)	Viruses are propagated individually in embryonated chicken eggs	Low speed centrifugation and filtration	Phosphate buffered saline
Hepatitis B	Recombovax HB	Recombinant antigen produced in yeast cells grown in complex media	Not disclosed	Suspension of HBsAg in aluminum sulfate suspension
Hepatitis A	HAVRIX (inactivated)	Virus propagated in MRC-5 human cells	Ultracentrifugation and chromatography followed by formalin inactivation	Adsorbed onto aluminum hydroxide
Yellow fever	YF-VAX (live attenuated)	Virus propagated in embryonated chicken eggs	Homogenization and centrifugation	Lyophilized containing gelatin and sorbitol

components on the capsule that enable the organism to resist phagocytosis; they also differ in their ability to induce antibodies. Antibodies to the capsular polysaccharides are protective. Prevnar® polysaccharide vaccine contains 2µg of each polysaccharide form serotypes 4, 9V, 14, 18C, 19F, and 23F, and 4µg of polysaccharide from type 6B per dose. Bacteria that represent each serotype present in the Prevnar® vaccine are grown in soy peptone broth and the polysaccharide from each strain is purified by a process that involves centrifugation, precipitation, ultrafiltration, and column chromatography. Each polysaccharide is chemically activated to form individual saccharides for direct conjugation through reductive amination to CRM_{197}, a nontoxic mutant of diptheria toxin. The individual glycoconjugated polysaccharides is purified by ultrafiltration and column chromatography and analyzed for saccharide-to-protein ratios, molecular size, free saccharide, and free protein.

Inactivated virus subunits (influenza)
Each influenza strain is identified by the hemagglutinin (HA) protein subtype (H1–H18) and neuraminidase (NA) subtype (N1–11). The vaccine antigens are composed of the HA and NA surface glycoproteins, which induce protective virus-neutralizing antibodies. The inactivated influenza vaccine contains antigens from two strains of influenza A viruses (e.g., A/H1N1 and A/H3N2) and a single strain of influenza B virus. Each year, a vaccine "cocktail" is formulated based on the worldwide incidence of disease caused by specific antigenic variants of the prevalent A and B viruses. The identified virus strains are provided to vaccine manufacturers by the CDC, World Health Organization (WHO), NIBSC, and the FDA's Center for Biologics Evaluation and Research (CBER). Virus master and working seeds for each of the three virus strains are grown in embryonated chicken eggs and characterized to ensure sterility, antigenic character, specificity, and infectivity. Individual embryonated chicken eggs are automatically inoculated with the virus and incubated for a specific time and at defined temperature to facilitate virus growth in the chicken embryonic tissues. The allantoic fluid is harvested from each egg and the virus in the fluids inactivated with formaldehyde, disrupted with detergent, purified by sucrose gradient ultracentrifugation, and sterile filtered. Potency of the HA antigen for each type is determined by agarose gel diffusion and formulated to provide 15 μg of each of the three HA vaccine components in a vaccine dose.

Inactivated virus (polio)
The inactivated polio vaccine (IPV) is a mixture of three polioviruses grown in cell culture. In 1976 Behring produced seeds from Sabin original material obtained from the FDA. These strains were donated to WHO, and since 1986 have been stored at NIBSC, which sends them out at the request of WHO. The virus strains used for vaccine production are Mahony (type 1), MEFI (type 2), and Saukett (type 3). These polio virus master seeds are approved for use and maintained by NIBSC on behalf of WHO. The vaccine manufacturer will prepare master and working seeds in primary monkey kidney cells, a continuous culture

of human diploid cells (MRC-5) or a continuous cell line of green monkey kidney cells (Vero). These seeds are validated to ensure identity, sterility, potency, and purity. Each of the viruses to be included in the final vaccine product is grown in monkey kidney cells growing on microcarriers in suspension culture. The cultures are infected with the virus and incubated for 3 to 4 days when cytopathic effects in the cells become evident. The supernatant fluid from the suspension culture is harvested, clarified, and concentrated by ultrafiltration. The the virus is purified by column chromatography, inactivated with formalin, and filtered to remove clumps of virus particles. Final formulation of the vaccine is expressed in the concentration of poliovirus D antigen as determined in an ELISA.

Live attenuated (measles)
Current measles vaccines use either the Edmonston, Moraten, or Schwatz strains of measles virus. The virus is grown in chicken embryo fibroblast cells (CEFs) in roller-bottles. The cells in monolayer culture on the surface of the roller-bottles are infected with the virus and incubated for several days. When optimal titers of the virus are obtained in the culture the cells are disrupted to release the virus. The cell-culture medium is clarified of intact cells and large cellular debris by centrifugation and the measles virus is purified by additional centrifugation, filtered, and stored frozen.

Measles vaccine has also been produced in suspension cultures of Vero cells growing in serum free medium. In this case, the cell-culture medium containing the measles virus is clarified of cellular debris by centrifugation and the measles virus treated with Benzonase® to digest cellular DNA. The measles virus is then concentrated and purified using tangential flow filtration (TFF) and diafiltration.

Inactivated virus vaccine development (yellow fever)

Yellow fever 17D vaccine viruses were grown in carrier suspension cultures of Vero cells and purified to produce a candidate inactivated vaccine. This model and the availability of published information describing this development provides an excellent example of vaccine development where different steps in downstream and upstream processes were employed to prepare vaccine suitable for a phase I human trial.

The yellow fever 17D strain used for production of the vaccine was obtained from a commercial lot (YF-VAX®, Sanofi Pasteur, Swiftwater, PA) and adapted to grow in Vero cells by 10 serial passages at terminal dilution. Master and working seeds were prepared in Vero cells. Working virus seed was used to infect Vero cells grown on Cytodex®-microcarrier beads (GE Healthcare) in a 50-L stirred bioreactor and the virus harvested and purified (Figure 11.4). Virus in the cell-culture harvest was partially purified and concentrated by depth filtration, digestion with nuclease (Benzonase®), ultrafiltration, and diafiltration followed by sterile filtration. The virus was inactivated with betapropriolactone and further purified by cellufine sulfate chromatography. The bulk drug substance was diluted to target potency, adsorbed to aluminum hydroxide adjuvant (Alhydrogel®) and filled into glass vials. The final filled bulk drug product XRX-001 met specifications for potency, identity, sterility, endotoxin level, residual Vero cell DNA, pH, osmolarity, appearance, and stability. This inactivated YF vaccine XRX-001 was approved by the FDA and used in a phase I clinical trial.

Definition

Nonclinical: Term proposed by the World Health Organization to describe all research undertaken prior to studies in humans. Most countries have adopted this term. The US FDA uses the term *preclinical*. The term *nonclinical* will be used in this chapter.

Animal models

Nonclinical vaccine immunogenicity and efficacy

Understanding the immunological principles of protection is critical in vaccine development, and establishment of appropriate animal infection models is essential to evaluate protective efficacy of new vaccine candidates. It is essential that animal models of infection are available that show sufficient promise for prevention of infection in humans or animals, under field conditions. Care must be taken in choice and refinement of animal models of infection to ensure the type of immunological response and protective immunity are representative of the disease and are valid to extrapolate to the target species.

Inbred mice are the most widely used animal in immunological research. There are advantages for the use of murine models because of the wide range of immunological reagents available, and it is possible to transfer immune cells between donor and recipient from an inbred colony. However, inbred and genetically modified mice often produce atypical immune responses to specific infections that are not representative of those in higher animals (including humans) and therefore are inappropriate when studying the vaccine responses to infection in human infections.

While there are limited immunological reagents to critically study immunity in outbred laboratory

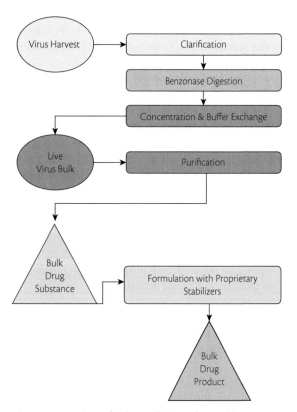

Figure 11.4 Scheme for the purification of a candidate inactivated yellow fever 17D virus vaccine produced in suspension cultures of Vero cells.

animals, they have the advantage that they can produce natural responses to specific infections. These constraints are becoming less limiting with development of additional reagents and monoclonal antibodies specific for different species of animals. Primates, guinea pigs, rabbits, cats, and ferrets have been used as experimental models of infection and provide models in which to study vaccine efficacy. Selection of the proper animal models that are to be used during the process of vaccine development is critical and an essential step in evaluation of vaccine efficacy as well as toxicity.

In vaccine efficacy studies, animal models of immunization and challenge are used to answer essential questions: (1) Does the vaccine induce a significant and appropriate immune response to the vaccine? (2) Do antibodies and immune cells stimulated by the vaccine provide protective immunity? (3) What is the correlate of immune protection and can the level of immune protection be correlated with seroprotection in clinical trials?

The golden hamster is used as a model for yellow fever virus (YFV) disease and for the immune response to immunization with both live and attenuated YFV vaccines. Golden hamsters vaccinated with the candidate YF XRX-001 vaccine developed significant titers of YFV neutralizing antibody and when challenged with virulent virus, 90% of animals with neutralizing antibody titers greater than 39 survived the challenge with a lethal dose of the wild-type virus. Additional passive antibody studies revealed animals with neutralizing antibody titers greater than 40 were completely protected from disease as evidenced by viremia, liver enzyme level, weight change, and death.

Nonclinical vaccine safety and toxicity

Studies to support safety of vaccines as biologics are significantly different from those designed to evaluate small molecules. Vaccines are produced by living cells and may undergo degradation during production. They can exaggerate pharmacological and toxicological responses and may be species specific. Regardless, the purpose of nonclinical toxicology/safety vaccine studies of small molecules and vaccines is the same. In the latter stages of vaccine development, when a process for preparation of vaccine for the phase I study has been confirmed, a toxicology/safety study needs to be conducted to determine safety of the vaccine for human studies. Vaccine toxicology studies are designed to identity target organs of toxicity and are ultimately used to establish safe starting doses of vaccine for clinical trials, as well as identify areas of concern for clinical safety monitoring. Vaccine toxicology studies are done with different types of products including inactivated /nonliving antigens and live attenuated organisms. Inactive non-replicating proteins or carbohydrates (e.g., tetanus toxoid, diptheria toxoid, *S. pneumoniae* polysaccharide) and inactivated organisms (e.g., inactivated polio virus) are given in repeated doses over a 3-week period with sacrifice 24 hours or 14 days after the final dose. In-life immunotox studies include analysis of proinflammatory cytokines and fibrogen production as well as tests for the production of antibody in the serum of the animals 14 days after the last dose of vaccine.

Toxicology studies with live attenuated (attenuated polio, measles, mumps, yellow fever) are usually conducted as safety studies. Live attenuated virus vaccines contain a minimum of virus and replicate in the host to infect multiple tissues and stimulate the immune response. Given that the live attenuated vaccine stimulates an immune response to the vaccine in the first 7 days after the first dose, it is unlikely that the virus will replicate efficiently in the immunized host and induce additional pathological changes. Therefore, toxicology tests with live attenuated vaccines are usually conducted as safety tests with blood samples taken during the in-life phase to evaluate proinflammatory cytokines and fibrogen as well as virus and virus-specific antibodies. Animals may be sacrificed 24 days after the first dose of vaccine is given to do a complete pathology analysis of body organs.

Good laboratory practices

As described elsewhere in this chapter and in Chapter 12, certain studies associated with nonclinical testing of candidate vaccines are required to be performed in compliance with regulations covering good laboratory practice (GLP). In the USA, FDA GLP regulations are specified in Title 21 of the Code of Federal Regulations, Part 58 (21 CFR 58). These studies may also be subject to other regulations, such as those covering work with biological "select agents," electronic records and electronic signatures (21 CFR 11), and animal welfare. Vaccine developers and testing facilities are also likely to consider other international documents, particularly the Organization for Economic Co-operation and Development (OECD) Principles on Good Laboratory Practice and their associated guidance, consensus, and advisory documents. The OECD GLP documents have been developed to promote mutual acceptance of safety testing data by different national regulatory authorities, thereby reducing duplication of testing that may otherwise be required for international product approvals.

The goal of the FDA GLP regulations is to "assure the quality and integrity of the safety data" [21 CFR 58.1(a)] derived from nonclinical studies supporting or intended to support vaccine (and other product) licensure by the FDA. GLP represents a comprehensive quality system that defines particular roles and responsibilities for personnel involved in performance or oversight of studies, and specifies other requirements related to operation of testing facilities, performance of studies, and generation of study reports. The regulations stipulate inspections of testing facilities by FDA personnel and include penalties for noncompliance. Unlike some other quality systems, there is no GLP certification process for facilities, equipment or methods. Assessment of GLP compliance comes via periodic FDA inspection, often after a particular study is concluded. Inspections are generally unannounced and facilities performing regulated studies must permit inspections or face refusal by FDA to review any data generated by the facility, or other actions. Due to their complexity, GLP studies are often performed by specialized testing facilities sometimes referred to as contract research organizations (CROs).

Originally, the GLP regulations were applicable primarily to safety studies, but compliance is also now required for pivotal studies associated with development of animal models and testing of product efficacy in those models under the Animal Rule. GLP as a quality system may also be applied to other nonclinical laboratory testing that supports early stage clinical trials, such as when a novel assay is required to measure a specific end point and that method may not be sufficiently developed to be employed in a clinical laboratory setting.

All personnel engaged in or supervising a regulated study must have documented education, training, and/or experiences demonstrating their ability to perform assigned tasks, but the FDA GLP regulations specify several key roles and associated responsibilities: testing facility management, a study director, and an independent QAU. Management is responsible for ensuring adequate resources (facilities, equipment, personnel) are available to perform a study, must appoint (and remove if necessary) a study director, must provide a QAU, and ensure that test and control articles have been adequately characterized prior to a study. In addition, management must ensure that personnel assigned to a study understand their roles and that any deviations identified by the QAU are reported to the study director and corrective actions are taken. Management must also approve the standard operating procedures (SOPs) used in the facility.

The study director is an individual with adequate training and/or experience who serves as the single point of control for a GLP study. The study director must be knowledgeable of both the scientific and regulatory requirements of the study. He or she is responsible for compliance with the GLP regulations, the study protocol, and associated SOPs, and must ensure that any deviations are documented and their impact on the study assessed. The study director is also responsible for interpretation, analysis, documentation, and reporting of the study results. In most cases, it is unlikely that any individual serving as a study director has expertise in all of these areas, so they will be assisted and advised by other technical staff and contributing scientists in the setup, performance, and reporting of a study. However, the study director is the individual ultimately responsible for these aspects and for the overall compliance of the study.

The QAU is responsible for maintaining a master schedule of all studies performed at a facility and copies of each study protocol. The QAU monitors each study, reporting to facility management on the compliance of all aspects of the study with the requirements of the regulations, and reviews study reports to ensure that they accurately reflect the actual methods and procedures used and the raw data generated during the study. Most importantly, the QAU must be entirely independent of the study to ensure no potential for conflict of interest and must have SOPs describing how it performs its functions.

The key element underpinning a GLP study is the study protocol. This document must be approved, usually by the study sponsor and the study director, and must indicate the objectives and all methods used for the performance of the study. The regulations stipulate several elements that must be included in the study protocol such as the details of test/control articles and the test system; experimental design; type and frequency of testing; proposed statistical methods; and records to be maintained. A study is considered to have commenced at the time the study director signs the protocol. If the study protocol is the master plan for the study, SOPs provide the specific detail for how study activities are performed. A testing facility must have written SOPs for all significant processes (i.e., those that could directly or indirectly impact the quality or integrity of a study). SOPs must be approved by management, must be immediately available in areas where those tasks are performed, and the facility must maintain a historical file showing all SOP revisions, the dates of those revisions, and evidence that personnel have been adequately trained on those SOPs that are relevant to their role.

The regulations stipulate few specific requirements for the facilities used for performance of GLP studies. They should be "of suitable size and construction" [21 CFR 58.41] and designed to allow separation of activities in order to prevent any adverse effects on a study. Facilities performing animal studies, a primary focus of the GLP regulations, should be designed with sufficient numbers of rooms to allow separation of species, isolation of individual studies (particularly if containment of hazardous materials or agents is required), quarantine of animals, and routine or specialized housing of animals. Designated areas should be set aside for diagnosis, treatment, and control of laboratory animal diseases that might otherwise impact outcomes of studies; for collection and disposal of wastes; and for storage of feed, bedding, supplies, and equipment. Separate areas must also be provided for receipt and storage of test/control articles, mixing of test/control articles with a carrier, and storage of mixtures, in order to "prevent contamination or mix-ups" [21 CFR 58.47(a)] and to preserve the integrity of the articles and mixtures.

Likewise, equipment must be "of appropriate design and adequate capacity to function according to the protocol" [21 CFR 58.61]. This means each piece of equipment must be independently assessed as to its suitability for the requirements of a particular study. The regulations stipulate that equipment should be adequately inspected, cleaned and maintained, and if used for generation measurement or assessment of data must be tested or calibrated to ensure correct function. Typically this assessment is accomplished via a process known as *equipment validation*, whereby the item is evaluated against criteria for correct installation and performance (often based on the manufacturer's specifications) as well as its specific operation as required for the study. SOPs must be developed for use, maintenance, and calibration of the equipment, and must specify who is responsible for each operation.

Definition

Good clinical practice (GCP): The regulations, guidance, and industry standards that contain the principles that provide assurance that the safety and well-being of human subjects participating in research have been protected and that the research yields quality scientific data. A trial conducted in full compliance gives the sponsor the ability to submit the data to regulatory authorities worldwide as the data was derived in accordance with a globally recognized standard.

The GLP regulations also specify requirements for handling and reporting of data and other key documents from studies. All study records, including appropriate equipment maintenance and personnel training records, as well as necessary wet specimens, samples of test/control articles and mixtures, and other specially prepared materials, must be retained in a dedicated, limited access archive, typically under the control of a dedicated archivist who is responsible for organization, storage, and security of the archive. These records must be readily retrievable if requested during a facility inspection, and minimum retention periods are specified under the regulations. For example, 21 CFR 58.195 specifies the shorter of (a) a 2-year period following approval of a research or marketing permit for the product, or (b) 5 years following the submission of data to the FDA for review in support of a research or marketing permit. If data are not submitted, study records must be retained for at least 2 years following completion of the study. A final report must be prepared on each study, and the regulations specify required information that must be included. Final reports must be reviewed by the QAU to ensure they are an accurate representation of the raw study data and records, and they must be signed by the study director. The study director's signature on the final report represents the conclusion of that study. Any subsequent additions or corrections to that report must be via formal amendments prepared by the study director.

The FDA is responsible for inspecting facilities that perform GLP studies supporting research/marketing applications for products to be sold in the USA, including facilities located in other countries, and the regulations specify penalties for noncompliance that can result in refusal to accept data from a particular study, disqualification of the testing facility from submitting data to the FDA, and/or civil or criminal penalties against the facility and/or individuals at the facility.

Summary

- The current product timeline for vaccines spans 8 to 10 years or longer and can cost $800 million or more.

- Knowledge of the gene sequence of a recognized immunogen from a known pathogen does not guarantee an immunogenic vaccine.

- Vaccine discovery and development tends to be an empiric trial-and-error process that has continued to improve with the integration of new technologies to understand vaccine antigens and the immune response.

- The basic processes of vaccine discovery and development depend upon systems for production and purification of new vaccine antigens with antigenic and immunogenic characterization of the immune response.

- Production and testing of a cGMP clinical lot of vaccine involves both upstream and downstream processes that are usually distinct for each vaccine.

- Measurable product characteristics that correlate with safety and efficacy must be defined. Chemical and biological safety testing of vaccines has been integrated into new biochemical and biological systems that facilitate rapid analysis.

- Efficacy testing of vaccines to demonstrate protection often requires development and use of animal models unique for each agent.

Further reading

Adamczyk- Poplawska M, Markowixz S, and Jagusztyn-Krynicka E (2011). Proteomics for development of vaccine. Journal of Proteomics 74, 2596–2616.

Anderson RM, Christi I, and Gupta S (1997). Vaccine design, evaluation, and community-based use for antigenicity variable infectious agents. Lancet 350, 1446–1470.

Barrett ADT and Beasley DWC (2009). Development pathway for biodefense vaccines. Vaccine 27, 2–7.

Barrett PN, Berezuk G, Fritsch S, Aichinger G, Hart MK, El-Amin W, Kistner O, and Ehlrich HJ (2011). Efficacy, safety, and immunogenicity of a Vero-cell-culture-derived trivalent influenza vaccine: a multicentre, double-blind, randomised, placebo-controlled trial. Lancet 377, 751–759.

Baylor NW and Midthun K. Regulation and testing of vaccines. In Vaccines, 5th edition (eds S Plotkin, W Orenstein, and P Offit), pp. 1611–1627. New York: Elsevier, 2008.

Bukland BC (2005). The process development challenge for a new vaccine. Nature Medicine 11, 16–19.

Code of Federal Regulations Title 21, Part 58 Good Laboratory Practice for Nonclinical Studies; viewable at http://www.accessdata.fda.gov/scripts/cdrh/cfdocs/cfcfr/cfrsearch.cfm?cfrpart=58.

Dasgupta G and BenMohamed L (2011). Of mice and not humans: How reliable are animal models for evaluation of herpes CD8+-T cell epitopes-based immunotherapeutic vaccine candidates. Vaccine 29, 524–536.

Gomez PL, Robinson JM and Rogalewicz J. Vaccine manufacturing. In Vaccines, 5th edition (eds S Plotkin, W Orenstein, and P Offit), pp. 45–58. New York: Elsevier, 2008.

Griffin JFT (2002). A strategic approach to vaccine development: animal models, monitoring vaccine efficacy, formulation and delivery. Advanced Drug Delivery Reviews 54, 851–861.

Hadler SC, Dietz V, Okwo-Bele J-M, and Cutts Felicity T. Immunization in developing countries. In Vaccines, 5th edition (eds S Plotkin, W Orenstein, and P Offit), pp. 1541–1571. New York: Elsevier, 2008.

Hoft DF, Brusic V, and Sakala IG (2011). Optimizing vaccine development. Cellular Microbiology 13, 934–942.

Julander JG, Trent DW, and Monath TP (2011). Immune correlates of protection against yellow fever determined by passive immunization and challenge in the hamster model. Vaccine 29, 608–6016.

Kwong PD and Shapiro L (2011). Vaccine design reaches the atomic level. Science Translational Medicine 91, 1–5.

Langfield LK, Walker HJ, Gregory LC, and Federspiel MJ. Manufacture of measles viruses. In Viral Vectors for Gene Therapy: Methods and Protocols, Methods (eds O Merten and M Al-Rubeai), pp. 345–366. New York: Humana Press, 2011.

Marshall V and Baylor NW (2011). Food and drug administration regulation and evaluation of vaccines. Pediatrics 127, 23–30.

Miller MA and Hinman AR. Economic analysis of vaccine policies. In Vaccines, 5th edition (eds S Plotkin, W Orenstein, and P Offit), pp. 1593–1609. New York: Elsevier, 2008

Monath TP, Fowler E, Johnson CT, Balser J, Morin M, Sisti M, and Trent DW (2011). An inactivated cell-culture vaccine against yellow fever. New England Journal of Medicine 364, 1326–1333.

Monath TP, Lee CK, Julander JG, Brown A, Beasley DW, Watts DM, Hayman E, Guertin P, Makowiecki J, Crowell J, Levesque P, Bowick GC, Morin M, Fowler E, and Trent DW (2010). Inactivated yellow fever vaccine: Development and nonclinical safety, immunogenicity and protective activity. Vaccine 28, 3827–3840.

Osorio JE, Huang CYH, Kinney RM, and Stinchcomb DT (2011). Development of DENVax: a chimeric dengue-2 based tetravalent vaccine for protection against dengue fever. Vaccine 29, 7251–7260.

Peeters CCAM, Langerman PR, deWeers O, Hoogerhout P, Beurret M, and Poolman JT. Preparation of polysaccharide-conjugate vaccines. In Methods in Molecular Medicine, Vaccine Protocols, Vol. 87, 2nd edition (eds A Robinson, MJ Hudson and MP Carnage), pp. 153–173. Totowa, NJ: Springer, 2003.

Quenee LE, Ciletti N, Berube B, Krausz T, Elli D, Hermanas T, and Schneewind O (2011). Plague guinea pigs and its prevention by subunit vaccines. American Journal of Pathology 179, 1689–1700.

Sanchez-Schmitz G and Levy O (2001). Development of newborn and infant vaccines. Science Translational Medicine 3, 1–7.

Tripp RA and Tompkins SM Animal models for evaluation of influenza vaccines. In Vaccines for Pandemic Influenza, Current Topics in Microbiology and Immunology, Vol. 33 (eds RW Compans and SM Tompkins), pp. 397–412. Berlin, Germany: Springer-Verlag.

12 The regulatory path to vaccine licensure

Dennis W. Trent

Office of Nonclinical Regulated Studies, University of Texas Medical Branch, Galveston, TX, USA

Abbreviations

ARTG	Australian Register of Therapeutic Goods	ICH	International Conference on Harmonisation
BLA	Biologics License Application		
CBER	Center for Biologics Evaluation and Research	IND	Investigational new drug
		IRB	Institutional review board
CDER	Center for Drugs Evaluation and Research	MHLW	Japanese Ministry of Health, Labor and Welfare
CFDA	China Food and Drug Administration	NDA	New Drug Application
CFR	Code of Federal Regulations	NDS	New drug submission
CMC	Chemistry manufacturing and controls	NIH	National Institutes of Health
CTD	Common technical document	OBRR	Office of Blood Research and Review
DBAP	Division of Bacterial, Parasitic and Allergenic Products	OCGT	Office of Cellular, Tissue and Gene Therapies
DBS	Division of Biological Standards	OVRR	Office of Vaccines Research and Review
DVP	Division of Viral Products		
DVRPA	Division of Vaccines and Related Product Applications	PFSB	Japanese Pharmaceutical and Food Safety Bureau
EMA	European Medicines Agency	PMDA	Japanese Pharmaceutical and Medical Device Agency
ERA	Environmental risk assessment		
FD&C	Federal Food, Drug, and Cosmetic Act	QA	Quality assurance
GLP	Good laboratory practice	QC	Quality control
GMO	Genetically modified organisms	US FDA	US Food and Drug Administration

Introduction

In Chapter 11, the use of animals in preclinical studies was presented. Animal studies to evaluate toxicity of the vaccine must be conducted under regulations designated good laboratory practice (GLP). In Chapter 15, clinical trials in humans will be described, which must also be conducted under the specifications of good clinical practice (GCP). Providing the vaccine shows efficacy with acceptable adverse events in clinical trials, the drug will be registered and manufactured for commercial sale under regulations that require compliance with good manufacturing practice (cGMP). The processes that are involved in each of these steps

Vaccinology: An Essential Guide, First Edition. Edited by Gregg N. Milligan and Alan D.T. Barrett.
© 2015 John Wiley & Sons, Ltd. Published 2015 by John Wiley & Sons, Ltd.

are governed by regulatory policy and overseen by regulatory authorities.

Definition

Good laboratory practice (GLP) regulations govern laboratory facilities, personnel, equipment, and operations. Compliance with GLPs requires procedures and documentation of training, study schedules, processes, and status reports, which are submitted to facility management and included in the final study report to the regulatory agency, such as the FDA.

The US Food and Drug Administration (US FDA) is one of the most comprehensive and transparent regulatory organizations in the world of drug and biologics regulation. In this chapter the emphasis will be on the process of regulatory approval and licensure. The first official step toward licensure of biologics is submission of an investigational new drug (IND) application to the US FDA and reviewed by the Center for Biologics Evaluation and Review (CBER), or the Center for Drug Evaluation and Review (CDER). Human clinical trials have the purpose of demonstrating safety and efficacy for human use. Upon completion of the human clinical trials the sponsor will prepare a Biologics License Application (BLA) that is submitted to the

US FDA and reviewed by CBER or CBER for marketing approval. Other countries have similar organizations that have similar regulatory processes for licensure of vaccines and biologics; these are discussed toward the end of this chapter.

Definition

The **investigational new drug application (IND)** is a submission to the US FDA for permission to initiate a clinical study with a new drug product in the USA. From a legal perspective, the IND is an exception from the Federal Food, Drug and Cosmetic (FD&C) that prohibits interstate commerce without an approved application. The IND application allows a company to ship an investigational drug. The IND allows a company to initiate and conduct clinical studies with an investigational new drug product. The safety of the clinical trial subject is the primary concern of the US FDA and when reviewing the IND, regardless of the phase of clinical study, the US FDA evaluates the protocol to ensure the safety of the participants.

In Figure 12.1 the vaccine/drug development process and the applicable regulatory steps are outlined. After the vaccine or drug is developed, basic research is conducted to determine the physical and chemical characteristics, purity, potency, and efficacy

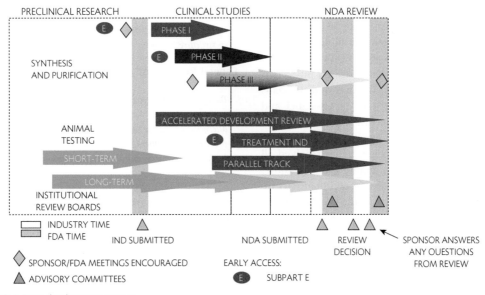

Figure 12.1 Drug development process.

in animal models. Before the vaccine can be administered to humans, the US FDA requires GLP-regulated safety testing of the product in an animal model. With the basic research and development information, a description of the manufacturing process, and detailed characterization of the vaccine product the sponsor is prepared to write an IND application. The IND is submitted to the US FDA and depending on its composition and mechanism of action is reviewed by CBER or CDER to determine if human testing of the vaccine is appropriate. Most human vaccines are reviewed by CBER, and therefore this center will be used as the model for regulatory vaccine review and licensure.

The CBER has 30 days to review the IND and to approve or deny the request to initiate a human clinical trial. If approved a phase I clinical trial may be conducted with the primary purpose to determine safety and limited consideration of vaccine dose and immunization schedule. Phase II human clinical trials are conducted with larger numbers of vaccinees with the primary purposes to confirm safety, to establish vaccine dose, and to determine the schedule to be used to immunize humans with the licensed product. The primary purpose of phase III clinical trials is to demonstrate vaccine efficacy in a larger number of vaccinees (2000 or more individuals) and to provide more information about vaccine safety. Upon completion of the phase III clinical trial(s) and definition of the processes for cGMP vaccine manufacture, the sponsor will organize the experimental information and write a Biologics License Application (BLA) that will be submitted to the US FDA/CBER for review. This review is conducted by scientists and physicians within the CBER plus selected scientists and clinicians working as an expert panel. The expert panel and scientists/physicians from the CBER will review the BLA and organize a meeting with the sponsor to discuss the BLA. When the sponsor has resolved all questions about the safety, immunogenicity, dose, schedule, immunogenicity, efficacy, and manufacture of the vaccine to the satisfaction of the US FDA review board and expert committee, the sponsor will be advised of the decision to grant or deny licensure of the vaccine and conditions for use of the vaccine. Based upon this decision, a license will be granted to the sponsor for commercial sale and use of the vaccine as approved by the review board.

Biologics license application (BLA)

Manufacturers of biologics for introduction into interstate commerce must hold a license for products, which are issued by the CBER. A BLA is used rather than an NDA, though the official BLA form is designated 365h and is identical to the NDA form. Compounds characterized as biologics are reviewed by the CBER. The CDER has certain responsibilities for certain therapeutic biologic products that were transferred from the CBER. The CBER regulates xenotransplantation and has a large regulatory role in vaccine development, tissue safety, and blood.

Regulation of biologics

The US FDA is organized into two centers with specific areas of responsibility: CBER and CDER. For this reason, vaccines are most often considered biologics and for regulatory review assigned to the CBER and more specifically the Office of Vaccines Research and Review (OVRR). Vaccines are considered by the US FDA to be biologics and are regulated by the US FDA as defined in the following statement:

Biological products, like other drugs, are used for the treatment, prevention, or cure of disease in humans. In contrast to chemically synthesized small molecular weight drugs, which have a well-defined structure and can thoroughly characterized, biological products are generally derived from living materials—human, animal, or microorganism—are complex in structure, and thus are usually not fully characterized.

Federal Regulations 21 CFR 600.3 state:

Biological product means any virus, therapeutic serum, toxin, antitoxin, vaccine, blood, blood component or derivative, allergenic product, or analogous product ... applicable to the prevention, treatment, or cure of diseases of conditions of human beings.

Biologics and government regulation of these products in the USA have an intense and focused history. Until the early 1900s, epidemics of smallpox, yellow fever, typhoid, cholera, and tuberculosis were rampant. Scientific investigation of these infectious diseases identified microorganisms to be the etiologic causes of these diseases, which defined fundamental concepts of infectious disease and development of related sciences, notably microbiology and immunology. Discovery of the etiologic cause of diseases motivated their application to the clinical practices of vaccination and therapeutic use of antitoxin. The success of these programs resulted in the development of companies that produced biologics. Biologics that were produced during this early period were manufactured employing crude processes and insensitive analytical methods with minimal quality control. Consequently, the efficacy and safety of these biologics were highly variable, resulting in products that were hazardous and unsuitable to be administered to humans. The lack of scientific information coupled with the absence of government and industry standards resulted in failure to ensure the safety and effectiveness of some biologics that were produced during this period.

A clinical tragedy involving a biologic motivated the federal government to establish laws that would regulate the production and use of biologics for treatment of human disease. It was determined that during a serious diphtheria epidemic in 1901, 10 children died after being treated with an antitoxin that was later discovered to be contaminated with live tetanus bacteria. No safety testing of the antitoxin had been done prior to administration to the children.

In response to this tragedy and concerns about manufacture of antitoxins, Congress introduced legislation mandating biologics be regulated. In 1902, The Biologics Control Act was signed into law with the following responsibilities: (1) authorize regulation of the sale of viruses, serums, toxins, and analogous products, (2) authorize the development of biologics regulations, (3) require licensure of manufacturing establishments and manufacturers, and (4) provide inspection authority to the federal government.

In 1903, federal authorities issued the first biologics regulations. Administered by the Public Health Service's (PHS) Hygienic Laboratory, these regulations formalized the concept of unannounced government inspections.

Not until 1906 did Congress pass the Pure Food and Drugs Act, which was enacted so federal authorities could regulate other drugs. This law required that drugs must not be mislabeled or adulterated, and meet standards of potency and purity. This law did not mention biologics or the Biologics Control Act of 1902, representing the first distinction between drugs and biologics.

In 1919 the biologics regulations were amended to require all licensed manufacturers to report changes in equipment, personnel, manufacturing methods, and quality control procedures. These regulations required that the manufacturer submit some product samples to the federal government for testing and approval before releasing batches of lots from which the samples were derived.

In 1930, the Randsell Act redesignated the Hygienic Laboratory as the National Institutes of Health (NIH) with expanded responsibilities. The NIH was reorganized in 1937, and the new Division of Biologics Control

The Cutter incident

The Cutter incident of epidemic poliovirus infection was due to the lack of regulatory supervision of companies that had no experience making inactivated polio vaccines, and serves as a lesson in vaccine safety. Two weeks after two lots of formalin-inactivated polio vaccine were released by Cutter Laboratories, the director of the Laboratory of Biologics received a series of telephone calls advising him that five children in California who had received the polio vaccine had become paralyzed. Based on this information, the Epidemic Intelligence Service of the Communicable Disease Center, a precursor of the Centers for Disease Control and Prevention, was asked to determine whether the polio vaccine was the cause of the paralysis.

Epidemiologic analysis revealed two production lots accounting for 120,000 doses of vaccine contained live polio virus. Among the children who received the vaccine from these lots, abortive polio developed in 70,000, 51 were permanently paralyzed, and 5 died. The vaccine initiated a poliovirus epidemic: 113 people in the children's families and/or in the communities where they lived were paralyzed, and 5 died.

Subsequent studies revealed cell debris and clumping of poliovirus particles prevented adequate exposure of the virus particles to formaldehyde and that filters used to remove the clumps of debris from the final product were changed without detailed investigation. As a result, federal requirements for production of the vaccine were revised, and between 1955 and 1962 more than 500 million doses of inactivated poliovirus vaccine were produced and distributed in the USA, resulting in a dramatic decrease in the incidence of poliomyelitis.

was assigned responsibility to regulate biologics. In 1948, the Division of Biologics Control was made part of the National Microbiological Institute, which later became the Institute of Allergy and Infectious Diseases. In 1955, the authority for biologics regulation was transferred to the Division of Biological Standards (DBS). This division regulated biologics until 1972, when the US FDA assumed this responsibility. After numerous reorganizations, as of 2012, the US FDA's CBER regulates all biological products in the USA.

The critical role of the US FDA in regulation of biologics is clearly defined by the carelessness of Cutter Laboratories and from the lack of scrutiny from the NIH Laboratory of Biologics Control, which trusted foundation reports. The Cutter incident was one of the worst pharmaceutical disasters in US history, where several thousand children thought to be given formalin-inactivated polio vaccine were exposed to live wild-type polio virus upon vaccination. The Cutter inactivated polio virus vaccine had been certified by the NIH Laboratory of Biologics Control despite warnings that monkeys inoculated with the vaccine had become paralyzed. Unfortunately, the director of the NIH refused to acknowledge this warning.

The biological IND

The IND application is a submission by the vaccine sponsor to notify the US FDA of its intention to conduct clinical studies. The IND document is a descriptive document that the sponsor must submit to the US FDA for review 30 days before beginning a phase I clinical trial in the USA. From a legal perspective, the IND is a request for exemption from the FD&C that prohibits introducing any new drug into interstate commerce without an approval application. The IND allows legal shipment an unapproved drug, or importation of the new drug from a foreign country.

The IND application allows a company to initiate and conduct clinical studies of an investigational new biologic or drug. This application provides the US FDA with the information necessary to determine if the new biologic or drug and the proposed clinical trial pose reasonable risk to human subjects who would participate in a clinical study. If the US FDA considers the proposed clinical trial to present an unreasonable risk to the safety of the subjects, it will act to place the clinical trial on hold until the safety issues can be resolved.

In reality, the IND is the product of successful non-clinical development designed to determine if pharmacological activity of the vaccine justifies commercial development and whether it is reasonably safe for initial human use. When a vaccine is identified as a candidate for further development, work focuses on gathering information to establish in the IND document that the vaccine is sufficiently safe to conduct a phase I clinical trial. Usually, information included in the IND defines three broad areas:

1. *Clinical protocols and investigator information.* Detailed protocols that outline a clinical study designed to determine whether the participants will be exposed to unnecessary risks in a phase I trial. The qualifications of the physicians and investigators designated to conduct the trial and ability to fulfill clinical trial duties are central to study approval.

2. *Manufacturing information.* Information that describes the composition, manufacturing process,

---

Definitions

Clinical protocol: A clinical protocol describes how a particular clinical trial is to be conducted. It describes the objectives of the study, the trial design, the selection of subjects, and the manner in which the trial is to be conducted. The IND is required to include a clinical protocol for the initial planned study; however, the phase I protocol in the IND may be less detailed and more flexible and can be modified by the FDA review prior to conduct of the trial. Clinical protocols for phase II and phase III studies are less flexible, and end points are defined.

Institutional review board: Prior to commencement of a clinical investigation a clinical protocol must be developed, proposed by the sponsor, and reviewed by an institutional review board (IRB). An IRB is required by regulation and is a committee of medical and ethical experts designated by an institution such as a university or medical center where the clinical study is to be done. The charge of the IRB is to oversee the study to ensure the rights of human test subjects are protected and that rigorous medical and scientific standards are maintained. The IRB must approve the proposed clinical study and monitor the research as it progresses.

product stability, and defines the controls used to characterize the vaccine as a drug substance and/or drug product that will permit an assessment of the company's ability to produce at scale consistent batches of the vaccine.

3. *Animal immunology and toxicology studies.* Nonclinical data to determine immunogenicity and efficacy in an appropriate animal model and an assessment of the product safety in an animal model to determine whether the vaccine is safe for initial testing in humans.

Content and format of the IND

The content and format of an initial IND is laid out in 21 CFR part 312 and numerous guidance documents published by the US FDA. This section outlines in limited detail the required content and format of an initial IND based on CFR requirements.

Introductory statement and general Investigational plan—section 312.23(a) (3)

This section should provide a brief, three- to four-page overview of the investigational vaccine and the sponsor's investigational plan for the coming year. The goal of this section is to provide a brief description of the vaccine and to outlay the development plan. For a phase I, first-in-person submission, two or three pages may be sufficient.

The introductory statement should begin with a description of the vaccine and the indications to be studied including the active ingredients, dosage form, and route of administration. This section should include the sponsor's plan for studies to be conducted during the following year and the rationale for the vaccine and research study proposed.

Investigator's Brochure—section 312.23(a) (5)

This section is described in 21 CFR section 312.23(a) (5) and in greater detail in the International Conference on Harmonisation (ICH). The Investigator's Brochure is provided to each clinical investigator and the institutional review board at each of the clinical sites. This provides investigators with the information necessary to understand the rationale for the proposed clinical trial and makes an unbiased risk-benefit assessment of the proposed trial.

The extent of the information provided in the Investigator's Brochure will depend on the stage of vaccine development but should contain the following:

(a) A brief summary of the chemistry–manufacturing–control information that will include the name of the vaccine, properties of the vaccine (inactivated, live attenuated, subunit, etc.), formulation in which the vaccine is provided and the storage and handling conditions.

(b) A summary of the relevant nonclinical animal studies including safety and toxicology, immunogenicity, efficacy and potency.

(c) If human studies have been conducted with the vaccine, a summary of information relating to safety and efficacy should be presented including information on dose response.

(d) A summary of data for guidance of the investigator in management of subjects during the trial. An overall discussion of the nonclinical data presented as relates to possible risks and adverse reactions associated with administration of the vaccine including special tests, observations and precautions that may be needed during the trial.

Clinical protocol—section 312.23(a) (6)

As with the Investigator's Brochure, the content and format of the protocol is described in 21 CFR Section 312.23.

A clinical protocol describes how a particular clinical trial is to be conducted. It describes the objectives of the study, the trial design, the selection of subjects, and the manner in which the trial is carried out. The initial IND is required to have a protocol for the phase I clinical trial; however, the protocol presented in this case may be less detailed with more flexibility than protocols for phase II and phase III studies. The protocol for phase I should be dedicated to providing an outline of the investigation: an estimate of the number of subjects; a description of safety exclusions; and a description of the dosing plan including duration and dose.

A protocol submitted for conduct of a phase I study and submitted as part of the IND should contain the following elements:

Statement of objectives and purpose:
(a) Name and address and a statement of qualifications for each investigator and each subinvestigator; name of each of the clinical facilities to be used; and address of each reviewing IRB.

(b) Criteria for patient selection and for exclusion; an estimate of the number of patients to be studied.

(c) Description of the study design, including the type of control group to be used, and methods to be used to minimize bias on part of the subjects and investigators.

(d) Method for determining the dose(s) to be administered with the planned maximum dosage to be used.

(e) A description of the observations and measurements to be made that will fulfill the objectives of the study.

(f) A description of clinical procedures, laboratory tests, or other measures to be taken to determine the effects of the vaccine on human subjects and to minimize risk.

Phase I, II, III, and IV clinical trials

Clinical trials: Clinical trials are divided into four phases. Each of the trials is conducted with a specific purpose to evaluate the safety and effectiveness of the drug in a defined population. The *phase I trial* is the first clinical experiment in which the drug is tested on the human body. The primary aim of the trial is to assess safety of the new drug. Other areas of study include pharmacokinetics (adsorption, distribution, metabolism, and excretion) and pharmacodynamics. The aim of a *phase II clinical trial* is to examine safety and effectiveness of the drug in a targeted disease group. A series of doses of varying strengths may be used. The control group is given either the current standard treatment or placebo that is determined by establishing the risk-benefit profile of the control. Another practice is to blind the trial, which means subjects are not privy as to whether they receive the placebo or drug. In some trials, the investigator is unaware of whether the subject is in the control or active group. The result of a *phase II trial* is information to determine the effective dose and dosing regimen of frequency and duration. After successful completion of the phase II trial, the objective of phase III is to confirm the efficacy of the drug in a large patient group. Phase III is the extension of phase II, and the trial is normally conducted in several hospitals in different demographic locations to determine the influence of ethnic responses, together with the incorporation of new criteria for fine-tuning the trial. Because results are critical to determine drug effectiveness, the appropriate phase II or III trial is referred as the *pivotal trial*. The *phase IV trial* is postlicensure efficacy and extended safety.

Chemistry manufacturing and controls (CMC) information—section 312.23(a) (7)

The IND presents quality information, describes composition of the vaccine, presents the manufacturing process and control oversight for the bulk drug substance and bulk drug product. The chemistry, manufacturing, and controls (CMC) section must provide in sufficient detail information to demonstrate the identity, quality, purity, and potency of the vaccine product. The amount of information needed to describe the vaccine will depend on the phase of the study, the duration of the study, dosage form of the investigation vaccine and the amount of additional information available. For vaccine to be used in a phase I study, CMC information for raw materials, vaccine substance, and vaccine product should be sufficiently detailed that the US FDA can determine the safety of the subjects participating in the trial. If regulators have a safety concern or there is a lack of data that makes it impossible for the US FDA to conduct an adequate safety evaluation, this presents justification for a clinical hold to be imposed based on the CMC section. Section 21 CFR 312.23(a) (7) identifies and outlines the CMC information that must comprise this section of the IND:

(a) *Drug substance.* The description of the drug substance will include its physical, chemical, or biological characteristics; name of the manufacturer; general method of manufacture; the acceptable limits and analytical methods used to ensure the identity, potency, quality, and purity of the drug substance; information to support stability of the drug substance during the toxicology studies and planned clinical studies.

(b) *Drug product.* A list of components, which may include alternatives, that have been used to manufacture the investigational drug product, including those components that are intended to be in the drug product and those that are not in the drug product but were used during the manufacturing process, and the quantitative composition for the investigational drug product. Also required are the name and address of the drug product manufacturer; a brief description of the manufacturing process; the acceptable limits and analytical methods to ensure identity, strength, quality, and purity of the drug product; and information to support stability of the drug substance during the toxicology and planned clinical studies.

(1) *Control*. A brief description of the composition, manufacture, and control of any placebo used in a controlled clinical trial.

(2) *Labeling*. A copy of all labels and labeling provided each investigator

(3) *Environmental analysis requirements*. A claim for categorical exclusion under 21 CFR 25.30 or 25.31.

Definition

Chemistry, manufacturing, and control (CMC): The IND describes the chemical structure and properties of the vaccine; the composition, manufacturing process, and control of the raw materials; drug substance; and drug product that ensure the identity, quality, purity, and potency of the vaccine. The ICH guidance refers to this as the Quality section of the file.

Pharmacology and toxicology data—section 21CFR 312.23(a) (8)

This module contains information on the nonclinical safety and efficacy of the vaccine in animal models. Safety of the vaccine is determined in a regulated GLP study conducted in an animal model. If the vaccine does not multiply in the host (e.g., inactivated or protein subunit vaccine) the animals are given multiple doses of the highest anticipated human dose by the anticipated route of immunization. If the vaccine replicates in the host after injection to increase the vaccine mass in the animals after inoculation, the vaccine is given as a single injection at the highest anticipated human dose. The decision to proceed with a phase I clinical trial with the investigational vaccine must include the conduct and review of data from nonclinical *in vivo* toxicology, immunology, and efficacy, as well as *in vitro* studies of antigenic structure, potency, sterility, chemical composition, and stability upon storage at various temperatures. These data must provide a high level of confidence that the new vaccine is reasonably safe for humans. The goals of nonclinical safety testing include characterization of toxic effects with respect to target organs, dose dependence, exposure duration and potential reversibility of a toxic effect. Nonclinical safety information is important in determining the initial starting dose for human trials and the parameters for clinical monitoring of adverse events.

The pharmacology and toxicology information in the safety section of the original IND should contain the following information: (1) pharmacology and drug disposition; (2) toxicology, which should be included in an integrated summary of the toxicological effects of the drug in animals; (3) a statement of compliance or noncompliance with GLP.

According to guidelines, the integrated toxicology summary should contain the following:

(a) A brief description of the design and dates of the trials and deviations from the design in conduct of the trial.

(b) A systematic presentation of the findings from the animal toxicology studies.

(c) Identification and qualifications of individuals who evaluated the animal safety data and concluded it was reasonably safe to begin the proposed clinical trial.

(d) A statement of where the animal studies were conducted and where the study records are available for inspection.

(e) A standard GLP declaration.

Previous human experience—section 21 CFR 312.23(a) (9)

This section should contain an integrated summary report of all previous human studies and experiences with the vaccine. This section should be indicated as not applicable if the planned study represents the first administration of the vaccine to human (so-called first-time in humans). If previous human studies have been conducted, the sponsor of the candidate vaccine should provide details of clinical protocols implemented so that the US FDA reviewer can assess the adequacy of the sponsor's conclusions regarding safety and efficacy. Summary information should describe the study design and indicate the following for each group: the product dose; route and schedule of administration; age, sex, general health, and the number of subjects studied; enumeration of the clinical and laboratory parameters that were monitored; and a relevant presentation of results.

The US FDA CBER IND review process

When a sponsor submits an IND to the US FDA, the agency assumes an important role in development of the biological product. Most sponsor activities beyond the nonclinical development phase are subject to some form of US FDA oversight because they involve human subjects and their health. When the IND is submitted to the US FDA for review the sponsor signs Form 1571 in the IND, which states the following:

I agree not to begin clinical investigations until 30 days after FDA's receipt of the IND unless I receive further notification by from the FDA that the studies may begin. I also agree not to begin or continue clinical investigations covered by the IND if those studies are placed on clinical hold. I agree that an Institutional Review Board (IRB) that complies with federal regulations will be responsible for the initial and continuing review and approval of each of the studies in the proposed clinical trial. I agree to conduct the investigation in accordance with all other applicable regulatory requirements.

Vaccine development involves processes that include nonclinical development, clinical development, licensing, and approval. The primary US FDA reviewing center for vaccines is the CBER, although it can vary depending upon the product type. Biologics that are well-characterized proteins, such as therapeutic monoclonal antibodies, growth factors, and enzymes, are reviewed by the CDER. For example, a vaccine produced and used in combination with another drug or device may be reviewed by CDER and Center for Devices and Radiological Health (CDRH). The US FDA does not require redundant product submissions to conduct review of a combination product.

Biological products regulated by CBER include the following:

- gene therapy products
- products composed of human or animal cells
- allergen patch tests
- allergenic diagnostic reagents
- monoclonal antibodies
- vaccines
- toxoids and toxins used for immunization
- antitoxins and antivenins
- *in vitro* diagnostics to screen donor blood, blood components, cellular products
- devices used to collect and process blood and blood products
- tissue—human cells for implantation or transplantation and xenotransplantation
- transplantation, implantation or infusion into a human recipient living cells, tissues, or organs from a nonhuman source or human body fluids, cells tissues, or organs

CBER organization structure

Within the CBER, the organizational structure for reviewing these diverse biological product submissions is divided into three main review offices:

1. Office of Blood Research and Review (OBRR)
2. Office of Cellular, Tissue and Gene Therapies (OCGT)
3. Office of Vaccine Research and Review (OVRR)
  (a) Division of Bacterial, Parasitic and Allergenic Products (DBAP)
  (b) Division of Viral Products (DVP)
  (c) Division of Vaccines and Related Product Applications (DVRPA)

Scientists in the office of OVRR review vaccine regulatory documents that describe a heterogeneous class of medical products containing antigenic substances capable of inducing specific, active, and protective host immunity against an infectious agent or pathogen. Vaccines for human use include live attenuated organisms, inactivated organisms, and subcomponents of purified immunogens, synthetic antigens, and polynucleotides such as DNA.

The CBER review process for INDs

The IND review process and the US FDA's analysis of the INDs represent a delicate balance between the federal government's responsibility to protect clinical trial subjects from unnecessary risk and its desire to avoid impeding progress of medical research that should promote the health of its citizens. Within the framework of these dual goals, federal law establishes that the US FDA must perform a safety review of the IND prior to the initiation of clinical trials and provides the agency 30 working days in which to reach a decision on whether the product should move forward.

The US FDA's principal goals during the IND review are (1) to determine if the available research data demonstrate that the product is reasonably safe for administration to human subjects and (2) determine if the protocol for the proposed clinical study will expose subjects to unnecessary risk.

After determining which of CBER's three product research and review offices has authority over an

IND, the Document Control Center forwards the submission to that office's application review division. Vaccine IND documents submitted to the US FDA are usually sent to the DVRPA within the OVRR for review.

Once within the relevant division, the IND is assigned to a primary reviewer, who first conducts an administrative review to determine whether (1) the IND contains sufficient information to justify a scientific review, (2) the submission contains all necessary completed forms, and (3) the product belongs under authority of CBER and the division to which the application has been forwarded. INDs describing viral vaccines are usually forwarded to the DVP; vaccines dealing with bacterial, fungal, or parasitic diseases are sent to the DBAP for review.

CBER's reputation for conducting highly qualified and informed reviews is related to the strong scientific base provided by these laboratory research and review divisions. Because they are staffed by physicians and scientists who are involved in both regulatory decision making and laboratory research, the individuals in these laboratories have the unique expertise to review even the most scientifically complex and advanced product.

During the initial 30-day review period, the IND reviewers will evaluate the application and confer with other reviewers assigned to the application. The primary reviewer then reconciles the various reviews and makes a determination on the IND in consultation with the applicable branch chief within DVRPA. Generally, the primary reviewer presents the go/no go decision at a weekly office-wide staff meeting, which provides other reviewers an opportunity to offer input on the IND. The division directors within DVRPA have the final authority over the fate of the IND in their respective divisions.

Despite the brevity of the 30-day time line, applicable to IND reviews, the CBER and IND applicants may have the opportunity to communicate during the period to address reviewer questions and possible issues with the submission. In many cases, members of the IND review team communicate directly with the applicant via facsimile and telephone. The US FDA does not use email for this notice as it informs the sponsor that they can begin a clinical trial, which is a legal statement and must be via facsimile and phone for short notice.

The IND and 30-day review clock

The US FDA has 30 calendar days in which to reach a decision on a pending biologic IND. An IND goes into effect 30 days after the US FDA receives the IND, unless the agency notifies the sponsor that the investigations described in the IND are subject to a clinical hold order; or upon earlier notification by the US FDA that the clinical investigations described in the IND may begin.

Definition

Clinical hold: An order issued by the US FDA to the sponsor to delay a proposed clinical study or suspend an ongoing clinical investigation. Subjects may not be given the investigational drug, or the hold may require that no new subjects be enrolled in the investigation. The hold may be issued before the end of the 30-day IND review period to prevent initiation of a proposed protocol, or any time during the life of the IND.

If CBER finds no significant deficiencies in the IND and determines the proposed clinical trials do not present any unnecessary risks to study subjects, the relevant center may "passively" approve the IND without issuing any communication to the sponsor at the conclusion of the 30-day review period. In this way, the INDs are not formally approved by the US FDA. Although not required, sponsors are encouraged to contact the relevant center before initiation of clinical trials.

Alternate licensure strategies

The "Animal Rule"

The US FDA's regulations concerning the approval of new drugs or biological products when human efficacy studies are neither ethical nor feasible are known as "the Animal Rule" (21 CFR 314.600 for drugs; 21 CFR 601.90 for biological products). The Animal Rule states that in selected circumstances, when it is neither ethical nor feasible to conduct human efficacy studies, the US FDA may grant marketing approval based on adequate and well-controlled animal studies when the results of those studies establish that the drug or biological product is reasonably likely to produce clinical benefit in humans. Demonstration of the product's safety in humans is still necessary.

To develop an animal model to demonstrate efficacy, the sponsor should obtain information on the natural biology of the disease in both humans and animals, on the etiologic agent, and on the proposed intervention. Data from human experience with the etiologic agent and/or intervention, if available may support application of the Animal Rule.

The Animal Rule states that the US FDA can rely on evidence from animal model studies to provide substantial evidence of effectiveness when (1) there is a reasonably well-understood pathophysiological mechanism for toxicity of the etiologic agent and its prevention or reduction by the proposed product; (2) the effect is demonstrated in more than one animal species expected to react with a response predictive for humans, unless the effect is demonstrated in a single animal species that represents a sufficiently well-characterized animal model to predict the human response; (3) the animal model is clearly related to the desired benefit in humans, generally survival; (4) the data on pharmacokinetics and pharmacodynamics of the product in animals and humans allow selection of an effective dose for humans [21 CFR 314.610(a) (1)-(4); 21CFR 601.91(a) (1)-(4)].

If these criteria are met, it is reasonable to expect the effectiveness of the product in animals to be a reliable indicator of its effectiveness in humans.

The Animal Rule allows approval based on a single animal species if the animal model is sufficiently well characterized; however, the usual exception is that the efficacy will be demonstrated in more than one species.

If another regulatory pathway to approval using human data is feasible and ethical, that pathway must be used (21 CFR 314.600 and 601.90). The Animal Rule allows development of products that would otherwise not have any route to approval; the rule reflects the agency's recognition that many treatments that appear to be effective in animals have not proven to be effective in humans. Consequently, developing animal models that will yield efficacy results that can be predicted to be predictive for humans is challenging.

Accelerated approval and priority review

Fast track

Fast track is a process designed to facilitate the development, and expedite the review, of drugs and biologics to treat serious disease and fill an unmet medical need. The purpose is to get important new drugs to the patient earlier. This process addresses a broad range of serious diseases.

Determining whether a disease is serious is a matter of judgment, but generally it is based on whether the drug will have a impact on such factors as survival, day-to-day functioning, and the likelihood that the disease, if left untreated, will progress to a more serious one.

The US FDA defines filling an unmet medical need as providing a therapy where none exists or providing a therapy that may be potentially superior to an existing therapy.

Any drug developed to treat or prevent a disease with no current therapy is directed at an unmet need. If there are existing therapies, a fast track drug must show some advantage over the available treatment, such as its ability to (a) show superior effectiveness; (b) avoid serious side effects; (c) improve diagnosis; (d) decrease a clinically significant toxicity of an accepted treatment.

Most drugs eligible for fast track designation are also eligible to receive priority review. Fast track designation must be requested by the drug company and can be initiated any time if the drug meets an unmet medical need in a serious disease.

Accelerated approval

When studying a new drug, it can require a long time to demonstrate efficacy and that the patient is living longer or feeling better. Realizing that obtaining data to support a clinical outcome can take a long time, the US FDA instituted the accelerated approval regulation, allowing earlier approval of drugs to treat serious diseases based on a surrogate end point.

A surrogate end point is a marker—a laboratory measurement or physical sign—that is used in clinical trials as an indirect measure that represents a meaningful outcome. The use of a surrogate end point can shorten the time required prior to receiving US FDA approval. For example, in cases where phase III clinical trials to demonstrate vaccine efficacy cannot be done, neutralizing antibodies stimulated by the vaccine may be designated a surrogate end point, knowing that antibodies to the infectious agent protect laboratory animals from infection. Based on antibody titer information from human immunization studies, the vaccine can be given accelerated approval after phase II clinical trials in which the vaccine dose and immune response to the vaccine have been determined. In this case, the sponsor is given accelerated approval to market the vaccine for human use with the provision that those individuals who receive the vaccine are monitored for protection against the infectious agent for which the vaccine was developed. In some cases, this will require several years to accomplish if the disease does not reoccur with a high incidence in the area where vaccinated individuals reside.

Priority review

Prior to approval, each drug marketed in the USA must go through a detailed US FDA review process. In 1991, the agency agreed to specific goals to improve drug review time and created a two-tiered system of review times: standard review and priority review.

Standard review is applied to drugs that offer, at most, only minor improvement over existing marketed therapies. It was agreed that a standard review of a new drug application be accomplished within a 10-month time frame.

Priority review is applied to drugs that offer major advances in treatment or provide a treatment where no adequate therapy exists. The US FDA goal for a priority review is 6 months.

Environmental risk assessment

Scope

Some countries have legislation covering the environment and issues related to the use of live organisms that are derived by recombinant DNA technology. These organisms are generally considered genetically modified organisms (GMOs). Similar genetic changes that involve genetic recombination between viruses or other organisms in nature and/or recombination by conventional means can result in genetic diversity.

This section of the chapter considers the environmental risk assessment (ERA) a GMO vaccine may have on the environment prior to regulatory approval and licensure. The ERA analyzes the risk that a GMO presents to the environment. It does not assess risk to the intended recipient of the vaccine; this is assessed in clinical trials with the recombinant vaccine. Nor

does the ERA assess the risk of infection with the virus to laboratory workers during development of the vaccine.

The environmental impact analysis is usually not the responsibility of the national regulatory authority but of other agencies. However, the national regulatory authority does receive a copy of the ERA and is involved in making licensure decisions based on information presented in the ERA to ensure steps are taken to protect the environment.

Principles and objectives

A live vaccine in which the genome has been genetically modified by recombinant DNA technology is considered a GMO. Shipment of such live recombinant vaccines, for research or commercial use, either intrastate, interstate, or across international boundaries, should comply with any relevant legislation or regulations of the producing and recipient countries regarding GMOs. In some countries, regulatory compliance with environmental regulations requires an ERA be undertaken if the live vaccine is to be tested in a clinical trial or prior to commercial distribution.

The objective of an ERA is to identify and evaluate, on a case-by-case basis, potential adverse effects of a GMO on public health and the environment, direct or indirect, immediate or delayed. This means that for each different live recombinant vaccine, a case-by-case ERA should be performed. *Direct effects* refer to primary effects on human health or on the environment that are a result of the GMO and that occur through a short causal chain of events. *Indirect effects* refer to effects occurring through a more extended causal chain of events, through mechanisms such as interactions with other organisms, transfer of genetic material, or changes in use or management. *Immediate effects* are observed during the period of the release of the GMO, whereas *delayed effects* refer to effects that may not be observed during the period of release of the GMO but become apparent as a direct or indirect effect either at a later stage or after termination of the release.

The ERA should be performed in a scientifically sound and transparent manner based on available scientific and technical data. Important aspects to be addressed in an ERA include the characteristics of the following: (a) the parental organism, (b) the recipient organism, (c) viral vector characteristics, (d) the donor sequence, (e) genetic modification, (f) the intended use, and (g) the receiving environment. The data needed to evaluate the ERA do not have to derive solely from experiments performed by the applicant; data available in the scientific literature can also be used in the assessment. Regardless of the source of the data, it should be both relevant and of an acceptable scientific quality. The ERA could be based on data of experiments previously performed for other purposes, such as product characterization tests, and nonclinical safety and toxicity studies.

Ideally, the ERA is based on quantitative data and expressed in quantitative terms. However, much of the information available for an ERA may be qualitative. For this reason quantification of the GMO impact is often hard to establish and may not be essential to making a decision. The level of detail and information required in the ERA will vary according to the nature and the scale of the proposed release. Information requirements may differ between licensure and clinical development and whether studies will be carried out in a single country or multiple countries.

Uncertainty is inherent in the concept of risk. Therefore, it is important to identify and analyze areas of uncertainty in the risk assessment. Since there is no universally accepted approach for addressing uncertainty, risk management strategies may be considered. Precise data on the environmental fate of the live vaccine in early clinical trials will, in most cases, be insufficient or lacking. However, at the market registration stage, the level of uncertainty is expected to be lower as identified gaps in available data should already have been addressed.

The need for risk management measures should be based upon the estimated level of risk. If new information on the GMO becomes available, the ERA may need to be re-performed to determine whether the estimated level of risk has changed. This also holds true if the risks for the participating subjects have changed as these aspects can be translated to other individuals. It should be noted that the ERA will not deal with medical benefit for the subject or scientific issues such as proof of principle.

Procedure for environmental risk assessment

Risk assessment involves identification of novel characteristics of the GMO that may have adverse effects (hazard), evaluating the consequences of each

Table 12.1 Environmental Risk Analysis for Release of a Genetically Modified Organism (GMO) Vaccine

Step 1	Identify characteristics of the genetically modified organism(s) (GMOs) in the vaccine that may cause adverse side effects.
Step 2	Evaluate potential consequences of each adverse event.
Step 3	Evaluate the likelihood of the occurrence of each potential adverse event.
Step 4	Estimate the risk posed by each identified characteristic of the GMOs in the vaccine.
Step 5	Apply management strategies for risks from the deliberate release of the GMOs into the environment.
Step 6	Determine the overall risk of the vaccine GMOs to cause adverse side effects.

potential adverse effect, estimation of the likelihood of the occurrence of adverse effects, risk estimation, risk management, and, in some methodologies, estimation of the overall risk for the environment (Table 12.1).

These processes should identify the potential adverse effects by comparing the properties of the GMO with non-modified organisms under the same conditions, in the same environment. The principles and methodology of an ERA should be applicable irrespective of the geographic location of the intended environmental release of the GMO. If live attenuated mosquito-borne virus vaccines are being considered, the ERA must take into account the specificities associated with the mosquito vector being endemic or non-endemic in the region in which vaccine trials will be carried out, and/or where licensure is being requested. Depending upon local regulatory requirements, the ERA may be undertaken by the applicant or by the local competent authority on the basis of data supplied. In all cases, the local competent authority should use the ERA as a basis for deciding whether any identified environmental risks are acceptable. However, the decision on whether any identified risks are acceptable may vary from country to country.

New Drug Application and Common Technical Document

The New Drug Application (NDA) is the vehicle through which drug sponsors formally propose the US FDA approve a new pharmaceutical for marketing and sale in the USA. To obtain government authorization, the sponsor must submit in an accepted NDA format, thousands of documents that contain nonclinical and clinical data with their analyses, drug chemistry information, descriptions of manufacturing procedures, and information on other significant issues in a format that has been revised and refined over the years.

To promote both international harmonization and encourage use of an "all-electronic submissions environment" the ICH has encouraged use of the Common Technical Document (CTD) format. Regardless of format structure, size, or complexity, the NDA or CTD must provide sufficient information, data, and analysis to enable US FDA reviewers to evaluate the data and make several key decisions that include:

1. Is the drug safe and effective for its proposed use, and do the benefits outweigh the risks?
2. Does the drug's proposed labeling contain the appropriate information?
3. Do the methods used to manufacture and formulate the drug adequately preserve the drug's strength, quality, and purity?

International Conference on Harmonisation (ICH) of technical requirements for registration of pharmaceuticals for human use

The ICH project brings together regulatory authorities from the USA, Europe, and Japan with experts from the pharmaceutical industry to discuss scientific and technical aspects of product registration. The purpose of ICH is to simplify processes to avoid duplication of regulatory required testing for registration, achieve harmonization of technical guidelines, and establish new guidelines for registration of pharmaceuticals. Harmonization of guidelines facilitates conservation of time, resources, and effort to eliminate unnecessary delay in global development and availability of new medicines, while protecting public health.

Common Technical Document

In mid-1997, members of the ICH agreed to develop a CTD that would harmonize the format in which all information needed for licensure could be organized. As a result of these efforts, the CTD format was developed. The CTD format strategy presents a common way that sponsors from many parts of the world can organize the information required in the NDA application. However, it does not modify the scope or detail of the information required in the NDA format. Since its introduction, use of the CTD format has significantly increased with the development of electronic Common Technical Document specifications (eCTD). Maximum benefit of this format is realized once an IND application is in electronic format and amendments can be submitted to the eCTD document over the life of the project.

Organization of the CTD is displayed as a pyramid composed of five separate domains (Figure 12.2). The five modules in the CTD format are:

1. *Module 1.* Administrative and prescribing information that includes product labeling and documents specific for each country. Also included are a comprehensive Table of Contents for each section and an index for entire submission.
2. *Module 2.* CTD summaries of the technical data in modules 3 through 5. This includes summary documents, an overall quality summary, nonclinical overview, nonclinical written and tabulated summaries, clinical overview, and clinical summary.
3. *Module 3.* Table of Contents for Module 3 only, and detailed technical information regarding CMC can be provided regarding the drug substance and drug product and literature references.
4. *Module 4.* Table of Contents for Module 4 only, and nonclinical study reports and literature references.
5. *Module 5.* Table of Contents for Module 5 only, and a tabular listing of all clinical studies, clinical study reports, and literature references.

Electronic submissions

Preparation of the NDA in an electronic format provides many advantages to the applicant as well as the regulatory agency review. Once in an electronic format, the document can be stored and managed using many different types of media. This reduces the

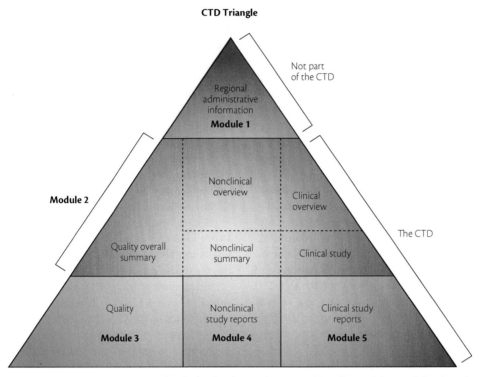

CTD Triangle

Figure 12.2 The Common Technical Document (CTD) triangle. The CTD is organized into five modules. Module 1 is region specific, and modules 2, 3, 4, and 5 are intended to be common for all regions.

amount of time required to review the documents because it is hyperlinked throughout the document and analyzed using software at the regulatory agency.

In addition to harmonizing requirements and format for submission of the NDA, the ICH initiative stimulated development of specifications for a common eCTD. The eCTD presents an interface between industry and regulatory agency for rapid and efficient transfer of regulatory information as well as creating a life cycle for management of applications throughout the cycle of their development and archival documentation.

Submission and review of the NDA

Once complete, the NDA sponsor prepares multiple copies of the document: (1) archival, (2) review, and (3) field copies for submission to the US FDA.

Archival copies contain all sections of the NDA document plus copies of all of the documents submitted

---

Definition

Common Technical Document (CTD): The CTD is a format for the preparation of a well-organized new drug/biologic license application (NDA/BLA) that will be submitted to regulatory authorities to support registration of pharmaceuticals for human use. The format was agreed upon by all parties of the ICH and is a joint initiative harmonizing the technical requirements for pharmaceuticals. The CTD "triangle" organizes the BLA/NDA application into five separate modules. Modules 2 through 5 are harmonized and contain the technical information required in a registration submission.

---

to the regulatory agency to support the license application. The review copy contains the technical sections of the NDA organized as appropriate technical sections. The field copy is used by US FDA inspectors during pre-approval inspections of facilities for manufacture and production of the product. If the NDA is submitted in eCTD format the agency may require only the archival copy since format field offices will have immediate access to the eCTD formatted document.

Once the NDA document has been submitted to the regulatory agency that will conduct the review, a review clock is started for the NDA. The US FDA has 60 days to decide whether to "file" or "not to file" this document for review. The document is received, logged in, and sent to the reviewing division for evaluation. The reviewing division sends the applicant a letter acknowledging receipt of the NDA with a number, the project manager's contact information, and date of receipt. The project manager performs a preliminary review of the documents to ensure that the NDA is complete. If problems with the document are identified, the division can issue a letter of refusal notifying the applicant of the deficiencies and may continue the review or place review of the document on hold until the deficiencies are corrected.

Once the NDA document is accepted by the division conducting the review, the project manager forwards sections of the document to different members of the review team. Review of the NDA is a demanding task requiring a team that includes clinicians, pharmacokineticists, pharmacologists, statisticians, microbiologists, and chemists. Each member of the team will review the technical section assigned to ensure the appropriate information has been included and that the information is adequate and sufficient to validate the sponsor's contention that the vaccine is safe and effective for its intended purpose. In addition, the reviewing division will organize pre-approval inspections of the drug manufacturing site and clinical sites as appropriate. These inspections will verify information in the NDA and confirm compliance with cGMPs and GCPs.

Once review of the NDA is complete, each member of the review team will write an evaluation of their section of the NDA document that contains data on specific topics presented in the NDA. Once written evaluations of the NDA, site inspections, and product label negotiations are complete, the reviewers and their supervisors are prepared to make a recommendation concerning the NDA. The recommendations can be: "approval," which means the drug is ready to be marketed under provisions of the FD&C Act. Under these circumstances the sponsor is entitled to manufacture the vaccine under the cGMP provisions described in the NDA, formulate and fill product for commercial sale, advertise and market the product, and provide physicians and certified public health workers vaccine to be administered to individuals as described in the NDA document. If the recommendation is "approvable," additional issues need to be resolved before the drug can be marketed. If the application is regarded as "nonapprovable," then the drug cannot be marketed and must be withdrawn from further consideration.

Maintenance of the NDA

Once the NDA is approved, the sponsor must conduct extensive post marketing surveillance of the drug to determine safety. The sponsor is required to review all adverse drug experience (ADE) about their drug from any source to determine safety of the drug for the proposed use in the population at risk.

Worldwide regulatory authorities

Many countries have national regulatory authorities (NRAs) that oversee and regulate the development, manufacture, clinical testing, and licensure of vaccines. At present there are more than 75 NRAs worldwide that regulate vaccines.

European Medicines Agency (EMA)

There are several avenues for drug approval in Europe that include:

1. *Centralized Procedure*: European Community Regulation 726/2004 and Directive 2004/27EC, the Centralized Procedure that is mandatory for medical products of the following types: (a) products produced by biotechnology and genetic engineering and (b) orphan medicines.

2. *Mutual Recognition Procedure*: A medicine that is recognized by a member state and for which the applicant can seek authorization through a mutual recognition procedure. The EMA mediates, and its decision is binding on all member states.

3. *Decentralized Procedure*: When an application has not been approved by any member state the applicant may apply for simultaneous approval by more than one EMEA member.

The EMA's key role in approval of medicines to be used within the European Union (EU) are to (1) protect public health, (2) provide quick access to new therapy, (3) encourage free distribution of medicines throughout all of the EU, (4) distribute information about new medication to patients and physicians, and (5) harmonize scientific requirements to harmonize compliance worldwide.

The EMA committee for human drug use receives applications according to an agreed upon procedure for review. If approved, clinical trials may be initiated with new medicines as appropriate. Clinical trials applications are not centralized and are made through individual states.

Japan's Ministry of Health, Labor and Welfare

The Ministry of Health, Labor and Welfare (MHLW) is responsible to ensure the quality, efficacy, and safety of drugs and medical devices in Japan. There are three main divisions that oversee this charter: (1) Pharmaceutical and Food Safety Bureau (PFSB), (2) Health Policy Bureau, and (3) the Pharmaceutical and Medical Device Agency (PMDA).

The Pharmaceutical and Food Safety Bureau is responsible for ensuring the safety and efficacy of drugs and medical devices, clinical trials, and importation of drugs into Japan. The Health Policy Bureau oversees the manufacture and distribution of all medicines within Japan. The PMDA reviews clinical protocols and deals with the manufacturers and distributors to ensure quality. In Japan, all new medicines are approved by the Pharmaceutical Affairs Department of the WHLW based on recommendations of the PSFB.

Foreign clinical trials are acceptable except where there are immunological and ethnic differences between Japanese natives and foreigners. In cases where there are differences, the MHLW may require the conducting of comparative clinical trials in Japan to establish equivalence with dose and immune response to establish efficacy.

All new drug applications in Japan are expected to be in the CTD format according to ICH guidelines. The standard processing schedule for a new drug is: (1) 1 year for review, (2) 1 year for applicant response, and (3) a total of 2 years for approval.

China Food and Drug Administration

The regulation of drugs in China is governed by the China Food and Drug Administration (CFDA), which is governed by the State Council. Through the CFDA, regulations are instituted to control registration, clinical trials, distribution, and marketing of new and generic drugs. The CFDA also regulates manufacturing, compliance, adverse events, and it prosecutes fraudulent drug manufacture. This agency also oversees compliance to GMP for medical products, GLP for nonclinical drug safety research, and GCP for clinical trials. There are many departments in the CFDA that control and regulate medical devices, drug safety, inspection, "Western drugs" imported into China, and traditional Chinese medications.

Australia's Therapeutic Goods Administration

In Australia, the Therapeutic Goods Administration (TGA) regulates prescription drugs, prescription medicines, over-the-counter medications, complementary medicines, and medical devices. The TGA has a regulatory role in the development, maintenance, manufacturing, adverse event reporting, surveillance activities, public inquires, and assessment of medicines for export.

All medicines in Australia are registered with the Australian Register of Therapeutic Goods (ARTG). The sponsor must apply to the ARTG to show scientific validity, safety, ethical acceptability, and efficacy of the drug in a CTD format.

Health Canada

All drugs sold in Canada must be authorized by Health Canada, which has several divisions that have the responsibility to oversee (1) therapeutic products, (2) biologics and genetic therapies, and (3) natural drug products. Manufacture of vaccines and biologics is regulated by the Directorate of Biologics and Genetic Therapies. In Canada, a Clinical Trial Application must be submitted to Health Canada seeking permission to conduct clinical trials. This application usually is submitted in the CTD format that includes information regarding characteristics, test data, animal studies, and a clinical protocol. After a drug has demonstrated efficacy in a phase III trial, a New Drug Submission (NDS) may be submitted to support the request for licensure. The NDS document is similar to the NDA and can be formatted in the eCTD format recognized by international regulatory authorities.

Summary

- Formulation of a regulatory strategy is one of the most important elements of product development.

- This strategy comprises the overall development plan that specifies the approach to pharmacological, toxicological, clinical testing, product development, and manufacturing.

- Regulatory strategy is based on the nature of the product under development.

- Product classification is critically important because of fundamental differences in the regulatory requirements for drugs and biologics.

- Vaccines are biologics composed of subunits of organisms, inactivated organisms, or live attenuated organisms. Regulatory requirements for vaccines of different types are specific and unique to enable immunization that will stimulate a protective immune response.

- From concept to product, regulatory strategy governs progress and must be in harmony with regulations specified by regulatory agencies. In the USA this process is regulated and reviewed by the CBER.

- Biologics approval requires the submission of a BLA, which primarily focuses on chemical, pharmacological, and toxicological characterization of the product, and demonstration of safety and effectiveness in humans.

- Vaccines are biologics and usually require only one adequate and controlled human trial to demonstrate safety and efficacy. Submission of an IND and BLA are important and critical steps in development of a new product for treatment, prevention, or diagnosis of disease. As discussed in this chapter, the critical responsibilities of the regulatory agency and IND sponsor have been addressed to show the path to licensure. The responsibilities and processes of regulatory approval are defined in a manner to enable understanding and stimulate compliance.

Further reading

Capen R, Shank-Retzlaff ML, Sings HL, Esser M, Sattler C, Washabaugh M, and Sitrin R (2007). Establishing potency specific antigen for vaccines. BioProcess International 5, 30–43.

CBER SOPP 8101.1. Scheduling and Conduct of Regulatory Review Meetings with Sponsors and Applicants May 2007.

FDA Consumer Information by Audience – Fast Track, Accelerated Approval and Priority Review, August 2011.

FDA Draft Guidance for Industry. Submitting Marketing Applications According to the ICH-CTD Format-General Considerations, August 2001.

FDA eCTD Table of Contents Headings and Hierarchy. Updated 2005. Accessed December 2007 at http://ww.fda.gov/Cder/regulatory/ersr/ectd/htm.

FDA Guidance for Industry. Content of Investigational New Drug Applications (INDs) for Phase 1 Studies of Drugs, Including Well-Characterized, Therapeutic, Biotechnology-Derived Products, November 1995.

FDA Guidance for Industry. Providing Clinical Evidence of Effectiveness for Human Drug and Biological Products, May 1998.

FDA Guidance for Industry. Content and Format of Chemistry, Manufacturing and Controls Information and Establishment Description Information for a Vaccine or Related Product. January 1999.

FDA Guidance for Industry. Formal Meetings with Sponsors and Applicants for PPDUFA Products, February 2000.

FDA Guidance for Industry. IND meetings for Human Drugs and Biologics. Chemistry, Manufacturing and Controls Information. May 2001.

FDA Guidance for Industry. Providing Regulatory Submissions to CBER in Electric Format- Investigational New Drug Applications (INDs), March 2002.

FDA Guidance for Industry. Fast Track Drug Development Programs—Designation, Development and Application Review, July 2004.

FDA Guidance for Industry. Fast Track Drug Development Programs-Designation, Development, and Application Review, January 2006.

FDA Guidance for Industry. Considerations for Development Toxicity Studies for Prevention and Therapeutic Vaccines for Infectious Disease Indications, February 2006.

FDA Guidance for Industry. Development of Preventive HIV Vaccines for Use in Pediatric Populations May 2006.

FDA Guidance for Industry. Characterization and Qualification of Cell Substrates and Other Biological starting Materials Used in the Production of Viral Vaccines for the

Prevention and Treatment of Infectious Diseases, September 2006.

FDA Guidance for Industry. Clinical Data Needed to Support the Licensure of Seasonal Inactivated Influenza Vaccines, May 2007.

FDA Guidance for Industry. Clinical Data Needed to Support the Licensure of Pandemic Influenza Vaccines, May 2007.

FDA Guidance for Industry. Integrated Summaries of Effectiveness and Safety: Location Within the Common Technical Document, June 2007.

FDA Guidance for Industry. Toxicity Grading Scale for Healthy Adult and Adolescent Volunteers Enrolled in Preventive Vaccine Clinical Trials, September 2007.

FDA Guidance for Industry. Considerations for Plasmid DNA Vaccines for Infectious Disease Indications, November 2007.

FDA Guidance for Industry. Providing Regulatory Submissions in Electronic Format-Human Pharmaceutical Product Applications and Related Submissions Using the eCTD Specifications, Revision 12, June 2008.

FDA Guidance for Industry. General Principles for the Development of Vaccines to Protect Against Global Infectious Diseases, September 2008.

FDA Guidance for Industry. Animal Models—Essential Elements to Address Efficacy Under the Animal Rule, January 2009.

FDA Guidance for Industry for the Submission of Chemistry, Manufacturing, and Controls Information for a Therapeutic Recombinant DNA-Derived Product or a Monoclonal Antibody Product for In Vivo Use, August 1996.

Federal Register Notice. New Drug and Biological Drug Products; Evidence Needed to Demonstrate Effectiveness of New Drugs When Human Efficacy Studies are Not Ethical or Feasible; Final Rule, May 2002, FR 67:37988-37998.

Gisonni-Lex L (2005). Meeting Report. Cancer Vaccine Consortium—Potency Testing Workshop. San Francisco, November 8, 2004. Part I: Historical perspective of vaccine potency tests. Biologicals: Journal of the International Association of Biological Standardization 33, 123–128.

Goldenthal KL, McVittie LD, Kleppinger C, and Geber A. The clinical evaluation of preventive vaccines for infectious disease indications. In Biologics Development: A Regulatory Overview, 3rd edition (ed M Mathieu), pp. 99–114. Waltham, MA: Parexel International Corporation, 2004.

Hamrell MR. What is an IND. In FDA Regulatory Affairs: A Guide for Prescription Drugs, Medical Devices, and Biologics, 2nd edition (eds DJ Pisano and DS Mantus), pp. 13–108. New York: Informa Health Care USA, 2008.

ICH. Harmonized Tripartite Guideline. Q5C. Quality of Biotechnology Products: Stability Testing of Biotechnological/Biological Products, November 1995.

ICH. Harmonized Tripartite Guideline. Q5B. Quality of Biotechnology Products: Analysis of the Expression Construct in Cells Use for Production of r-DNA Derived Products, November 1995.

ICH. Harmonized Tripartite Guideline. E6(R1). Guideline for Good Clinical Practice, June 1996.

ICH. Harmonized Tripartite Guideline. Q5D. Derivation and Characterization of Cell Substrates Used for Production of Biotechnological/Biological Products, July 1997.

ICH. Harmonized Tripartite Guideline. 6S. Preclinical Safety Evaluation of Biotechnology-Derived Pharmaceuticals, July 1997.

ICH. Harmonized Tripartite Guideline. Q6B. Specifications: Test Procedures and Acceptance Criteria for Biotechnological/Biological Products, March 1999.

ICH. Harmonized Tripartite Guideline. Q5A (R1). Viral Safety Evaluation of Biotechnology Products Derived from Cell Lines of Human and Animal Origin, September 1999.

ICH. Harmonized Tripartite Guideline. M4E (R1). Clinical Overview and Clinical Summary of Module 2; Module 5: Clinical Study Reports, September 2002.

ICH. Harmonized Tripartite Guideline. M4Q (R1). Quality Overall summary of Module 2; Module 3: Quality, September 2002.

ICH. Harmonized Tripartite Guideline. M4S (R2). Nonclinical Overview and Nonclinical Summaries of Module 2; Organization of Module 4, December 2002.

ICH. Harmonized Tripartite Guideline. M4Q. Implementation Working Group Questions and Answers (R1), July 2003.

ICH. Harmonized Tripartite Guideline. M4S Implementation of Working Group Questions and answers (R4), November 2003.

ICH. Harmonized Tripartite Guideline. M4(R3). Organization of the Common Technical Document for the Registration of Pharmaceuticals for Human Use, January 2004.

ICH. Harmonized Tripartite Guideline. M4. Implementation Working Group Questions and Answers (R3), June 2004.

ICH. Harmonized Tripartite Guideline. M4E. Implementation Working Group Questions and Answers (R4), June 2004.

ICH. Harmonized Tripartite Guideline. Q5E. Comparability of Biotechnological/Biological Products Subject to Changes in their Manufacturing Process, November 2004.

Mathieu M. The biological IND review Process. In Biologics Development: A Regulatory Overview, 3rd edition, (ed

M Mathieu), pp. 53–97. Waltham, MA: Parexel International Corporation, 2004.

Mathieu M. The biological license application (BLA) review process. In Biologics Development: A Regulatory Overview, 3rd edition (ed M Mathieu), pp. 187–218. Waltham, MA: Parexel International Corporation, 2004.

Mathieu M, Whisenand TD, Spaulding A, and Kane K. The biological license application (BLA). In Biologics Development: A Regulatory Overview, 3rd edition, (ed M Mathieu), pp. 133–169. Waltham, MA: Parexel International Corporation, 2004.

Monahan C and Babirz JC. The new drug application. In FDA Regulatory Affairs: A Guide for Prescription Drugs, Medical Devices and Biologics, 2nd edition (eds DJ Pisano and D Mantus), pp. 69–108. New York: Informa Healthcare, 2008.

Ng R. Regulatory Authorities. In Drugs from Discovery to Approval, 2nd edition (ed R Nig), pp. 208–230. Hoboken, NJ: John Wiley & Sons, 2009.

Ng R. Regulatory Applications. In Drugs from Discovery to Approval, 2nd edition (ed R Nig), pp. 231–277. Hoboken, NJ: John Wiley & Sons, 2009.

Novak JM, Ruckman J, and Trent DW. The US Food and Drug Administration pre-IND and IND process for vaccines. In Vaccines for Biodefense and Emerging and Neglected Diseases, 1st edition (eds AD Barrett and LR Stanberry), pp. 172–189. London, UK: Elsevier, Inc., 2009.

Offit AP (2005). The Cutter incident, 50 years later. The New England Journal of Medicine 352, 1411–1412.

Petriccani J, Egan W, Vicari G, Furesz J, and Schild G (2007). Potency assays for therapeutic live whole cell cancer vaccines. Biologicals: Journal of the International Association of Biological Standardization 35, 107–113.

Schalk JACK, deVries CGJCA, and Jongen PMJM (2007). Potency estimation of measles, mumps and rubella trivalent vaccines with quantitative PCR infectivity assay. Biologicals: Journal of the International Association of Biological Standardization 35, 107–113.

United States Pharmacopeia, General Chapter <1041> Biologics.

United States Pharmacopeia, General Chapter <1045> Biotechnology Derived Articles.

World Health Organization Guidance. WHO Guidance on Nonclinical Evaluation of Vaccines, November 2003.

World Health Organization Guidance. WHO Guidance on the Quality, Safety and Efficacy of Dengue Tetravalent Vaccines (Live, Attenuated), October 2011.

13 Veterinary vaccines: regulations and impact on emerging infectious diseases

A. Paige Adams

Kansas State University, Olathe, KS, USA

Abbreviations

APHIS	Animal and Plant Health Inspection Service	GMP	Good manufacturing practice
APVMA	Australian Pesticides and Veterinary Medicine Authority	MUMS	Minor use/minor species
		NVS	National veterinary stockpile
CFR	Code of Federal Regulations	OIE	World Organization for Animal Health
CVB	Center for Veterinary Biologics	ORV	Oral rabies vaccine
CVMP	Committee for Veterinary Medicinal Products	USDA	US Department of Agriculture
		VBPL	Veterinary biological product license
DOI	Duration of immunity	VICH	International Cooperation on Harmonization of Technical Requirements for Registration of Veterinary Medicinal Products
EMA	European Medicines Agency		
EPAA	European Partnership for Alternative Approaches to Animal Testing	WHO	World Health Organization

Global veterinary vaccine market

When considering the history of vaccine development, Edward Jenner was the first to recognize the close relationship between human and animal infectious diseases when he described the inoculation of humans with the cowpox virus to confer protection against the related human smallpox virus, later naming this practice "vaccination" from the Latin term *vacca* (meaning "cow"). Nearly 100 years later, the discovery of the first veterinary vaccine occurred in 1880 by Louis Pasteur for fowl cholera (causative agent, *Pasteurella multocida*), in which he also discovered the technique of attenuation by extending culture intervals. From these early discoveries, the number of veterinary vaccines has expanded and now comprises at least 23% of the global market for animal health products, some of which have the potential to reduce the estimated 17% of annual production losses that are associated with infectious diseases.

Overall, the veterinary vaccine market is expected to grow even further in the future due to several different factors, including new technological discoveries in vaccine development, the continuous development

Vaccinology: An Essential Guide, First Edition. Edited by Gregg N. Milligan and Alan D.T. Barrett.
© 2015 John Wiley & Sons, Ltd. Published 2015 by John Wiley & Sons, Ltd.

of drug resistance by pathogens, and the unpredictable emergence of new infectious diseases. The growing population and its need for the nutrients of food-producing animals, the recognition of unrelenting animal epidemics, and the increasing public concern for animal welfare are additional factors that will contribute to the growth of the global veterinary vaccine market. There is also increased awareness that veterinary vaccines can have a significant impact on public health through the control and prevention of food-borne and zoonotic diseases. For example, the incidence of human salmonellosis in the UK rapidly decreased after the implementation of a vaccination program in poultry (which included other preventive practices) in 1998. Vaccines can also decrease the use of antibiotics for treating infections, which was effectively demonstrated in Norwegian salmon production following the introduction of fish vaccines for vibriosis and furunculosis in the early 1990s.

In 2004, the global veterinary vaccine market was worth an estimated $3.1 billion, where 41% of the market was based in the Americas, 37% in Europe, and 22% for the rest of the world. Based on recent market reports, the global market for veterinary vaccines is forecast to reach $5.6 billion by 2015, in which livestock vaccines represent the largest product segment in the market.

Veterinary versus human vaccine development

When compared to human vaccine development, animal vaccine development has many advantages, especially when it comes to regulatory issues. Overall, veterinary vaccines have less rigorous regulatory and nonclinical trial requirements and associated costs, which results in a shorter time to reach the market and a quicker return on the investment for research and development of the product. With the less stringent regulatory requirements, veterinary vaccines can be at the forefront of testing and commercialization of innovative technologies before those of human vaccines. A major advantage of veterinary vaccine development over human vaccine development is that research can be performed on the relevant target species (including dose-response studies and challenge inoculations) rather than having to rely on animal models during nonclinical development, which may or may not respond as a human would to a vaccine candidate.

However, a major disadvantage of veterinary vaccine development when compared to human vaccines is related to the economics of vaccine development. Since the market for veterinary vaccines is spread across a large number of animal species, the potential returns for animal vaccine producers are significantly less than those for human vaccines. Since commercial vaccine production focuses on diseases that generate revenue that cover the cost of development (in addition to some profits), the development of vaccines for animal diseases that are less widespread usually require the financial support of the public or special interest groups. In addition to the smaller market size, veterinary vaccines generally have lower sales prices, which result in a much lower investment in research and development for these vaccines when compared to human vaccines. For example, the global market size for the human vaccine against papillomavirus (Gardasil® and Cervarix®), a major cause of cervical cancer, is estimated to be greater than $1 billion per year, while the most successful vaccines in animal health have a *combined* market size that is a fraction (10–20%) of this figure. Unfortunately, the contrast in market sizes between veterinary and human vaccines fails to reflect the complexity and wide range of hosts and pathogens that are involved in veterinary medicine.

Veterinary vaccine regulations: an overview

The time frame for veterinary vaccine development from discovery to licensure is approximately 5–8 years

---

Definitions

Companion animal: Domesticated or domestic-bred animals whose physical, emotional, and social needs can be readily met as companions in the home, or in close daily relationships with humans; the more usual word is "pet."

Food-producing animal: Animals used in the production food for humans, including meat-, egg-, and milk-producing animals.

for an estimated cost of $50 million to $100 million. However, the length of time and the costs associated with vaccine development depend on several factors. First, the time required to develop an effective vaccine varies across species. Companion animal vaccines generally cost less and require less time to develop when compared to food-producing animal vaccines, which usually require more cost and time to address safety issues. In addition, the length of time for the field trials, any modifications that are made to the product or application, and the time the pharmaceutical company takes to respond to correspondence with the regulatory authorities can influence the time frame and the associated costs related to vaccine development. Lastly, the nature of the pathogen itself can also affect how efficiently a vaccine can be developed and manufactured.

The policies and regulations for registering and licensing veterinary vaccines vary among countries, which can also affect the time frame for developing and licensing veterinary vaccines. This factor also has implications on the regulations regarding the importation and exportation of vaccines between countries. Since some countries use different quality standards for the approval of the use of a vaccine, imported vaccines during nonemergency situations may be required to go through a conventional licensing process, which can be costly and time consuming. There has been some effort by different organizations to harmonize the testing procedures used by different countries to prevent duplicate testing of imported vaccines that are undergoing registration. To ensure the release of a high-quality product, some countries have adopted specific standards in manufacturing (i.e., good manufacturing practice [GMP] compliance), which may be mutually recognized by other countries. In the USA, European Union (EU), Australia, and other countries that are currently developing and licensing vaccines for use in animals, the overall objective of their regulations are essentially the same: to license a veterinary biologic (also called an *immunological veterinary medicinal product*) that is pure, safe, potent, and efficacious. Table 13.1 provides a general overview of the research and development phases for a veterinary vaccine, from documentation to licensure. The development and implementation of these regulations can be unique to different countries, some of which are discussed in more detail below.

Veterinary vaccine regulations: USA, European Union, and Australia

Definition

Veterinary biologic: Vaccine and other product intended for use in animals, which work primarily through the stimulation of the immune system in order to prevent, treat, or diagnose diseases in animals.

United States of America

In the USA, the regulation of veterinary biologics, including vaccines, began with the passage of the 1913 Virus-Serum-Toxin Act (Title 21 of the US Code Parts 151-159) by the US Congress, which provides the legal basis for the regulation of veterinary biologics. This act was later amended in 1985 by the Food Security Act to include distribution of all veterinary biologics (both interstate and intrastate) in the USA and those intended for export. Within the US Department of Agriculture (USDA) Animal and Plant Health Inspection Service (APHIS), the Center for Veterinary Biologics (CVB), which is located in Ames, Iowa, regulates veterinary biological products, including, but not limited to, vaccines, bacterins, toxoids, antibodies, and antitoxins. The USDA is also responsible for regulating diagnostic kits for use in animals.

To manufacture and sell veterinary biologics in the USA, a pharmaceutical company (or sponsor) must have two licenses as issued by the USDA: (1) Veterinary Biological Product License through Title 9 of the Code of Federal Regulations (9 CFR) and (2) Veterinary Biologics Establishment License. The Veterinary Biological Product License can be either a "conventional" (also called "regular" or "full") license or a "conditional" license for specific situations or under certain conditions. Conditional licenses usually have additional requirements, including annual renewal, special labeling, and restricted use or administration of the veterinary biologic. For companies or individuals wishing to market an imported veterinary biological product in the USA, a US Veterinary Biological Product Permit is required.

The Veterinary Biologics Establishment License requires proof that the sponsor is a competent and responsible organization capable of creating safe, potent, and high-quality products. This license also requires that the staff members must be experienced

Table 13.1 Overview of the Research and Development Phases for a Veterinary Vaccine[a]

1. Documentation	2. Feasibility	3. Predevelopment	4. Development	5. Registration	6. Commercialization
a. Product profile	a. Establishment of experimental batch b. Formulation testing c. Antigen selection d. Proof of concept studies	a. Establishment of prototype batch b. Formulation testing c. Production process initiation d. Control tests e. Dose-effect (safety and efficacy) studies f. Pre-stability studies	a. Establishment of pilot batch b. Production process validation c. Control test validation d. Safety studies, efficacy studies e. Stability studies f. Field trials for: — Directions for use — Indications — Contraindications — Safety — Efficacy	a. Compilation and submission of registration materials (dossier) to regulatory authorities b. Response to comments/requests by regulatory authorities c. License approval	a. Sales and marketing b. Pharmacovigilance

[a]Table adapted from Heldens et al. (2008).

and qualified, especially research scientists and management staff. Facility blueprints with legends must be provided that explain what is kept in different rooms and laboratories to rule out any concerns for cross-contamination of different products. The establishment must also be ecologically responsible with waste and water, usually requiring a water quality statement from local authorities.

USDA regulatory program responsibilities

(1) Review of all data developed by manufacturers in support of each product and product claim.

(2) Inspection of manufacturing processes and practices, including equipment, facilities materials, personnel, production, quality control, and records.

(3) Confirmatory testing of manufacturers' biological seeds, cells, and product.

(4) Post-licensing monitoring system of inspection and random testing of product.

(5) Postmarketing epidemiological surveillance of product performance under normal conditions of use (i.e., pharmacovigilance).

The current USDA regulatory program consists of the following: (1) review of all data developed by manufacturers in support of each product and product claim, (2) inspection of manufacturing processes and practices, including equipment, facilities, materials, personnel, production, quality control, and records, (3) confirmatory testing of manufacturers' biological seeds, cells, and product, (4) post-licensing monitoring system of inspection and random testing of product, and (5) postmarketing epidemiological surveillance of product performance under normal conditions of use (i.e., pharmacovigilance).

For the approval of a Veterinary Biological Product License, the pre-licensing data evaluation and review procedures of the USDA are designed to assess the purity, safety, potency, and efficacy of each product and determine if the product supports all label claims. This includes the complete characterization and identification of seed material and ingredients, laboratory and host animal safety and efficacy studies, demonstration of stability, and monitoring of field performance.

Definitions

Purity: The quality or state of being pure, including the freedom from contamination.
Safety: Does not cause harm.
Potency: Term used in reference to the dosage of a drug or vaccine necessary in order to produce a desired result.
Efficacy: Capacity or power to produce a desired effect.
Good manufacturing practice (GMP): A guidance that outlines the aspects of production and testing that can impact the quality of a product.

All product components must meet standards of purity and quality. Master seed, master cell stock, primary cells, ingredients of animal origin, and final products must be tested and shown to be free of extraneous microorganisms. There is no official GMP requirement for veterinary biologics in the USA; however, the USA is considered to have a GMP-like environment when it comes to manufacturing veterinary biologics. The implementation of a GMP standard for veterinary products in the USA remains controversial in that some pharmaceutical companies of veterinary biologics feel that this requirement is too expensive and would result in vaccines that are too costly for their customers.

For safety, all master seeds and master cell stocks must be fully identified and characterized. Master seeds for live products should be tested for shed, spread, and reversion to virulence through back passage studies in rodents and/or target animals. Other safety studies may be required, including the safe use of the product in pregnant animals, environmental safety, safety of adjuvants in the product in food-producing animals, and field safety studies.

For efficacy and potency, all products must be shown to be effective according to the claims indicated on the label. Each batch (or serial) of each product must demonstrate potency at least equal to that of the reference serial(s). Efficacy is generally demonstrated by statistically valid host animal vaccination-challenge studies and must be correlated to the product potency assay. Immunogenicity studies must be conducted with minimal levels of antigen at the highest passage level from the master seed that is permitted for production. Challenge methods or criteria for evaluating protection will vary with the immunizing agent, but tests are conducted under controlled conditions using seronegative animals of the youngest age recommended on the label. Duration of immunity (DOI) data are required for some existing products (e.g., rabies) as well as for all newly licensed antigens. Field efficacy studies may be considered where laboratory animal challenge models are not well established; however, serology data can be used to establish efficacy when serology results are indicative of protection (i.e., correlate of protective immunity). Data are required for *each* species for which the product is recommended and for *each* route, dose, and regimen of administration. For products with two or more components (e.g., multivalent vaccine), data demonstrating no antigenic interference are required, and stability studies are required to set the expiration date on the label. Based on the outcomes of the efficacy studies, the USDA has formulated a hierarchy of efficacy claims for the label statement, which include (1) prevention of infection, (2) prevention of disease, (3) aid in disease prevention, (4) aid in disease control, and (5) other claims, such as the control of infectiousness through the reduction of pathogen shedding.

Definition

Correlate of protective immunity: A specific immune response to a vaccine that is closely related to protection against infection, disease, or other defined end point.

A product catalog of currently approved US veterinary biologics is available on the APHIS-USDA website. This listing also provides a listing of approved licensees, subsidiaries, divisions, and manufacturing establishments for veterinary biologics (www.aphis.usda .gov/animal_health/vet_biologics/vb_licensed_ products.shtml).

European Union (EU)

In the EU, the European Commission (EC) codified requirements for medicinal product registration in a series of directives, which were initiated in 1965. These directives are outlined in a document titled, "The Rules Governing Medicinal Products in the European Union." In 2001, the requirements for veterinary

medicinal products were consolidated in Directive 2001/82/EC, which are detailed in Volume 6 of "The Rules." Quality standards of general application as well as the requirements for specific products have also been published in the *European Pharmacopoeia*. In the EU, manufacturing of all medicinal products for sale must comply with the standards of GMP that, for veterinary products, were described in 1991 by Directive 91/412/EEC. Therefore, any application for marketing authorization (i.e., product license) must be accompanied by a certificate of GMP compliance issued by the responsible authority of a member state (country) of the EU. Compliance is validated by periodic inspections of the manufacturing facilities, conducted by the member state within which the facility is located, and the other member states must mutually recognize these inspections. The mutual recognition of GMP standards also exists between the EU and some non-EU countries (e.g., Australia and New Zealand).

Registration of a medicinal product for animals or humans within two or more member states of the EU can be achieved by several procedures. The centralized procedure, operated through the European Medicines Agency (EMA), leads to a community marketing authorization that is valid for all member states. All products based on genetic engineering must be registered through the centralized procedure, but the EMA will also consider products containing a new active agent, or which use novel technology, for registration via this route. The mutual recognition procedure relies on an initial registration (marketing authorization) by one member state, which is then submitted to as many member states as the applicant requires, for mutual recognition and the eventual registration by each selected member state. If a member state fails to mutually recognize the application, the EMA provides independent arbitration through the work of the Committee for Veterinary Medicinal Products (CVMP), which provides a final recommendation to the EC. For the recently introduced decentralized procedure, the data file (or most often referred to as the "dossier") is sent to one member state, which carries out a scientific assessment and compiles a draft assessment report. The dossier and draft assessment report are then sent to all concerned member states for a collective mutual agreement and market authorization, thus skipping the first step of the mutual recognition procedure. All conventional products and varieties of existing products are now registered via the decentralized procedure. There is also a national procedure, in which each member state has its own competent licensing authority in the form of an independent government agency or a department within the ministry of health and/or agriculture. Therefore, if a company wishes to license a veterinary product in just one member state (e.g., for a local disease or species), it can submit an application for marketing authorization to the recognized national authority.

There are specific requirements regulating the registration of veterinary immunological products in the EU, and the *European Pharmacopoeia* monograph "Vaccines for Veterinary Use" describes in detail the basic standards for quality that is applicable to all veterinary vaccines. It also describes the requirements for specific types of vaccines and vaccines for major target species. Similar to the pre-licensing requirements of the USA, the data provided for registration of a veterinary vaccine in the EU should address: (1) safety for the target species and the environment, (2) efficacy in compliance with the claims made for the product, (3) quality in terms of purity, manufacturing consistency, potency, safety, and stability, and (4) labeling. Overall, these data must provide evidence that supports the claims made about the vaccine in the product literature. The presentation of the dossier is required to follow the format described in Volume 6 of "The Rules," in which the documentation within the dossier is presented in four parts. Part I includes details of the manufacturing facility and evidence of GMP compliance, draft product literature including a "Summary of Product Characteristics," and "Expert Reports" on the manufacture, control, safety, and efficacy of the product. Part II addresses any issues concerning the manufacture and quality of the product. Part III addresses issues relating to safety. Part IV provides evidence that the vaccine meets the claims made for it when used as recommended.

Like the US requirements, master seed lots that have been fully characterized and stored under stable conditions must be used to initiate the production batches (termed *serials* in the USA), and all subsequent handling of the seed lots must be GMP compliant with a limitation on the number of consecutive *in vivo* passages between the master seeds and final product. Every commercial batch of vaccine must be shown to be safe in the target species and meet the potency standard established in the efficacy studies. The potency test that is applied to the vaccine must certify that any batch, when used as recommended, will be as efficacious as that demonstrated in the controlled challenge studies that are detailed in the registration dossier.

In compliance with the EU requirements, the assessment of safety should be performed in the target species at the highest potency at which the vaccine will be manufactured. The interpretation of this requirement is the subject of the EMA guideline "EU Requirements for Batches with Maximum and Minimum Titer or Batch Potency for Developmental Safety and Efficacy Studies (2002)." Similar to the USA, safety tests should also be conducted in the target species of the youngest age at which the vaccine is to be used, which also includes the assessment of the animal as follows: (1) during 21 days after administration of the recommended dose, (2) after a 10-fold overdose, and (3) after at least one repeated dosing. Reproductive performance or any possible interference with immunological functions should be considered when evaluating the possibility of adverse effects. Safety studies must also examine the potential for live attenuated vaccines to spread to non-vaccinated individuals of the target species. As an EU requirement for all live attenuated vaccines, feces, urine, milk, eggs, oral, nasal, and other secretions should be tested for the presence of the organism postvaccination and in the appropriate target species. Freedom from reversion to virulence should also be demonstrated in live attenuated vaccines by conducting at least six consecutive *in vivo* passages without selection pressure in the target host. The possibility of, and potential consequences arising from, recombination or genomic reassortment with wild-type strains in the environment should also be evaluated. The environmental safety of the vaccine and the possibility of the accumulation of chemical residues in the tissues of food-producing animals must be addressed in the dossier. Finally, laboratory-derived safety evidence should be supported by the results of field trials, similar to what has been described for the pre-licensing requirements of US vaccines. Although not required for registration in the EU, a substantial amount of commercial value can also be obtained in field trials that are designed to evaluate the economic benefit of vaccination.

Australia

In Australia, chemicals and biologics, including vaccines, for use in animals must be registered with the Australian Pesticides and Veterinary Medicine Authority (APVMA). Prior to 1993, each state and territory government in Australia had its own system of registration of agricultural and veterinary chemical products, but in 1993, the APVMA was established to centralize the registration process for the entire country. Similar to the regulations set forth by the USA and EU, the APVMA requires that all veterinary biologics are safe and effective before they are licensed for use in animals. Similar to the EU, GMP requirements for manufacturing veterinary biologics are in place in Australia (and New Zealand) and are considered equivalent to those in the EU and vice versa. To register a vaccine, the APVMA must assess a comprehensive data package that is provided with the application, which includes the studies previously described for pre-licensing of veterinary vaccines in the USA and EU. Once veterinary vaccines are registered and licensed in Australia, the APVMA does not have regulatory authority over their use; instead, each state and territory becomes responsible for this regulation.

With regard to the DOI studies that are required for licensing veterinary vaccines, most published research studies suggest the DOI for live attenuated vaccines are longer than 1 year. Since most DOI studies only support 12-month revaccination intervals, there is growing interest in Australia and other countries in increasing the revaccination intervals for these vaccines. In order for a longer revaccination interval to be specified on the vaccine label, an increasing number of registrants are presenting additional DOI studies to confirm that their vaccine candidates are effective for longer periods of time.

Animal testing during vaccine development

While animal testing is essential at various stages during vaccine development, minimizing the number of animals that are required at each stage has become highly favorable in the USA and other countries. In the EU, the guidelines set forth in the *European Pharmacopoeia* publication provide specific information about what animal tests are required for licensing in order to try to decrease unnecessary animal experimentation. Similarly, in an effort to prevent duplicate testing, the International Cooperation on Harmonization of Technical Requirements for Registration of Veterinary Medicinal Products (VICH) was formed in 1996 with the EU, Japan, and the USA to ensure standard testing procedures were accepted globally. With its efforts to harmonize some of these regulatory requirements, this forum has the potential to agree on alternative approaches to animal testing that would minimize the number of animals required for product licensing. In 2005, this approach was supported even further when the European Partnership to Promote Alternative Approaches to Animal Testing (EPPAA) was formed between the EC, European trade associations, and companies from seven industry sectors to pool knowledge and resources in order to accelerate the development, validation, and acceptance of alternative approaches that would eventually lead to further replacement, reduction, and refinement of animals for regulatory testing.

Impact of veterinary vaccines in public health

According to the World Health Organization (WHO), nearly 15 million (approximately 25%) of the 57 million annual deaths worldwide are the direct result of infectious diseases. Globalization, climate change, and the opening of previously closed ecosystems have changed the patterns of endemic and enzootic infectious diseases and contributed to the emergence of new agents that are pathogenic for humans and animals. There are other factors that can contribute to

---

Definitions

Emerging infectious diseases: A subcategory of infectious diseases, which can be defined as infections that have newly appeared in a population or have existed but are rapidly increasing in incidence or geographic range.

Zoonoses: Any infectious diseases that can be transmitted from nonhuman animals, both wild and domestic, to humans; the primary source of emerging infectious diseases. In some instances, these include infectious diseases that can also be transmitted by an invertebrate vector (e.g., mosquitoes and ticks).

the emergence of infectious diseases. With the high global demand for animal protein as a food source, the husbandry practice of housing a large number of food-producing animals in a confined area often leads to stress, increasing the likelihood of shedding of viral and bacterial pathogens, some of which may be zoonotic. This demand also runs the risk of introducing pathogens into a herd or flock if proper biosecurity precautions have been overlooked during large-scale animal rearing and production. Extended periods of flooding and drought also impact how well invertebrate vectors are able to transmit pathogens to areas with naïve human and animal hosts. Globalization and the ease of international travel have provided a new way to efficiently transport infected humans, animals, and vectors to uninfected areas, potentially resulting in outbreaks with devastating outcomes and high economic losses. Political unrest and natural disasters also impact human and animal health when government services and regulations are interrupted. With the encroachment of wildlife habitats, humans and domesticated animals run the risk of being exposed to novel pathogens; conversely, wildlife animal species may be vulnerable to new pathogens associated with humans and domesticated animals. Lastly, the pathogens themselves have the ability to evolve, developing new ways to evade the host's immune system, often resulting in increased virulence.

Of the 1415 pathogens known to affect humans, 61% are zoonotic, and of the zoonotic emerging infectious diseases, 72% are caused by pathogens with a wildlife animal origin (Figure 13.1). Nipah virus in the genus *Henipavirus* is one example of this. In 1999, this virus emerged from Pteropid fruit bats (also called "flying foxes") in Perak, Malaysia, causing high case fatalities in humans due to severe encephalitis. Not only was this outbreak devastating due to the loss of human lives, the economic repercussions of this disease were considerable. However, the impact of emerging infectious diseases can vary widely and depend on different factors, including virulence of the pathogen, mode of transmission, incubation period, host immunocompetence, and cross-protective immunity. The economic losses due to the Nipah virus outbreak were relatively minor ($350 million to $450 million) when compared to severe acute respiratory syndrome coronavirus (SARS-CoV). In 2003, SARS-CoV emerged from palm civets in Guangdong Province, China, causing a near pandemic of severe respiratory disease in humans with an estimated economic loss of $40 billion to $50 billion.

In the past, vaccines for animals have mainly been developed to protect animal health and increase animal welfare by preventing suffering as a result of an infectious disease, but as discussed above, the impact of some of these animal-based diseases can have profound effects on human populations as well as national and global economies. As a result, this factor has stimulated the implementation of vaccination programs against zoonotic diseases, and it has challenged scientists to develop effective veterinary vaccines that prevent the transmission of disease to humans.

For some of infectious diseases listed by the World Organization for Animal Health (OIE), slaughter policies are required to limit the spread of disease and to decrease the associated economic losses. For example, the foot-and-mouth disease (FMD) outbreak in the UK in 2001 lead to the depopulation of over 10 million head of cattle, sheep, pigs, and goats at an estimated cost to the UK economy of over £8 billion ($13 billion). However, these figures fail to reflect the mental anguish experienced by the producers, their families, and communities during the mass slaughter of otherwise healthy animals to control the outbreak. For this reason, public opinion in the UK and elsewhere will likely disapprove of this policy for future outbreaks, potentially leading to its eventual elimination as a control measure. This factor also adds to the growing need for veterinary vaccines that are not only protec-

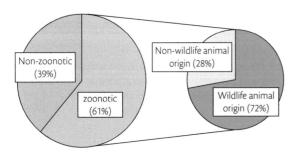

Figure 13.1 Charts showing the relative contribution of zoonotic pathogens to human emerging infectious diseases. Emerging infectious diseases are dominated by zoonoses, where the majority of these zoonotic diseases originate from wildlife. Adapted from Jones et al. (2008).

tive, but, ideally, efficiently marked to distinguish them from natural disease exposure, thereby making it easier to more effectively control outbreaks in the future.

Since the 1940s, the number of emerging infectious disease events caused by pathogens originating from wildlife animal species has increased significantly with time, constituting 52% of these events from 1990 to 2000. Geographic maps of the global distribution of emerging infectious diseases have been generated, indicating the relative risks of the emergence of zoonotic pathogens from wildlife species, zoonotic pathogens from non-wildlife species, drug-resistant pathogens, and vector-borne pathogens. Maps of these "hotspots" of emerging infectious disease events have been recently incorporated into a website (http://www.healthmap.org/predict/), which delivers real-time information from a number of different sources to provide users a comprehensive view of the current global state of emerging infectious diseases and their effects on human and animal health.

Depending on the animal target, some veterinary vaccines are more effective than others in preventing human disease. This is another factor that should be considered when developing veterinary vaccines against zoonotic pathogens. For example, although a vaccine was developed to prevent Nipah virus (*Henipavirus*) infection in pigs, the effect of this vaccine was minimal in countries like Bangladesh, where humans are directly infected by the reservoir host (Pteropid fruit bats). In contrast, a veterinary vaccine that has effectively prevented human disease in the USA is the one for the domestic dog–coyote variant of the rabies virus. Rabies virus (family *Rhabdoviridae*, genus *Lyssavirus*) is most commonly transmitted by a bite from an infected animal, where 97% of human rabies cases that occur worldwide are from dog bites. Rabies virus infections cause approximately 55,000 human deaths per year worldwide and are fatal if postexposure prophylaxis (PEP) is not administered prior to the onset of symptoms. In the USA, animal control and vaccination programs have virtually eliminated the domestic dog–coyote variant. A key factor in the elimination of the domestic dog–coyote variant was the oral rabies vaccine (ORV) program, which involved the mass vaccination of free-ranging wildlife animals. Initiated in Texas in 1995, the program was also determined to be economically beneficial. Unfortunately,

other wildlife rabies reservoirs (and their variants) continue to be plentiful in the USA, including raccoons, bats, skunks, and foxes, and account for more than 80% of reported rabid animals in the USA. Given the success of the ORV program for the domestic dog–coyote variant, more ORV programs are currently underway in the USA that target other rabies variants. In Europe, a similar program has been overwhelmingly successful in the large-scale elimination of rabies in foxes. Unfortunately, human rabies in the USA has now become primarily associated with the exposure to rabid bats. This presents a new challenge since rabies control in bats by conventional methods is not currently feasible. Instead, prevention must rely on (1) health education to avoid exposure, (2) proper exclusion of bats from living quarters, (3) careful assessment in the event of exposure, and (4) the judicial administration of PEP.

Response of national authorities to animal disease threats

Since the emergence or introduction of certain animal diseases into a country could devastate agriculture, threaten the food supply, harm the economy, and potentially threaten public health if zoonotic, a rapid response to the most serious animal disease threats is crucial. In the USA, the National Veterinary Stockpile (NVS), as part of the USDA-APHIS Veterinary Services division, exists to provide the resources (including supplies, equipment, field tests, vaccines, and response support services) to respond to the most serious animal disease threats. Operational since 2006, the NVS can be deployed within 24 hours of notice for at least 17 major diseases, including African horse sickness, African swine fever, bovine spongiform encephalopathy (BSE), classical swine fever, *Coxiella burnetii* (Q fever), Venezuelan and eastern equine encephalitis, *Ehrlichia ruminentium* (heartwater disease), exotic Newcastle disease, FMD, highly pathogenic avian influenza (HPAI), Japanese encephalitis, Nipah and Hendra virus infection, Rift Valley fever, and rinderpest.

Since conventional evaluations of veterinary biologics may not be possible during the emergence of a new animal disease agent, agrobioterrorism, or unintentional introduction of a significant exotic animal disease agent, most national regulatory authorities also have various mechanisms for expedited product approval or may provide an exemption of products for some or all regulatory requirements for conventional product approval.

Future challenges

With the ever-present threat of new, emerging, and potentially zoonotic diseases in companion and food-producing animals, research and development of safe and effective vaccines for these diseases require a significant amount of time and cost before they become available for use. The issue of vaccine availability is especially challenging for less common animal species or for those with less common conditions (often referred to as minor use/minor species [MUMS]). In these cases, public funding is usually required to develop a vaccine or test existing vaccines for efficacy and safety in minor species. Overall, scientists, pharmaceutical companies, and regulatory authorities must work together to efficiently develop, license, and market veterinary vaccines against threatening pathogens, including those that directly affect human health. New advances in vaccine design and formulations should provide innovative ways for developing safer vaccines while achieving selective induction of effective immune responses.

Summary

- Veterinary vaccines are the most effective means in controlling animal infectious diseases, and they must be proven to be pure, safe, potent, effective, and support all label claims before they can be considered for licensing for animal use.

- Veterinary vaccines have a positive indirect effect on human health by preventing the nutritional and economic losses that are associated with infectious diseases of food-producing animals.
- Emerging infectious diseases that are caused by zoonotic pathogens represent an ever-increasing and very significant threat to global health; the economic impact of these diseases can be devastating for the affected countries.
- The control of zoonotic diseases by veterinary vaccines effectively limits the spread of disease to humans for which no vaccines or therapeutics are readily available.

Further reading

Elsken LA, Carr MY, Frana TS, Brake DA, Garland T, Smith K, and Foley PL (2007). Regulations for vaccines against emerging infections and agrobioterrorism in the United States of America. Revue Scientifique et Technique (International Office of Epizootics) 26, 429–441.

Heldens JGM, Patel JR, Chanter N, ten Thij GJ, Gravendijck M, Schjns VEJC, Langen A, and Schetters ThPM (2008). Veterinary vaccine development from an industrial perspective. Veterinary Journal (London, England: 1997) 178, 7–20.

Jones KE, Patel NG, Levy MA, Storeygard A, Balk D, Gittleman JL, and Daszak P (2008). Global trends in emerging infectious diseases. Nature 451, 990–993.

O'Brien D and Zanker S (2007). Animal vaccination and the veterinary pharmaceutical industry. Revue Scientifique et Technique (International Office of Epizootics) 26, 471–477.

Paul-Pierre P (2009). Emerging diseases, zoonoses, and vaccines to control them. Vaccine 27, 6435–6438.

Todd JI (2007). Good manufacturing practice for immunological veterinary medicinal products. Revue Scientifique et Technique (International Office of Epizootics) 26, 135–145.

14 Vaccine manufacturing

Dirk E. Teuwen[1] and Alan D.T. Barrett[2]

[1]UCB Pharma S.A., Brussels, Belgium

[2]Sealy Center for Vaccine Development, University of Texas Medical Branch, Galveston, TX, USA

Abbreviations

AA	Adventitious agents	HBsAg	Hepatitis B surface antigen
ACIP	Advisory Committee on Immunization Practices	HBV	Hepatitis B virus
		Hib	*Haemophilus influenzae* type b
BWG	Biotechnology Working Group	HPV	Human papillomavirus
CBER	Center for Biologics Evaluation and Research	ICH	International Conference of Harmonisation
CBS	Cell bank system	IPV	Inactivated polio vaccine
CCL	Cold chain and logistics	MDCK	Madin–Darby canine kidney
CDC	US Centers for Disease Control and Prevention	MMR	Measles, mumps, and rubella
		MMRV	Measles, mumps, rubella, and varicella
CEF	chicken embryo fibroblasts	MSB	Master cell bank
CFDA	China State Food and Drug Administration	MSL	Master cell lot
CFR	Code of Federal Regulation	MSV	Monovalent seed virus
CHMP	Committee for medicinal products for human use	MSVC	Monovalent split virus concentrate
		MV	Measles virus
CL	Cell line	NYVAC	New York City Board of Health
CLL	Continuous cell line	OPV	Oral polio vaccine
COG	Cost of goods	PMDA	Japanese Pharmaceutical and Medical Devices Agency
DHSS	US Department Health and Human Services		
		PriCC	Primary cell cultures
DTaP	Diphtheria, tetanus, acellular pertussis vaccine	ProCC	Production cell culture
		QC	Quality control
DTwP	diphtheria, tetanus, whole-cell pertussis	VLP	Virus-like particle
EC	European Commission	VWG	Vaccine Working Group
eIPV	Enhanced-potency inactivated vaccine	WHO	World Health Organization
GCCP	Good cell culture practice	WSB	Working cell bank
GMP	Good manufacturing practice	WSL	working seed lot

Vaccinology: An Essential Guide, First Edition. Edited by Gregg N. Milligan and Alan D.T. Barrett.

© 2015 John Wiley & Sons, Ltd. Published 2015 by John Wiley & Sons, Ltd.

Introduction

The development and use of vaccines to prevent infectious diseases has been one of the greatest successes of personal and public health since their introduction in early 19th century. Vaccination is considered to be one of the most cost-effective health interventions. The first vaccines were based on partially purified live attenuated (weakened) viruses (e.g., smallpox, rabies) or inactivated bacteria (e.g., whole-cell pertussis). The first vaccine used whole live virus or human-to-human or animal-to-human transfer, such as the early smallpox vaccine by Edward Jenner who used cowpox (*vaccinia*) pus inoculation in 1796.[1] Bacterial vaccines were created by Louis Pasteur in the 1880s, including vaccines for chicken cholera and anthrax using weakened bacterial cultures and, most importantly, the development of a live attenuated rabies viral vaccine grown in brain culture.

Even though vaccines have been developed for a limited number of human pathogens, the actual number of vaccine products is considerably higher due to the manufacture and administration of multiple combinations of vaccines. Indeed, there are demands for specific combination vaccines, formulations, and presentations for different age target groups and selected geographical regions. Many vaccine candidates have been developed over time but few make it to become licensed products. One of the major challenges in vaccine development is the "scale-up," i.e., how to manufacture a vaccine candidate at large scale to make it economically feasible? Unfortunately, several vaccine candidates cannot be produced at large scale for various reasons (expression, technical, etc.). Once a candidate vaccine is in the nonclinical development phase, joint teams of laboratory, scaling-up, and industrial manufacturing staff are created to investigate on how to plan the manufacture of pilot lots at satisfactory volume in a consistent manner before additional major investments are made.

The history of vaccine development is associated with the discovery and isolation of those human pathogens. Initially the manufacture of vaccine was mastered through the conventional manufacturing technology of sequential attenuation or inactivation by chemical treatment (e.g., formaldehyde for tetanus toxoid extracted from fermentations of *Clostridium tetani*) and adsorbed onto an adjuvant. Subsequently, the development of purified polysaccharide, e.g., *Haemophilus influenzae* type b (Hib) extracted from fermenter culture of *H. influenzae* and conjugated to carrier proteins, created a broader platform, and more recently, modern technologies, e.g., recombinant virus-like particles for hepatitis B or human papilloma virus vaccines have been applied to manufacturing. A history of those milestones is summarized in Table 14.1; the table also includes actions by regulatory authorities regarding safety (in italics).

Manufacturing principles

Manufacturing steps

The manufacturing of vaccines may be summarized in six major steps.

A first step is the maintenance of viral and bacterial master seed lot (MSL), working seed lot (WSL), and master cell bank (MSB) system for the anticipated lifetime of the vaccines. This is challenging for some older vaccines as no MSL or WSL materials remain. Preparing for new MSL and WSL implies an elaborated testing for characterization and adventitious agents, plus clinical evaluation of seeds to ensure the vaccines are consistent with previously produced vaccine.

A second step is the generation of an adequate antigen. This step involves the amplification of the pathogen itself (for subsequent inactivation or isolation of the subunit) or the generation of a recombinant protein derived from the pathogen. Viruses are grown in different cell cultures, either in primary cells, e.g., leucosis-free chicken embryos, embryonated chicken eggs, or in continuous cell lines, e.g., MRC-5 or WI-38 human diploid lung fibroblasts. Note, few continuous cell lines are approved for the manufacture of human vaccines due to the need to extensively characterize the cells for adventious agents and the potential to be oncogenic. Bacterial pathogens are

[1] In fact, the word "vaccination" originated from this first vaccine since it was derived from a virus "pertaining to cows, from cows" from Latin *vaccinus* "from cows," from *vacca* "cow" (*bos* being originally "*ox*")

Table 14.1 Historic Dates and Events Related to Vaccines, Licensing, and Events

1796	Smallpox vaccination by vaccine using animal-to-human cowpox inoculation (Edward Jenner)
1879	Chicken cholera by live attenuated bacterial vaccine (Louis Pasteur)
1884	Rabies by live attenuated viral vaccine grown in brain tissue (Louis Pasteur)
1896	Diphtheria and tetanus toxoid vaccine (Emil von Behring and Shibasaburo Kitasato)
1897	Bubonic plague vaccine prepared from horse serum (AlexandreYersin)
1902	*US Biologics Control Act includes regulation of vaccine and antitoxin manufacturers and outlines both licensing and inspections of manufacturing sites. The standards imposed by the 1902 Act resulted in the bankruptcy of nearly 30% of companies manufacturing antitoxins and vaccines.*
1915	Whooping cough pertussis vaccine by whole-cell formaldehyde inactivated bacteria
1921	Tuberculosis through serial attenuation of the *Mycobacterium bovis* (Albert Calmette and Camille Guérin)
1923	Influenza and mumps
1931	Smallpox freeze-dried vaccine approved in USA
1935	Yellow fever vaccine in embryonated chick eggs (Max Theiler and Hugh Smith)
1937	*Division of Biologics Control was formed within the US National Institute of Health*
1945	Influenza A/B inactivated vaccine
1949	Combination diphtheria–tetanus–whole-cell pertussis [(DTwP) vaccine]
1949	*In-vitro cultivation of polio virus in non-neural human cells (John F. Enders)*
1952	Typhoid heat-phenol inactivated vaccine
1954	Polio virus replication *in vitro* with non-neural human cells (John F Enders and Thomas Peebles)
1955	Polio inactivated viral vaccine (IPV) produced *in vitro* on primary monkey kidney cells (Jonas Salk)
1961	Polio live attenuated viral vaccine type 1 and type 2 (OPV) produced *in vitro* on primary monkey kidney cells (Albert Sabin)
1962	Polio live attenuated viral vaccine type 3 (OPV) produced *in vitro* on primary monkey kidney cells (Albert Sabin)
1963	Edmonston live attenuated measles strain vaccine on chick embryo cell cultures developed byJohn F. Enders in 1961
1965	Schwartz (further) live attenuated measles strain vaccine, derived from Edmonston measles strain
1967	Jeryl Lynn, live attenuated mumps strain vaccine (Maurice Hilleman)
1968	Moraten (further) live attenuated measles strain vaccine, derived from Edmonston measles strain
1969	Rubella, live attenuated vaccines, i.e., HPV-77 grown in dog kidney cells, HPV-77 grown in duck embryo culture, and Cendehill grown in rabbit kidney cells
1974	Monovalent group C meningococcal polysaccharide vaccine
1977	Pneumococcal 14-valent vaccine
1979	Rubella RA27/3 strain grown in human diploid fibroblast with the discontinuation of all other live attenuated rubella virus strains (Stanley Plotkin)
1981	Quadrivalent groups A, C, Y, and W_{135} meningococcal vaccine

(Continued)

Table 14.1 (*Continued*)

1981	Hepatitis B vaccine, plasma-derived
1985	*Haemophilis influenzae* type b (Hib) polysaccharide vaccine
1986	*National Childhood Vaccine Injury Act enacted by US Congress with the establishment of the Vaccine Adverse Event Reporting System (VAERS), coadministered by the US FDA and CDC to record all suspected adverse events, in all age groups.*
1986	Hepatitis B vaccine, recombinant surface antigen subunit using recombinant DNA technology
1987	*Haemophilus influenzae* type b (Hib) protein-conjugated vaccine
1988	*US National Vaccine Injury Compensation Program*
1989	Typhoid live, oral vaccine
1990	Polio, enhanced-potency inactivated vaccine (eIPV)
1991	Diphtheria tetanus acellular pertussis vaccine (DTaP)
1992	Japanese encephalitis inactivated virus vaccine
1993	Combined *H influenzae* type b whole-cell pertussis diphtheria tetanus vaccine
1994	Typhoid Vi polysaccharide inactivated injectable polysaccharide vaccine
1994	Hepatitis A inactivated vaccine
1995	Varicella, live attenuated OKA strain vaccine (Michiaki Takahashi), although already licensed in Japan in 1986
1996	Combined *H influenzae* type b hepatitis B vaccine
1996	Combined *H influenzae* type b, diphtheria, tetanus, and acellular pertussis vaccine
1998	Rotavirus live oral tetravalent vaccine, subsequently withdrawn on October 16, 1999
1998	Lyme recombinant OspA vaccine, discontinued on February 25, 2002
2000	Pneumococcal 7-valent conjugate vaccine
2001	*US Institute of Medicine (IoM) called for creation of a national vaccine authority "to advance the development, production, and procurement of new and improved vaccines of limited commercial potential but of global public health need."*
2001	Combined hepatitis A – hepatitis B vaccine
2001	*The Bill and Melinda Gates Foundation supports the development and production of meningitis vaccines (Menococcal serotype A vaccine) tailored for children and adults living in Africa.*
2002	Combined diphtheria, tetanus, acellular pertussis, inactivated polio, and hepatitis B vaccine
2003	Influenza nasal spray live attenuated A and B strain
2003	*US Bio Shield Act for development of vaccines, drugs and other biomedical countermeasures for biological, nuclear, chemical, and radiological weapons*
2005	Combined meningococcal groups A, C, Y, and W$_{135}$ polysaccharide diphtheria toxoid conjugate vaccine
2005	Development of cell-culture based influenza vaccine supported by Department Health and Human Services (DHHS)
2005	Combined measles, mumps, rubella, and varicella vaccine

Table 14.1 (*Continued*)

2006	Rotavirus live attenuated oral pentavalent vaccine
2006	Herpes-zoster vaccine
2006	Human papilloma (types 6, 11, 16, and 18) vaccine
2007	Avian influenza H5N1 vaccine
2007	Smallpox vaccine based on purified "live" New York City Board of Health (NYVAC) vaccinia strain, freeze-dried
2008	Rotavirus live attenuated oral
2008	Combined diphtheria, tetanus, acellular pertussis, inactivated polio vaccine
2009	*DHHS awards $1 billion for development of novel vaccines for H1N1 influenza*
2009	Production of monovalent measles, monovalent mumps, and monovalent rubella vaccines will not resume.
2010	*Advisory Committee on Immunization Practices (ACIP) recommends universal influenza vaccination for those 6 months of age and older*
2010	Combined Meningococcal groups A,C,W, and Y conjugate vaccine approved in Europe
2013	Multi-component meningococcal group B vaccine licensed in Europe. First vaccine developed using "reverse vaccinology."
2013	First recombinant protein, highly purified, egg-free seasonal influenza vaccine

grown in bioreactors using different media, e.g., Mueller and Miller medium or Eagle MEM modified medium. Recombinant proteins can be manufactured in bacteria, vertebrate cell culture, insect cell culture, or *Sacchoromyces cerevisiae* yeast. The different technologies used in the vaccine manufacturing and some examples can be found in Table 14.2.

The third step is the harvesting of the vaccine antigen from the substrate and segregating the antigen from the culture material. It may involve an isolation of free virus from cells, secreted proteins from cells, or cells containing the antigen from the culture.

The purification of the antigen is a fourth step and, depending of the vaccine type, may involve chromatography, ultrafiltration, removal of any residual medium for inactivated vaccines, or a combination of procedures.

The fifth step relates to the formulation, stabilization, and adjuvanting of the vaccine, designed to optimize the potency of the antigen through appropriate adjuvants, the stability to provide an optimum shelf life or storage conditions, or preservatives to allow

Steps in manufacturing a vaccine

1. Maintenance of viral and bacterial master seed lot (MSL), working seed lot (WSL), and master cell bank (MSB) system.
2. Generation of an adequate vaccine antigen.
   a. Amplification of the pathogen itself (for subsequent inactivation or isolation of the subunit).
   b. Generation of a recombinant protein derived from the pathogen.
3. Harvesting of the vaccine antigen from the substrate and segregating the antigen from the culture material.
4. Purification of the vaccine antigen.
5. Formulation, stabilization, and adjuvanting of the vaccine.
6. Design of the appropriate delivery device, and the capacity and logistics, including cold-chain surveillance, to supply the vaccine to the site of use.

Table 14.2 Manufacturing Process and Examples of Vaccines

Manufacturing Process	Vaccines Examples
Live attenuated virus	Smallpox, polio, measles, mumps, rubella, varicella, rotavirus, herpes zoster, influenza, yellow fever
Inactivated purified virus	Polio, Japanese encephalitis, hepatitis A, influenza, rabies
Live attenuated bacterium	Tuberculosis, typhoid
Whole-cell inactivated bacterium	Whole-cell pertussis
Purified protein	Acellular pertussis
Purified protein toxoid	Tetanus, anthrax, diphtheria
Purified virus-like particles (VLP)	Hepatitis B, human papilloma[1]
Purified polysaccharide	Pneumococcal, typhoid
Polysaccharide conjugated to carrier proteins	Pneumococcal, *H. influenzae* type b, *N meningitidis*
Plasmid DNA	GTU®-encoded protein HIV vaccine candidate
Adenovirus DNA delivery	HIV vaccine candidate

[1]VLP reassembled from type 16 and 18 type specific L1 proteins expressed and purified from insect cells infected with a recombinant baculovirus or HPV 6, 11, 16 and 18 type specific L1 proteins expressed and purified from yeast containing L1 expression plasmids.

for multidose vials to be used in field conditions in the developing world. The formulation step for combined vaccines demands further skills in mixing, mastering potential interference in the final container, and when the immune response will be elicited after administration.

The sixth and last step involves the design of the appropriate delivery device, and the capacity and logistics, including cold chain and logistics surveillance, to supply and distribute those vaccines across the world.

Cold chain and logistics

Cold chain and logistics (CCL) is a temperature-controlled distribution chain, essential for temperature-sensitive vaccines, such as live attenuated vaccines. The management of the cold-chain demands strict temperature-regulated storage (between narrow temperature ranges) and logistics.

CCL surveillance includes a highly performing information technology system to capture and report manufacturing, inventory, transportation, supply, and delivery data, as well as highly trained staff to monitoring variations in temperature that might affect the potency of different vaccines.

Manufacturing definitions

A number of important definitions in the manufacturing process of viral and bacterial vaccines can be found in Table 14.3.

Examples of cell substrates

The following are examples of routinely used as well as novel cell substrates (Hess et al., 2012).

Primary cell culture

Primary cells are established directly from tissues of animals. Chicken embryo fibroblasts (CEFs) as well as kidney, lung, or ovary cells from dogs, monkeys, rabbits, and hamsters have been used in the manufacturing of vaccines.

Diploid cell line

Diploid cells from human (e.g., WI-38 or MRC-5) or monkey origin (e.g., FRh1-2) have a finite capacity (i.e., a limited number of passages) for serial propagation that ends in senescence. The cells have the cytological characteristic of a low frequency of chromosomal abnormalities.

Continuous cell line

Continuous cell lines (CCLs) have the advantages of being immortalized and easily obtained through serial subcultivations leading to spontaneous transformation of primary cells, e.g., Madin–Darby canine kidney (MDCK) cells and African green monkey continuous cell line (Vero). Targeted manipulation of primary cells by either activation of proto-oncogenes or transforma-

Table 14.3 Some Definitions in the Manufacturing Process

Adventitious agents (AA)	Contaminating microorganisms of the virus or cell substrate or materials used in their cultures, which may include bacteria, fungi, mycoplasmas, and endogenous and exogenous viruses that have been unintentionally introduced.
Cell bank system (CBS)	A system whereby successive final lots (batches) of a product are manufactured by culture in cells derived from the same master cell bank are used to prepare a working cell bank. The cell bank system is validated for the highest passage level achieved during routine production.
Cell lines (CL)	Cultures of cells that have a high capacity for multiplication *in vitro*.
Master cell bank (MCB)	A culture of cells distributed into containers in a single operation, processed together, and stored in such a manner as to ensure uniformity and stability and to prevent contamination. A master cell bank lot in liquid is usually stored at −70°C.
Master seed lot (MSL)	A culture of a microorganism distributed from a single bulk into containers and processed together in a single operation in such manner as to ensure uniformity and stability and to prevent contamination. A master seed lot in liquid is usually stored at −70°C.
Primary cell cultures (PriCC)	Cultures of cells obtained by trypsination of a suitable tissue or organ. The cells are essentially identical to those of the tissue or origin and are no more than five *in vitro* passages from the initial preparation.
Production cell culture (ProCC)	A culture of cells intended for use in production; it may be derived from one or more containers of the working cell bank or it may be a primary cell culture.
Working cell bank (WCB)	A culture of cells derived from the master cell bank and intended for use in the preparation of production cell cultures.
Working seed lot (WSL)	A culture of a microorganism derived from a master seed lot and intended for use in production. WSLs are distributed into containers and stored usually at −70°C

Source: European Pharmacopoeia online 8.1. 5.2.1. Terminology used in monographs on biological products. 01/2008:50201, corrected 6.0. Consulted on May 5, 2014.

tion through oncogenic genes or oncogenic viruses also results in the transformed phenotype and immortalization of cells.

Novel cell substrates

Novel cell substrates are derived predominantly from human (e.g., HEK 293 and PER.C6) and avian (e.g., EB66 and CR) sources.

HEK 293

Human embryonic kidney cell 293 cell line was generated in the late 1970s by transformation of embryonic kidney cells with sheared DNA of human adenovirus type 5 (Ad5). The adenovirus-derived genes contain early transforming genes and immortalize the cell, hence resulting in continuous cell growth.

PER.C6

The PER.C6 cell line is a human retina-derived cell line that also possesses the E1A and the E1B genes of Ad5. The PER.C6 cell line is able to complement the growth of replication incompetent adenoviruses (which lack the Ad5 E1 region).

EB66

The EB66 cell line is a duck embryonic stem cell-derived substrate engineered for the expression of monoclonal antibodies.

CR

The *Cairina retina* cell line is derived from Muscovy duck retinal tissue subsequently transfected with Ad5 E1 genes and Ad5 pIX gene, resulting in AGE1.CR.pIX.

HEK 293 and PER.C6 could be considered a cell substrate for the manufacture of live attenuated viral vaccines because they produce high virus yields, which is important from a manufacturing perspective.

Vaccine manufacturing: overview

In considering vaccine manufacturing it is important to evaluate the different industrial and technical technologies. A selected production method of a vaccine can significantly influence the manufacturing capacity and cost of goods (COGs) and hence the availability at the local or global level. Oral polio vaccine (OPV) belongs to the category of traditional low-cost live attenuated vaccines, as the three Sabin vaccine strains in the vaccine (polio serotypes 1, 2, and 3) grow very well in culture to high titers, even though in-process and final preparation demands complex and lengthy quality control (QC) procedures. Multivalent glycoconjugate pneumococcal or meningococcal vaccines and multivalent recombinant human papilloma virus-like particles (VLPs) vaccines are more complex as the separate components need to be produced independently with component specific yields, and require more complex QC on the separate and final vaccines. Consequently, the OPV (and similar vaccines) can be produced in significant quantities with low COGs and hence can be supplied and distributed worldwide, whereas more complex vaccines can be produced only in more limited quantities, resulting in significantly lower global capacities and higher COGs.

At each of the different steps of the manufacturing process, various assays, high-performing QC, and compliance are required. Determination of the physicochemical properties includes pH, osmolality, characterization, identification and functionality of the components, excipients and adjuvants, search for impurities that are process related or component related, microbiological testing for sterility, concentration and potency testing, and animal-based testing for toxicity. To that effect, different assays are available such as chromatography, electrophoresis, mass spectrometry, nuclear magnetic imaging, sterility tests, bacterial endotoxin assay, pyrogen (a substance capable of inducing fever such as bacterial lipopolysaccharide) assay, amino acid analysis, capillary electrophoresis, isoelectric focusing, polyacrylamide gel electrophoresis, dot-blot, Western blot, and enzyme-linked immunosorbent assay (ELISA), among many others.

Different national regulatory authorities may demand country-specific release criteria in addition to the standard armamentarium of testing assays and tests.

Example: quality control (QC) testing for diphtheria toxoid vaccine

Diphtheria toxoid vaccine bulk requires tests for all properties mentioned in the text, including animal testing over at least 6 weeks to illustrate absence of residual toxicity.

Diphtheria toxoid in a combination vaccine, such as diphtheria, tetanus, and acellular pertussis (DTaP) or diphtheria, tetanus, acellular pertussis, inactivated polio and hepatitis B (DTaP-IPV-HBV) will require additional QC tests after blending of the different antigens. The manufacturer is required to demonstrate sterility, stable physicochemical properties, and that all individual components are identifiable and at the recommended concentration and potency. When considering the pentavalent DTaP-IPV-HBV vaccine, it requires a significant amount of time to complete the appropriate testing, including a residual toxicity testing in animals, adding easily another 6 weeks to the release time.

Source: Smith et al., 2011

After the completion of the manufacturing, single syringes and/or multidose vials containing either freeze-dried or stabilized liquid in appropriate packages and with proper labeling need to be stored in adequate cold-chain conditions before shipment, according to the World Health Organization's (WHO) published guidelines on international packaging and shipping of vaccines.

After shipment, the local warehouse will need to wait until the regulatory authorities have completed their sampling and testing before finally releasing the vaccine to the marketplace.

Examples of vaccine production

Each manufacturer has developed processes that are somewhat different; however, all those processes result in vaccines standardized to ensure an adequate and comparable immunogenicity. The following examples provide an overview of the complexity of the manufacturing processes for traditional and new vaccines.

Inactivated vaccine: influenza vaccine

The first influenza vaccine was manufactured in 1937 as an inactivated whole virus vaccine, whereas the first commercial vaccines were approved in the USA in 1945. Progress at the manufacturing level was led by an ability to grow large quantities of the influenza virus in eggs, and by the development of chemical inactivation, which made it feasible to consider preparing an adequate number of doses of vaccines.

The influenza vaccine contains two strains of influenza A viruses (currently H1N1 and H3N2) and a single influenza B virus, as determined early every year by the WHO, US Centers for Disease Control (CDC), and US Food and Drug Administration Center for Biologics Evaluation and Research (CBER). The two influenza A viruses are characterized by the hemagglutinin (H or HA) and neuraminidase (N or NA) glycoproteins.

Each of the three influenza virus strains in the vaccine is replicated individually in substrates of animal origin. The substrate most commonly used by producers of influenza vaccine is the 11-day-old embryonated chicken egg. The material of each selected influenza strain is received from either WHO, CDC, or CBER and is passaged in those eggs. The inoculated eggs are placed in huge incubators for a specific time and at a specific temperature, and the virus replicates in the allontoic fluid. The fluids are harvested and tested for infectivity, concentration, specificity, and sterility. These fluids constitute the monovalent seed virus (MSV) and are controlled by the national regulatory authority where the vaccine is manufactured.

Thereafter, the MSV is introduced into eggs by automated inoculators kept at specific temperatures until harvesting starts. Purification is accomplished by high-speed centrifugation on a sucrose gradient or by chromatography, yielding a monovalent split virus concentrate (MSVC). The splitting of the influenza virus by detergents is performed before the final filtration. The influenza virus is inactivated using formaldehyde or β-propiolactone either prior to or during the primary purification step, depending on the manufacturer.

Finally, the MSVC of the three strains are blended at the appropriate concentrations as to generate the final bulk of the trivalent types A and type B influenza split virus vaccine.

Note that multiple types of influenza vaccine are manufactured: not only inactivated whole virus, but also split virus, live attenuated, subunit surface antigens derived from virus, and recombinant baculovirus expressed protein.

Live attenuated: measles virus vaccine

In 1954, the measles virus (MV) was isolated by John Enders and Thomas Peebles and characterized as a member of the genus *Morbillivirus* in the family *Paramyxoviridae*. Vaccine development started very quickly with the Edmonston strain, named after the person from whom the virus was isolated.

The Enders-Edmonston B strain of measles virus was passaged at 95–96°F (35–36 °C) 24 times in primary kidney cells, 28 times in primary human amnion cells, and followed by 6 passages in chicken embryos to be finally passaged in chicken embryo cells. The initial vaccine was associated with a high rate of fever and rash.

Subsequently, the Edmonston strain of measles virus was further attenuated to generate additional strains, such as the currently available Schwarz and Moraten strains by passage in chick embryo fibroblasts (CEFs), and the AIK-C strain by passage in human kidney, sheep kidney, and CEFs. Note there are also other non-Edmonston–derived measles strains used as vaccine, such as the Leningrad-16, Shanghai-191, CAM-70, and TD-97 strains.

The manufacturing process starts with specific pathogen-free (SPF) embryonated chicken eggs incubated for several days. The embryos are removed from the eggs, dissociated into single cell suspension with trypsin, clarified, and centrifuged as cell substrate prior to virus infection. This preparatory work is performed in strict aseptic conditions, as required.

The CEFs are suspended in roller bottles or stainless steel tanks, using fetal calf sera and M199 Hanks media for optimization of the cell growth. An appropriate volume of thawed measles stock is added to the seeding medium, stirred and incubated for culture of the virus. The cell sheets are rinsed and refed with medium several times, and the virus is harvested (measles harvested virus fluids [HVFs]).

The manufacturing process follows the specification and acceptance criteria for the critical process parameters and critical quality attributes. Those specifications and acceptance criteria are based on historical process data and new manufacturing specifications of the monovalent measles vaccine, subject to the approval of the national regulatory authority.

After completion of all quality control tests, the measles vaccine is formulated either alone or with mumps and rubella (MMR vaccine) or mumps, rubella, and varicella (MMRV vaccine). The vaccine is lyophilized to provide a high degree of stabilisation.

The vaccine needs to be reconstituted just before use.

Recombinant: hepatitis B vaccine

The discovery that the hepatitis B surface antigen (HBsAg) was the key component to conferring protection to hepatitis B virus (HBV) infection and allowing for the development of hepatitis B vaccines.

The first available hepatitis B vaccines were manufactured by harvesting HBsAg from the plasma of persons with chronic HBV infection. These 22-nm particles were highly purified, and any residual infectious particles were inactivated by various combinations of urea, pepsin, formaldehyde, and heat.

With the availability of recombinant DNA technology in the 1970s it became feasible to insert the 226-amino acid HBsAg gene product into an expression vector, such as genetically engineered *Saccharomyces cerevisiae* yeast. Recombinant HBV vaccines containing the pre-S1 and pre-S2 proteins, in addition to the S protein, have also been produced. The S gene of the HBV is cloned in a functional expression plasmid for introduction into *S cerevisae*.

A first recombinant HBV vaccine involves yeast cells that are grown in stirred tank fermenters supplemented by a complex fermentation medium, consisting of soy peptone, dextrose, amino acids, and mineral salts. After fermentation, the yeast cells are disrupted; residual solids are precipitated or separated by hydrophobic interaction and size-exclusion chromatography. The resulting HBsAg is assembled into lipoprotein particles 22 nm in diameter. The purified protein is treated in a phosphate buffer with formaldehyde,

sterile filtered, and then coprecipitated with aluminium sulphate to form a bulk vaccine adjuvanted with amorphous aluminium hydroxyphosphate sulphate (a version of alum).

A second recombinant HBV vaccine involves yeast cells that are also grown in stirred tank fermenters but the downstream processing differs. After fermentation, the yeast cells are disrupted through gel permeation chromatography, ion exchange chromatography, and caesium chloride gradient ultrafiltration, and soluble contaminants are removed through diafiltration. The HBsAg is formulated as a suspension of antigen absorbed on aluminium hydroxide (a version of alum).

Each lot of HBV vaccine is tested for potency, for safety in mice and guinea pigs, and for stability, and by assessing the ability of the vaccine to induce antibodies against HBsAg in mice. QC product testing for purity and identity includes numerous chemical, biochemical, and physical assays on the final product to ensure thorough characterization and lot-to-lot consistency.

HBV vaccines are prepared as a sterile suspension for intramuscular injection. They contain thimerosal, a mercury-derived preservative at 1:20,000 or 50 μg/mL concentration as well as aluminium (provided as with amorphous aluminium hydroxyphosphate sulphate) at less than 0.5 mg per milliliter of vaccine.

Because recombinant HBV vaccines are extensively characterized and have demonstrated a satisfactory safety profile in a lot-to-lot comparison, CBER allows an exception for the HBV vaccine for the lot-to-lot release.

Today, close to 10 manufacturers produce HBV vaccines worldwide, either as a monovalent vaccine or combined with other antigens, such as diphtheria, tetanus, polio, acellular pertussis, whole-cell pertussis and/or *H influenzae* type b antigens.

Analytical aspects

The manufacturing process for a vaccine candidate also demands the development of new or refinement of existing analytical methods (see Table 14.4). Techniques are developed for measuring the vaccine antigens, its potency, and any impurities to ensure lot-to-lot consistency.

Table 14.4 Some examples of Assays Used in Quality Control of Vaccines

Assays	Descriptions
Chromatography	Laboratory methods to separate and or analyze complex mixtures into their individual components, based on the principle that the different components will stick to the solid surface or dissolve in a film or liquid to different degrees
GC	Gas chromatography
HPLC	High pressure liquid chromatography
IEC	Ion exchange chromatography
AC	Afffinity chromatography
Electrophoresis	Method in which different molecules, e.g., DNA or proteins, can be sorted by size or other factors. Molecules are placed on a gel and moved or sorted through electrophoresis
PAGE	Polyacrylamide gel electrophoresis
IEF	Iso-electro focusing
CE	Capillary electrophoresis
Immunological	
Immunodiffusion	Technique involving diffusion of antigen or antibody through a semisolid medium, usually agar or agarose gel
Immunoelectrophoresis	Technique combining separation of antigens by electrophoresis with immunodiffusion against an antiserum
Dot-blot	Technique for detecting, analyzing, and identifying proteins by spotting through circular templates directly onto the membrane or paper substrate
Western blot	Technique detecting specific proteins using a gel electrophoresis to separate native or denatured proteins by the length of the protein
ELISA	Enzyme-linked immunosorbent assay (ELISA) uses an enzyme linked to an antibody or antigen as a marker for the detection of a specific protein
RIA	Radioimmunoassay used for measurement of minute quantities of specific antibodies or antigens against which specific antibodies can be raised
Enzyme activity	
Protein characterization	
Peptide mapping	
Amino acid mapping	
N- or C-terminal mapping	
Others	
NMR	Nuclear magnetic resonance
Cytogenic analysis	

An example of the complexity and the extent of required testing is illustrated in the recently approved recombinant human papillomavirus virus-like particle (HPV VLP) vaccine.

The recombinant HPV VLP vaccine is a sterile liquid vaccine preparation that contains purified VLPs composed of the recombinant major capsid proteins of one or more HPV serotypes and formulated with a suitable adjuvant. The HPV VLP vaccines are to be used for prophylactic use. The manufacturing requirements for this vaccine were detailed by WHO. The recommended international name for the vaccine is "Recombinant human papillomavirus virus-like particle vaccine" followed in parenthesis by the serotype specificity and the name of the recombinant protein (e.g., serotype 16 L1 protein, serotype 18 L1 genotype).

The application of new assays and tests in the control of the manufacturing process of the HPV VLP vaccine is significant and illustrated below. In addition to the standard manufacturing requirements, the manufacturing of HPV VLP vaccines should comply as follows:

1. Production steps involving manipulations of recombinant HPV L1 VLP types are to be conducted at a biosafety level consistent with the recombinant production microorganism.

2. QC procedures should ensure segregation of the different HPV L1 VLP types during bulk manufacturing steps.

3. Antigen manufacturing process should be validated to demonstrate production consistency, including an evaluation of critical quality parameters and their corresponding attributes. Examples of process quality attributes are nucleic acid and host cell protein contamination or cumulated population doubling level and column loading as key process operating parameters. The process validation of antigen batches should meet compliance with the preestablished antigen quality control specifications for the HPV antigens, such as antigen identity and antigen purity.

The HPV antigen characterization is performed on lots produced during vaccine development, including the process validation batches. The protein composition should be established by different techniques, e.g., sodium dodecyl sulphate polyacrylamide gel electrophoresis (SDS-PAGE) under reducing conditions or mass spectrometry. Bands should be identified by sensitive staining techniques and, where possible, by specific antibodies or mass spectrometry to confirm the presence of expected products of the HPV L1 protein. The identity should be established by peptide mapping and/or terminal amino acid sequence analysis.

Because of the importance of the conformational epitopes in the efficacy, it is critical to determine the morphological characteristics of the VLPs and the degree of aggregation. Protein, lipid, nucleic acid, and carbohydrate content should be measured when applicable, and VLP characterization may be done by atomic force and transmission electron microscopy, dynamic light scattering, epitope mapping, and reactivity with neutralizing monoclonal antibodies.

The level of residual host cell protein derived from insect cells and/or novel cell substrate should meet acceptable safety in nonclinical and clinical studies.

The control of source materials applies to all levels in the manufacturing process as follows:

1. *Control of cell cultures for manufacturing of antigen.* Only cell cultures, based on the principle of a cell bank system, should be used for vaccine production and specifically, only cells approved by the national regulatory authority. In addition, depending on the selected manufacturing process, the yeast cells or the insect cells should be fully described. In the case of yeast cells, information on the absence of adventitious agents and on gene homogenicity for the master and the working cell banks should be provided. In the case of insect cells, the cell substrates and the cell banks should conform to the WHO criteria for "Requirements for use of animal cells as *in vitro* substrates for the production of biologicals."

2. *Control of cell culture medium.* If serum is used for the propagation of cells, it should be tested to demonstrate freedom from bacteria, fungi, and mycoplasma, as well as for phage and endotoxin. Validated molecular tests for bovine viruses may replace the cell culture tests of bovine sera. The acceptability of the source(s) of any component of bovine, porcine, sheep, or goat origin used should be approved by the national regulatory authority.

If trypsin is used for preparing cell cultures and aiding in virus infection, it should be tested and demonstrated free of bacteria, fungi, mycoplasmas, and infectious viruses, especially bovine or porcine parvo-viruses, as appropriate. The methods should be approved by the national regulatory authority.

3. *Control of master and working cell banks.* Depending on the selected manufacturing process, an important number of tests are required to validate the master (MCB) and working cell banks (WCB) of the yeast cells or the insect cells.

In the case of yeast, an absence of adventitious bacteria, fungi, and mycoplasma should be documented. Cells must be maintained in a frozen state that enables recovery of viable cells without alteration of genotype.

In the case of insect cells for recombinant baculovirus expression system, tests must show that the MWB and WCB are free of bacteria, fungi, mycoplasma, *Mycobacterium* spp., and adventitious agents relevant to the species and in its derivation. For insect cell lines a special emphasis is required on potential insect-borne human pathogens (e.g., arboviruses [arthropod-borne viruses], including bunyavirus, flavivirus, togavirus, reovirus [such as orbivirus], rhabdovirus, and asfavirus). Because of the novel approach of using insect cells, additional tests may be needed to identify other potential adventitious agents. PCR, electron microscopy, and cocultivation may be used to identify such pathogens; further monitoring of the importance of invertebrates or vertebrates viruses is required.

4. *Control of recombinant baculovirus master seeds and working seeds.* The recombinant baculovirus expression vector contains the coding sequence of the recombinant HPV protein, and segments of the expression construct must be analyzed, including the use of nucleic acid techniques, among others. Genetic stability must be ensured from the baculovirus MSL seed lot up to the highest level used in production.

The identity of each baculovirus MSL and WSL should be identified by HPV type of the inserted gene or origin, using appropriate methods, e.g., PCR. Each baculovirus seed lot must be tested for potential bacterial, fungal, and mycoplasmal contamination, as well as for insect mollicutes (mycoplasma), such as spiroplasma, entomoplasma, and mesoplasma.

The baculovirus cell cultures should be assessed for the absence of adventitious viruses that may have been present during the production, including those that may be present in the source materials used at each production step.

With the objective to determine the recombinant baculovirus concentration, each seed lot will be assayed for infectivity in an insect cell culture system.

5. *Control of HPV antigen vaccine.* Depending on the selected manufacturing process, an important number of tests are required to evaluate the single harvest of the yeast expression system or the recombinant baculovirus in insect cells expression system.

In the case of yeast, the microbial purity in each fermentation run should be monitored at the end of the production run.

In the case of recombinant baculovirus, specific parameters need to be tested on the single harvest, such as presence of adventitious viruses in the control cell culture, presence of hemadsorbing viruses and testing for the identity of insect cells. For the latter, the suitable methods are, but not limited to, biochemical tests (e.g., isoenzyme analyses), cytogenetic tests (e.g., chromosomal markers), and tests for genetic markers (e.g., DNA fingerprinting).

6. *Control of purified monovalent antigen bulk.* The purification process can be applied to a single harvest, a part of a single antigen harvest, or a pool of single antigen harvest. It may require several purification steps based on different principles and may involve disassembly and reassembly of VLPs. The tests include (a) identity of the HPV antigen type; (b) purity; (c) protein content; (d) antigen content; (e) sterility test for bacteria and fungi; (f) percentage intact HPV L1 monomer; (g) VLP size and structure; (h) presence of potentially hazardous agents used during manufacture; (i) absence of residuals from the antigen expression system; and (j) validation to eliminate (by removal and/or inactivation) adventitious viruses (during the manufacturing process validation).

7. *Control on adsorbed monovalent antigen bulk.* The individual HPV VLP antigen may be absorbed onto a mineral vehicle, such as aluminium salt. Its use and concentration must be approved by national regulatory authorities. Different tests on the adsorbed monovalent antigen bulk are approved by the national regulatory authority and include (a) sterility tests for bacteria and fungi; (b) bacterial endotoxin; (c) identity; (d) concentration of adjuvant; (e) pH; and (f) antigen content.

8. *Control on final vaccine bulk.* The final bulk should be aseptically prepared in combinations of adsorbed monovalent antigen bulks that have successfully passed the control tests of the monovalent antigen bulk. Different tests on the final vaccine bulk include (a) sterility tests for bacteria and fungi; (b) content of adjuvants; (c) the completeness of adsorption of each antigen present in each final vaccine bulk; (d) preservative content, if added; (e) *in vivo* potency tests may be used on the final bulk or the final vaccine lot, whereas *in vitro* potency tests should be performed on every lot of final vaccine lot; and (f) filling and containers.

9. *Control on final vaccine lots.* Samples taken from each final vaccine lot should be tested. These tests are approved by the national regulatory authorities and include (a) inspection of containers; (b) appearance through a visual inspection; (c) identity of the different individual HPV VLP antigens; (d) sterility for bacteria and fungi; (e) pH and osmolarity; (f) preservatives; (g) test for pyrogenic substances; (h) adjuvant content; (i) protein content; (j) degree of adsorption; and (k) potency of each final vaccine lot.

10. *Control of records, retained samples, distribution, and labeling.* The archiving of manufacturing process records and of samples retained for further testing must be performed according to good manufacturing practice (GMP) for biological products. The same GMP requirements also apply for the distribution and transport of the vaccine lots.

The labeling on the carton, the container, or the package insert should also meet the recommendation of the national regulatory authorities authorizing the vaccine onto the market.

Good manufacturing practices

Good manufacturing practices

In the USA, national requirements are codified in the Code of Federal Regulations (CFR) title 21, parts 200 and 600. Additional recommendations are documented by US Food and Drug Administration's "Points to Consider" and "Guidance to Industry." As new analytical and preparative methodologies are introduced and validated, they are included in the respective pharmacopoeias. Late 2011, the *US Pharmacopeia* adopted USP 1235 ("Vaccines for Human Use – General Considerations"), USP 1037 ("Virology Test Methods"),

and USP 1050 ("Viral Safety Evaluation of Biotechnology Products Derived From Cell Lines of Human or Animal Origin"). In 2010 the "Guidance for Industry" on characterization and qualification of cell substrates and other biological starting material used in the production of viral vaccines for the prevention and treatment of infectious disease was finalized.

The European Commission (EC) describes the GMP provisions for biological medicinal products in *EudraLex* Volume 4 and describes in different parts the guidelines and requirements for GMPs for medicinal products for human and veterinary use, as well as the required GMP documentation. The *European Pharmacopeia* also provides principles and guidelines of GMP in specific subsections. In addition, the European Medicines Agency (EMA) clarifies through documents and concept papers authored by the Biotechnology Working Group (BWG) and the Vaccine Working Group (VWG) of the Committee for Medicinal Products for Human Use (CHMP) new guidelines on vaccine-related topics, such as the need to swiftly integrate new testing methods and their standardization and analytical tests for influenza vaccines, or guidance for DNA vaccines (http://wwweuropa.eu/ema).

Moreover, the International Conference of Harmonisation (ICH) and WHO also provide guidance documents that are generally adopted by most regulatory authorities worldwide. The guidance document "Derivation and Characterization of Cell Substrates Used for Production of Biotechnological/Biological Products" (Q5D) provides a description of potential biosafety issues and outlines a standardized algorithm of the characterization of cell substrates.

Different health authorities, such as the China Food and Drug Administration (CFDA) and the Japanese Pharmaceutical and Medical Devices Agency (PMDA) also issue their own guidelines. In Japan, the provisions in Article 42-1 of the Pharmaceutical Affairs Law enable setting the necessary standards for manufacturing, properties, and quality described as the "minimum requirements for vaccines, antitoxins, and blood products."

Good cell culture practices

In 1999, good cell culture practices (GCCPs) were initiated at the Third World Congress on Alternatives and

Animal Use in Life Sciences and relate to the quality control of cell substrates and cell cultures.

Good distribution and supply practices

After the licensing of vaccines by the national regulatory authority, the vaccines can be distributed. It should be recognized that vaccines can be licensed directly in those countries with competent national regulatory authorities, while other countries need to rely on licensure in the country of manufacture, followed by review and approval by the final country of use. Provided vaccines are required in all countries worldwide, WHO developed a "prequalification" process to ensure that vaccines meet global standards of quality, safety, and efficacy in order to optimize local health resources and improve health outcomes. The process consists of a transparent, scientific, and technical assessment, which includes dossier review, consistency testing or performance evaluation, and site visits to manufacturers. Based on the outcome of the prequalification process and licensing in the country of manufacture, procurement of vaccine can be performed by United Nations agencies. Currently, a total of 37 vaccines are considered prequalified, but not all manufacturers of a particular vaccine will be qualified; each manufacturer has to seek WHO prequalification for a specific vaccine. In addition, there is a specific mechanism to accelerate manufacturing of new vaccines that address an emerging medical need in certain countries for a vaccine that will be manufactured but not used in the country of origin.

The planning for the production of monovalent and combined vaccines, process and timing of testing, country-specific logistical requirements for distribution, packaging, and labeling, etc., is highly complex and very intensive. In the USA, access to vaccine is usually via the health care professionals who order directly from the manufacturer or the distributor; some vaccines can be available through retail channels (e.g., the influenza vaccine). The European Union member states apply different distribution policies even though manufacturers ship to distribution centres and wholesalers. In almost all member states, price controls are imposed and in some countries vaccines are procured by government tender. In addition, vaccine-preventable disease outbreaks may impact production planning and demand flexibility of manufacturers, as illustrated by the 2007–2008 yellow fever outbreak in Paraguay with an unplanned shipment of over 6 million doses of yellow fever vaccine.

It is critical to ensure the maintenance of the cold chain between the manufacturer and the end user. This step in the supply chain demands a robust and reliable process with routine monitoring for possible deviations.

Future outlook

New technologies

Modern vaccine development is currently exploring a wide range of novel technologies to create safer and more efficacious vaccines.

These technologies include viral vectors produced in animal cells, VLPs produced in yeast or insect cells, polysaccharide conjugation to carrier proteins, DNA plasmids produced in *E. coli*, and therapeutic vaccine candidates created by *in vitro* activation of patient leucocytes.

New technologies also address purification steps (e.g., membrane adsorption, precipitation), analytical methods (e.g., microsphere multiplex assays, RNA microarrays), and novel adjuvants (e.g., monophosphoryl lipid A [MPL], MF59 squalene).

Vaccine safety

Health care providers, regulatory authorities, and manufacturers are required to investigate early signals of vaccine safety thoroughly and report those findings to the public and the media.

The perceptions of the risks of vaccination are readily seen and comprise concerns over adverse events, use of preservatives, adjuvants, additives, and presumed or real manufacturing residuals, such as inactivating agents, antibiotics, yeast proteins, and egg proteins. These perceived risks are a universal phenomenon, with similar questions and concerns for the mother of a child who will potentially receive a particular vaccine, be it in the USA, the Democratic Republic of Congo, Japan, or Belgium. It is the task of the partners mentioned above to engage in resolving the many challenges.

Mucosal vaccination

The mucosal immune system is an attractive target site for vaccines since many pathogens infect the host at microfold cells (M cells) in the mucosal surface. Mucosal delivery without the need for a needle is already used for several vaccines, i.e., the live attenuated influenza vaccine given in a nasal spray. This route of administration may contribute to a heterologous cross-protection by inducing a broader immunity. Vaccination at mucosal surfaces can induce local protection at the potential infection sites as well as inducing a systemic immunity; however, the direct delivery only induces a poor immune response.

Further work is required to examine whether the promising results of the coadministration or fusing of a particular vaccine antigen with a strong mucosal adjuvant or particle-mediated delivery systems with an incorporated adjuvant can be confirmed when tested in further clinical trials.

Elimination of preservatives

The elimination of preservatives should be recognized as an extension of the request for higher vaccine purity and the perception of the public of vaccine safety. Several preservatives are routinely used and include thimerosal, phenol, benzethonium, formaldehyde, and 2-phenoxyethanol. Those products have bactericidal and/or bacteriostatic properties and have been necessary when addressing the safety of vaccines in the past. In addition, preservatives are used in multidose vials to prevent contamination of future doses during the extraction of the first doses from the vial. The risk of an infection or sepsis due to a dose from a contaminated, unpreserved vial is considered to be far greater than the potential risk of an adverse event from the preservative itself.

In light of the public concern, manufacturers are exploring how to eliminate preservatives or to reduce the concentration of the preservative, as these are used also for inactivation agents in the manufacturing process.

Influenza viral drift

Influenza viruses continuously go through antigenic drift resulting in the need to routinely monitor circulating influenza strains and annually update the influenza vaccine formulation. The monitoring of the emergence of a new influenza strains is a global effort including a network of over 110 National Influenza Centers in more than 90 countries and four WHO Collaborative Centres for Reference and Research on Influenza in Atlanta, London, Tokyo, and Melbourne (http://www.who.int/topics/influenza/en/). These centers determine the antigenic and genetic properties of the clinical isolates in circulation each year and provide the basis for the WHO recommendation of the annual influenza strains to be included in vaccines. These decisions take place in February for the Northern hemisphere influenza vaccine and in September for the Southern hemisphere influenza vaccine. These dates are set because of the need to allow sufficient time for manufacturers to prepare and produce sufficient vaccine for the annual influenza season (see Figure 14.1 for the time line to generate the annual seasonal influenza vaccine).

The timely access to the identified influenza vaccine is critical, especially for the Northern hemisphere where there is a capacity request of 400 million doses to be manufactured, formulated, filled, packaged, released, shipped, and administered.

Summary

- Delivering human vaccines on a global scale demands the application of complex and diverse production methods, high-standard quality control, and vast and reliable distribution channels to ensure the vaccines are effective at the point of delivery and administration.

- The current and new technologies for the manufacturing of different types of vaccines should impact vaccine cost and number of vaccines administrations required, enabling improved access in developing countries reducing the number of vaccine-preventable diseases and deaths.

- Vaccine formulations and presentations tailored to the specification in different countries should serve their target populations.

- Vaccine manufacturing in appropriate quantities and at realistic prices is essential for both the individual and public health as a whole.

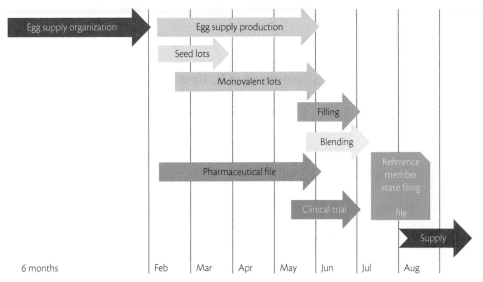

Figure 14.1 Seasonal influenza vaccine manufacturing time line.

Further reading

Gomez PL, Robinson JM, and Rogalewicz JA. Vaccine manufacturing. In Vaccines, 6th edition (eds SA Plotkin, WA Orenstein and PA Offit), pp. 44–57. Philadelphia: Elsevier Saunders, 2013.

Guidance for Industry. Characterization and qualification of cell substrates and other biological materials used in the production of viral vaccines for infectious disease indications. U.S. Department of Health and Human Services, Food and Drug Administration, February 2010.

Guidelines to assure the quality, safety and efficacy of recombinant human papillomavirus virus-like particle vaccines. Expert Committee on Biological Standardization. WHO/BS/06.2050 – Final 2006.

Hess RD, Weber F, Watson K, and Schmitt S (2012). Regulatory, biosafety and safety challenges for novel cells as substrates for human vaccines. Vaccine 30, 2715–2727.

Immunization Action Coalition. Historic dates and events related to Vaccines and immunization. 2012. http://www.immunize.org/timeline

Josefsberg JO and Buckland B (2012). Vaccine process technology. Biotechnology and Bioengineering 109, 1443–1460.

Langfield KK, Walker HJ, Gregory LC, and Federspiel MJ. Manufacture of measles viruses. In Viral Vectors for Gene Therapy: Methods and Protocols, Vol. 737, Methods in Molecular Biology (eds O-W Merten and M Al-Rubeai), pp. 345–366. New York: Humana Press, 2011.

Smith J, Lipsitch M, and Almond JW (2011). Vaccine production, distribution, access and uptake. Lancet 378, 428–438.

15 Clinical evaluation of vaccines

Richard E. Rupp and Bridget E. Hawkins

Sealy Center for Vaccine Development, University of Texas Medical Branch, Galveston, TX, USA

Abbreviations

APEC	Asia-Pacific Economic Cooperation	IEC	Independent Ethics Committee
ASEAN	Association of Southeast Asian Nations	IFPMA	International Federation of Pharmaceutical Manufacturers & Associations
CBER	Center for Biologics Evaluation and Research	IND	Investigational new drug
CFR	Code of Federal Regulations	IRB	Institutional Review Board
CPE	Japanese Center for Product Evaluation	MHLW	Japanese Ministry of Health, Labor and Welfare
CTN	Australian Clinical Trials Notification	NDA	New Drug Application
CTX	Australian Clinical Trials Exemption	NHMRC	National Health and Medical Research Council
DHHS	Department of Health and Human Services		
DMC	Data Monitoring Committee	OHRP	Office for Human Research Protections
DSMB	Data and Safety Monitoring Board		
DSMP	Data and Safety Monitoring Plan	PAFSC	Japanese Pharmaceutical Affairs and Food Sanitation Council
EEA-EFTA	European Economic Area European Free Trade Association	PAL	Japanese Pharmaceutical Affairs Law
EFPIA	European Federation of Pharmaceutical Industries and Associations	PANDRH	Pan American Network on Drug Regulatory Harmonization
EGE	European Group on Ethics in Science and New Technologies	PhRMA	Pharmaceutical Research and Manufacturers of America
EMA	European Medicines Agency	PMDA	Japanese Pharmaceuticals and Medical Devices Agency
GCC	Gulf Cooperation Council		
GCG	Global Cooperation Group	SADC	South African Development Community
GCP	Good clinical practice		
GLP	Good laboratory practice	TGA	Therapeutic Goods Administration
HREC	Human Research Ethics Committee	US FDA	US Food and Drug Administration
ICH	International Conference on Harmonisation of Technical Requirements for Registration of Pharmaceuticals for Human Use	VRBPAC	Vaccines and Related Biological Products Advisory Committee
		WHO	World Health Organization

Vaccinology: An Essential Guide, First Edition. Edited by Gregg N. Milligan and Alan D.T. Barrett.
© 2015 John Wiley & Sons, Ltd. Published 2015 by John Wiley & Sons, Ltd.

Introduction

Clinical trials are arguably the most important step in the development process for any human vaccine candidate. The research prior to this point only provides data for an educated prediction about the action of the investigational vaccine in humans. In our current state of science, the only way to actually determine the safety and efficacy of a candidate vaccine in humans is by conducting clinical trials. Very few vaccine candidates proceed as far as clinical evaluation, with most vaccines failing because they do not have the ability to translate good immunogenicity data in small animals, such as mice, to large/higher animals, such as nonhuman primates. In addition, some vaccine candidates have safety issues due to the components, or purity of components in the vaccine. Accordingly, few vaccines obtain the investigational new drug (IND) status needed to proceed to clinical evaluation.

Studies testing the safety and effectiveness of drugs and biologics such as vaccines in humans are known as *clinical trials* or *clinical research*. The written plan for the clinical trial is referred to as the *protocol*. The protocol contains the objectives, design, and detailed procedures for the conduct of the trial. Examples of objectives include developing a profile of adverse effects, determining optimum dosing, and determining immunogenicity in a certain age group. The trial design includes details such as the use of control groups, blinding, and a statistical analysis demonstrating that the objectives can be accomplished with the projected study population. The protocol also includes specifics about the production, handling, and storage of the investigational vaccine, method of delivery such as type and site of injection/route of administration, needle size, etc., and the obtaining, processing, and storage of laboratory specimens. In short, the protocol contains the blueprint for running the entire trial.

A data and safety plan (DSMP) is an important part of the protocol. The DSMP includes how subject safety will be monitored and evaluated and how adverse events will be addressed and reported to regulatory agencies. A part of the DSMP may be a data monitoring committee (DMC) or data and safety monitoring board (DSMB). The DMC/DSMB comprises a group of experts independent from the sponsor and investigator. The group monitors and evaluates patient safety and treatment efficacy data while a clinical trial is ongoing. This is especially important in blinded studies where the sponsor and investigator do not know which subjects are receiving the candidate vaccine or drug. The DMC/DSMB may halt the trial if the candidate appears unsafe or their data demonstrate a lack of efficacy.

The person, company, institution, or organization taking responsibility for the clinical trial is known as the *sponsor*. Essentially, the sponsor is responsible for every aspect of the trial including study design, management, and financing. The actual location where subjects receive the study vaccine is a *clinical site*. Multisite or multicenter trials are conducted at more than one clinical site. The coordinating or lead investigator is responsible for organizing and coordinating the different centers. The *investigator*, also known as the *principal investigator*, is the individual at the local site under whose direct supervision the investigational vaccine is given. Subinvestigators, coinvestigators, or collaborators are individuals (scientists and/or physicians) at the local site designated and supervised by the investigator to perform trial related duties.

Subjects or *volunteers* are the people who participate in the clinical trial, whether they receive the active intervention (the vaccine) or serve as controls. Their contribution should never be downplayed; it is critical, as the volunteers are placing their own physical well-being at risk for the conduct of the clinical trial.

Phases of clinical trials

An overview of the vaccine development pipeline is shown in Figure 15.1. Clinical trials are performed in a stepwise manner to minimize both the number of subjects placed at risk as well as minimize risk to individual subjects. These steps are called *phases*. In vaccine clinical trials there are usually four phases. The first three are performed to demonstrate safety and efficacy (phases I, II, and III). The fourth phase is conducted after licensure and marketing to gather more information about the vaccine or expand indications. The latter is important as often multiple vaccine companies market very similar products for a particular vaccine and the question arises whether or not the vaccines can be "mixed and matched." For example, there are two live attenuated rotavirus vaccines. One requires

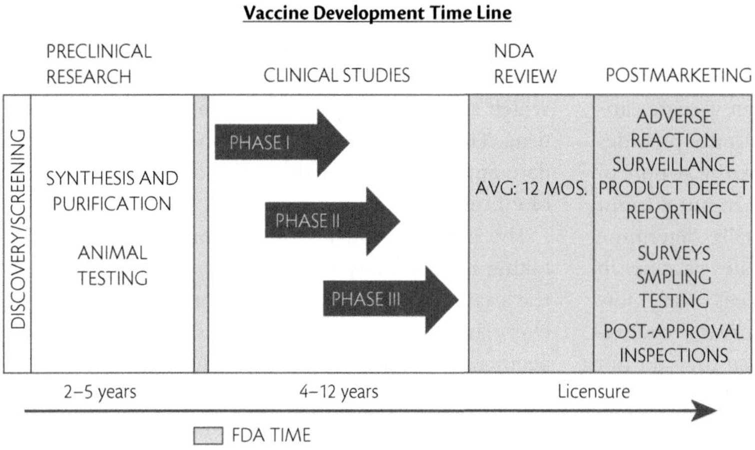

Vaccine Development Time Line

Figure 15.1 An overview of the vaccine development time line.

two doses and the other requires three doses, and questions arise such as can you take dose 1 and 3 of vaccine company A and dose 2 of vaccine company B? This is important, as vaccine company A has optimized its vaccine and schedule for its own product, while vaccine company B has done the same for its product. The situation becomes more complicated with the increasing number of combination vaccines used today. Table 15.1 provides an overview of the phase of vaccine clinical trials.

Phase I

Phase I studies are the first examination of the vaccine in humans. The primary goal is to assess the tolerability and safety of the investigational vaccine. Secondary objectives may include measuring markers of the immune response. In phase I studies, the vaccine is given to a small number of subjects (typically 20–80). The subjects are usually adults 18–45 years of age in excellent health because such individuals are the most likely to recover in the case of an adverse effect such as inflammation of the heart or a severe drop in blood pressure. An exception to using healthy subjects in phase I studies is made for toxic drugs with very specific indications. For example, a drug known to damage heart muscle in animals may be tested in terminal patients to see if it has an effect on their cancer.

Phase I trials are often performed in an environment where the subjects can be closely monitored and

Key terms in the vaccine clinical trials process

- **Blinding:** A clinical trial is *blind* if participants are unaware whether they are in the experimental or control arm of the study; also called *masked*.
- **Clinical site:** Geographic location(s) where the investigational vaccine is administered.
- **Clinical trials or research:** Studies testing the safety and/or effectiveness of a vaccine in human subjects.
- **Control groups:** The standard by which experimental observations are evaluated. In many clinical trials, one group of patients will be given an experimental drug or treatment, while the control group is given either a standard treatment for the illness or a placebo.
- **Investigational vaccine:** A vaccine candidate with a safety and/or efficacy profile that has yet to be fully researched.
- **Investigator(s):** The individual(s) at the clinical site under whose direct supervision the study vaccine is given; this could be a scientist or researcher or both.
- **Protocol:** Written document that contains experiment and vaccine information necessary to complete the clinical trial.
- **Sponsor:** The person, company, institution, or organization taking responsibility for the clinical trial.
- **Subjects or Volunteers:** People that participate in the clinical trial.

Table 15.1 Vaccine Clinical Trial Phases

	Objectives	Subjects
Phase I	Tolerability, safety, pharmacokinetics, and pharmacodynamics; may include dose ranging.	20–80 Healthy
Phase II	IIa: Demonstrate safety and first signs of efficacy or immunogenicity. IIb: More extensive study used to establish dose, overall efficacy, and safety properties in order to establish benefit-to-risk ratio. Used to determine design of phase III studies.	80–300 May include intended target population
Phase III	IIIa: Additional evidence of efficacy and to better understand safety and adverse effects. IIb: Conducted after submission for marketing approval. Purposes include differentiation from other treatments, data from additional patient populations, establishing new indications, and exploring adverse events.	300 to several thousands Target population
Phase IV	Postmarketing studies that examine additional indications and may include certain populations, such as pregnant women.	

emergency care is readily available in case of a severe immediate reaction such as anaphylaxis (a life-threatening allergic reaction marked by airway swelling and low blood pressure). These trials are usually conducted in a slow deliberate manner. Frequently, the first subjects are only administered a small dose of the vaccine. The subjects are monitored for several weeks for signs of illness before the next subjects are tested at a higher dose. This stepwise progression continues until the likely effective dose is tested.

Phase II

Phase II trials only begin after the data demonstrating safety and tolerability are available from the phase I trial and approval of the national regulatory authority. These studies are designed to assess vaccine immunogenicity or efficacy, as well as to continue the safety assessments on a larger group of subjects. Typically, phase II trials are conducted with 80 to 300 subjects. The criteria for subjects are not as restrictive as phase I trials, and subjects may be the actual group targeted for the vaccine such as children or the elderly. Investigational vaccines often fail during phase II trials when they are discovered not to be immunogenic or have to have poor efficacy. If this happens, oftentimes the trial will end, and the vaccine will undergo modifications and further preclinical testing or the project

may end due to scientific issues or financial concerns.

Phase II trials are often subdivided in to two types. Phase IIa studies are designed to look for signs of immunogenicity and/or efficacy while the objective of phase IIb studies include finding the optimum dose. Data from phase IIb studies establish the benefit-to-risk ratio and help to determine the design of the phase III studies. Some protocols mix aspects from both phase I and phase II studies. Such phase I/II studies attempt to establish both safety and immunogenicity or efficacy in the very first human trials. This may happen when an improvement on a currently licensed vaccine is being evaluated.

Phase III

Most phase III studies are randomized, controlled, multicenter trials utilizing much larger groups of subjects (300–3000). Some phase III studies may have larger numbers of subjects. For example, the live rotavirus vaccine candidates that were subsequently licensed each involved over 70,000 subjects, due to concerns of intussusception identified with an earlier vaccine shortly after licensure, which was withdrawn from the market. The quadrivalent human papillomavirus (HPV) vaccine was evaluated in over 60,000 subjects. Such studies are aimed at demonstrating the actual efficacy or immunogenicity of the vaccine. As in phase I and II studies, safety data are collected. Phase III trials are the most expensive due to their size and long duration. Phase III studies are also subdivided. Phase IIIa studies provide evidence of efficacy and safety for the New Drug Application (NDA), which indicates an application for licensure. Phase IIIb trials are often launched after other study data has been submitted to the national regulatory authority

for licensure. Possible objectives for phase IIIb trials include expansion of the target population, differentiating the investigational vaccine from other similar vaccines, adding new indications and further exploration of specific adverse events.

Phase IV

Examples of the goals for phase IV trials include collecting data on rare side effects, looking at the duration of protection, studying effects on herd immunity, investigating if younger and/or older individuals can receive the vaccine, or the effect of utilizing similar but not identical vaccines from different companies when repeated dosing is necessary. Phase IV studies may be long, lasting many years. The remainder of the discussion will be limited to the premarketing phases.

Some well-designed phase II/III clinical trials are referred to as *pivotal* in that the data are very important for licensure by the national regulatory authority. Pivotal trials must be of adequate size to clearly demonstrate efficacy or immunogenicity and usually utilize a randomized, double-blinded design. In some countries, such as the USA or the UK, if a drug or vaccine is found to be effective and well tolerated, the US Food and Drug Administration (US FDA) or European Medicines Agency (EMA) can choose to expedite the approval process by allowing vaccine licensure to occur after Phase II thereby allowing postmarketing surveillance (typically referred to as Phase IV) to occur in Phase III.

Some phase II and most phase III vaccine trials are controlled, randomized, and double blinded.

- Controlled studies use an agent in addition to the investigational vaccine. In some studies the control may be a placebo such as saline but it may also be a licensed vaccine. For example, infants in a conjugate pneumococcal vaccine study received either the licensed vaccine (a 7-serotype vaccine) or the investigational vaccine (a 13-serotype vaccine). The use of a control helps maintain blinding as well as determine the significance of data. If volunteers develop headaches at the same rate in both the investigational vaccine and placebo groups then it is unlikely the investigational vaccine is the cause of the headaches.
- Volunteers are randomized into the different arms of a research protocol. Randomization is performed to remove selection bias. Both researchers and volunteers are subject to selection bias. For example, researchers might place "sicklier" volunteers in the investigational arm believing the less healthy volunteers might benefit the most from the investigational arm. Such a selection bias could make it appear that the investigational vaccine has more side effects if the selected individuals are more prone to infections, fevers, headaches, and other symptoms.
- Blinding is used to keep volunteers and researchers from biasing the study results. During a single-blinded study the volunteers are unaware of whether they are receiving the investigational vaccine. Double-blinded studies are those where both the investigators and volunteers are unaware which volunteers are receiving the investigational vaccine. Studies are "unblinded" upon completion so the data can be analyzed. The investigators notify the subjects as to whether they received the investigational vaccine after unblinding.

There are four phases of vaccine clinical trials:

- Phase I: Tolerability and safety of investigational vaccine and typically includes 20–80 healthy adults.
- Phase II: (a) Examines signs of immunogenicity and/or efficacy; (b) optimum dose; typically includes 80–300 subjects; may be combined with Phase I.
- Phase III: (a) Efficacy and safety evidence is obtained; (b) expansion of target population; typically includes 300–3000 (or more) subjects; may be combined with Phase II.
- Phase IV: Postmarketing surveillance that examines effects of vaccine on entire target population; may also include certain populations like pregnant females.

Government jurisdiction

In the USA, two governmental agencies within the Department of Health and Human Services (DHHS) have jurisdiction over the conduct of clinical trials. Each has its own set of regulations that govern different aspects of clinical trials. The first agency, the Office for Human Research Protections (OHRP), oversees and ensures the rights, welfare and well-being of research subjects.

The second agency, the US FDA, is responsible for protecting public health by ensuring the safety, efficacy, and security of human and veterinary drugs, biologic products, medical devices, food supply, cosmetics, and products that emit radiation. Because of its wide-ranging responsibilities, the US FDA has centers of expertise regulating different areas such as food, drugs, devices, veterinary medicine, toxicological research, and tobacco. Vaccines are regulated by the Center for Biologics Evaluation and Research (CBER). US FDA regulations are designed to ensure the quality and integrity of the data collected in clinical trials as well as ensure the rights and safety of research subjects. The data from the clinical trials must demonstrate a favorable risk-benefit profile for the US FDA to license a vaccine. The roles of both OHRP and the US FDA are further discussed later in this chapter. The Vaccines and Related Biological Products Advisory Committee (VRBPAC) provides advice to the commissioner of food and drugs on the safety, effectiveness, and appropriate use of vaccines. The committee consists of 12 core voting members that are appointed by the commissioner. The members provide expertise in the fields of immunology, virology, bacteriology, epidemiology, preventive medicine, infectious diseases, pediatrics, microbiology, and biochemistry.

Clinical research is regulated in a roughly parallel manner in the European Union (EU) and the European Economic Area European Free Trade Association (EEA-EFTA) countries (Iceland, Liechtenstein, and Norway). Ethical issues related to the conduct of clinical trials are addressed through legislation and directives from the European Parliament, based on proposals from the European Commission, which in turn is advised by the European Group on Ethics in Science and New Technologies (EGE). Similar to the US FDA, the European Medicines Agency (EMA) is responsible for the scientific evaluation and marketing authorization of new medicines, including vaccines. Unlike the US FDA, the EMA is a scientific agency with powers that are decentralized, relying on a network of about 3500 experts throughout the EU. This chapter focuses primarily on the conduct of clinical trials in the USA, but it should be kept in mind that the regulations and processes are very similar in the countries of the EU (EMA), Japan (Pharmaceuticals and Medical Devices Agency [PMDA]) and Australia (Therapeutics Goods Administration [TGA]).

In Japan, after nonclinical tests have been performed in animals, clinical trials may begin by following the same Phase I–IV plan as the USA and EU. Once the clinical trials have been completed, an application for product approval (similar to the USA's NDA) gets submitted to Japan's PMDA, which consults external expert reviewers regarding the safety and efficacy of the vaccine and then submits their report to the Japanese Ministry of Health, Labor and Welfare (MHLW). Specifically, the Office of Biologics II, a division of the Center for Product Evaluation (CPE) within the PMDA, deals with applications for vaccine approval. All forms need to be submitted in Japanese and must be in accordance with Japan's Pharmaceutical Affairs Law (PAL). The MHLW consults with the Pharmaceutical Affairs and Food Sanitation Council (PAFSC), and then, if the candidate vaccine is deemed safe and efficacious, the MHLW will issue an approval to the applicant. Postmarketing safety measures are put into place, and the MHLW/PMDA also has implemented a system of relief for those affected by adverse health effects.

Australia's system for vaccine approval utilizes the same Phase I–IV plan as the USA, EU, and Japan, with a few exceptions. Investigators have their choice of two options for vaccine clinical trial approval: (1) clinical trials notification (CTN) or (2) clinical trials exemption (CTX) application. The CTN scheme, which is preferred for Phase I–IV vaccine studies that have enough preclinical (animal) safety and efficacy data to indicate that the vaccine would be safe for human usage, allows for expedited regulatory review because the applicant only has to submit a "notification of intent to conduct a clinical trial" form to the TGA's Office of Scientific Evaluation before beginning a clinical trial. If there is insufficient or conflicting safety data or in cases of some medical devices, the CTX application route is preferred as it requires the TGA to review the investigational vaccine's safety data and provide advice to the investigator about what is needed to show evidence of safety. Under Australia's National Health and Medical Research Council (NHMRC), the TGA's only task is to review the safety of drugs, biologicals, and medical devices. The institution (approving authority) where the clinical trial will take place assumes the responsibility for vaccine approval. The institution's Human Research Ethics Committee (HREC) at that institution approves the trial protocol and assumes responsibility for monitoring the conduct of the clinical trial, which is different from that in the USA, where the sponsor monitors the conduct of the clinical trial. Interestingly, all vaccine clinical trials must have an Australian sponsor to be conducted in Australia.

Governmental entities with jurisdiction over clinical trials

In Australia:
- National Health and Medical Research Council (NHMRC)
  - Therapeutic Goods Administration (TGA)
    - Office of Scientific Evaluation

In European Union countries:
- European Parliament and European Commission
  - European Group on Ethics in Science and New Technologies (EGE)
  - European Medicines Agency (EMA)

In Japan:
- Japanese Ministry of Health, Labor and Welfare (MHLW)
  - Pharmaceuticals and Medical Devices Agency (PMDA)
    - Center for Product Evaluation (CPE)
      - Office of Biologics II
  - Pharmaceutical Affairs and Food Sanitation Council (PAFSC)

In the USA:
- Department of Health and Human Services (DHHS)
  - Office for Human Research Protections (OHRP)
  - US FDA with advice from the Vaccines and Related Biological Products Advisory Committee (VRBPAC)
    - Center for Biologics Evaluation and Research (CBER)

The investigational new drug process

Clinical trials are conducted in a heavily regulated and regimented manner. In the USA, the sponsor is required to follow the investigational new drug (IND) process. It is in the best interest of the sponsor to engage in a dialogue with the US FDA through the entire clinical research process, from early protocol design through filing for licensure. The dialogue helps ensure the process progresses as smoothly and efficiently as possible.

The first step requires the sponsor to file an application for an IND with the US FDA. The IND application requires information necessary for the US FDA to evaluate whether the trials will expose subjects to unwarranted risks. The application covers three general areas: (1) preclinical data permitting consideration as to whether the product is reasonably safe for initial testing in humans (this may include previous experience with vaccine clinical trials in foreign countries); (2) manufacturing information for the assessment of the composition, stability, and controls required to ensure the sponsor can produce and supply consistent batches of the investigational vaccine; and (3) detailed protocols for proposed clinical trials.

The vaccine sponsor must wait 30 days after filing the IND application before initiating a clinical trial. During this period, the US FDA assesses the application and decides whether to issue an IND number. If the period lapses without an inquiry from the US FDA, the sponsor may start the trial on the presumption an IND number is not required. This is unlikely as the US FDA requires most, if not all, trials of unlicensed vaccines to have an IND number.

The US FDA usually requests more information or clarification of information already provided, making it improbable that any clinical trial may be initiated within 30 days of filing. Once the US FDA requests the information, it may issue an IND number or place the application on *hold*. There are several reasons why a hold may be issued, including: (1) the sponsor does not have sufficient data to completely assess risks to subjects; (2) the risk to the subjects appears significant; (3) the Investigator's Brochure is misleading, erroneous, or materially incomplete (see details on the Investigator's Brochure later in the chapter); (4) clinical investigators are not qualified by scientific training or experience; (5) the protocol design makes it unlikely to achieve the stated objectives. The US FDA may place certain requirements on the sponsor in order to lift the hold such as performing further preclinical studies, modifying the protocol, or obtaining investigators with appropriate expertise. Depending on the length of time it takes to meet the requirements, it may take months or even years to gain final US FDA approval of the IND application.

After the IND number is issued, the clinical trials may commence. During the trials, the sponsor is responsible for keeping the US FDA aware of any serious adverse problems that may jeopardize the subjects' safety. Such reports may result in the US FDA placing a hold on the clinical trial. Once again, the hold may be lifted once further information is obtained or the protocol is modified to improve subject safety. The safety concerns may be of such a magnitude that the trial is permanently suspended.

In the USA, the sponsor also must register phase II and phase III clinical trials on the government's clinical trials website www.clinicaltrials.gov. (Note that the EMA has the EU Clinical Trials register [www.clinicaltrialsregister.eu/].) The trial is then given a unique ClinicalTrials.gov identifier number to track the progress of the trial from recruitment to reporting the results.

If the sponsor feels the clinical trials demonstrate adequate vaccine efficacy and safety, the sponsor submits the results to the US FDA as part of a New Drug Application (NDA). The US FDA considers the NDA primarily by examining the risk-benefit ratio. If the risk-benefit ratio is favorable, the US FDA approves the NDA for specific populations and indications supported by the provided data. The US FDA licensure of the quadrivalent HPV vaccine illustrates this practice. The vaccine was initially licensed in females aged 9 to 26 years old for the prevention of genital warts along with cervical, vulvar and vaginal dysplastic lesions, and cancer. At the time, the licensure did not include older women, males, or other diseases such as anal cancer. Although it was reasonably assumed the vaccine could benefit older women and males, and the vaccine could prevent other diseases related to HPV, the NDA did not include the data to support such indications. Once licensed, the vaccine may be marketed to consumers for only the approved indications.

During the IND process, the US FDA may inspect and audit the clinical research sites for several different reasons. Some audits are random surveillance to help ensure compliance with the protocol and regulations. Other audits may be "for cause" to investigate a complaint or the cause of a serious adverse event or unanticipated problem.

Important terms to know

- **Contract research organization (CRO):** A company that can be contracted to perform one or more of the clinical trials' related duties.
- **Good clinical practice (GCP):** Set of guidelines that standardize how clinical trials are performed.
- **Good laboratory practice (GLP):** Set of guidelines that standardize how preclinical testing of potential test articles (future approved drugs and vaccines) are performed.
- **Good manufacturing practice (GMP):** Set of guidelines that standardize how potential test articles (future approved drugs and vaccines) are produced.
- **Human Research Ethics Committee (HREC)/ Independent Ethics Committee (IEC)/Institutional Review Board (IRB):** A committee charged with the responsibility to examine ethical issues of a clinical study.
- **International Conference on Harmonisation of Technical Requirements for Registration of Pharmaceuticals for Human Use (ICH):** International committee charged with minimizing conflicting regulatory requirements of each country in order to expedite the approval process of drugs and vaccines in multiple countries.
- **Investigator's Brochure (IB):** A collection of the preclinical and clinical data that exist for a given candidate drug or vaccine.
- **Investigational new drug (IND):** Application filed with the US FDA that contains preclinical data and manufacturing information that helps the US FDA determine if the candidate drug or vaccine is safe to administer to humans; required prior to initiation of clinical trial in the USA.
- **New Drug Application (NDA):** Application filed with the US FDA that contains clinical trial data and is required prior to marketing and sales of a drug or vaccine.

A common trigger for an audit is the NDA. In this case, the primary objective is to verify the validity and veracity of the data by ensuring they were recorded, analyzed, and accurately reported according to the protocol, good clinical practice (GCP), and the regulatory requirements.

Good clinical practice (GCP)

The first International Conference on Harmonisation of Technical Requirements for Registration of Pharmaceuticals for Human Use (ICH) was held in 1990 due to the realization that drug and vaccine development had become a truly global enterprise. The group sought to minimize differing government regulatory requirements that made it difficult for the pharmaceutical industry to perform global clinical trials. The conference brought together the government drug regulatory authorities and pharmaceutical industry of three regions: Europe, Japan, and the USA. Over time, this group developed a set of guidelines known as *good clinical practice* (GCP) that standardizes the way in which clinical trials are performed.

ICH harmonization activities are governed by the Steering Committee. Currently the committee membership is composed of two representatives from each of the sponsoring agencies. These sponsors include the European Commission, representing the EU; the European Federation of Pharmaceutical Industries and Associations (EFPIA); the Japanese MHLW; Japan Pharmaceutical Manufacturers Association (JPMA); the US FDA; and the Pharmaceutical Research and Manufacturers of America (PhRMA). The International Federation of Pharmaceutical Manufacturers & Associations (IFPMA) provides the ICH Secretariat and also participates as a nonvoting member of the Steering Committee. The Secretariat is responsible for the day-to-day management of ICH, including the organization of committee and working group meetings and the associated documentation. There are three organizations with observer status and they include WHO, Health Canada, and the EFTA (representing Iceland, Liechtenstein, Norway, and Switzerland). In 1999, the ICH Steering Committee formed a subcommittee known as the Global Cooperation Group (GCG) to spread GCP harmonization to other regions by working with other groups and countries

such as the Asia-Pacific Economic Cooperation (APEC), the Association of Southeast Asian Nations (ASEAN), the Gulf Cooperation Council (GCC), the Pan American Network on Drug Regulatory Harmonization (PANDRH), the South African Development Community (SADC), Australia, Brazil, China, Chinese Taipei, India, South Korea, Russia, and Singapore.

The standardization of research practices ensures that effective, high-quality medicines and vaccines are developed in a resource-efficient manner without compromising safety. In other words, following ICH-GCP standards ensures the validity and integrity of the data so that information from trials in other countries can be used for licensure. For example, prior to ICH-GCP, it was not uncommon for the FDA or EMA to refuse to consider data derived from trials outside their jurisdiction while requiring similar or nearly identical trials be performed in their own countries. Reducing duplication helps control the expense of research and development while minimizing the delay in making safe and efficacious new treatments available. At the same time, such standards keep human volunteers from being placed at needless risk due to poorly designed and performed clinical trials that may produce data that are not interpretable or reliable. Following ICH-GCP ensures quality data. Additionally, the elimination of duplication helps reduce the number of subjects burdened or placed at risk through participation in clinical trials.

GCP outlines the responsibilities of the sponsor, the investigator, and the independent ethics committee or institutional review board.

The sponsor

Table 15.2 shows an overview of the responsibilities of the sponsor. The sponsor is accountable for the conduct of the entire clinical trial. Sponsors are responsible for filing all of the necessary regulatory paperwork as well as establishing all necessary contracts and agreements. For example, the sponsor may need to contract a qualified laboratory to determine antibody levels or perform safety blood work. Other contracts may be with the clinical sites, investigators, vaccine suppliers, shippers, etc.

Protocol design is another important sponsor responsibility. Qualified medical and scientific experts

Table 15.2 GCP Sponsor Responsibilities

GCP Sponsor Responsibilities
• Ensure the quality of the clinical trial
• Obtain agreements between appropriate entities (e.g., university, research sites, laboratory, manufacturer)
• Employ appropriate expertise (e.g., physicians, scientists, biostatisticians)
• Design trial
• Manage the trial including data handling and record keeping
• Select investigators (sites) based on expertise and ability to perform study
• Gain approval/ notify regulatory authorities (e.g., US FDA, EMA)
• Confirm IRB approval
• Maintain Investigator's Brochure (IB)
• Manufacture, package, label, and code investigational product (IP)
• Ensure the supply and handling of investigational product
• Guarantee record access for audits (e.g., IRB, US FDA)
• Maintain safety information
• Report adverse events
• Report study site noncompliance (e.g., IRB, US FDA)
• Monitor and audit sites

must be involved in the design and conduct of the trial. Medical expertise is important to safeguard the safety of subjects and to handle health-related issues that may arise during the clinical trial. The sponsor is also held accountable for timely reporting of any adverse event that occurs to a subject while on study.

The sponsor must control the consistency and quality of the study vaccine through each step, from manufacturing through administration to the subject. Shipping is often difficult as packages may be exposed to temperature extremes while vaccine quality usually depends on the product remaining within a narrow temperature range. The distribution and storage of the vaccine within the required temperature range is referred to as the *cold chain*. The sponsor is responsible for documentation that the cold chain remained unbroken during the study. They are also responsible for the unused/returned investigational study vaccine.

Sponsors are accountable for each clinical site and must monitor them. Before the trial may begin at a site, the sponsor performs a site activation visit. The purpose of the visit is to ensure the site is prepared to store and handle study vaccine, properly enroll subjects, document study data, and handle laboratory specimens. Once the site is enrolling subjects, regular monitoring visits are made to confirm that the rights and well-being of subjects are being protected and that the trial data are accurate, complete, and verifiable. Finally, the sponsor is obligated to ensure that all sites, source documents, and data are available for inspection and auditing by appropriate domestic and foreign regulatory authorities. Retention of records including source documents, data, and samples are required to be retained 2–16 years after the completion of the study, depending on the circumstances and the regulatory agency. Completion of the study is signified by either the approval of a marketing application/license or the disapproval or termination of the clinical trial.

Sometimes the sponsor may hire a contract research organization (CRO) to perform one or more of a sponsor's trial related duties or functions. A CRO may be a commercial or academic organization or an individual. A sponsor may choose to use a CRO because the sponsor lacks the expertise to manage all of the aspects of a clinical trial or because it may be more cost-effective to outsource the work.

Sponsors are also expected to maintain document called the *Investigator's Brochure (IB)*. The IB is a compilation of the preclinical and clinical data that exist for the vaccine. The IB is a living document that grows in length as the results of more studies become available and are added. The purpose of the IB is to keep those involved with the trial apprised of all the information available on the candidate vaccine. If the results from the clinical trials are positive, the information in the IB becomes part of the NDA.

The investigator

Table 15.3 shows an overview of the responsibilities of the investigator. The investigator is the person responsible for the conduct of the clinical trial at a trial site. In the event that the trial is conducted by a team, the investigator is the leader of the team. Usually, the investigator is a physician possessing

Table 15.3 GCP Investigator Responsibilities

- Knowledgeable of investigational product, protocol, and Investigator's Brochure
- Ensure sufficient personal time to properly conduct the trial
- Permit monitoring and auditing (sponsor, IRB, US FDA)
- Delegate significant trial-related duties only to qualified persons
- Recruit the required number of suitable subjects within the agreed recruitment period
- Employ a qualified physician responsible for all trial-related medical decisions (usually the investigator fills this position)
- Ensure adequate medical care is provided to a subject for any adverse events related to the trial
- Inform a subject when medical care is needed for intercurrent illness unrelated to the trial
- Conduct the trial in compliance with the protocol agreed to by the sponsor and approved by the IRB
- Document and explain any deviation from the approved protocol

Table 15.4 Common Mistakes Leading to Noncompliance

- Poor supervision and training of study staff
- Insufficient involvement in study conduct
- Inappropriate delegation of study tasks to unqualified persons
- Failure to adequately protect study subjects
- Overworked investigator and study staff

the medical expertise and required licensure to make medical decisions and provide medical care if necessary. The investigator leads the clinical trial team and delegates critical trial procedures to other members of the group. The first and foremost of the investigator's responsibilities is to be thoroughly familiar with the protocol and to comply with the protocol. The only time it is acceptable to break from the protocol is when the well-being of a subject is immediately threatened. The investigator must obtain approval for the trial from an institutional review board (IRB) or independent ethics committee (IEC). The investigator is required to ensure that all subjects have provided their informed consent. The investigator must ascertain the accuracy of all data and maintain the appropriate documentation as required by regulations. The investigator must report all adverse events as specified in the protocol to the IRB and sponsor. Table 15.4 provides an overview of common mistakes leading to noncompliance.

In the USA, the US FDA requires the investigator to sign a Form 1572. The EMA, TGA, and the PMDA do not require this type of form. Signing the form indicates the investigator's commitment: (1) to personally conduct or supervise the trial; (2) to ensure all members of the team are informed of their obligations; (3) that all subjects have provided informed consent; (4) that IRB approval is maintained; and (5) that adverse events are reported to the sponsor and appropriate regulatory authorities. Investigators can face significant penalties for failure to live up to their commitment. Penalties include warning letters from the US FDA, restrictions and debarments in conducting US FDA regulated research, and criminal prosecution resulting in prison and fines. The US FDA provides the investigator an opportunity to explain deviations prior to decisions on penalties. In the case of penalties, the investigator is held responsible by the national regulatory authority for not following GCP, while for GLP the head of the organization is held responsible by the regulatory authorities.

Institutional review boards and independent ethics committees

Table 15.5 provides an overview of the responsibilities of institutional review boards and independent ethics committees. The committee charged with examining the ethical issues of a clinical study is known in the USA as an *institutional review board (IRB)* and commonly in Europe as an *independent ethics committee (IEC)*. The IRB/IEC must approve the conduct of the study for a given clinical trial site. Most universities and medical organizations have their own IRBs but some may utilize an IRB that is outside of their organization, which is often referred to as an *external* or *central IRB*. Such external IRBs are often run by commercial entities, but others are supported by govern-

Table 15.5 Institutional Review Board Responsibilities

- Safeguard the rights, safety, and well-being of all trial subjects, paying special attention to trials that include vulnerable subjects
- Ensure the qualifications of the investigator
- Review both the amount and method of payment to subjects to ensure that neither presents problems of coercion or undue influence on the trial subjects
- Render an opinion on a clinical trial such that it is either approved, approved with modifications, deferred, or disapproved
- Conduct continuing review of each ongoing trial at intervals appropriate to the degree of risk to human subjects, but at least once per year

mental agencies in order to maintain a high degree of expertise. An example of the latter is the US National Cancer Institute Central IRB that maintains panels of oncology experts from across the nation.

In the USA, the Office for Human Research Protections (OHRP) oversees the rules for operating an IRB as set forth in the Code of Federal Regulations for the Protection of Human Subjects (CFR 45 Part 46). The regulations state that an IRB must consist of at least five members with the expertise to complete an adequate review of all aspects of the research activities. The membership must include a scientist as well as a non-scientist, and at least one of the members must not be affiliated with the institution. The committee should be diverse, including members of different races, genders, and cultural backgrounds. The goal is to represent a number of views that will reflect community values and protect individual rights.

IRB members participating as an investigator or collaborator in a study or with financial interest in a protocol are considered to have a conflict of interest. Members are not allowed to participate in committee discussions or decisions related to protocol with which they have a conflict. The one exception is that the IRB may request specific information from the member with a conflict if the member has expertise related to the subject.

An IRB has the authority to approve, require modifications to secure approval, or disapprove protocols. In order to approve a protocol, the IRB must determine that all of the following requirements are met: (1) risks to subjects are minimized to the greatest extent possible; (2) risks to subjects are reasonable in relation to anticipated benefits; (3) selection of subjects is equitable; (4) informed consent will be sought from each prospective subject or the subject's legal representative; (5) the research plan makes adequate provision for monitoring the data collected to ensure the safety of subjects.

Ensuring informed consent is one of the most important responsibilities of the IRB. To put it clearly, the individual has the right to know what participation entails and what the possible risks and benefits may be. Based on this information, the individual has the right to participate or not.

The IRB also has a duty to protect vulnerable individuals participating in clinical research. These individuals may be unable to freely give informed consent or may be at higher risk of physical, psychological, or economic damage. The classic vulnerable populations are pregnant women, fetuses, infants, children, the mentally incapacitated (also referred to as *decisionally impaired*), and prisoners. For instance, pregnant women require special safeguards because an investigational product may lead to birth defects in the fetus. At times, other groups may be considered vulnerable, such as socioeconomically disadvantaged individuals, for example, who may ignore risks just to receive compensation because they are desperate for money.

Five key requirements must be met for IRB approval

1. Risks to subjects are minimized to the greatest extent possible
2. Risks to subjects are reasonable in relation to anticipated benefits
3. Selection of subjects is equitable
4. Informed consent will be sought from each prospective subject or the subject's legal representative
5. The research plan makes adequate provision for monitoring the data collected to ensure the safety of subjects

Conclusion

Clinical trials are an important step in vaccine development. Governmental agencies heavily regulate clinical trials in an effort to protect the rights and safety of human subjects and ensure the validity of the study data.

Summary

- The testing of investigational vaccines in humans is called *clinical trials* or *clinical research*.

- Clinical trials are conducted in a highly structured manner and are heavily regulated.

- There are four phases of clinical trials. The first three are performed to demonstrate safety and efficacy (phases I, II, and III). The fourth phase is conducted after licensure and marketing to gather more information about the vaccine or expand indications.

- Governmental bodies such as the US Food and Drug Administration and the European Medicines Agency regulate the conduct of clinical trials.

- The International Conference on Harmonisation of Technical Requirements for Registration of Pharmaceuticals for Human Use (ICH) seeks to minimize differing government regulatory requirements that make it difficult for the pharmaceutical industry to perform global clinical trials. The ICH has created guidelines for the conduct of clinical trials known as *good clinical practice* (GCP).

- The ICH-GCP guidelines outline the responsibilities of the clinical trial sponsor, the principal investigator, and the independent ethics committee/institutional review board.

Further reading

Code of Federal Regulations, Title 45, Public Welfare, Department of Health and Human Services, Part 46, Protection Of Human Subjects. Last revised January 15, 2010. http://www.hhs.gov/ohrp/humansubjects/guidance/45cfr46.html.

European Medicines Agency. 2014. http://www.ema.europa.eu/ema/index.jsp?curl=pages/about_us/general/general_content_000091.jsp&murl=menus/about_us/about_us.jsp&mid=WC0b01ac0580028a42&jsenabled=true.

FDA Investigational New Drug (IND) Application. Page last updated: October 18, 2013. http://www.fda.gov/Drugs/DevelopmentApprovalProcess/HowDrugsareDevelopedandApproved/ApprovalApplications/InvestigationalNewDrugINDApplication/default.htm.

FDA Guidance on Investigator Responsibilities. 2009. http://www.fda.gov/downloads/drugs/guidancecomplianceregulatoryinformation/guidances/ucm187772.pdf.

International Conference on Harmonisation. 2014. http://www.ich.org/home.html.

16 Vaccine recommendations and special populations

Richard E. Rupp and Bridget E. Hawkins

Sealy Center for Vaccine Development, University of Texas Medical Branch, Galveston, TX, USA

Abbreviations

AAFP	American Academy of Family Physicians	IND	Investigational new drug
AAP	American Academy of Pediatrics	JCVI	UK Committee on Vaccination and Immunization
ACIP	Advisory Committee on Immunization Practices	JE	Japanese encephalitis
ATAGI	Australian Technical Advisory Group on Immunization	MMR	Measles, mumps, and rubella
		MMRV	Measles, mumps, rubella, and varicella
CBRN	Chemical, biological, radiological, and nuclear	NIC	Australian National Immunization Committee
CDC	US Centers for Disease Control and Prevention	PMDA	Japanese Pharmaceuticals and Medical Devices Agency
EMA	European Medicines Agency	TGA	Therapeutic Goods Administration
HHS	Health and Human Services	US FDA	US Food and Drug Administration

What happens after a vaccine is licensed?

Most countries have a regulatory body whose duty it is to determine whether to approve and license a vaccine or not. The US Food and Drug Administration (US FDA) licenses vaccines for human use in the USA while the European Medicines Agency (EMA) performs the same function for the European Union (EU). Japan's Ministry of Health, Labor and Welfare's Pharmaceuticals and Medical Devices Agency (PMDA) and Australia's National Health and Medical Research Council's Therapeutic Goods Administration (TGA) also approve the use of vaccines in their respective countries. Each country mentioned above has established similar pathways for vaccine licensure in order to streamline the approval process, making it quicker

and easier for international companies to obtain global approval for their products. The US FDA and EMA have issued a "General Principles" statement on parallel scientific advice for those submitting applications to both the USA and EU for vaccine approval. This mechanism makes it easier for US FDA and EU officials to converse with each other regarding any regulatory issues that may arise during the drug or vaccine development process, thus avoiding unnecessary duplication of tests, which makes the vaccine development and approval process more efficient.

The vaccine license itself contains specific indications for vaccine usage based on clinical trial data provided by the pharmaceutical company. A vaccine may not be licensed for all population groups or possess indications for which there is no evidence of

Vaccinology: An Essential Guide, First Edition. Edited by Gregg N. Milligan and Alan D.T. Barrett.
© 2015 John Wiley & Sons, Ltd. Published 2015 by John Wiley & Sons, Ltd.

safety or efficacy, and this is particularly true if such clinical trials have not been completed. Pharmaceutical companies may only market the vaccine based on the approved indications. Marketing is not allowed based on anecdotal evidence or studies not accepted by the licensing agency. On the other hand, physicians are not limited to the licensed indications and may use the vaccine for non-approved purposes based on medical judgment. Utilization of a vaccine in a non-approved manner is termed *off-label use*.

Definition

Licensed indication and usage: A licensed indication is a legally valid reason for using a vaccine product. Approved indications are very specific and may include an age group, gender, and purpose. The original approval of the quadravalent human papillomavirus (HPV) vaccine in the USA was for the use in females aged 9 to 26 years old for the prevention of cervical, vaginal and vulvar dysplasia, and cancer and genital warts caused by human papillomavirus types 6, 11, 16, and 18. Some physicians used the vaccine off-label by vaccinating high-risk men (those having sex with other men) in the belief that the men would benefit from vaccination although the studies were not complete at the time. Eventually such trials were completed and presented to the US FDA, and the indications were expanded to include males and the prevention of anal dysplasia and anal cancer.

Recommendations

Vaccine licensure by itself does not guarantee vaccine utilization or marketability. Recommendations made by various governmental and nongovernmental organizations play a key role in the uptake (use) of a vaccine. In making their recommendations, these organizations take into account disease severity and epidemiology, vaccine efficacy, and safety profile along with the cost-effectiveness of each vaccine (Table 16.1).

The most influential body making vaccine recommendations in the USA is the Advisory Committee on Immunization Practices (ACIP). This committee provides advice and guidance to the Secretary of the Department of Health and Human Services (HHS), the Assistant Secretary for HHS, and the Director of the Centers for Disease Control and Prevention (CDC),

Table 16.1 Factors Considered in Making Universal Vaccine Recommendations

Disease	Likelihood of a Universal Recommendation	
	Less	**More**
Incidence	Rare	Common
Morbidity	Trivial	Significant
Mortality	Low	High
Treatable	Easy	Difficult (untreatable)
Vaccine		
Frequency adverse effects	Common	Rare
Severity adverse effects	Serious	Minor
Efficacy	Low	High
Costs		
Disease	High	Low
Vaccination	Low	High

regarding the appropriate use of vaccines. ACIP provides written recommendations for the routine administration of vaccines to children and adults in the civilian population. These recommendations form the basis for the immunization schedules that are used throughout the USA.

Definition

Licensed indications versus recommendations: *Licensed indications* are quite rigid, as they are based on clinical data presented to the licensing agency. On the other hand, *recommendations* take into account clinical data as well as established knowledge and actual circumstances. This is illustrated by the case of the meningococcal conjugate quadrivalent vaccines. The licensed indication is for a single dose in normal risk individuals 2–55 years of age, while the initial ACIP recommendation was for a single dose in 11–12 year olds. The recommendation was based on the belief that protection would last approximately 10 years, thereby covering the high-risk early college years. In 2011, when it appeared that protection may only last 3–5 years, ACIP broadened its recommendation to include a second "booster" dose at age 16. While the recommendation has changed on this subject, the licensed indication and usage has not.

ACIP comprises 15 experts in fields associated with immunization and are appointed by the Secretary of HHS, 8 *ex officio* members representing other federal agencies responsible for immunization programs (e.g., Indian Health Service, National Vaccine Program Office, Center for Medicaid), and 26 nonvoting representatives who act as liaisons for organizations with immunization expertise (e.g., American Academy of Pediatrics, National Association of County and City Health Officials, American Medical Association). The participation of these nongovernmental organizations in ACIP deliberations is essential for several reasons. One reason is that harmonization of recommendations from the organizations sends a clear, unambiguous message. Secondly, many physicians are often hesitant to follow new vaccine recommendations without the endorsement of their professional associations.

The Australian Technical Advisory Group on Immunisation (ATAGI) serves a similar function as the USA's ACIP. ATAGI consults with the National Immunization Committee (NIC) to provide recommendations for immunizations for young children through older adulthood. This advisory group is composed of technical experts, consumers, and general practitioners.

The Joint Committee on Vaccination and Immunisation (JCVI) is the UK's advisory group that provides statements, advice, and recommendations concerning vaccines. Members of this committee are appointed on merit by the Appointment Commission of the Department of Health. JCVI makes recommendations to the Ministry of Health about which vaccines should be administered, and these recommendations are the basis for determining the immunization schedules for the UK.

Japan's government has an opt-in immunization policy where it is an individual's choice to receive vaccinations, and if they choose to do so, they should first consult their physician. The physicians have a list of suggested vaccinations, similar to the immunization schedules of the USA and EU, but with a few modifications. Japan does not recommend hepatitis A or B, *Haemophilus influenza* type b (Hib), human papillomavirus, *Meningococcus*, mumps, *Pneumococcus*, rotavirus, and varicella vaccines. Japanese encephalitis (JE) virus vaccine is recommended in Japan, whereas it is not in the USA and Europe. This is an example of a vaccine recommendation in one country (Japan) where the disease (JE) is endemic but not in the USA or Europe where the disease is not found. However, both the USA and Europe recommend the vaccine for travelers to Asia.

The WHO has a set of universal recommendations for childhood and adult vaccines for countries to use as a guide in developing their own recommendations (Figure 16.1). As stated above, individual countries have specific recommendations made by their national Ministry of Health.

A case of disparate recommendations

During the 1980s it became apparent that individuals would require a second dose of the measles, mumps, rubella vaccine (MMR) to control the spread of measles. The American Academy of Pediatrics (AAP) recommended the second dose at approximately 11–12 years of age while the Advisory Committee on Immunization Practices (ACIP) and American Academy of Family Physicians (AAFP) recommended the dose be given at 4–6 years of age at the time of school entry. Both recommendations were based on sound reasoning. The existence of two different recommendations led to some confusion among health care providers and the populace that likely led to lower vaccination rates. Recognizing this, the AAP brought its recommendations in line with the other organizations.

Mandates

Some vaccines may have such a substantial potential for impacting public health that their use is mandated by governmental bodies. In many countries, the responsible entity is the ministry of health. In the USA, the power to enact laws requiring vaccination for daycare or school attendance and even employment in certain fields lies with the individual states. Generally, vaccines that are not mandated have poor uptake, while vaccination rates are much higher for mandated vaccines. In this era, the unfamiliarity of the general public in developed nations with the dreadfulness of many vaccine-preventable diseases such as measles, polio, and diphtheria contributes to a lack of motivation to receive vaccinations. Mandates provide an additional incentive for vaccination, as most families desire their children to attend daycare and schools. Additionally, mandates are often associated with public monies for vaccinating underinsured populations.

Antigen		Children (see Table 2 for details)		Adolescents	Adults	Considerations (see footnotes for details)
Recommendations for all						
BCG[1]		1 dose				Exceptions HIV
Hepatitis B[2]		3–4-doses (see footnote for schedule options)		3 doses (for high-risk groups if not previously immunized) (see footnote)		Birth dose Premature and low birth weight Co-administratiion and combination vaccine Definition high-risk
Polio[3]		3–4 doses (at least one dose of IPV) with DTP				OPV birth dose Type of vaccine Transmission and importation risk criteria
DTP[4]		3 doses	Booster (DTP) 1–6 years of age	Booster (Td) (see footnote)	Booster (Td) early adulthood or pregnancy	Delayed/interrupted schedule Combination vaccine
Haemophilus influenzae type b[5]	Option 1	3 doses, with DTP				Single dose if ≥ 12 months of age Not recommended for children > 5 yrs old Delayed/interrupted schedule Co-administration and combination vaccine
	Option 2	2 or 3 doses, with booster at least 6 months after last dose				
Pneumococcal (Conjugate)[6]	Option 1	3 doses, with DTP				Vaccine options Initiate before 6 months of age Co-administration HIV + and preterm neonates booster
	Option 2	2 doses before 6 months of age, plus booster dose at 9–15 months of age				
Rotavirus[7]		Rotarix: 2 doses with DTP RotaTeq: 3 doses with DTP				Vaccine options Not recommended if > 24 months old
Measles[8]		2 doses				Combination vaccine; HIV early vaccination; Pregnancy
Rubella[9]		1 dose (see footnote)		1 dose (adolescent girls and/or child bearing aged women if not previously vaccinated; see footnote)		Achieve and sustain 80% coverage Combination vaccine and co-administration Pregnancy
HPV[10]				3 doses (girls)		Vaccination of males for prevention of cervical cancer is not recommended at this time

Figure 16.1 The 2014 WHO-recommended immunization chart for routine immunization. This table summarizes the WHO vaccination recommendations. It is designed to assist the development of country-specific schedules and is not intended for direct use by health care workers. Country specific schedules should be based on local epidemiologic, programmatic, resource, and policy considerations. While vaccines are universally recommended, some children may have contraindications to particular vaccines. Refer to http://www.who.int/immunization/documents/positionpapers/ for the footnotes and most recent version of this table. This version was updated February 26, 2014.

What are vaccination schedules?

Vaccination schedules are a tabular form of the vaccine recommendations for different populations. The most commonly utilized schedules are for different age groups. In the USA, ACIP has schedules for the 0–18 years of age (Figure 16.2) and adult (Figure 16.3) age groups. In addition to the routine schedules there are "catch-up" schedules created for individuals who did not get vaccinated on the routine schedule or their vaccination record is lost or no longer available (Figure 16.4). Catch-up schedules take into account that fewer doses may be required in older individuals as well as minimal vaccination intervals. For example,

vaccination for *Haemophilus influenzae* type b routinely requires a four-dose series with the first at 2 months of age, while a child starting the series between 12 and 14 months requires two doses, and a child starting between 15 and 59 months of age requires only one dose. Unvaccinated individuals over the age of 6 years are considered immune, and it is not recommended they receive the vaccine at all. Similarly, routine measles, mumps, rubella (MMR) vaccination is performed routinely at 12–15 months of age and repeated at 4–6 years of age. In the catch-up schedule for an older individual with no record of vaccination, the second vaccination is given only 4 weeks after the first dose.

Antigen	Children (see Table 2 for details)	Adolescents	Adults	Considerations (see footnotes for details)
Recommendations for certain regions				
Japanese Encephalitis[11]	*Live attenuated vaccine*: 1 dose Booster after 1 year *Mouse brain-derived vaccine*: 2 doses, and booster after 1 year and then every 3 years	*Mouse brain-derived vaccine*: booster every 3 years up to 10–15 years of age		Vaccine options
Yellow Fever[12]	1 dose, with measles containing vaccine			
Tick-Borne Encephalitis[13]	3 doses (> 1 yr FSME-Immun and Encepur: > 3 yrs TBE-Moscow and EnceVir) with at least 1 booster dose (every 3 years for TBE-Moscow and EnceVir)			Definition of high-risk Vaccine options; Timing of booster
Recommendations for some high-risk populations				
Typhoid[14]	*Vi polysaccharide vaccine*: 1 dose; *Ty21a live oral vaccine*; 3–4 doses (see footnote). Booster dose 3–7 years after primary series			Definition of high-risk Vaccine options
Cholera[15]	*Dukoral (WC-rBS)*: 3 doses ≥ 2–5 yrs, booster every 6 months; 2 doses adults/children > 6 yrs, booster every 2nd year; *Shanchol & mORCVAX*: 2 doses ≥1 yrs, booster dose after 2 yrs			Minimum age Definition of high-risk
Meningococcal[16] — MenA conjugate	1 dose (1–29 years)			Definition of high-risk; Vaccine options
Meningococcal[16] — MenC conjugate	2 doses (2–11 months) with booster 1 year after 1 dose (≥ 12 months)			
Meningococcal[16] — Quadrivalent conjugate	2 doses (9–23 months) 1 dose (≥ 2 years)			
Hepatitis A[17]	At least 1 dose ≥ 1 year of age			Level of endemicity; Vaccine options; Definition of high risk groups
Rabies[18]	3 doses			Definition of high-risk; Booster
Recommendations for immunization programmes with certain characteristics				
Mumps[19]	2 doses, with measles containing vaccine			Coverage criteria > 80% Combination vaccine
Influenza (inactivated)[20]	First vaccine use: 2 doses Revaccinate annually: 1 dose only (see footnote)	1 dose from 9 yrs age. Revaccinate annually (see footnote)		Priority targets Definition of high-risk Lower dosage for children

Figure 16.1 (*Continued*)

Definition

Vaccine exemptions: Individual states in the USA vary widely on their vaccine exemption policies. All states allow for exemptions based on medical reasons while 48 allow exemptions for religious reasons (Mississippi and West Virginia do not). Fifteen states allow exemptions for philosophical objections as well. Medical exemptions usually require documentation from a health care provider. Some states make religious and philosophical exemptions more convenient by allowing a parent (or legal guardian) to fill out a simple single-use form to opt-out of immunizations while other states may discourage exemptions by requiring annual certification from health departments or school officials.

Are there any exceptions for certain people (special populations)?

Different groups within the population may require special consideration when vaccine recommendations are made. These considerations involve immune competency and risk of disease.

Children

Newborns and infants are highly susceptible to infectious diseases due to the immaturity and naivety of their immune system. The innate weaknesses in the infant immune system have yet to be well characterized and understood. The very same limitations that leave infants and young children vulnerable also decrease the efficacy of vaccination resulting in an extensive vaccine schedule (Figure 16.2). Infants and children require repeated doses and boosters in order to obtain and then maintain protective immunity. The vaccination schedule is actually the basis for the well-child health visits (i.e., routine infant and child exams). In the USA, vaccination is routinely performed at 2, 4, 6, 9, 12, 15, 18, and 24 months of age. Even with such an intensive schedule, effective vaccines for

Vaccine	Birth	1 mo	2 mos	4 mos	6 mos	9 mos	12 mos	15 mos	18 mos	19–23 mos	2–3 yrs	4–6 yrs	7–10 yrs	11–12 yrs	13–15 yrs	16–18 yrs
Hepatitis B[1] (HepB)	1st dose	← 2nd dose →					← 3rd dose →									
Rotavirus[2] (RV) RV1 (2-dose series); RV5 (3-dose series)			1st dose	2nd dose	See footnote 2											
Diphtheria, tetanus, & acellular pertussis[3] (DTaP: < 7 yrs)			1st dose	2nd dose	3rd dose			← 4th dose →				5th dose				
Tetanus, diphtheria, & acellular pertussis[4] (Tdap: ≥ 7 yrs)														(Tdap)		
Haemophilus influenzae type b[5] (Hib)			1st dose	2nd dose	See footnote 5		← 3rd or 4th dose See footnote 5 →									
Pneumococcal conjugate[5] (PCV13)			1st dose	2nd dose	3rd dose		← 4th dose →									
Pneumococcal polysaccharide[5] (PPSV23)																
Inactivated poliovirus[7] (IPV) (<18 yrs)			1st dose	2nd dose			← 3rd dose →					4th dose				
Influenza[5] (IIV; LAIV) 2 doses for some: See footnote 8							Annual vaccination (IIV only)						Annual vaccination (IIV or LAIV)			
Measles, mumps, rubella[9] (MMR)							← 1st dose →					2nd dose				
Varicella[10] (VAR)							← 1st dose →					2nd dose				
Hepatitis A[11] (HepA)							← 2-dose series, see footnote 11 →									
Human papillomavirus[12] (HPV2: females only; HPV4: males and females)														(3-dose series)		
Meningococcal[13] (Hib-MenCY ≥ 6 weeks; MenACWY-D ≥ 9 mos; MenACWY-CRM ≥ 2 mos)						See footnote 13								1st dose		Booster

Range of recommended ages for all children

Range of recommended ages for catch-up immunization

Range of recommended ages for certain high-risk groups

Range of recommended ages during which catch-up is encouraged and for certain high-risk groups

Not routinely recommended

Figure 16.2 Recommended immunization schedule for persons aged 0 through 18 years—United States, 2014. This schedule includes recommendations in effect as of January 1, 2014. For those who fall behind or start late, see the catch-up schedule in Figure 16.4. The recommendations must be read along with the footnotes (found at: http://www.cdc.gov/vaccines/schedules/hcp/imz/child-adolescent.html).

VACCINE ▼ AGE GROUP ▶	19–21 years	22–26 years	27–49 years	50–59 years	60–64 years	≥ 65 years
Influenza[2,*]	1 doses annually					
Tetanus, diphtheria, pertussis (Td/Tdap)[3,*]	Substitute 1-time dose of Tdap for Td booster; then boost with Td every 10 yrs					
Varicella[4,*]	2 doses					
Human papillomavirus (HPV) Female[5,*]	3 doses					
Human papillomavirus (HPV) Male[5,*]	3 doses					
Zoster[6]					1 dose	
Measles, mumps, rubella (MMR)[7,*]	1 or 2 doses					
Pneumococcal 13-valent conjugate (PCV13)[8,*]	1 dose					
Pneumococcal polysaccharide (PPSV23)[9,10]	1 or 2 doses					1 dose
Meningococcal[11,*]	1 or more doses					
Hepatitis A[12,*]	2 doses					
Hepatitis B[13,*]	3 doses					
Haemophilus influenzae type b (Hib)[14,*]	1 or 3 doses					

*Covered by the Vaccine Injury Compensation Program

[Shaded box] For all persons in this category who meet the age requirements and who lack documentation of vaccination or have no evidence of previous infection; zoster vaccine recommended regardless of prior episode of zoster

[Shaded box] Recommended if some other risk factor is present (e.g., on the basis of medical, occupational, lifestyle, or other indication)

[Empty box] No recommendation

Report all clinically significant postvaccination reactions to the Vaccine Adverse Event Reporting System (VAERS), Reporting forms and instructions on filling a VAERS report are available at www.vaers.hhs.gov or by telephone, 800-822-7967.

Information on how to file a Vaccine Injury Compensation Program claim is available at www.hrsa.gov/vaccinecompensation or by telephone, 800-338-2382. To file a claim for vaccine injury, contact the U.S. Court of Federal Claims, 717 Madison Place. N.W., Washington, D.C. 20005; telephone, 202-357-6400.

Additional information about the vaccines in this schedule, extent of available date, and contraindications for vaccination is also available at www.cdc.gow/vaccines or from the CDC-INFO Contact Center at 800-CDC-INFO (800-232-4636) in english and spanish, 8:00 a.m. – 8:00 p.m. Eastern Time, Monday - Friday, excluding holidays.

Use of trade names and ssommercial cources is for identification only and does not imply endorsement by the U.S. Department of Health and Human Services.

The recommendations in this schedule were approved by the Centers For Disease Control and Prevention's (CDC) Advisory Committee on Immunization Practices (ACIP), the American Academy of Family Physicians (AAFP), the American College of Physicians (ACP), American College of Obstetricians and Gynecologists (ACOG) and American College of Nurse-Midwives (ACNM).

Figure 16.3 Recommended Adult Immunization Schedule—United States, 2014. The figure below provides adult vaccination schedules according to age. Always use this table in conjunction with their respective footnotes (found at: http://www.cdc.gov/vaccines/schedules/downloads/adult/adult-schedule.pdf).

Persons aged 4 months through 6 years

Vaccine	Minimum Age for Dose 1	Minimum Interval Between Doses			
		Dose 1 to dose 2	Dose 2 to dose 3	Dose 3 to dose 4	Dose 4 to dose 5
Hepatitis B[1]	Birth	4 weeks	8 weeks and at least 16 weeks after first dose; minimum age for the final dose is 24 weeks		
Rotavirus[2]	6 weeks	4 weeks	4 weeks[2]		
Diphtheria, tetanus, & acellular pertussis[3]	6 weeks	4 weeks	4 weeks	6 months	6 months[3]
Haemophilus influenzae type b[5]	6 weeks	4 weeks if first dose administered at younger than age 12 months / 8 weeks (as final dose) if first dose administered at age 12 through 14 months / No further doses needed if first dose administered at age 15 months or older	4 weeks[6] if current age is younger than 12 months and first dose administered at < 7 months old / 8 weeks and age 12 months through 59 months (as final dose)[6] if current age is younger than 12 months and first dose administered between 7 through 11 months (regardless of Hib vaccine [PRP-T or PRP-OMP] used for first dose); OR if current age is 12 through 59 months and first dose administered at younger than age 12 months; OR first 2 doses were PRP-OMP and administered at younger than 12 months. / No further doses needed if previous dose administered at age 15 months or older	8 weeks (as final dose) This dose only necessary for children aged 12 through 59 months who received 3 (PRP-T) doses before age 12 months and started the primary series before age 7 months	
Pneumococcal[6]	6 weeks	4 weeks if first dose administered at younger than age 12 months / 8 weeks (as final dose for healthy children) if first dose administered at age 12 months or older / No further doses needed for healthy children if first dose administered at age 24 months or older	4 weeks if current age is younger than 12 months / 8 weeks (as final dose for healthy children) if current age is 12 months or older / No further doses needed for healthy children if previous dose administered at age 24 months or older	8 weeks (as final dose) This dose only necessary for children aged 12 through 59 months who received 3 doses before age 12 months or for children at high risk who received 3 doses at any age	
Inactivated poliovirus[7]	6 weeks	4 weeks[7]	4 weeks[7]	6 months[7] minimum age 4 years for final dose	
Meningococcal[13]	6 weeks	8 weeks[13]	See footnote 13	See footnote 13	
Measles, mumps, rubella[9]	12 months	4 weeks			
Varicella[10]	12 months	3 months			
Hepatitis A[11]	12 months	6 months			

Persons aged 7 through 18 years

Vaccine	Minimum Age for Dose 1	Dose 1 to dose 2	Dose 2 to dose 3	Dose 3 to dose 4	Dose 4 to dose 5
Tetanus, diphtheria; tetanus, diphtheria & acellular pertussis[4]	7 years[4]	4 weeks	4 weeks if first dose of DTaP/DT administered at younger than age 12 months / 6 months if first dose of DTaP/DT administered at age 12 months or older and then no further doses needed for catch-up	6 months if first dose of DTaP/DT administered at younger than age 12 months	
Human papillomavirus[12]	9 years	Routine dosing intervals are recommended[12]			
Hepatitis A[11]	12 months	6 months			
Hepatitis B[1]	Birth	4 weeks	8 weeks (and at least 16 weeks after first dose)		
Inactivated poliovirus[7]	6 weeks	4 weeks	4 weeks[7]	6 months[7]	
Meningococcal[13]	6 weeks	8 weeks[13]			
Measles, mumps, rubella[9]	12 months	4 weeks			
Varicella[10]	12 months	3 months if person is younger than age 13 years / 4 weeks if person is aged 13 years or older			

Figure 16.4 Catch-up immunization schedule for persons aged 4 months through 18 years who start late or who are more than 1 month behind—United States, 2014. This figure provides catch-up schedules and minimum intervals between doses for children whose vaccinations have been delayed. A vaccine series does not need to be restarted regardless of the time that has elapsed between doses. Use the section appropriate for the child's age. Always use this table in conjunction with the accompanying childhood and adolescent immunization schedule (Figure 16.2) and their respective footnotes (found at: http://www.cdc.gov/vaccines/schedules/downloads/child/0-18yrs-child-combined-schedule.pdf).

certain important pathogens (e.g., influenza, meningococcus) in the first 6 months of life remain elusive.

Combination confusion

Combination vaccines from different pharmaceutical companies often cover different mixes of pathogens. This may lead to difficulty interpreting vaccination records and ordering correct vaccines.

As an example, infants routinely receive injections against diphtheria, tetanus, pertussis, poliovirus, *Haemophilus influenzae* type b, hepatitis B, and pneumococcus. The GlaxoSmithKline product, Pediarix®, covers diphtheria, tetanus, pertussis, poliovirus and **hepatitis B**, whereas Sanofi Pasteur's Pentacel® covers diphtheria, tetanus, pertussis, poliovirus, and ***Haemophilus influenzae* type b**. Sometimes an infant may receive one product at one visit and the other product at another visit. A health provider needs to pay particular attention to counting doses for individual pathogens to ensure the child is protected. There is also the issue of mixing and matching. If multiple visits are needed for immunization, can the health care provider administer the first dose with the vaccine of one manufacturer and then use the vaccine of a different manufacturer for the second dose?

The children's vaccination schedule is full of intricacies. Most children in the USA are routinely vaccinated against 14 different pathogens during the first 2 years of life. This may require as many as five separate immunizations (injections) during some visits and even more if the child is behind on vaccination. Many parents are hesitant to have their children undergo so many injections. Combination vaccines have been developed to limit the number of injections. For example, the live attenuated viruses for measles, mumps, and rubella (MMR) was given as one vaccine but following the introduction of the varicella vaccine resulted in a tetravalent formulation (MMRV) that may all be delivered in the same vaccine.

Health care providers must be knowledgeable about dosing when vaccinating children. Many people are surprised to find out that the dose for many vaccines is the same for infants as older children and adults. For example, both a 2-kg infant and a 75-kg teen receive 10 μg of the hepatitis B vaccine, Engerix-B™ made by GlaxoSmithKline. At other times, vaccine doses differ. For diphtheria, tetanus, and pertussis vaccines the infant actually receives more of some components than an adult. The Sanofi Pasteur product for infants, Daptacel® and the product for older children and adults, Adacel®, contain identical amounts of tetanus toxoid, filamentous hemagglutinin, pertactin, and fimbriae antigens. The infant vaccine contains more than the older children and adult product of the diphtheria toxoid (15 Lf vs. 2 Lf) and pertussis toxin (10 μg vs. 2.5 μg). On the other hand, children younger than 3 years of age usually receive half the adult dose of the injectable influenza vaccine.

Another complexity is that vaccination regimens differ between some of the products for children. A case in point is the rotavirus products. The GlaxoSmithKline product Rotarix® is given at 2 and 4 months of age while the Merck product, Rotateq®, is given at 2, 4, and 6 months of age.

The meaning of Lf

Toxoids, such as diphtheria and tetanus, are quantified using Lf units. Lf units describe the level of antigenic strength and purity of the toxoid by its flocculation value. Vaccine manufacturers use the flocculation test to standardize lots of vaccine made at different times during the production process. This flocculation test is an immunological binding assay that determines the number of antitoxin units it takes to produce an optimally flocculating mixture, when combined with the sample. Visible flocculation occurs when the antigen and antibody form a complex. The Lf or "Limit of Flocculation" is defined as the antigen content forming a 1:1 ratio against 1 unit of antitoxin.

Adults

In the USA, there are no legal mandates for adult vaccination except for those entering the military (see discussion below regarding occupational risk). Some employers may require vaccination for occupations that are at risk such as hepatitis B and influenza vaccine for health care workers or hepatitis A vaccine for food handlers. Laws in other countries vary.

Aging adult population

Although there are no adult mandates in the USA, ACIP has recommended vaccinations throughout adulthood (Figure 16.3). Of special concern are older individuals since their general immunity may be waning. Immunosenescence, age-related changes in immunity, may predispose them to developing illnesses such as influenza and pneumonia, and it may take more boosters of a vaccine to confer the same level of protection as in younger adults. Older adults may wish to obtain seasonal influenza (annually) and pneumococcus (one-time) immunizations to lessen the chance of developing debilitating infections. Recently, a higher dose flu vaccine has become available for seniors. They are also recommended to be vaccinated against varicella zoster (shingles) over the age of 60 and against pneumococcus over the age of 65.

Pregnant women

Historically, pregnancy was a contraindication for vaccination except for the case of tetanus (a subunit toxoid vaccine with no live components). The driving force was the theoretical risk posed to the fetus by live virus vaccines such as the MMR vaccine; in addition, it was felt that other vaccine components may endanger the fetus as well. Over the past 5 decades, many pregnant women have been unintentionally vaccinated because of mistakes and the difficulty of ensuring that women are not pregnant or do not become pregnant shortly after vaccination. There is no evidence from the multitude of cases that there is an increased risk to mother or fetus from any currently available live vaccine. Even so, live virus vaccines remain contraindicated. If they are inadvertently given to a pregnant woman or if a woman becomes pregnant within 4 weeks after vaccination, she should be counseled about the potential effects on the fetus, but vaccination is not ordinarily an indication to terminate the pregnancy. Additionally, no evidence exists of risk to the fetus from immunization with inactivated virus or bacterial or toxoid vaccines.

Several vaccines are recommended for pregnant women who do not have up to date immunizations, such as the inactivated influenza (but not live attenuated influenza vaccine); hepatitis B; and tetanus, diphtheria, and acellular pertussis (Tdap) vaccine. In addition, pregnant women at risk of certain diseases due to travel or exposure are recommended to be vaccinated for pathogens such as meningococcus and rabies.

Newborns

Immunization of the mother during pregnancy with inactivated influenza vaccine (not live influenza vaccine) has been shown to protect the baby. Cocooning is also recommended for influenza, especially because infants under 6 months of age are not vaccinated. Pertussis is usually a minor illness in older children and adults but frequently hospitalizes infants and may result in infant death. Since infants cannot be vaccinated for pertussis until they reach 2 months of age, it is recommended that mother, father, grandparents, and others around the child be vaccinated against pertussis to prevent exposure. Protecting vulnerable individuals by vaccinating those around them is referred to as *cocooning* or *ring immunization*. It is particularly important in the case of pertussis because of its contagiousness and the fact that vaccination is not completely protective in young infants. Maternal antibodies typically last until the infant is 4–6 months of age.

Due to recent pertussis outbreaks, vaccination of women against pertussis during each pregnancy is recommended in the USA. Vaccination is advised during the period from 27 to 36 weeks of pregnancy. The mother should have a strong antibody response about 2 weeks following vaccination. This is expected to maximize transplacental antibody transfer to the infant prior to delivery at 38 to 40 weeks. In addition to cocooning, the maternal antibodies will theoretically provide additional protection for the infant during the first several months of life.

Altered immunocompetence

Having a primary or secondary immune deficiency places individuals at higher risk for certain vaccine preventable diseases. Specific vaccines are recommended for persons with these conditions. The type and degree of immune deficiency may be such that live vaccines may be contraindicated. Individuals may be immunocompromised due to medications and/or radiation given for the treatment of malignancies; due to medications used for treatment of autoimmune or other inflammatory diseases (e.g., corticosteroids, alkylating drugs, or antimetabolites); to prevent rejection in the case of organ transplantation; due to infection by human immunodeficiency virus (HIV) (symptomatic HIV infection or asymptomatic HIV infection when accompanied by evidence of impaired immune function); or the removal or absence of the spleen or thymus.

Vaccines often are less effective during periods of altered immunocompetence.

Administration of live vaccines might need to be deferred until immune function has improved. Inactivated vaccines administered during the period of altered immunocompetence might need to be repeated after immune function has improved. A thorough discussion of the topic of vaccination and altered immune response is beyond the scope of this chapter; thus it will be limited to a brief discussion on vaccination and more common conditions.

Asplenia

Individuals may have a congenital absence of their spleen or lose it due to trauma. Other diseases, such as sickle cell disease, render the spleen nonfunctional. Persons with anatomic or functional asplenia are at higher risk for infections caused by encapsulated organisms such as *Streptococcus pneumoniae*, *Neisseria meningitidis*, and *Haemophilus influenzae*.

Children with asplenia have a 20-fold to 100-fold higher rate of pneumococcal infection compared with healthy children. Children younger than 5 years of age with asplenia should receive an age-appropriate series of pneumococcal conjugate vaccine. Persons older than 2 years of age should receive one dose of the child pneumococcal vaccine along with two doses of the 23-valent pneumococcal polysaccharide vaccine separated by 5 years. There appears to be some indication that having an influenza infection increases the chance that an asplenic person will develop a pneumococcal infection. For this reason, annual influenza immunizations are also recommended for asplenic individuals. Asplenic adults older than age 50 should receive inactivated vaccine as the live vaccine is not currently approved for those aged 50 years and older while healthy children and adults may receive either inactivated or live attenuated influenza vaccines.

Individuals with asplenia infected with *Neisseria meningitidis* are two to three times more likely to succumb to the illness than the general population. Because of this, a quadrivalent meningococcal conjugate vaccine is recommended for individuals with asplenia who are 2 years and older, with a second dose within 3 years for those who received their first dose at 2–6 years of age. Individuals who received their first dose at 6 years of age (or older) are recommended to receive their second dose 8–12 weeks apart, followed by a booster every 5 years afterward.

It is recommended that when elective splenectomy is planned, pneumococcal, meningococcal, and *Haemophilus influenzae* type B vaccinations should be administered, if possible, at least 14 days prior to surgery. If the vaccinations are not administered before surgery, they should be administered after the procedure as soon as the patient's condition is stable.

Thymectomy

Removal of the thymus (thymectomy) does not necessarily result in T-cell immunodeficiency, but it may result in decreased robustness of immune system potency in older adults, particularly if the thymectomy occurred in childhood. In a recent study involving thymectomized children, it was shown that even though they did not have higher infection rates than their non-thymectomized peers, they had decreased levels of CD4+ and CD8+ T cells, which diminished their response to vaccinations.

Human immunodeficiency virus (HIV)

HIV-positive individuals have an increased risk of contracting infectious diseases as their immune systems begin to fail. Of the vaccine-preventable diseases, HIV-positive individuals are known to be at particular risk of complications if infected with wild-type varicella or measles viruses. If possible, individuals with HIV should receive all of their necessary vaccines prior to becoming severely immunocompromised for two reasons: (1) increasing immune system dysfunction may decrease the vigor of the response to vaccination; (2) live attenuated vaccines may pose a threat to severely immunocompromised individuals. HIV-positive individuals who are significantly immunocompromised and untreated may benefit from awaiting vaccination until started on antiretroviral therapy, and their immune function improves. Health care providers should make decisions about the level of immunosuppression and vaccination based on CD4+ T-lymphocyte counts and HIV disease symptoms. For example, for live attenuated yellow fever vaccine, the vaccine is contraindicated when there is symptomatic HIV infection or CD4+ T-lymphocytes are less than $200/mm^3$ (or less than 15% of the total in children

Table 16.2 Typical Travel-Related Vaccines

Vaccine	Recommendation
Hepatitis A	Travel to intermediate- to high-endemicity areas that occur primarily in developing countries
Japanese encephalitis	Travel to endemic rural areas in most of Asia and parts of the western Pacific during transmission season
Meningococcal	Visiting the parts of sub-Saharan Africa known as the "meningitis belt" during the dry season (December–June).
Rabies	Travelers spending a lot of time outdoors in rural areas, involvement in any activities that might result in direct contact with bats, carnivores, and other mammals, or significant occupational risk (such as veterinarians)
Typhoid	Travel to areas in which there is a risk of exposure to *S. Typhi*, mainly to developing countries in Asia, Africa, the Caribbean, and Central and South America
Yellow fever	Travel to areas of countries at risk for transmission in tropical South America and Africa

From http://apps.who.int/immunization_monitoring/en/globalsummary/scheduleselect.cfm

age younger than 6 years). The response to some vaccines can be checked by measuring antibody titers. If titers remain low, repeated vaccination may be indicated.

Other chronic conditions

Although not considered immunocompromised in a classical sense, chronic conditions place individuals at increased risk of complication from several vaccine-preventable diseases. As a result, there are vaccination recommendations for these conditions. Individuals with chronic heart disease, chronic lung disease, diabetes mellitus, and cochlear implants are all recommended to receive pneumococcal vaccination. Those with chronic heart or lung disease; cognitive, neurologic, or neuromuscular disorders; or diabetes mellitus are also targeted for influenza vaccination.

Travelers

International travel places people at risk for many vaccine-preventable diseases. It is important that all routine recommended vaccines are current as travel may expose the traveler to diseases that have been effectively eliminated in their home country, such as measles, diphtheria, and polio. Travel to certain regions of the globe may also expose the traveler to tropical diseases such as JE and yellow fever.

The only vaccine required by International Health Regulations is yellow fever vaccination for travel to certain countries in sub-Saharan Africa and tropical South America. Meningococcal vaccination is required by the government of Saudi Arabia for annual travel during the hajj. Other vaccines are recommended to protect travelers based on a number of factors including destination, time spent in rural areas, the season, age, health status, and previous immunizations (see Table 16.2 for a list of typical travel-related vaccines). Hepatitis A and typhoid vaccinations are recommended for those traveling to countries (such as countries in South America and Africa) that have a moderate to high prevalence for hepatitis A infections and typhoid fever from contaminated food and water. Rabies vaccination is recommended for persons working with animals or for people who plan to be in a high-incidence region of a country for an extended period of time. It is important that travelers only receive the vaccines that they need. For example, although JE is endemic in Asia, the disease is very rare in Singapore and so JE vaccine is not recommended for those visiting Singapore unless the individual is planning to visit adjacent jungle areas.

Behavioral and occupational risks

Adults may face increased risks of exposure to certain diseases based on their behavior and occupation. For instance, people who work with livestock and in meat processing plants may have an increased risk of exposure (over the general adult population) to developing anthrax and Q-fever and may need to be vaccinated to prevent this from occurring. Veterinarians, animal technicians, and people working with wild animals at zoos and refuges may also need to receive a prophylactic rabies vaccination. Certain exotic pets, such as prairie dogs, have also been known to transmit disease, such as monkeypox, to their human companions. As there are no monkeypox vaccines available, people have been given smallpox vaccines, since it is a similar virus and confers some cross-protection.

Health care and lab workers may be exposed to bodily fluids that may contain pathogens. Workers who are at risk for exposure to blood-borne pathogens should receive immunizations against tetanus and hepatitis B. Since hospital staff are routinely exposed to people who have active infections and to people who may be immunocompromised, they may also need to receive influenza vaccinations and, depending on the population they work with and their own health needs, may wish to receive hepatitis A, meningococcal, pertussis, and pneumococcal vaccines as well. Medical aid workers may also need polio and MMR immunizations if they will be traveling to a country where polio is circulating. Vaccinations serve to not only protect the individual, but also their patients, from developing disease symptoms.

Military members and college students living in dorms or close quarters are strongly advised, if not required, to be up to date on their routine vaccinations and be vaccinated against meningitis, as bacterial meningitis can spread very quickly among these groups and can result in morbidity and death. Members of the US military are also required to receive influenza and hepatitis A vaccines and, depending on their deployment and job function, may also receive immunizations against anthrax, smallpox, yellow fever, JE, typhoid, rabies, and hepatitis B. Biomedical researchers may also receive one or more of those vaccinations, depending on what animals, tissues, and pathogens they are working with and their potential exposure levels. Military members and biomedical researchers may also require protection from potential biothreat agents. Some of these countermeasures may not have received full regulatory approval from the US FDA, which would allow marketing of these drugs and vaccines for that particular indication, but may be allowed under investigational new drug (IND) status under the Project BioShield Act.

The Project BioShield Act has three main provisions: (1) relaxing procedures for some chemical, biological, radiological, and nuclear (CBRN) terrorism-related spending, including hiring and awarding research grants; (2) guaranteeing a federal government market for new CBRN medical countermeasures; and (3) permitting emergency use of unapproved countermeasures. The USA has used this mechanism to acquire countermeasures against anthrax, botulism, radiation, and smallpox for military personnel.

Conclusion

Various governmental and nongovernmental organizations may recommend or mandate the use of specific vaccines for certain populations. Vaccine appropriateness is dependent on many factors such as disease prevalence in that particular country, occupational needs and the health status of the individual receiving the vaccine. Each regulating authority has different criteria for making choices about vaccines, but overall the standard schedule for immunizations is similar among countries of the EU, Australia, Japan and the USA.

Summary

- Vaccines are licensed for certain indications. Marketing of vaccines is limited to those indications. Physician use of a vaccine outside of the indications is termed *off-label*.
- Governmental and nongovernmental agencies make recommendations about how a vaccine should be

(Continued)

used. These recommendations are important for the creation of public policy and obtaining the buy-in from physicians.

- Governments may legally mandate vaccination for daycare, school attendance, and certain occupations.
- Vaccination schedules are the tabular form of the recommendations. Health care providers follow the schedules to ensure patients are vaccinated appropriately.
- Special consideration is given when making recommendations for certain populations. These populations include children, adults, those with altered immunocompetence, travelers, and the military.

Further reading

Advisory Committee on Immunization Practices (ACIP). Vaccine Recommendations of the ACIP. http://www.cdc.gov/vaccines/hcp/acip-recs/index.html.

Centers for Disease Control and Prevention. CDC Health Information for International Travel 2012. The Yellow Book (ed GW Brunette). New York: Oxford University Press, 2011.

Centers for Disease Control and Prevention. Travelers' Health. http://wwwnc.cdc.gov/travel/destinations/list.

Doshi P and Akabayashi A (2010). Special Section: International Voices 2010: Japanese Childhood Vaccination Policy. Cambridge Quarterly of Healthcare Ethics 19, 283–289.

European Medicines Agency. http://www.ema.europa.eu/ema/.

Ministry of Health, Labour and Welfare (Japan). http://www.mhlw.go.jp/english/.

Prelog M, Wilk C, Keller M, Karall T, Orth D, Geiger R, Walder G, Laufer G, Cottogni M, Zimmerhackl Lothar B, Stein J, Grubeck-Loebenstein B, and Wuerzner R (2008). Diminshed response to tick-borne encephalitis vaccination in thymectomized children. Vaccine 26, 598–600.

Smith JC (2010). The structure, role, and procedures of the U.S. Advisory Committee on Immunization Practices (ACIP). Vaccine 21, 339–345.

Stephenson JE and Anderson AO. Ethical and research dilemmas in biodefense research. In Medical Aspects of Biological Warfare (ed MK Lenhart), pp. 559–577. Washington, DC: Borden Institute, 2007. ISBN- 978-0-16 -079731-8.

Therapeutic Goods Administration (Australia). http://www.tga.gov.au/.

World Health Organization. http://www.who.int/topics/vaccines/en/.

17 Vaccine safety

Dirk E. Teuwen[1] and Alan D.T. Barrett[2]

[1]UCB Pharma S.A., Brussels, Belgium
[2]Sealy Center for Vaccine Development, University of Texas Medical Branch, Galveston, TX, USA

Abbreviations

AAP	American Academy of Pediatrics	NCVIA	National Childhood Vaccine Injury Act
ACIP	Advisory Committee on Immunization Practices	NDA	New Drug Application
		NHS	British National Health Service
AEFI	Adverse events following immunization	NVIRS	Australian National Centre for Immunization Research and Surveillance
BLA	Biologics License Application		
CAEFISS	Canadian Adverse Event Following Immunization Surveillance System	PAES	Post-authorization efficacy study
		PAS	Post-authorization study
CDC	US Centers of Disease Control and Prevention	PASS	Post-authorization safety study
		PHAC	Public Health Agency of Canada
CIRID	Centre for Immunization and Respiratory Infectious Disease	PLA	Product License Application
		RCA	Rapid Cycle Analysis
CISA	Clinical Immunization Safety Assessment	SORD	Surveillance and Outbreak Response Division
CPRD	Clinical Practice Research Datalink	SYSVAK	Norwegian National Electronic Immunization Register
ELA	Establishment License Application		
ENCePP	European Network of Centres for Pharmacoepidemiology and Pharmacovigilance	TIV	Trivalent influenza vaccine
		TP	Thrombocytopenic Purpura
		UMC	Uppsala Monitoring Centre
EPI	World Health Organization Expanded Programme on Immunization	US FDA	US Food and Drug Administration
		VAERS	Vaccine Adverse Event Reporting System
GBS	Guillain–Barré syndrome		
HMO	Health maintenance organization	VAR	Vaccine Administration Record
IMPACT	Immunization Monitoring Program-Active	VCIP	National Vaccine Injury Compensation Program
IND	Investigational new drug	VENICE II	Vaccine European New Integrated Collaboration Effort
IRB	Institutional review board		
MAH	Marketing Authorization Holder	VIS	Vaccine Information Statements
MCO	Managed care organizations	VSD	Vaccine Safety DataLink
MMR	Measles, mumps, rubella	WHO	World Health Organization

Vaccinology: An Essential Guide, First Edition. Edited by Gregg N. Milligan and Alan D.T. Barrett.
© 2015 John Wiley & Sons, Ltd. Published 2015 by John Wiley & Sons, Ltd.

Introduction

Vaccine pharmacovigilance is defined as the science and activities relating to the detection, assessment, understanding, prevention, and communication of adverse events following immunization (AEFI) or of other vaccine- or immunization-related issues.

Monitoring health problems after vaccination by health care professionals, patients, and consumers is essential to ensure that vaccines are held to the highest standard of safety. Because vaccines are administered to healthy children and adults, a higher standard of safety is generally expected compared to other medical treatments or interventions. The acceptance of adverse reactions to pharmaceutical products given to healthy persons, e.g., vaccines and contraceptives, to prevent certain conditions is much lower than to products used in the treatment of sick people, e.g., antibiotics or chemotherapy.

Safety monitoring is carried out during clinical development and after vaccine licensure, with slightly different objectives. In general, the different monitoring systems in different countries have several objectives, as follows:

- To thoroughly review safety data obtained in the pre-licensure phase I, phase II, and phase III clinical trials
- To actively monitor the safety of marketed vaccine in post-licensure phase IV clinical trials

- To continuously monitor the safety of marketed vaccines
- To identify timely increases in the frequency or severity of previously identified vaccine-related reactions
- To identify previously unknown AEFI that could possibly be related to the vaccine

Vaccine safety in vaccine development

Vaccine manufacturers follow a standard set of steps in the vaccine development process, as also performed by manufacturers of pharmaceutical drugs.

Initial exploratory discovery and nonclinical phase

The exploratory stage is characterized by fundamental laboratory research for the appropriate antigen. These antigens may include virus-like particles, weakened/attenuated or killed viruses or bacteria, weakened/attenuated bacterial toxins, or subunits, among others.

The nonclinical phase may use tissue-culture or cell-culture systems and will require animal testing to assess the safety of the vaccine candidate, its immunogenicity, or ability to induce an optimal immune response. Different animal species are selected and may include mice, rabbits, and rhesus macaque monkeys, among others. As challenge studies are rarely performed in humans, animal challenge studies are unique because they provide an insight into the immune response after infection with the target pathogen. Those studies provide data on the potential cellular responses to be expected in humans, an appropriate starting dose, and route of administration for the subsequent administration to humans.

As discussed in detail in Chapter 12, when a decision is reached to proceed with the human clinical development, the sponsor will proceed with an application for an investigational new drug (IND) to the US Food and Drug Administration (US FDA). The IND describes the manufacturing, production, and testing processes; summarizes the laboratory reports; and describes the safety profile of the vaccine candidate and the proposed study. An institutional review board (IRB), representing an institution where the clinical trial will be conducted, must approve the clinical trial protocol. Once the IND application has been approved by the regulatory authority, the vaccine candidate is subject to three phases of clinical evaluation (discussed in Chapter 15).

Clinical studies with human subjects

Phase I trials

A phase I trial assesses a vaccine candidate in a small group of adults, usually between 20 and 80 subjects with the objective to assess the safety of the vaccine candidate and to determine the type and extent of immune response that the vaccine candidate induces. Such trial may be open-label (not blinded) in that the clinicians and perhaps the subjects know whether a vaccine candidate or placebo is used.

Phase II trials

In phase II trials, a larger group of some hundred individual participants is included with the objective study the vaccine candidate's safety profile, immunogenicity, proposed doses, schedule of immunizations, as well as method of delivery. Some of the individuals may belong to groups at risk of acquiring the disease. These trials are randomized and well controlled, and include a placebo group.

Phase III trials

Phase III trials may involve from thousands to tens of thousands of people with the objective to evaluate vaccine safety and efficacy in such a large group of people. Certain rare adverse events might not surface in the smaller groups of subjects tested in phase I and phase II. These phase III trials are randomized and double-blind and involve the vaccine candidate—in its final composition and formulation—being tested against a placebo or control vaccine. The efficacy is also evaluated based on different criteria, such as (a) does the vaccine candidate prevent disease; (b) does the vaccine candidate prevent infection with the pathogen; (c) does the vaccine candidate induce antibodies or other types of immune responses related to the pathogen; and (d) does the vaccine candidate not interfere with the immune response of other vaccines?

Intussusception following receipt of rotavirus vaccine

A newly approved tetravalent *rhesus* rotavirus vaccine was introduced in the USA in August 1998 and was administered to over 600,000 infants in the first 9 months of the routine immunization program. In July 1999, intussusception was reported to occur in the first 2 weeks after administration of the first dose of the tetravalent *rhesus* rotavirus vaccine. The mechanism of this adverse event was never clearly elucidated, and the exact risk, which was calculated to be 1 in 10,000 vaccine recipients, remains a point of discussion. The vaccine was withdrawn by the manufacturer.

Subsequent analyses by different teams indicated that the risk was age related. The vaccine was offered to children at the time of their routine immunization at 2, 4, and 6 months of age, and catch-up immunization was provided any time up to 7 months of age. Most of the cases of intussusception occurred in the catch-up children who were older than 90 days at the time of immunization. The risk of infants who received their vaccine on schedule was subsequently estimated at 1 in 30,000–50,000, a risk 10-fold to 20-fold less than that reported when the vaccine was withdrawn.

As natural intussusception is not observed in infants in the first 3 months of life, the next generation of vaccine candidates needed to be tested with first doses administered almost exclusively to babies aged less than 90 days. Table 17.1 provides a summary of the study population on the efficacy trials of two rotavirus vaccines (i.e., attenuated human monovalent vaccine [Rotarix®, GlaxoSmithKline] and bovine–human pentavalent reassortant vaccine [RotaTeq®, Merck]). In addition, new vaccine candidates needed to be tested in phase III trials recruiting at least 30,000 vaccinees and 30,000 controls (see Table 17.2).

(Continued)

Table 17.1 Summary of Efficacy Trials of Two Rotavirus Vaccine Candidates

Vaccine	Site	# Patients Enrolled		# Outcomes			Effectiveness (95% CI)
		Vaccine	Control	Gastroenteritis	Vaccinated	Control	
Monovalent	Finland	245	123	Any	13	23	72 (42–87)
				Severe	3	10	85 (42–97)
	Brazil, Mexico, Venezuela	464	454	Any	15	49	70 (46–84)
				Severe	5	34	86 (63–96)
	Latin America	10,159	10,010	Severe	Not available	Not available	84.7 (71.7–92.4)
				Admission			85.0 (69.6–93.5)
Pentavalent	USA, Finland	2,834	2,839	Any	83	315	74.0 (66.8–79.9)
				Severe	1	51	98.0 (88.3–100.0)
	USA	650	660	Any	15	54	72.5 (50.6–85.6)
				Moderate/ severe	10	42	76.3 (52.0–89.4)
				Severe	0	6	100 (13.0–100.0)

Table 17.2 Summary of Vaccine Safety Trials With an Emphasis on Intussusception, With the Relative Risk of the Condition Following Receipt of the Rotavirus Vaccine Candidate or Control

Vaccine	Site	Follow-up Period	# Patients Enrolled		# Cases Intussusception			Relative Risk (95% CI)
			Vaccine	Control		Vaccinated	Comtrol	
Monovalent	Europe, Asia	31 days	~31,500	~31,500	Total	6	7	~0.86 (0.29–2.55)
	Latin America				Dose 1	1	2	~0.50 (0.05–5.51)
					Dose 2	5	5	~1.00 (0.29–3.45)
	Latin America	1 year	10,159	10,010	Total	4	14	0.28 (0.10–0.81)
Pentavalent	USA, others	42 days	~35,150	~35,150	Total	6	5	~1.20 (0.37–3.93)
					Dose 1	0	1	~0 (0–17.30)
					Dose 2	4	1	~4.00 (0.45–35.79)
					Dose 3	2	3	~0.67 (0.11–3.99)
		1 year	~35,150	~35,150	Total	12	15	~0.80 (0.35–1.71)

Source: Glass RI, Parashar UD, Bresee JS, et al. (2006). Rotavirus vaccines: current prospects and future challenges. Lancet 368, 323–332.

Vaccine safety post-approval

Approval process

In the USA, the sponsor, following completion of the clinical development program, including phase III trials, will prepare and submit an electronic Biologics Marketing Application according to the US FDA Guidance for Industry [Biologics License Application (BLA), Product License Application (PLA)/Establishment License Application (ELA), and New Drug Application (NDA)]. The US FDA will proceed with an inspection of not only the manufacturing site but also approval of the labeling of the vaccine candidate.

After licensure, the US FDA will continue to monitor the production of the vaccine, including inspection of manufacturing facilities and review of the manufacturer's tests of lots of vaccines for potency, safety, and purity. Those inspections will also include a review of the safety data management and timely reporting of adverse events to the US FDA. In addition, the US FDA may proceed with the testing of manufacturers' vaccines.

In other countries similar procedures for submission and inspections are applicable.

Post-licensure safety and efficacy monitoring of vaccines

In the postmarketing period, a much larger and likely more diverse population will be exposed to the vaccine compared to clinical studies. The fact that vaccines are administered to healthy people has implications for the continued reassessment of the overall risk-benefit evaluation for the vaccine. Monitoring of the safety profile of marketed vaccines is supported by passive and active surveillance and/or the conduct of surveillance studies.

Passive and active surveillance system

Definitions

Passive surveillance: Passive reporting from all potential sources of clinical conditions observed after the administration of a compound.
Active surveillance: Proactive request of reporting from specific health care professionals or other sources of clinical conditions observed after the administration of a compound.

In the USA, the National Childhood Vaccine Injury Act (NCVIA) of 1986 was enacted to facilitate compensation of patients suffering from vaccine-related injuries. The Act established the National Vaccine Injury Compensation Program (VICP) as well as the Vaccine Adverse Event Reporting System (VAERS), the new Vaccine Administration Record (VAR) rules, and the requirements around providing Vaccine Information Statements (VIS) for each vaccine. The VIS for each vaccine is available on the US Centers for Diseases Control and Prevention (CDC) website (http://www.cdc.gov/vaccines/pubs/vis/default.htm).

The VAERS is the national vaccine safety surveillance system cosponsored by the CDC and the US FDA, established in 1990. A first objective is to collect information about adverse events (possible side effects) that occur after the administration of the vaccines newly licensed in the USA, reported by health care professionals, manufacturers, and consumers. Other objectives are (a) detecting new, unusual, or rare vaccine adverse events; (b) monitoring of potential changes in frequency of known adverse events; (c) identification of potential patient subpopulations with risk factors for particular types of adverse events; and (d) identification of vaccine lots with an increased number or type of reported adverse events. The safety data are recorded, reported, analyzed, and thereafter made available to the public. VAERS is also the system to distribute vaccine-related information, including vaccine safety signal, to parents and guardians, health care professionals, state vaccine programs, and other constituencies. A Web-based electronic reporting was implemented in 2002, and VAERS data, following removal of personal identifiers, can be reviewed by the public by accessing http://www.vaers.org.

In 2011, the US FDA worked with the World Health Organization (WHO) Uppsala Monitoring Centre (UMC) to upload the VAERS data and a total of 245,454 reports (up to the year 2007) were uploaded and integrated in the UMC VigiSearch database. The US data account for 46% of the total of vaccine adverse event reports.

Other countries also have organized passive surveillance system for monitoring immunization safety. Examples are Norway with a national electronic immunization register (SYSVAK) established in 1995; Australia with a National Centre for Immunization Research and Surveillance (NVIRS) established in

1997; Canada with the Canadian Adverse Event Following Immunization Surveillance System (CAEFISS) reporting system established in 1987 supplemented with the active, 12 pediatric hospitals surveillance system, i.e., Immunization Monitoring Program-Active (IMPACT); among several others.

The differences in the passive surveillance programs across the various countries and continents do not facilitate a uniform collection, interpretation, and reporting of vaccine-associated adverse events. Efforts to introduce standardized definitions have been fostered by the Brighton Collaboration group (https://brightoncollaboration.org/public). The group is committed to developing standardized, widely disseminated, and globally accepted case definitions for an exhaustive number of AEFIs; and definitions intended to enhance data comparability within and across clinical trials, surveillance systems, and post-licensure clinical studies. A Vaccine European New Integrated Collaboration Effort (VENICE II) project, sponsored by the European Commission's Directorate General for Health and Consumers, intends to collect and share experience and expertise on national vaccination programs through a network of health care professionals and to create a knowledge-based platform to improve the performance of immunization programs. This should enable a systematic comparison of safety results across European countries.

Although passive reporting systems have methodological limitations or weaknesses, particularly for ascertaining reliable rate of occurrence of adverse event rates, for investigating causal relationship, absence of necessary confirmatory laboratory data, signals may be identified in the different data sets, warranting further investigations (see box).

How effective are passive and active surveillance systems?

In 1998, IMPACT identified an unexpected high rate of disseminated Bacille Calmette–Guérin (BCG) infection among aboriginal infants resulting in a review of the routine use of BCG vaccine for tuberculosis control on American Indian reservations and consideration of population immunity investigations.

Source: Schiefele DW, Halperin SA, Members of CPS/ Health Canada, Immunization Monitoring Program, Active (IMPACT) (2003). Immunization monitoring programme, active: a model of active surveillance of vaccine safety. Pediatric Infectious Disease Journal 14, 213–219.

In 1999, VAERS identified intussusception (a bowel obstruction in which one segment of the bowel becomes enfolded within another segment) among children vaccinated with the tetravalent rhesus-based rotavirus vaccine (RotaShield®). In addition, other gastrointestinal problems, such as bloody stools, vomiting, diarrhea, abdominal pain, and gastroenteritis, may also have been more frequently observed.

Source: CDC (1999). Intussusception among recipients of rotavirus vaccine—United States 1998-1999. MMWR 48, 577–81.

In 1996, reports of ideopathic thrombocytopenic purpura (TP) in VAERS resulted in further investigations of a potential association between TP and childhood vaccines, especially to measles, mumps, rubella (MMR) vaccines (Beeler et al., 1996). Follow-up investigations in VAERS yielded no consistent outcome with TP being reported after the administration of inactivated as well as live attenuated viral vaccines (Woo et al., 2011). Nevertheless, other researchers using 2000–2005 data from five managed care organizations report that TP is likely only associated with MMR vaccine, although further investigations are required for a possible association of TP and hepatitis A; varicella; and diphtheria, tetanus, acellular pertussis (DTaP) vaccine in older children (O'Leary et al., 2012).

Sources: Beeler J, Varrechio F, Wise R (1996). Thrombocytopenia after immunization with measles vaccines: review of vaccine adverse events reporting system (1990-1994). Pediatric Infectious Disease Journal 15, 88–90.
O'Leary ST, Glanz JM, McClure DL et al. (2012). The risk of immune thrombocytopenic purpura after vaccination in children and adolescents. Pediatrics 129, 248–55.
Woo EJ, Wise RP, Menschik D et al. (2011). Thrombocytopenia after immunization: case reports of the US Vaccine Adverse Event Reporting System, 1990-2008. Vaccine 29, 1319–23.

Active surveillance through studies

Alongside with the post-authorization passive/active surveillance and reporting of adverse events, post-authorization safety and/or efficacy studies may be requested or organized by the vaccine manufacturer or Marketing Authorization Holder (MAH).

The MAH may conduct phase IV trials to further test the safety profile and efficacy in the real world or to explore other objectives, such as the effect of changes in vaccine formulation, changes of vaccine strain, introduction of a new seed lot, number and timing of the administration of the vaccine doses, coadministration with other vaccines, immune interference with other vaccines or drugs, or other study populations, among others.

Possible phase IV studies

Case control studies: A type of epidemiological study designed to identify factors that may contribute to a medical condition by comparing a group of patients with the condition to a group of patients without the condition. They are intended for identifying risk factors for rare diseases or conditions.

Cohort studies: A type of epidemiological study designed to have a large number of patients to distinguish cause from effect. These are also called *follow-up studies, incidence studies, longitudinal studies,* or *prospective studies.*

PAES: A post-authorization efficacy study; any study that aims to clarify the efficacy for a medicine on the market, including in everyday medical practice.

PASS: A post-authorization safety study; any study relating to an authorized medicinal product conducted with the aim of identifying, characterizing, or quantifying a safety hazard; confirming the safety profile of the medicinal product; or of measuring the effectiveness of risk management measures with strict principles for the implementation, execution, and reporting of the study and the results.

In the USA, the US FDA may request a post-authorization safety study (or studies) and have the MAH perform a study (or studies) (PASS) at the time of approval. Other countries have that authority to demand a PASS. Recently, definitions of post-authorization research studies have been provided by the Health Authority in Europe. A PASS is defined as any study relating to an authorized medicinal products

conducted with the aim to identifying, characterizing, or quantifying a safety hazard; confirming the safety profile of the medicinal product; or of measuring the effectiveness of risk management measures with strict principles for the implementation, execution, and reporting of the study and the results. A post-authorization efficacy study (PAES) aims to clarify the efficacy for a medicine on the market, including in everyday medical practice.

There are two types of pharmacoepidemiological studies, i.e., case-control studies and cohort studies. Case control studies are one type of epidemiological study designed used to identify factors that may contribute to a medical condition by comparing a group of patients with the condition to a group of patients without the condition. They are intended for identifying risk factors for rare diseases or conditions. Cohort studies are another type of epidemiological study designs involving a large number of patients and proceed from cause to effect. These are also called *follow-up studies, incidence studies, longitudinal studies,* or *prospective studies.* Three subtypes can be identified (1) prospective; (2) retrospective; and (3) historical retrospective.

Large linked databases, such as Vaccine Safety DataLink project

The Vaccine Safety DataLink (VSD) project is a collaborative effort between the CDC's Immunization Safety Office and eight managed care organizations (MCOs). It was established to monitor immunization safety and address gaps in scientific and medical knowledge about rare and serious AEFIs. The VSD project includes a large linked database that uses administrative data sources at each MCO. Each MCO prepares computerized data files by using a standardized data dictionary containing demographic and medical information on its members, e.g., age and gender, health plan enrollment, vaccinations, hospitalizations, outpatient clinic visits, emergency department visits, urgent care visits, and mortality data, as well as additional birth information (e.g., birth weight) when available. Other information sources, such as medical chart review, member surveys, and pharmacy, laboratory, and radiology data, are often used in VSD studies to validate outcomes and vaccination data. The VSD project allows for planned immunization safety studies, i.e., evaluation of serious neurologic, allergic, hematologic, infectious, inflammatory, and metabolic conditions as well as *ad hoc* investigations of hypotheses that arise from the review of medical literature or from potential signals identified in VAERS. In addition, through changes in data-collection procedures, the creation of near real-time data files, and the development of near real-time postmarketing surveillance, newly licensed vaccines or changes in vaccine recommendations can be monitored appropriately. Recognized as an important resource in vaccine safety, the VSD is working toward increasing transparency through data sharing and external input. With its recent enhancements, the VSD provides scientific expertise, continues to develop innovative approaches for vaccine-safety research, and may serve as a model for other patient safety collaborative research projects.

Examples VSD studies

Hepatitis B vaccine and risk of auto-immune thyroid disease

A possible link between hepatitis B vaccine and autoimmune thyroid disease such as Graves' disease and Hashimoto thyroiditis had been suggested by a study conducted in Europe and by single reports to VAERS. Supplementing interviews and medical record data with routinely collected automated data, the VSD was able to investigate this alleged relationship through a multisite case-control study. The study analyzed 335 vases of Graves' disease, 418 cases of Hashimoto thyroiditis, and 1102 frequency-matched controls, which revealed that having ever received hepatitis B vaccine did not increase the risk of either Graves' disease or Hashimoto thyroiditis.

The study results reveal the ability to collect comprehensive vaccine information and to accurately identify and confirm cases through alternative data collection methods.

Safety of trivalent inactivated influenza vaccine in children aged 6 to 23 months

VSD conducted a retrospective population-based trivalent influenza vaccine (TIV) study enrolling 45,356 children receiving a total of 69,359 influenza vaccinations between January 1, 1993, and May 31, 2003. Self-control case series were used for the analysis. Cycle files were analyzed to identify medically attended events seen in clinic, emergency department, or hospital settings after vaccination with TIV. Preliminary analyses revealed that gastritis/duodenitis was more likely to occur in the

14 days after TIV (matched odds ratio [ORs]: 5.50 [95% CI 1.22–24.81] for control period 1 [0–3 days] and 4.33 [95% CI 1.23–15.21] for control period 2 [1–14 days]). No other significant associations with medically attended events were found. Further analysis including chart review and a subanalysis of 28,820 children with no underlying medical conditions that would put them at increased risk of complications of influenza vaccination revealed that children vaccinated with TIV were not at increased risk of gastritis/duodenitis compared to the entire study population.

The study supported the Advisory Committee on Immunization Practices (ACIP) vaccination recommendations by providing reassurance to support the safety of universally immunizing all children aged 6 to 23 months with influenza vaccination.

Early thimerosal exposure and neuropsychological outcomes at 7 to 10 years

Thimerosal is a mercury-containing preservative that was used to enhance stability and extend the shelf life of a vaccine. In 1999, the Public Health Service and the American Academy of Pediatrics (AAP) called on vaccine manufacturers to remove thimerosal from vaccines. The decision to remove thimerosal was a precautionary measure, and subsequent studies have found no significant association between thimerosal and neuropsychological deficits. A retrospective cohort study with extensive assessments and interviews among study populations and their parents was initiated. A total of 1047 children, aged 7 to 10 years, were enrolled in four MCOs. Standardized tests assessed 42 neuropsychological outcomes, including speech and language measures, verbal memory, fine motor coordination, tics, and behavioral regulation. Only 5% of the statistical tests (19 out of 378) showed significant associations, 12 tests revealed a positive association, and 7 tests revealed a negative association. The vast majority of the tests revealed no association, and the 5% who showed associations could be explained by chance observation alone. The results added to accumulated evidence that thimerosal does not cause neuropsychological deficits in children.

The study illustrated the ability of VSD to supplement administrative data with data of other sources to conduct rigorous studies and test vaccine-safety hypotheses.

Source: Baggs J, Gee J, Lewis E et al. (2011). The vaccine safety datalink: a model for monitoring immunization safety. Pediatrics 127, S45–S53.

Rapid cycle analysis (RCA) studies

The size of the population covered by the VSD project, now with 8.8 million members annually, also allows separation of the risks associated with individual vaccines from those associated with vaccine combinations, whether given in the same syringe or simultaneously at different body sites. Such RCA studies are especially valuable in view of combined pediatric vaccines.

VSD is also conducting rapid cycle analysis (RCA) studies. The safety of different vaccines, such as RotaTeq® (rotavirus), Menectra® (meningococcal men-

---

Examples of RCA studies

Menectra® and Guillain–Barré syndrome

Between March 2005 and September 2008, more than 570,000 Menectra® doses were delivered to participating MCOs and no case reports of Guillain–Barré syndrome (GBS) after medical records review were observed among vaccine recipients aged 11 to 19 years within a 6-week time period after vaccination. During the same period, five unconfirmed case reports of GBS were identified among an unvaccinated comparison group of over 900,000 people aged 11 to 19 years.

The results of the study do not suggest an association of the serious AEFI with Menectra®.

Intussusception and RotaTeq®

Between May 2006 and May 2008 more than 205,000 doses of RotaTeq® were administered orally to infants aged 2, 4, and 6 months in VSD monitored MCOs. Only five cases of intussusception within 30 days of vaccination were reported; in contrast, on the basis of historical background rates, 6.75 cases were expected to occur by chance alone.

The results of the study suggested that there was no evidence that RotaTeq® vaccine was associated with an increased risk of intussusception or other pre-specified events.

Source: Baggs J, Gee J, Lewis E et al. (2011). The vaccine safety datalink: a model for monitoring immunization safety. Pediatrics 127, S45–S53.

---

ingitis), Gardasil® (human papillomavirus) Adacel® (tetanus toxoid, reduced diphtheria toxoid and acellular pertussis vaccine, adsorbed, produced by Sanofi Pasteur), and Boostrix® (tetanus toxoid, reduced diphtheria toxoid and acellular pertussis vaccine, adsorbed, produced by GSK), ProQuad® (measles, mumps, rubella, and varicella) were also tested.

Clinical Immunization Safety Assessment (CISA) network

The Clinical Immunization Safety Assessment (CISA) network is a US national network of six medical research centers with expertise in immunization safety and conducting clinical research on immunization associated health risks. CISA was established in 2001 as a collaborative project between the US CDC Immunization Safety Office, six medical research centers, and America's Health Insurance Plans.

The mission of CISA is (1) to conduct focused clinical research about vaccine adverse events and the role of individual variation; (2) to provide clinicians with vaccine-based counsel and empower individuals to make informed immunization decisions; (3) to assist domestic and global vaccine safety policy makers in the recommendation of exclusion criteria for at-risk individuals; and (4) to enhance public confidence in sustaining immunization benefits to all populations.

The goals of CISA are to (1) study the pathophysiologic basis of AEFI using hypothesis-driven protocols; (2) study risk factors associated with developing an adverse event following immunization using hypothesis-driven protocols, including genetic host-risk factors; (3) provide clinicians with evidence-based vaccinations or revaccination guidelines; and (4) serve as a regional referral center to address complex vaccine safety inquiries.

Because many AEFIs are rare, it is difficult to have an adequate number of cases to appropriately evaluate risk factors, including genetic risk factors. As a result, the CISA Network initiated a postimmunization adverse event clinical registry and specimen repository, i.e., the Immunization Safety BioBank. This will enable the CISA Network to bank sufficient biological specimens and associated clinical information in anticipation of future studies to assess genetic

Examples of CISA studies

Dryvax® and evaluation of active telephone surveillance to evaluate adverse events

A total of 825 recipients of Dryvax® vaccine were interviewed by telephone to characterize and actively monitor adverse events after Dryvax® vaccinia vaccination in civilian health care workers and first responders (those involved in response to use of a biological weapon). Although 12.5% reported missing work because of AEFIs, most AEFIs were anticipated and of short duration.

Transverse myelitis and vaccines

Working with a team of neurologists, CISA Network investigators developed a standardized algorithm for identification and assessment of possible causes of acute transverse myelitis (a neurological disorder caused by inflammation across both sides of one segment of the spinal cord). An ongoing study will determine if there is an association between vaccines and idiopathic transverse myelitis and will compare the clinical characteristics of idiopathic transverse myelitis with onset in the 6-week period after vaccines with transverse myelitis not temporally associated with vaccines.

Role of genetics in the immune response to varicella vaccine

This assessment of immune responses to varicella vaccine within sibling pairs was conducted by CISA Network investigators. The evaluation revealed that post-varicella immunization antibody titers within sibling pairs clustered more often than in non-sibling pairs, which supports the hypothesis that genetic factors play a role in the antibody response to the varicella vaccine.

Recurrent sterile abscesses after immunization

The study examined three children with recurrent sterile abscesses after immunization and proposed a role of aluminum adjuvant in the development of sterile abscesses after immunization.

Source: LaRussa PS, Edwards KM, Dekker CL et al. (2011). Vaccine-safety system and vaccine-safety studies. Understanding the role of human variation in vaccine adverse events: the clinical immunization safety assessment network. Pediatrics 127, S65–S73.

and immunologic host factors that may predispose people to selected AEFIs.

European Network of Centres for Pharmacoepidemiology and Pharmacovigilance (ENCePP)

Definition

EudraVigilance: EudraVigilance is a central computer database created by the European Medicines Agency in December 2001. It contains adverse reaction reports to medicines licensed across the European Union that are received from the regulatory agencies and from pharmaceutical companies within the European Union. http://eudravigilance.ema.europa.eu/human/EVBackground(FAQ).asp

ENCePP aims to support quality pharmacoepidemiological studies and to stimulate innovation that benefits patients and public health at large. The overview document and Web resource (www.encepp.eu) provides methodological guidance. Four different approaches to data collection have been described and include (1) secondary use of data, e.g., HMO database, claims database, Clinical Practice Research Datalink (CPRD), a new National Health System observation data and interventional research service designed to maximize the way de-identified NHS clinical data can be linked to enable different types of observational research; (2) primary data collection, with data obtained through case control studies or case control surveillance networks; (3) research networks, with the ENCePP databases of Research Resources or the HMO Research Network in the USA; and (4) spontaneous report database, with the EudraVigilance database or VAERS database.

Most importantly, an e-Register of studies can be accessed through the ENCePP website.

Causality assessment

Vaccines and drugs are different at several levels. Vaccines as biological compounds are sensitive to temperature variation and sunlight. The traditional knowledge on pharmacokinetics and pharmacodynamics of drugs are replaced by information of cellular and humoral immune response. Most vaccines are used in preventive health care, and administrated by trained staff using a uniform dosing and recommended frequency. Due to the availability of combination vaccines (i.e., multiple antigens and/or multiple vaccines given in one dose), the causality assessment to a particular antigen may be difficult or impossible. Vaccines require a stringent lot-to-lot surveillance and access to adequate vaccine distribution data is critical in the interpretation of the relative reporting rates. As vaccines are part of larger immunization programs (childhood and occupational immunization programs, e.g., hepatitis B and health care professionals, and multiple vaccines in the military) programmatic errors need to be monitored. Vaccines are also used in the World Health Organization Expanded Programme on Immunization (EPI) in many countries with limited support for the monitoring and reporting of adverse events.

Nevertheless, causality assessment of AEFI is an important task to be performed by the MAH, as most case reports concern *suspected* adverse reactions. Causality assessment is considered complex, because in most cases there are no specific tests to prove a causal association between a vaccine and an AEFI. Still, three guiding principles can be applied: (1) Can it? With the subsequent questions can the vaccine cause the event, at least in certain people under certain circumstances? (2) Will it? With the subsequent questions how frequently will vaccine recipients experience the adverse event as a result of the vaccination? and (3) Did it? With the subsequent question was the adverse event cause by the vaccine?

For drugs, adverse reactions are rarely specific for the medicinal product, diagnostic tests are usually absent, and rechallenge is rarely ethically acceptable. As a result, few adverse reactions are "certain" or "unlikely"; most are somewhere in between these limits, i.e., "possible" or "probable." None of these systems, however, have been shown to produce a precise, reliable, and reproducible quantitative estimation of the likelihood of a relationship.

Causality assessment for drugs

Certain
- Event or laboratory test abnormality, with plausible time relationship to vaccine administration
- Cannot be explained by disease or other drugs
- Response to withdrawal plausible (pharmacologically, pathologically)
- Event definitive pharmacologically or phenomenologically (i.e., an objective and specific medical disorder or recognised pharmacological phenomenon)
- Rechallenge satisfactory, if necessary

Probable to likely
- Event or laboratory test abnormality, with reasonable time relationship to vaccine administration
- Unlikely to be attributed to disease or other drugs
- Response to withdrawal reasonable (pharmacologically, pathologically)
- Rechallenge not required

Possible
- Event or laboratory test abnormality, with reasonable time relationship to vaccine administration
- Cannot also be explained by disease or other drugs
- Information on drug withdrawal may be lacking or unclear

Unlikely
- Event or laboratory test abnormality, with a time to drug intake that makes a relationship improbable
- Disease or other drugs provide plausible explanation

Conditional to unclassified
- Event or laboratory test abnormality
- More data for proper assessment required
- Additional data under examination

Unassessable to unclassifiable
- Report suggesting an adverse reactions
- Cannot be judged because information is insufficient or contradictory
- Data cannot be supplemented or verified

Source: The use of the WHO-UMC system for standardised case causality assessment. http://www.who.int/medicines/areas/quality_safety/safety_efficacy/WHOcausality_assessment.pdf. Accessed July 14, 2012.

In case of AEFI, the Public Health Agency of Canada (PHAC) supported the Canadian Vaccine Safety Blueprint in close collaboration with other partners, such as Centre for Immunization and Respiratory Infectious Disease (CIRID), Surveillance and Outbreak Response Division (SORD), and the Vaccine Safety Section. The Vaccine Vigilance Working Group proposed a causality grid and compared the quality of the causality assessment of reports collected through an active and through a passive reporting system.

Examples of vaccine fears

It is recognized that confidence in vaccine safety is of paramount importance to national immunization strategies and to global public health. Vaccine safety issues have increasingly had an impact on the acceptance of vaccines by the general public, as well as by some health care professionals. Concern over liability has limited the development of vaccine candidates for maternal immunization against important diseases, such as group B *streptococcus*. It is of concern that certain acute and chronic conditions are very easily linked to immunizations. It will be important to build capacities and capabilities for detecting, reporting, and responding to AEFI in all countries, including in the developing world. Scientific and medical responses are the only approach to respond to alleged claims.

Vaccines and mad cow disease

Background
By July 2000, at least 73 people in the UK developed a progressive neurological disease called *variant Creutzfeld-Jacob disease*. The condition is likely associated from eating meat prepared from cows with "mad-cow" disease, a disease caused by proteinaceous infectious particles (prions).

Situation analysis
• In the manufacturing process of some vaccines bovine serum (growth factor for cell culture) and/or gelatin (stabilizing vaccines) are being used.
• These are obtained from cows from the United Kingdom or from other countries at risk of "mad cow" disease and hence these *may* obtain prions.

Bovine-derived products are *not* likely to contain prions, as

• Fetal bovine serum and gelatin are obtained from blood and connective tissue, respectively; neither sources that have been found to contain prions.
• Fetal bovine serum is highly diluted and eventually removed from cells during the growth of vaccine viruses.
• Prions are propagated in mammalian brains and not in cell cultures used to make vaccine.
• Transmission of prions occurs from either eating brains from infected animals or, in experimental studies, directly inoculating preparations of brains from infected animals of experimental animals.
• Transmission of prions has not been documented after inoculation into the muscles or under the skin.

Considering the above, the chance that currently licensed vaccines contain prions is essentially zero. In addition, vaccine manufacturers have further reduced and/or removed fetal bovine serum and gelatin from their manufacturing cycles.

Measles, mumps, rubella vaccine causes autism
Autism is a chronic developmental disorder characterized by problems in social interaction, communication, and responsiveness, and by repetitive interests and activities. Although the causes of autism are largely unknown, family and twin studies suggest that genetics plays a fundamental role. In addition, overexpression of neuropeptides and neurotrophins has been found in the immediate perinatal period among children later diagnosed with autism, suggesting that prenatal or perinatal influences or both play a more important role than postnatal insults. However, because autistic symptoms generally first become apparent in the second year of life, some scientists have focused on the potential role of MMR vaccine.

Concern over the role of MMR vaccine was heightened in 1998 when a UK study based on 12 children proposed an association between the vaccine and the development of ileonodular hyperplasia, nonspecific colitis, and regressive developmental disorders.

Significant concerns about the validity of the study included the lack of appropriate control or comparison group, inconsistent timing to support causality (some children presented autistic symptoms before the bowel syndrome), and the lack of an accepted definition of the syndrome. Subsequently, population-based studies of autistic children in the UK found no association between MMR and the autism onset or developmental regression. In addition, a VSD study investigated whether measles-containing vaccine was associated with inflammatory bowel disease and found no relationship. Several studies have also refuted the notion that MMR vaccine caused autism. In 2004 the initial article reporting the suspect study was retracted.

Vaccines cause cancer

Background
Simian virus 40 (SV40) was present in monkey kidney cells used in the manufacturing of inactivated polio vaccine, live attenuated polio vaccine, and inactivated adenovirus vaccines in the late 1950s. At the time of the discovery the manufacturing was stopped.

Situation analysis
In 2004, investigators found SV40 DNA in biopsy specimens obtained from patients with certain unusual cancers (e.g., mesothelioma, osteosarcoma, and non-Hodgkin lymphoma), leading some to a hypothesis of a link between vaccination and subsequent development of cancer.

The observations required further in-depth investigations, which found:

• Genetic material of SV40 was present in cancers of people who either had or had not been vaccinated with a SV40-contaminated polio vaccine
• People with cancers who had never received SV40-contaminated polio vaccine were found to have SV40 genetic material in the cancerous cells
• Epidemiologic studies did not show en increased risk of cancer in those received polio vaccine between 1955 and 1963 and those who did not receive polio vaccine

Based on the above, the hypothesis that SV40 virus contained in polio vaccines administered before 1963 caused cancers was ill founded.

Oral polio vaccine trials in Belgian Congo and the origin of HIV

Background
The idea that the origin of AIDS could be traced to a certain polio vaccine that was administered in the Belgian Congo between 1957 and 1960 was first reported in a popular press magazine article and a book.

Situation analysis
• Inactivated and live attenuated polio vaccine are grown in monkey kidney cells.
• Chimpanzees are carriers of the simian immunodeficiency virus, SIV_{cpz}, the precursor of HIV
• American and Belgian researchers used kidney cells of chimpanzees for the growth of CHAT polio virus type 1 (the vaccine strain was named "CHAT" after "Charlton," the name of the child who was the donor of the virus from which the vaccine was derived), kidney cells containing the SIV_{cpz}
• The CHAT polio virus vaccine was administered to people and were inadvertently inoculated with SIV_{cpz}, which then progressed to HIV and caused the AIDS epidemic

The reasoning is problematic and based on erroneous assumptions.

• SIV_{cpz} is not found in kidney cells
• Kidneys of rhesus macaque monkeys are used in the cell culture of polio vaccine; kidneys of chimpanzees are not
• SIV_{cpz} and HIV are not close genetically and mutation would likely require decades, not years
• Samples of the original CHAT vaccine retained at the Wistar Institute (Philadelphia, PA, USA) and the Karolinska Institute (Stockholm, Sweden) were tested and contained genetic material from rhesus macaques monkeys, and did not contain SIVcpz or genetic material from chimpanzees

Although sufficient data were available to reject the hypothesis, the idea continued to persist. As a consequence, research was initiated to recover human tissue samples from the Democratic Republic of Congo. Initially, samples from the Provincial Medical

Laboratory of Kisangani were obtained. The selected samples could be tested for human and viral material, and after completing successfully the proof of concept, further collection of samples was attempted. In 2006, a selection of samples from 1958 to 1961 was obtained from the histopathology department of the University of Kinshasa and tested at the University of Arizona. A lymph node collected from a 28-year-old woman collected in January 1960 tested positive for a HIV-1 M group subtype A/A1. It was computed that the virus evolved from a common ancestor circulating in the African population near the beginning of the 20th century.

The scientific data provided above enabled the rejection of the oral polio vaccine hypothesis. Unfortunately, the story that an oral polio vaccine could cause AIDS will continue to live its life and be an obstacle to eliminating polio in several countries in Africa; it will also impact the acceptance of other vaccines as well.

Communication perspective in vaccine safety

Because of the nature of preventive vaccination programs, the viability of these public health interventions is particularly susceptible to public perceptions. This is because vaccination relies on a concept of *herd immunity*, success of which requires rational public behavior that can only be obtained through full and accurate communication about the risks and benefits.

Communication of health risk has traditionally consisted of messages designed to encourage positive behavior that reduces individual and societal risk. When hundreds of thousands of people contracted vaccine-preventable diseases such as poliomyelitis, measles, or whooping cough, few people stopped to ask about vaccine-associated adverse events. Now that vaccines have been successful in controlling and eliminating some infectious diseases so that these diseases are virtually unheard of, people affected by AEFI may outnumber the cases of diseases that do still occur. This has resulted in people scrutinizing the adverse events, not knowing or forgetting about those important diseases with recognized morbidity and mortality that vaccines have successfully defeated.

For some people, risks ensuing from specific actions—such as receiving a vaccine—are viewed as worse than risks that occur "on their own," such as an infection with a vaccine-preventable disease. (The distinction is sometimes referred to as an *act of commission* vs. an *act of omission*). It remains challenging for parents and patients assimilating and interpreting risk-benefit information for both research and treatment. This is due, in part, to the manner in which risks, benefits, and risk-benefit profiles are communicated and to the literacy and numeracy abilities of the individual, as well as the absence of cases of the natural wild-type infectious disease.

When preparing for good communication some elements should be considered: (1) risk communication is a dynamic process in which several individuals participate—persons influenced by a wide range of circumstances, education, information, and information needs; (2) the objective of risk communication is to have concerned parties join toward an informed medical decision making; (3) reducing the continuous uncertainty about the estimates of vaccine and vaccination-associated risks and allow all individuals, presented with risk statistics and comparisons between risks and benefits, to reach an informed medical decision; and (4) describing potential consequences of reduced vaccination coverage. The combination of these elements should have a beneficial impact on parental or patient beliefs about immunizations. Fear, misconception, and misinformation can erode very quickly the confidence in vaccines and the providers. It is therefore that the science of effective risk communication has emerged as an important skill for managers of immunization programs worldwide and health care professionals who administer vaccines.

Risk perception and irrational behavior
Fears motivating irrational behavior are intrinsically human; and media coverage may heighten a sense of risk.

Vaccine providers, policymakers, health care professionals, parents, and patients should endeavor to understand the different factors shaping the safety and risk perceptions in order to improve the communication among themselves as well as the general public. The influential role of the media should also be embraced. Communication should reflect reasoned assessment of benefit and risks and potential courses

Sensational headline: "Baby falls ill as scare widens across US."

During the anthrax scare in 2001 a US newspaper published an article with a sensational headline "Baby falls ill as scare widens across US." Although actual anthrax cases were limited to clusters in Boca Raton; New York City; and Washington, DC (though spores were found in distant locations such as Indianapolis and Kansas City, a fact not overlooked by the media) the threat was perceived to be much greater. According to an Institute of Medicine report, "the widespread reporting of anthrax contamination in the weeks after September 11, 2001, served to expand those events from several localized incidents into a potential generalized threat." The result was striking: According to an article in the *Journal of the American Medical Association*, more than 30,000 people are estimated to have received antibiotics related to the anthrax scare. Beyond supply issues, overuse of the antibiotic Ciprofloxacin has threatened the effectiveness of the drug for a number of conditions. "In case of anthrax, less than 20 cases resulted in thousands of people taking antibiotics that were not indicated. Perhaps 20% of these individuals experienced some side effects. The antibiotics changes the bacteriological environment and may have rendered some organisms resistant" to the antibiotic.

of action. If the assessment is not available and communicated, such as during the anthrax scare, fear will motivate a refusal of vaccination rather than encourage acceptance. Thereafter the basic problem for the public remains: Lack of adequate information may result in irrational behavior, motivated by misconception of risks. Sensational media reports may enhance noncompliance as the low level of perceived risk of possibly contracting a vaccine-preventable disease makes vaccine safety issue more weighty for parents, often amplified by a strong antivaccination movement and their multiple Internet sites.

As adverse events are identified after immunization, health care providers should recognize that parents establish their beliefs on their own observations and the temporal association between vaccination and signs and symptoms, e.g., fever, rash, etc. In addition, it should be recognized that parents have relatively limited confidence in the institutions that shape immunization policy (and the distrust of official institutions is not limited to vaccine matters only). When a serious adverse event occurs, parents often question whether the vaccine-preventable disease was so serious and should their child, now suffering from an adverse event, have been vaccinated.

The challenges of these findings are also the opportunities to address vaccine safety concerns.

Definition

Herd immunity: A situation where protective immunity is achieved through attaining a high enough level of immunity to a disease in a population (through vaccination) to make exposure to the organism to those not protected extremely unlikely.

Public health and public communication

No vaccine is 100% effective. The success of vaccination programs relies on a concept known as *herd immunity*, wherein the protection is achieved through attaining a high enough level of immunity to a disease so as to make exposure to the organism that causes the disease extremely unlikely. If a critical mass of people is immune, then those who refuse vaccination remain protected through the herd immunity. So long as the level of vaccination is attained, those who are not vaccinated are nonetheless protected through the unlikelihood that they will ever be exposed to the pathogen. This is the cornerstone of trust: Individuals who seek exemption from mandatory childhood vaccination will be protected from contracting vaccine-preventable diseases through herd immunity, gaining this protection as a direct result of the widespread vaccination of others, while assuming no (real or perceived) risk of adverse reactions to the vaccines themselves. If exemptions to vaccination continue to increase and threaten the herd immunity, exposure to vaccine-preventable disease could be found in those exempted, those excluded from vaccination for medical reasons, and those vaccinated who did not respond adequately and remain susceptible to the disease. As growing numbers of parents are seeking exemption to childhood vaccination on behalf of their children, dramatic reemergence of highly communicable diseases, e.g., measles and mumps, have been reported in many countries.

With the objective of engaging parents and patients about vaccine safety concerns in an open dialogue, empathy, patience, scientific curiosity, and reliable data are required.

Measles, mumps vaccine-associated aseptic meningitis: an introduction to vaccine safety

In 1986, a case report of aseptic meningitis in a young child having received a newly introduced measles, mumps vaccine with isolation of a mumps virus in the cerebrospinal fluid 13 days post-vaccination triggered concerns over the safety profile. Several actions were considered so as to confirm the observation, including collecting the mumps strain from the provincial laboratory at some 500 km from the office. A visit to the reporting neurologist was also planned; our invitation was only accepted reluctantly. The initial contact was strained, and after sharing in-house safety data, reviewing jointly the patient's medical records, expanding on the ongoing scientific research work performed at the company, the neurologist supported our offer for help to investigate this particular case. Subsequently, the company encouraged the publication of the different observations.

It is important to create a "communication pathway" with a blueprint to different steps to accomplish, as gathering and conveying health information may mitigate crises created through fear.

A first communication step is the gathering of scientific and medical objective data in case of a single case report or cluster of case reports, including securing biological samples for further testing. This may require field visits to the reporting person and an open discussion. A second communication step is the seeking of advice and review from qualified experts, including experts from health authorities or other sources such as scientific experts in the specific area of the suspected adverse event, including experts from industry. A third communication step is the publication (or communication at a national or international conference) of single case reports so as to share the observation with the broader scientific community and public; even though the interpretation of single case reports or geographical or timely cluster of reports remains challenging, these reports are nonetheless informative. A fourth communication step is the execution of laboratory investigations and/or epidemiological studies and to communicate of the results to the health authorities. After an evaluation of the risk and benefit, a fifth communication step may be completed with a broader distribution of the scientific data together with an interpretation tailored at the different target groups.

It is important to recognize the importance of the communication with the specialized and public media

Health care professional guidance for discussions with parents about childhood immunizations

What can physicians do to keep parental confidence in vaccines high?

1. Be respectful and solicit questions:
   "What questions do you have about childhood vaccinations?"

2. Be emphatic if parents have concerns:
   "I understand your concern" or "I know your child is the most important thing in the world to you" or "taking decisions on immunizations can be confusing."

3. Educate the parent before the day of the child's immunization:
   "Here is a brochure describing the immunization process that may be helpful, and if you have questions please let me know at your next visit."

4. Give information tailored to the parent's concern, if possible:
   "If I use medical words that are too complicated, please interrupt me."

5. Be informed about current vaccine safety allegations, misconceptions, or misinformation so that you can address with confidence and respect:
   "Oh yes, I read the article posted on Internet on vaccines and cancer. But I would like to share the conclusion of the American Academy of Pediatrics. A panel of pediatricians reviewed the available scientific evidence and concluded that vaccines do not cause cancer. Let me give you their website so you can have a look yourself, and if you have questions please let me know at your next visit.

6. Recommend vaccines:
   I believe in immunization; my children are immunized.

to (re)build credibility and trust with reporters and the public by illustrating that scientific and medical expertise was applied to the investigations, that honesty and transparency were fostered with experts and health authorities, and that contacts with parents with children with adverse events were established.

Parents want to participate in the decision-making process of the immunization for their children; therefore, vaccine providers, policymakers, and health care professionals should provide appropriate information at an appropriate time. Whereas the content of the information is important, the timing of sharing the information is equally important. Parents should have the time to read the information and not being stressed to proceed with the immunization of their child. Health care professionals may benefit from some questions listed below creating an improved parent–health care professional relationship, which is the cornerstone for improving vaccine acceptance and controlling vaccine-preventable disease.

- epidemiologic studies or creation of registries to reassure the public about the safety of existing and future vaccines in the population at large or certain at risk subsets of populations.

- Best practices may be copied from other industries in order to create a "communication pathway" to minimize risk, establish benefits, and communicate scientific data in vaccine safety matters to all layers of the society.

Summary

- Few public health interventions have been as successful as immunizations to prevent untimely deaths and reduce morbidity from numerous childhood and other diseases. Vaccines are highly cost-effective improvements to human health, and particularly to that of children. As childhood immunization programs mature, vaccine safety has become critical in determining success or failure of those national vaccine-preventable disease programs.

- Vigilance is of the essence to detect early potential adverse events in every corner of the world, in developing and developed countries alike, especially as adverse publicity travels fast through the Internet.

- Access to electronic health care services in the different continents shall facilitate the conduct of

Further reading

Guideline on good pharmacovigilance practices (GVP). Module VIII Post-authorisation safety studies (9 July 2012). EMA/330405/2012.

Grabenstein JD. Vaccine safety. In Vaccines for Biodefense and Emerging and Neglected Diseases (eds ADT Barrett and LR Stanberry), p. 1478. London: Academic Press, 2009.

Hill R (2011). New vaccine reports from FDA to the Uppsala Monitoring Centre. International Journal of Risk and Safety in Medicine 23, 177–178.

May T (2005). Public perceptions, risk perception, and the viability of preventive vaccination against communicable diseases. Bioethics 19, 407–421. 1467-8519 (online).

National Childhood Vaccine Injury Act (NCVIA) (Public Law 99-660).

Offit P and DeStefano F. Vaccine safety. In Vaccines, 6th edition (eds SA Plotkin, WA Orenstein, and PA Offit, Chapter 76, pp 1464–1480. Philadelphia: Saunders Elsevier 2013.

Woo EJ, Ball R, Bostrom A, et al. (2004). Vaccine risk perception among reporters of autism after vaccination: vaccine adverse event reporting system 1990-2001. American Journal of Public Health 94, 990–995.

Worobey M, Gemmel M, Teuwen DE, et al. (2008). Direct evidence of extensive diversity of HIV-1 in Kinshasa by 1960. Nature 455, 661–665.

18 Understanding and measuring the dynamics of infectious disease transmission

Christine M. Arcari

Department of Preventive Medicine and Community Health, University of Texas Medical Branch at Galveston, Galveston, TX, USA

Abbreviations

ACIP	Advisory Committee on Immunization Practices	R	Effective reproductive number
ARI	Acute respiratory illness	R_0	Basic reproductive number
CDC	Centers for Disease Control and Prevention	SAR	Secondary attack rate
HIT	Herd immunity threshold	SIR	Susceptible, infected, and recovered
ILI	Influenza-like illness	VE	Vaccine efficacy
MIDAS	Models of Infectious Disease Agent Study	WNV	West Nile virus
		β	Transmission probability

Concepts of infectious disease transmission

Epidemiologists study the distribution and determinants of infectious diseases in populations. *Distribution* refers to the frequency and pattern of infection and disease in a population, and *determinants* refers to the factors that are associated with increased risk of infection and disease. The application of epidemiologic knowledge allows us to implement prevention and control measures, evaluate the effectiveness of health services, plan health care delivery systems, and guide public health policy.

Distribution and determinants of infectious diseases

Distribution refers to the frequency and pattern of infection and disease in a population, and *determinants* refers to the factors that are associated with increased risk of infection and disease.

Epidemiologic triad

A model of infectious disease causation known as the epidemiologic triad is shown in Figure 18.1. The triad consists of the infectious *agent*, the cause of disease; the *host*, an organism, usually human or animal, which is susceptible to the infectious agent; and the *environment*, the surroundings and conditions external to the host that allow the infectious agent and host to interact. Disease transmission depends on the complex interplay among characteristics of the infectious agent, host factors, and environmental influences. A *vector* may also be part of the infectious disease process. A vector is a living organism, such as an arthropod, that is capable of transmitting the infectious agent from an infected host to a susceptible host. The epidemiologic triad is important for understanding transmission of disease. Importantly, the disruption of any link of the epide-

Vaccinology: An Essential Guide, First Edition. Edited by Gregg N. Milligan and Alan D.T. Barrett.
© 2015 John Wiley & Sons, Ltd. Published 2015 by John Wiley & Sons, Ltd.

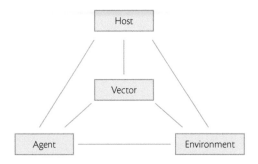

Figure 18.1 Epidemiologic triad of disease causation.

miologic triad can prevent disease. Vaccines disrupt the link between the infectious agent and the host.

Characteristics of infectious agents, hosts, and environments

Important characteristics of infectious agents are infectivity, pathogenicity, virulence, and immunogenicity. From an epidemiological perspective, *infectivity* is the ability of an infectious agent to enter, survive and multiply in a host. *Pathogenicity* is the ability of an infectious agent to induce infection. *Virulence* is the severity of the disease after infection occurs. Pathogenicity and virulence are often used interchangeably to refer to the severity of the disease. *Immunogenicity* is the ability of an infectious agent to produce a host immune response after an infection. The situation where an immune response has been induced that is capable of providing protection against reinfection with the same or similar organism in the host is called *protective immunity*. Protective immunity is normally lifelong in response to a natural infection. Following vaccination, it may be lifelong as is the case for some live vaccines (e.g., yellow fever) or short-lived (months) following administration of some inactivated vaccines (e.g., influenza). In addition, protective immunity may be sterilizing and prevent multiplication of the agent on reinfection, or it may allow for multiplication of the organism following reinfection but prevent clinical disease.

Characteristics of infectious agents

- **Infectivity** is the ability of an infectious agent to enter, survive, and multiply in a host.
- **Pathogenicity** is the ability of an infectious agent to induce infection.

- **Virulence** is the severity of the disease after infection occurs.
- **Immunogenicity** is the ability of an infectious agent to produce a host immune response after an infection.

Host factors are the intrinsic factors that determine a host's exposure, susceptibility, and response to an infectious agent. These include demographic characteristics (e.g., age, gender, and race or ethnicity); biological characteristics (e.g., gene, blood group, immunological response); social and economic characteristics (e.g., education, occupation, income and housing); and behaviors (e.g., nutrition, exercise, alcohol and drug use).

The greatest influence on host susceptibility is host immunity to a particular infectious agent. Diseases such as measles and chickenpox, caused by infectious agents with high immunogenicity, confer protective immunity after a single infection. However, other diseases caused by infectious agents with low immunogenicity such as influenza and gonorrhea, do not confer protective immunity, and leave the host susceptible to reinfection. There are active and passive mechanisms for acquiring immunity. Active immunity is protection that is produced by a person's own immune system, usually following natural infection. The goal of a vaccine is to produce active immunity similar to that acquired through natural infection but without the risk of disease. Passive immunity is acquired through the transfer or administration of antibody from an exogenous source. The most common form of passive immunity is the transfer of natural antibodies from mother to newborn child. This type of passive immunity diminishes over time, with antibodies against some diseases (e.g., measles, rubella, tetanus) providing longer protection than others (e.g., polio, pertussis). Other sources of passive immunity include almost all blood and blood products, immunoglobulins, and antitoxins.

Environmental factors are the extrinsic factors that affect the interaction between an infectious agent and a host. These can be categorized into three areas: physical (e.g., geography, climate, weather); biological (e.g., flora and fauna, presence of vectors and reservoirs), and social (e.g., culture, urbanization, laws, availability of health services). Environmental factors

305

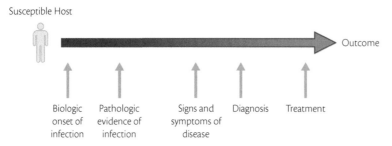

Figure 18.2 Natural history of disease.

facilitate the survival and infectivity of an infectious agent and the setting in which transmission occurs.

Mode of transmission

The mode of transmission refers to the mechanism by which an infectious agent is spread to a host. There are different ways to categorize the modes of transmission. Generally, infectious agents are transmitted through either direct or indirect contact. Direct contact refers to the immediate transfer of the infectious agent from the reservoir to the susceptible host. A reservoir is any person, animal, arthropod, plant, soil, or substance (or combination of these) in which an infectious agent normally lives and multiplies, on which it depends primarily for survival, and where it reproduces itself so that it can be transmitted to a susceptible host. Transmission by direct contact requires physical contact with blood or body fluids between an infected host and a susceptible host and the resulting transfer of the infectious agent. This includes human to human (skin and sexual), perinatal (mother to child), and droplet spread (large particles expelled from respiratory secretions). Pathogens that spread exclusively by direct contact are unable to survive for significant periods of time away from a host. Alternatively, indirect contact occurs when the infectious agent is carried from the reservoir to the susceptible host by ingestion of contaminated food and water products (food-borne or waterborne), inhalation of contaminated air (airborne), or transmission by a vector (vector-borne). Modes of transmission are characteristic of an infectious agent but are not mutually exclusive; some infectious agents can be transmitted by more than one mode of transmission. For example, West Nile virus (WNV) is normally transmitted indirectly by the bite of a virus-infected mosquito,

but it has been demonstrated that WNV can be spread to blood donor recipients by viremic individuals who donate blood.

Natural history

Natural history describes the progression of an infectious disease in an individual, over time, in the absence of intervention (see Figure 18.2). The start of the natural history time line is the successful infection of a susceptible host by an infectious agent. At some point after infection, pathologic evidence of infection is detectable, meaning the host may not know he/she is infected but a laboratory test, such as a test for antibodies, demonstrates infection. As the natural history of disease progresses, signs and symptoms of disease are visible. *Symptoms* refer to characteristics associated with feeling unwell (e.g., fever, coughing) while *signs* refer to measurable characteristics of being unwell (e.g., body temperature, mean hemoglobin level). If the signs and symptoms are severe enough, the host will seek medical care, receive a diagnosis, and start treatment if available. *Outcome* refers to the resolution of infection. The infection can continue, or the host can recover from the disease and develop immunity, or become a disease carrier, or the host can die.

Infection and disease are distinct concepts. *Infection* is the introduction and multiplication of an infectious agent within a host, while *disease* is the physiological dysfunction characterized by identifiable signs or symptoms. For a specific infectious disease, an infected individual may or may not have disease, but a diseased individual is always infected.

To illustrate the relationship between infection and disease, the stages of each are shown side by side in Figure 18.3. Both begin with a susceptible host who is not yet infected by the infectious agent. The *latent*

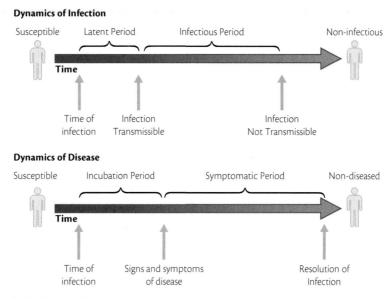

Figure 18.3 Stages of infection and disease.

period is the interval between the time of infection and the time when an infected host is able to transmit infection, or becomes infectious. The infectious period is the interval during which the infectious agent can be transmitted and infect another host or vector. The final stage in the infection process is when the infected host is no longer able to transmit the infectious agent, because the infection has cleared due to effective treatment or immune response, or because the host has died. Other possibilities not illustrated in the figure are for the host to become noninfectious while still harboring the infectious agent. The host may also become a carrier, recovered from the disease but still infectious (asymptomatically infected) (e.g., herpes, hepatitis B, syphilis, and malaria).

The stages of disease also begin with a susceptible host. The *incubation period* is the time from initial infection to the onset of symptoms and/or signs of clinical illness. Each infectious disease has a characteristic incubation period, dependent upon the rate of multiplication of the pathogen in the host, dose of the infectious agent, portal of entry, and host immune response. Because of the interplay of these factors, the incubation period for an infectious agent varies among individuals and is usually reported as a range. The symptomatic period is the time during which symptoms and/or signs of the disease are evident. The prob-

ability of a host developing symptomatic disease after becoming infected is based on the pathogenicity of the infectious agent and its interaction with the host.

The importance of distinguishing between the stages of infection and disease

The relation of the time lines for infection and disease is specific to each infectious agent and can have important epidemiologic implications that affect public health.

For example, HIV has a short latent period, usually 1–3 months, and a long incubation period, averaging 8–10 years. Therefore, people infected with HIV can infect many people before becoming aware of their HIV status and practicing safe behaviors to minimize chances for transmission to another person.

On the other hand, *Plasmodium falciparum*, one of the organisms that cause malaria, has an incubation period of about 14 days, but the infectious stage does not appear until about 10 days after the first symptoms of disease. Thus, early identification of disease and treatment of symptoms with a drug that prevents infectious stages can reduce transmission.

While the disease process and its associated time line are important to the infected person and clinician, the dynamics of infection are important for the propagation of the infectious agent and public health.

Measures of disease transmission

Transmission from an infected host to a susceptible host is an essential survival strategy for infectious agents; therefore, interrupting transmission between an infected host and a susceptible host is a prime goal for prevention and control measures. The *transmission probability*, the *secondary attack rate*, and the *basic reproductive number* are measures of disease frequency used by infectious disease epidemiologists to assess the transmissibility of an infectious agent.

Measures of disease transmission

The **transmission probability** (β) is the probability, in a population, that contact between an infectious case and a susceptible individual in the population will result in the successful transfer of the infectious agent and infection.

The **secondary attack rate** (SAR) is a special case of the transmission probability. The secondary attack rate measures the frequency of new cases of infection among susceptible contacts of known infectious cases in a defined population over a specified period of time.

The **basic reproductive number** (R_0) is an alternative method of measuring the transmissibility of an infectious agent. R_0 is also called the *basic reproductive rate*; however, it is technically not a rate. The importance of R_0 is it measures the effectiveness of an infectious agent to spread in a population. R_0 is the expected number of secondary cases (successful transmissions) produced when a single primary case is introduced into a totally susceptible population.

Transmission probability (β) and secondary attack rate

The transmission probability (β) is the probability, in a population, that contact between an infectious individual and a susceptible individual will result in the successful transfer of the infectious agent and result in infection.

The formula for the transmission probability is

$$\text{Transmission Probability } (\beta) = \frac{\begin{array}{c}\text{Number of infections that}\\\text{occur in a population during}\\\text{contacts between infectious}\\\text{and susceptible individuals}\end{array}}{\begin{array}{c}\text{Total number of contacts made}\\\text{between infectious and}\\\text{susceptible individuals}\\\text{in a population}\end{array}} \times 100$$

The secondary attack rate (SAR) is a special case of the transmission probability. It is the probability that an infectious agent will be transmitted in a small group, such as a household or a school class. The SAR measures the frequency of new cases of infection among susceptible contacts of known infectious cases in a defined population over a specified period. The primary case is the first case of an infection in a population, and the secondary cases are infections directly attributable to the primary case.

The formula for the SAR is

$$\text{Secondary Attack Rate (SAR)} = \frac{\begin{array}{c}\text{Number of susceptible individuals}\\\text{in a defined population who}\\\text{become infected following}\\\text{contact with a primary case}\\\text{during a specified period of time}\end{array}}{\begin{array}{c}\text{Total number of susceptible}\\\text{individuals exposed in a}\\\text{defined population during}\\\text{a specific period of time}\end{array}} \times 100$$

The definition of a contact of the primary case will vary and should always be clearly stated so the denominator is clear. For example, in a household study of SAR, contacts with a primary case could be defined as "eating and sleeping in the same house as a primary case during a specific period of time." In a school study of secondary attack rate, contact with a primary case could be defined as "attendance in the same class as a primary case during a specified period of time."

A specified period is necessary to determine the appropriate counts in the numerator and denominator of the SAR. The period often used is the maximum incubation period or the duration of infectiousness of the infectious agent. The secondary attack rate can be used to describe the transmission potential of an infectious disease within subgroups of a population defined by characteristics such as age, gender, and type of contact. The SAR is a measure of infectivity of an infectious agent.

The mode of transmission of the infectious agent determines which types of contact lead to a potentially infectious exposure. The SAR is generally used for diseases that are spread by direct contact with a short period of infectiousness, such as measles and chickenpox. If the period of infectiousness is long, such as for tuberculosis, the duration of exposure becomes important, and the denominator for the SAR is computed in person-time (person-weeks, person-months, or person-years) of exposure instead of total number of persons exposed.

To calculate the SAR directly, detailed information is needed on the number of susceptible individuals exposed to a primary case and the number of secondary cases within the population. These data are best obtained during outbreak investigations conducted by epidemiologists. It is possible to estimate the SAR indirectly using routine surveillance data that distinguishes between primary and secondary cases and estimating the number of exposed susceptible persons using data on the mean size of the population.

Secondary attack rates can be used to estimate the effectiveness of vaccination and other control measures and the effect of vaccination on reducing infectiousness in breakthrough cases, infections in newly vaccinated people by the same infectious agent that the vaccine was designed to protect against. Factor-specific (e.g., age- and gender-specific) SARs that show greatly increased risk of infection among subgroups in the population are often used to develop recommendations for the targeted use of a vaccine. The SAR can also be used to measure post-licensure vaccine effectiveness. Vaccine efficacy (VE) must be demonstrated, usually in a randomized trial, before a vaccine can be licensed for use. After licensure, effectiveness of both the vaccine and the vaccination program must continue to be monitored. This is sometimes called a *phase IV clinical trial*. One way to do this is to compare the secondary attack rates in vaccinated and unvaccinated persons in a household with a primary case of the disease under study.

Measles vaccine efficacy determined from secondary attack rates

In 1974, an epidemic of measles occurred on Native American reservations in North and South Dakota. There were 71 cases of measles and 3 deaths, and the overall attack rate was 9 cases per 1000 persons. Secondary attack rates in households were used to assess vaccine efficacy in part to control for uniformity of exposure among vaccinated and unvaccinated populations.

A primary case was defined as "fever, the occurrence of a rash on the face and body, and either a cough, red eyes, or a runny nose," and a secondary case was defined by the same signs but with the onset of symptoms one incubation period (7 to 18 days) after the index case.

Secondary attack rates in vaccinated (21 cases per 1000 persons) and unvaccinated (800 cases per 1000 persons) household contacts, under 9 years of age, were used to calculate a vaccine efficacy (VE) of 97.3% (95% confidence interval [CI] 80.1% to 99.9%).

The calculation of the secondary attack rate is based on a number of assumptions. The SAR depends on accurately identifying and quantifying susceptible individuals in a population. The means of identifying susceptible individuals varies according to the disease being studied and the time and resources available. Often, susceptible individuals are defined as persons who report no previous history of or vaccination against the disease. In special instances where the population is unvaccinated or the disease does not confer lifelong immunity, all members of the population are assumed to be susceptible. It is also assumed that all individuals in the population are equally susceptible. If these assumptions are not met, the calculation of the SAR may be subject to considerable error.

However, in fact it may not be possible to exactly identify who is or is not susceptible, and susceptibility may vary according to a number of characteristics of the exposed persons, such as age and gender. Counting as susceptible some individuals of the population who are actually immune to the disease will underestimate the SAR, because individuals who are not susceptible will artificially increase the size of the denominator and lower the estimate. Another assumption that is often made is that each secondary case derives from a single primary case. However, co-primary cases mistakenly counted as secondary cases or transmission from outside the population would inflate the numerator and cause an overestimation of the measure. The presence of asymptomatic cases in the population can lead to distortions of the estimate by including asymptomatic cases as susceptible (thereby inflating the denominator) or not counting as cases (thereby decreasing the numerator).

Pandemic (H1N1) 2009 early outbreak and disease characteristics and vaccination

When the pandemic (H1N1) 2009 flu outbreak was first detected in mid-April 2009, the US Centers for Disease Control and Prevention (CDC) began working with states to collect, compile, and analyze information regarding the outbreak. From April 12 to July 23, 2009, states reported a total of 43,667 laboratory-confirmed infections of pandemic influenza A (H1N1) infection. Of these, there were 5009 people who were hospitalized, and 302 people who died.

Investigations showed that reports of laboratory-confirmed infections greatly underestimated the burden of disease. A model was developed by the CDC to estimate the total number of pandemic (H1N1) 2009 flu cases in the USA. The model adjusted the count of laboratory-confirmed cases reported by states to account for known sources of underestimation (not all individuals with influenza seek medical care; not all persons who seek medical care have specimens collected by their health care provider; not all health care providers submit specimens for confirmation; laboratory detection of pandemic [H1N1] 2009 is not perfect; and not all confirmed cases are reported). Using this approach, which is commonly used to calculate the impact of food-borne illness in the USA, it was estimated that 3 million (range: 1.8 million to 5.7 million) symptomatic cases of pandemic (H1N1) 2009 and 14,000 (range: 9000 to 21,000) hospitalizations due to pandemic (H1N1) 2009 actually occurred between April and July 2009 in the USA.

Acute respiratory illness (ARI) is defined as two or more of the following four symptoms: fever, cough, sore throat, and rhinorrhea (runny nose). Influenza-like illness (ILI) is defined as fever and cough or sore throat. Epidemiologic field studies in several states found a secondary attack rate in household contacts for ARI was 18% to 19% and for ILI, 8% to 12%. Overall, the household secondary attack rates for pandemic (H1N1) 2009 were lower than household secondary attack rates for seasonal influenza. The use of antiviral medications for treatment of the index case and prophylaxis of household contacts may have decreased secondary attack rates.

Vaccines against pandemic (H1N1) 2009 infection were produced using methods similar to those used for seasonal influenza vaccine development, and vaccine distribution began in October 2009. The vaccine was recommended by the CDC Advisory Committee on Immunization Practices (ACIP) for five initial target groups: pregnant women, persons who live with or provide care for infants aged younger than 6 months, health care and emergency medical services personnel, children and young adults aged 6 months to 24 years, and persons aged 25–64 years with medical conditions that put them at higher risk for influenza-related complications. Among all persons aged older than 6 months, (H1N1) 2009 vaccine coverage was 27.0% (95% CI 26.6–27.4%). As a result of the vaccination campaign, CDC estimated 713,000 to 1.5 million cases; 3900 to 10,400 hospitalizations; and 200 to 520 deaths were averted.

Basic reproductive number (R_0)

The basic reproductive number (R_0) is an alternative method of measuring the transmissibility of an infectious agent. R_0 (pronounced *R-naught* or *R-zero*) is also called the basic reproductive rate; however, it is a dimensionless number and technically not a rate. R_0 measures how effective an infectious agent is at spreading in a population: R_0 is the expected number of secondary cases (successful transmissions) produced when a single primary case is introduced into a totally susceptible population.

In theory, it should be possible to measure R_0 directly by counting the number of infectious secondary cases that are produced after a primary case of infection is introduced into a totally susceptible population. However, this situation rarely occurs in reality. Instead, R_0 is calculated as the product of the transmission probability per contact (β), the product of the number of contacts per unit time (N), and the mean duration of infectiousness ($1/\gamma$). It can be very difficult to obtain reliable estimates of these parameters.

Basic Reproductive Number (R$_0$)

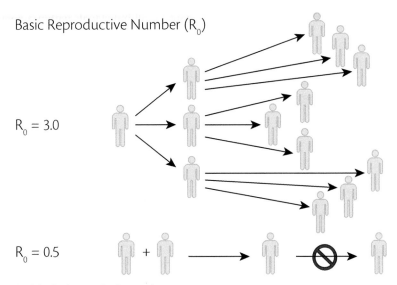

$R_0 = 3.0$

$R_0 = 0.5$

Figure 18.4 Schematic of the basic reproductive number.

The formula for the basic reproductive number is

Basic
Reproductive = Transmission probability per contact
Number   × number of contacts per unit time
              × duration of infectiousness

$$R_0 = \beta N * 1/y$$

R_0 reflects the transmission potential of a specific infectious agent within a specific host population at a particular time. If the basic reproductive number of an agent in a specific population is known, the expansion of the infectious agent in that population can be predicted (see Figure 18.4). It is influenced by the number of contacts made by the infectious case during the infectious period. Therefore, R_0 is not constant for a specific infectious agent.

If $R_0 = 1$, on average, each infectious primary case will produce one infectious secondary case and the incidence of disease in the population will remain static. If $R_0 < 1$, on average, each infectious primary case will produce less than one infectious secondary case, the incidence of disease will decrease, and the disease will eventually be eliminated from the population. The infectious agent cannot invade the population; therefore infection control measures will not be cost-effective and are unnecessary. If $R_0 > 1$, on average, each case will produce more than one infectious secondary case, the incidence of disease in the population will increase, and the infectious agent will invade the population. Control measures are therefore warranted to prevent or delay an epidemic. A larger value for R_0 is associated with a greater population density, which increases the number of contacts per unit time; high levels of infectivity, which increase the transmission probability per contact; and a longer duration of infectiousness. Ranges of R_0 for well-known infectious diseases are shown in Table 18.1.

The basic reproductive number assumes all interactions of the primary case are with a susceptible population. However, this scenario is unusual. More commonly, some individuals in the population will be already infected or immune, and the expected number of secondary cases produced by a single primary case will be less than estimated by R_0. The effective reproductive number (R) is the average number of secondary infections produced by one infected individual when that individual is introduced into a population where some of the individuals are not susceptible, either because they are immune from past infection or vaccination or the subjects are practicing control measures to limit transmission.

If all individuals in a population mix together at random (homogeneously), so that infectious cases are likely to make contact with those who are susceptible

Table 18.1 Values of R_0 for Well-Known Infectious Diseases

Disease	R_0
Measles	12–18
Pertussis	12–17
Diphtheria	6–7
Smallpox	5–7
Polio	5–7
Rubella	5–7
Mumps	4–7
HIV/AIDS	2–5
SARS	2–5
Influenza	2–3
Ebola	1.3–2.0
Yellow fever	1.2–6.8

as well as those who are not, R is the product of R_0 and the proportion of the population that is susceptible (x).

The formula for the effective reproductive number is

Effective
Reproductive = Basic reproductive number
Number   × proportion of the population
          susceptible

$$R = R_0 x$$

For an infectious agent to be transmitted within a population, susceptible individuals must be exposed to a source of infection. The continued transmission of an infectious agent in a population is dependent on the number of infectious and susceptible individuals in the population and the effective contact between these individuals. For an infectious agent to persist there must be an adequate number of susceptible individuals in the population because the probability of making effective contact that will enable transmission is dependent on the abundance of susceptible individuals. While the mode of transmission determines the transmission probability per contact, population size and behavior determine the rate at which effective contacts may occur.

There are two important assumptions for the use of R_0 and R: the assumption that transmissibility is constant for all individuals within a population, and the assumption of homogeneous mixing. If people in a population mix randomly, each person will have an equal chance of making contact with any other person, and so every susceptible person will have chance of being exposed to infection. However, in most populations people do not mix at random, but have complex contact patterns through social, professional, and familial networks.

Example of influences on the basic reproductive number (R_0) for a sexually transmitted hepatitis B virus infection

$$R_0 = \beta N * 1/\gamma$$

Influences

B   Hepatitis B vaccine, condom use
N   Health education, negotiating skills
$1/\gamma$ Case ascertainment, screening, partner notification, treatment, compliance, health-seeking behavior, accessibility to health services

---

Herd immunity

Vaccination programs can reduce the transmission probability of an infectious agent by reducing the proportion of people who are susceptible (x) in the population and increasing the proportion of people who are immune ($1-x$). *Herd immunity* is the resistance of a population to invasion and spread of an infectious agent based on the resistance of a high proportion of individual members in the population to the infection. If a sufficient number of individuals in a population is immune to an infectious agent, the effect of herd immunity may lead to the protection of susceptible individuals in the population and if insufficient numbers of susceptible individuals are available, the infectious agent may be eliminated from the population.

At a certain threshold, called the *herd immunity threshold* (HIT), each case will only be able to transmit the infection to one other case ($R_0 = 1$). Below this threshold, R_0 will be less than 1 and transmission will be interrupted. Thus, the HIT is the minimum proportion of the population that needs to be immune in order to control transmission. The larger R_0, the greater

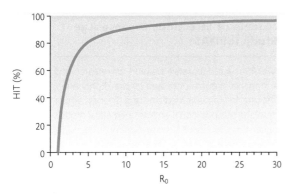

Figure 18.5 Relationship between herd immunity threshold and R_0.

Table 18.2 Values of the Herd Immunity Threshold for Well-known Infectious Diseases

Disease	Herd immunity threshold (%)
Malaria	99
Measles	90–95
Pertussis	90–95
Chicken pox	85–90
Mumps	85–90
Rubella	82–87
Poliomyelitis	82–87
Diphtheria	82–87
Scarlet fever	82–87
Smallpox	70–80

the proportion of immune individuals required to achieve herd immunity is (see Figure 18.5). R_0 can be used to estimate the proportion of the population that needs to be immune to ensure that the disease becomes stable.

The formula for herd immunity threshold is

Herd
Immunity $= 1 - (1/R_0) = (R_0 - 1)/R_0$
Threshold

If vaccination conferred complete and lifelong immunity to all those vaccinated, the HIT would be the proportion of the population that needs to be vaccinated to stabilize transmission. The proportion of the population vaccinated would need to be even greater to reduce transmission of the infectious agent to a level where it will eventually die out. The proportion of the population that would have to be vaccinated to make $R_0 < 1$ increases if the vaccine does not provide full immunity to all vaccinated individuals or if immunity is short-lived (such as influenza vaccination, which needs to be given each year). Table 18.2 shows the values of the HIT for some well-known infectious diseases.

The basic reproductive number can be used to help predict the effects of public health interventions on the transmission of an infectious agent in a population. Public health strategies to reduce the duration of infectiousness, the transmission probability per contact or the contact rate should lower R_0 and therefore decrease transmission in the population.

Ruining it for the rest of us

A radio segment on "This American Life" (Episode 370: Ruining It for the Rest of Us) (http://www.thisamericanlife.org) discusses an outbreak of measles in San Diego in 2008 that terrified the community. The outbreak began in January 2008 when an unvaccinated 7-year-old boy visited Switzerland with his family and unknowingly contracted the virus. He returned to the USA and attended school during the incubation period before the onset of symptoms. After becoming symptomatic, he visited a pediatrician's office and a hospital's emergency room before finally being diagnosed with measles. For at least some of the time before and after onset of symptoms he was infectious.

Eleven children in the county were diagnosed with measles, including the index patient's siblings, five children in his school, and four additional children who had been in the pediatrician's office at the same time. Approximately 70 additional infants and children exposed to the 12 measles cases were placed under home quarantine for 21 days because their parents had either declined measles vaccination or they were too young to be vaccinated.

This outbreak serves as an illustration of the principles and assumptions of herd immunity and as a reminder that unvaccinated persons remain at risk for measles. Measles virus is highly infectious, and vaccination coverage levels of greater than 90% are needed to interrupt disease transmission.

Introduction to infectious disease modeling

Models can be used to understand the epidemiology of infectious diseases, to predict the impact of infectious disease control programs, and increasingly to guide public health policy. Models aim to re-create the transmission dynamics of an infection using the smallest number of parameters and assumptions possible in an attempt to simplify a very complex system. A model is always "wrong" in the sense that it is simplified, but it allows conceptual studies of empirical data that would otherwise be difficult or impossible to conduct using traditional lab- and field-based methods.

In a virtual laboratory, models are created to mimic a real population. The model can be manipulated to study problems not easily examined in real life, such as the introduction and spread of a specific infectious agent. Modeling is used to understand the relative importance of critical factors on the spread of disease, elucidate the research questions that need to be answered, detect important data needs and gaps, compare the relative effects of different prevention and control policies on the spread of disease, and identify new research questions that are critical to better understanding the infectious agent.

Models are useful to researchers, public health workers, economists, and policy makers. Modeling can provide useful insight into the epidemiology of an infectious disease and predict future numbers of cases, critical levels of vaccination coverage based on herd immunity, and the impact of vaccination strategies and other control measures in populations. This information can be used to design cost-effective control strategies and guide public health policy decisions.

There are two types of models: stochastic and deterministic. Stochastic models allow for chance variation by simultaneously considering the probability of each possible value of a variable at each moment in time. Stochastic models are generally preferred over deterministic models because they show variability in outcomes that is also present in the real world. Stochastic models are the basis for advanced modeling techniques and beyond the scope of this chapter.

Basic principles of modeling are more easily understood in the context of deterministic models. Deterministic models describe what happens on average in a population. The parameters of a deterministic model

Models of Infectious Disease Agent Study (MIDAS)

MIDAS is a collaborative network of research and informatics groups sponsored by the US National Institute for General Medicine and Science, which develops computational and mathematical models to understand infectious disease dynamics. The MIDAS network develops models that are used to plan for infectious disease threats and detect and respond to outbreaks. MIDAS researchers have focused on influenza, methicillin-resistant *Staphylococcus aureus* (MRSA), cholera, dengue fever, malaria, and tuberculosis.

One of the first MIDAS projects addressed the public health community fear that an influenza strain emerging in Southeast Asia soon would spread worldwide. To help prepare and prevent such an event, MIDAS scientists modeled a flu pandemic. Their initial models examined the potential effectiveness of different interventions, including vaccinating people before an outbreak, distributing antiviral medications, closing schools, and quarantining infected individuals. The results suggested that a combination of measures, if implemented early and in a particular way, might contain spread.

This early work helped MIDAS scientists use models to study H1N1 or "swine flu," the first actual pandemic flu strain since 1968. Beginning in April 2009, they used incoming data to simulate spread, identify at-risk groups, and evaluate the potential health impact with and without intervention. Their work indicated that early vaccination of schoolchildren best reduced disease, while vaccinating elders became more important later on in the pandemic, indicating that the effectiveness of different vaccination strategies may vary during different phases of a pandemic. The model also indicated that people at risk for serious complications—including those who are pregnant or have certain preexisting health problems—should be given antivirals to take at the first signs of illness.

are fixed and the outcome predetermined; there is no element of chance. The majority of deterministic models are compartmental models. Compartmental models stratify individuals into broad epidemiologically meaningful categories, which depend on the disease, and describe the transitions between these categories. Compartmental models can be set up using differential equations.

Suspectible, Infected, and Recovered (SIR) model

The SIR model is one of the simplest and most fundamental of all epidemiologic models and appropriate for infectious diseases transmitted by direct contact, e.g., respiratory, fecal–oral, or sexual contact, but not indirect contact, e.g., infection via a bite from a mosquito or tick. It is based on compartmentalizing the population in one of three classes based on epidemiologic status: (1) susceptible to infection, (2) infected and therefore infectious, or (3) recovered and no longer infectious, and determining the rates of transition between these classes. The SIR model describes the progress of an epidemic through large populations, in which small fluctuations at the individual level are assumed not to have an important effect on the dynamics of disease transmission. SIR models are appropriate for directly transmitted infections that confer lifelong immunity. The SIR model is a deterministic model and describes what happens on average in a large population. However, these models are unlikely to provide a reliable answer to questions involving small populations, where chance might play an important role in the outcome.

Basics of the SIR model

$S + I + R = N$

S: Susceptible	Individuals in the population able to be infected. The susceptible period is the period prior to infection. A susceptible individual is not protected by any genetic or immune mechanism.
I: Infected	Individuals in the population able to transmit an infectious agent to another individual. The infectious period, also known as the period of communicability, is the period of the infection process during which the infected individual can transmit the infectious agent to another individual.
R: Recovered	Individuals in the population no longer able to transmit the infectious agent, either because they have cleared the infection through an effective immune response or treatment, or because they have died.
N: Population	Total number of individuals in the population.

The SIR model is a mathematical model using differential equations to describe the transmission dynamics of an infection in a population:

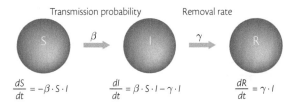

The compartments S, I, and R are variables that change with time. Shown are the basic differential equations for the SIR variables that give the rate of change of the proportion in each compartment with time. In the above equations, the input parameters β, the transmission probability, and γ, the removal rate, determine how the compartments change with time. β is the most common parameter in infectious disease models and also the most difficult to estimate. It is commonly referred to as "transmission probability," "transmission coefficient," "transmission parameter," and "transmission rate." It is the probability, in a population, that contact between an infectious individual and a susceptible individual will result in the successful transfer of the infectious agent, followed by infection. It is the effective contact between two specific individuals per unit time, and it may decrease over time as the result of interventions and behavior change. The inverse of the mean duration of infectiousness is γ. It is the average time at which individuals recover from an infectious disease. The average latent and infectious periods are usually known for vaccine-preventable infections.

The general predictions of the SIR model show the fundamental parameter that governs epidemic behavior is the basic reproductive number, R_0. At the end of an epidemic, a proportion of the population remains susceptible, and an infectious agent cannot spread within a population when the population of susceptibles is reduced below the HIT.

The SIR model makes several assumptions. It assumes that the population is fixed and all individuals in the population are represented by one of the three classes: susceptibles, infectious, or recovered. The only way a person can leave the susceptible group is to become infected. The only way a person can leave the infected group is to recover and become immune (or die from the disease). There is no in-migration and out-migration or deaths from other causes. There is no inherited immunity. Age, sex, social status, and race or ethnicity do not affect the probability of being infected. The members of the population mix homogeneously, individuals are as likely to contact people of different ages, gender, and social groups, as they are to contact people of their own age, gender, and social group.

SIR model dynamics

The SIR model predicts an epidemic that follows recognized patterns: The number of cases initially increases exponentially until the proportion of susceptibles in the population has been sufficiently depleted that the growth rate slows; this process continues until the epidemic can no longer be sustained and the number of cases drops, eventually leading to the extinction of the spread of infection.

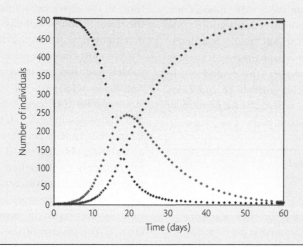

Typical disease examples for which a SIR model is used include measles, mumps, and chickenpox, infections that confer lifelong immunity. Variations of the SIR model through the removal and/or addition of compartments have been developed to incorporate different stages of the natural history of disease. For example, the SIS model is used for infections, such as rotavirus and gonorrhea, which do not confer long-lasting immunity and therefore do not have a recovered state; individuals become susceptible again after infection. The SIRS model is more suitable for infections such as pertussis where individuals initially recover but the immunity acquired by infection wanes with time so they become susceptible again. Another variation takes into account diseases in which individuals can be infected but not yet infectious. During the latent period, the individual is in compartment E (for exposed). There is the SEIS (no immunity) model, used for tuberculosis, and the SEIR (with immunity) model, used for smallpox. For some diseases, such as measles, infants are not born into the susceptible compartment but are immune to the disease for the first few months of life due to protection from maternal antibodies. The MSIR model adds an M compartment (for maternally derived immunity) at the beginning of the model.

Variations of the SIR model

The SIS model assumes there is no lasting immunity to the infection. Individuals recover with no immunity to the infectious disease; therefore they are immediately susceptible once they have recovered.

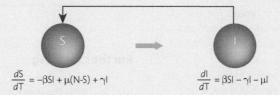

$$\frac{dS}{dT} = -\beta SI + \mu(N\text{-}S) + \gamma I \qquad \frac{dI}{dT} = \beta SI - \gamma I - \mu I$$

The SIRS model is simply an extension of the SIR model. The only difference is that it allows members of the recovered class to be free of infection and rejoin the susceptible class.

$$\frac{dS}{dT} = -\beta SI + \mu(N-S) + fR \qquad \frac{dI}{dT} = \beta SI - \gamma I - \mu I \qquad \frac{dR}{dT} = \gamma I - \mu R - fR$$

The SEIS model takes into consideration the exposed or latent period of the disease, creating an additional compartment, E. In this model there is no lasting immunity to the infection; thus individuals who have recovered return to being susceptible again.

$$\frac{dS}{dT} = B - \beta SI - \mu S + \gamma I \qquad \frac{dE}{dT} = \beta SI - (\epsilon + \mu)E \qquad \frac{dI}{dT} = \epsilon E - (\gamma + \mu)I$$

The SEIR model also takes into consideration the exposed or latent period of the disease creating an additional compartment, E. However, in this model there is lasting immunity to the infection.

$$\frac{dS}{dT} = B - \beta SI - \mu S \qquad \frac{dE}{dT} = \beta SI - (\epsilon + \mu)E \qquad \frac{dI}{dT} = \epsilon E - (\gamma + \mu)I \qquad \frac{dR}{dT} = \gamma I - \mu R$$

The MSIR model is used to describe diseases where an infant is born with passive immunity from its mother.

$$\frac{dM}{dT} = B - \delta MS - \mu M \qquad \frac{dS}{dT} = \delta MS - \beta SI - \mu S \qquad \frac{dI}{dT} = \beta SI - \gamma I - \mu I \qquad \frac{dR}{dT} = \gamma I - \mu R$$

Summary

- Many of the various mechanisms of infectious diseases are well understood, from the molecular aspects of the infectious agent to the interaction of the infectious agent, host, and environment. This level of understanding has enabled effective prevention and control measures to be developed for many infectious diseases.

- The success of vaccination programs in the prevention and control of infectious diseases is due to the disruption of disease transmission. Vaccination reduces the pool of susceptible individuals, and when vaccination coverage in a population is greater than the herd immunity threshold, an infectious disease cannot spread within the population. This is good news, as it is not necessary to vaccinate everyone to prevent an epidemic; disease elimination may even be possible! Models can be used to predict the outcome of an epidemic process or the impact of control measures.

- Models are an explanatory tool to elucidate fundamental principles of infectious disease transmission and are important for understanding population dynamics of the transmission of infectious agents and the potential impact of infectious disease control programs.

- The design and complexity of infectious disease transmission models depends on the questions to be answered. Models are used to illustrate general concepts and make disease predictions that can be used to design effective prevention and control measures and inform public health policy. It is important to remember that without a good statistical estimation of input parameters from epidemiologic data, models cannot be used as a predictive tool.

Further reading

Breman JG, de Quadros CA, Dowdle WR, Foege WH, Henderson DA, John TJ, and Levine MM (2011). The role of research in viral disease eradication and elimination programs: lessons for malaria eradication. PLoS Medicine 8, e1000405.

Moss WJ and Griffin DE (2012). Measles. Lancet 379, 153–164.

Nathanson N and Kew OM (2010). From emergence to eradication: the epidemiology of poliomyelitis deconstructed. American Journal of Epidemiology 172, 1213–1229.

Osterholm MT, Kelley NS, Sommer A, and Belongia EA (2012). Efficacy and effectiveness of influenza vaccines: a systematic review and meta-analysis. The Lancet Infectious Diseases 12, 36–44.

Sáfadi MA and McIntosh ED (2011). Epidemiology and prevention of meningococcal disease: a critical appraisal of vaccine policies. Expert Review of Vaccines 10, 1717–1730.

Tan TQ (2012). Pediatric invasive pneumococcal disease in the United States in the era of pneumococcal conjugate vaccines. Clinical Microbiology Reviews 25, 409–419.

19 | Vaccines from a global perspective

Alan D.T. Barrett and Bridget E. Hawkins

Sealy Center for Vaccine Development, University of Texas Medical Branch, Galveston, TX, USA

Abbreviations

ADIP	Accelerated Development and Implementation Plan	IFFIm	International Finance Facility for Immunization
AMC	Advance Market Commitments	IFPMA	International Federation of Pharmaceutical Manufacturers and Associations
AMP	Agence de Médecine Préventive		
APHIS	Animal and Plant Health Inspection Service	IPV	Inactivated polio virus
BCG	Bacillus Calmette–Guérin	IVR	Initiative for Vaccine Research
CDC	Centers for Disease Control and Prevention	NCL	National Control Laboratories
		NRA	National regulatory authorities
EMA	European Medicines Agency	OIE	World Organization for Animal Health (formerly the Office International des Epizooties)
EPI	Expanded Program on Immunizations		
ERA	Environmental risk assessment		
FAO	Food and Agriculture Organization	OPV	Oral polio vaccine
GACVS	Global Advisory Committee on Vaccine Safety	PATH	Program for Appropriate Technology in Health
GAVI	Global Alliance for Vaccines and Immunization	PDP	Product Development Partnerships
		PPP	Private–Public Partnerships
GIVS	Global Immunization Vision and Strategy	QSS	Quality, Safety, and Standards
GMO	Genetically manipulated organism	SAGE	Strategic Advisory Group of Experts on Immunization
GMP	Good Manufacturing Practices		
Hib	*Haemophilus influenza* type b	UN	United Nations
HIV	Human immunodeficiency virus	UNICEF	United Nations Children's Fund
HPV	Human papillomavirus	US FDA	US Food and Drug Administration
HVI	HIV Vaccine Initiative		
ICH	International Conference on Harmonisation	USDA	US Department of Agriculture
		WHO	World Health Organization

Vaccinology: An Essential Guide, First Edition. Edited by Gregg N. Milligan and Alan D.T. Barrett.
© 2015 John Wiley & Sons, Ltd. Published 2015 by John Wiley & Sons, Ltd.

The global perspective

There are four major factors pertaining to global vaccine development:

- Diseases
- Economics
- Infrastructure
- Regulatory affairs

The world is often divided in to three categories: developed countries (e.g., USA, Britain, France, Germany, and Australia), middle-income countries (e.g., Russia, Mexico, China, and India), and developing countries (e.g., many countries in Africa and Asia). Vaccine development is traditionally seen as a process that takes place in developed countries; however, this is not the true situation. Infectious diseases are a global problem and not surprisingly vaccine development takes place on a global scale. The human population is approximately 7 billion today and is predicted to rise to 9.5 billion by 2050. Thus there is a global need for vaccines. There is no doubt that vaccines are very successful and are second only to clean, safe drinking water as the most effective public health intervention of all time in reducing mortality and helping population growth in the 20th century. The World Health Organization (WHO) has estimated that vaccines prevent more than 2.5 million deaths of children each year.

There are four major factors pertaining to global vaccine development: diseases, economics, infrastructure, and regulatory affairs.

Diseases

Priority diseases for vaccine development

In addition to information on currently available vaccines, the WHO plays a very active role in vaccine development with respect to the future implementation of vaccines in advanced development. The WHO has identified 68 diseases where vaccines can reduce the morbidity and/or mortality (Table 19.1). This is a large list and includes diseases where no commercial vaccines exist and vaccines that are already available but not utilized to maximum effect in developing countries. Currently, the WHO has vaccine position papers on 21 of these diseases and agents (tuberculosis, cholera, diphtheria, Hib, hepatitis A, human papillomavirus (HPV), influenza, Japanese encephalitis, measles, meningococcal disease, mumps, pertussis, pneumococcus, polio, rabies, rotavirus, rubella, tetanus, typhoid, varicella, and yellow fever).

Examples of current global vaccine preventable diseases

Bacterial
Diphtheria
Haemophilus influenza
Meningitis
Neonatal tetanus
Tetanus
Tuberulosis

Viral
Hepatitis B
Measles
Mumps
Poliomyelitis
Rotavirus
Rubella and chronic rubella syndrome
Yellow fever

There are 24 diseases for which vaccine development is a priority, either as improved vaccines or as new vaccines (Table 19.2). For some of these diseases we already have vaccines (e.g., rabies and Japanese encephalitis), but the current vaccines are not affordable or cannot be manufactured at the large number of doses required for mass immunization campaigns. For example, the birth cohort in Asia is 500 million per year, and there is a target to immunize all against Japanese encephalitis. For other diseases, there are no vaccines currently available (e.g., respiratory syncytial virus), or there are vaccine candidates available that need further clinical development (e.g., malaria).

The research and development of vaccines used in developing countries cannot be based on experiences in developed countries. The burden of disease, epidemiology, health and nourishment of vaccinees, and immunogenicity in developed countries will all be different from that in developing countries. Different

Table 19.1 Diseases for Vaccine Research and Development[a]

Bacterial diseases	• Buruli ulcer *(Mycobacterium ulcerans)* • **Diphtheria** • Group A *Streptococcus*-associated diseases • Group B *Streptococcus*-associated diseases • ***Neisseria meningitidis*** meningitis (groups **A**, **B**, **C**, **Y**, **W135**) • **Pertussis** • *Staphylococcus aureus* associated diseases • Stomach cancer (Helicobacter pylori) • **Tetanus** • Trachoma
Enteric diseases	• Norovirus associated diarrhoea • Campylobacter diarrhoea • **Cholera** • Enterotoxigenic *Escherichia coli* (ETEC) diarrhea • **Rotavirus** diarrhea • Shigellosis • **Typhoid** fever
Hepatitis	• **Hepatitis A** • **Hepatitis B** • Hepatitis C • **Hepatitis E**
Parasitic diseases	• Amoebiasis • Hookworm disease • Leishmaniasis • Malaria (pre-erythrocyte, blood and sexual stages) • Schistosomiasis
Respiratory diseases	• ***Haemophilus influenzae B*** pneumonia and invasive disease • **Influenza** • **Measles** • **Mumps** • Parainfluenza-associated pneumonia (PIV-3) • **Pertussis** • Respiratory syncytial virus (RSV) pneumonia • Severe Acute Respiratory Syndrome (SARS) • ***Streptococcus pneumoniae*** pneumonia and invasive disease • **Tuberculosis**
Sexually transmitted diseases	• Cervical cancer (**human papillomavirus**) • *Chlamydia trachomatis*-associated genital diseases • Gonorrhea • Herpes simplex type 2 genital ulcers • HIV/AIDS

(Continued)

Table 19.1 (*Continued*)

Vector-borne viral diseases	• Dengue • **Japanese encephalitis** • **Tick-borne encephalitis** • West Nile virus-associated disease • **Yellow fever** • Cervical cancer (**human papillomavirus**) (see sexually transmitted diseases) • Gastric cancer (Helicobacter pylori) • Liver cancer (**Hepatitis B**) • Liver cancer (Hepatitis C) • Nasopharyngeal cancer (Epstein–Barr virus)
Zoonotic diseases	• Anthrax • Crimean–Congo hemorrhagic fever • Ebola hemorrhagic fever • Hepatitis E diarrhea • Lassa fever • Leishmaniasis • Leptospirosis • Lyme disease • Marburg hemorrhagic fever • Plague • **Rabies** • Rift Valley fever • Tularaemia
Other viral diseases	• **Mumps** • **Poliomyelitis** • **Rubella** • **Smallpox**

Modified from www.who.int/vaccine_research/diseases/portfolio/en/index.html.
[a]Diseases in bold font have vaccines commercially available.

Table 19.2 Priority Areas for Research and Development of New or Improved Vaccines

Diarrheal diseases	Malaria
Acute respiratory infections	Measles
Caliciviruses	Meningococcal vaccines
Campylobacter	Parainfluenza
Cholera	*Streptococcus pneumoniae*
Dengue	Rabies
Enterotoxigenic *Escherichia coli* (ETEC)	Rotavirus
Haemophilus influenzae	Respiratory syncytial virus (RSV)
Human immunodeficiency virus (HIV)	*Shigella*
Human papillomavirus	Tuberculosis
Influenza	Typhoid
Japanese encephalitis	

serotypes are found for a number of bacteria, viruses, and parasites in different geographical locations such that immunogenicity and vaccine components need to be evaluated by region. For example, meningococcal A conjugate (e.g., MenAfriVac in Africa) and rotavirus serotypes vary by geographic region. Consequently, clinical trials are needed in both developed and developing countries, and it is for this reason that clinical trials continually increase in numbers with 65,000–70,000 participants for the rotavirus vaccine clinical trials and up to 130,000 participants for the new meningococcal conjugate vaccines.

Meningitis vaccine project

Meningococcal meningitis, an infection of the membrane that surrounds the brain and spinal cord, is caused by bacteria that are transmitted via nasal and oral secretions from infected individuals. *Neisseria meningitides* is one species of bacteria with multiple serotypes (serotypes A, B, C, W135, X, and Y) that can cause meningitis. Each country's risk of an outbreak differs according to which serotype is prevalent in that region. The "meningitis belt" in sub-Saharan Africa has the highest incidence of meningitis worldwide. Polysaccharide vaccines for serotypes A, C, Y, and W135 have been in use since 1966 but with limited effectiveness in Africa. Nearly 80% of the cases there were attributed to the serotype A. In 1996, a particularly bad meningitis outbreak occurred that prompted the WHO to recommend that a conjugate MenA vaccine be developed. Since MenA primarily affects low-income countries, the large pharmaceutical companies could not find a viable market for the vaccine and would not be able to offer it at a low enough cost for the low-income countries to afford to adopt it. Subsequently, a partnership between the WHO and the Program for Appropriate Technology in Health (PATH) formed (supported by the Bill and Melinda Gates Foundation) and a MenA conjugate vaccine was created under a 10-year partnership called the Meningitis Vaccine Project (MVP). The MVP put together a product development partnership involving a Developing Country Vaccine Manufacturing Network company called the Serum Institute of India to manufacture the vaccine. The Serum Institute of India and Synco BioPartners in the Netherlands supplied the raw materials of the group A polysaccharide antigen and the protein tetanus toxoid protein, where the toxoid

acted as an adjuvant for the conjugate vaccine. The conjugation technology was provided by a partnership with the US Food and Drug Administration (US FDA) Center for Biologics Evaluation and Research (CBER) who transferred the technology to the Serum Institute of India at no cost. Thus, each vaccine dose costs less than $0.50. This low cost per dose makes it easier for poorer countries to adopt it into their routine immunization schedules. This new MenA conjugate vaccine (MenAfriVac™) was introduced in 2010 to a few countries in Africa, and these countries noticed a dramatic decrease in the number of meningitis cases attributed to serotype A. It is said to be more effective at preventing the spread of bacteria by carriers and is also more immunogenic so confers longer lasting protection against MenA infection. It is the main goal of the MVP to eliminate epidemic meningitis in Africa, and by 2016 they hope to have all of the countries in the "meningitis belt" immunizing their children and adults with this conjugate MenA vaccine.

Eradication of infectious diseases

Examples of diseases that we can eradicate with vaccination

- Smallpox
- Polio
- Measles
- Mumps
- Rubella
- Chickenpox
- Hepatitis B

Infectious agents that have a host other than humans (e.g., zoonotic diseases transmitted by insects or rodents) cannot be eliminated as they will always have a reservoir. However, in theory, any infectious agent that infects only humans can be eradicated by vaccination, but in reality this can be achieved for virus diseases only, as viruses need cells to multiply while other infectious agents can survive outside cells. Examples are measles, mumps, rubella, chickenpox, smallpox, hepatitis B, and poliomyelitis. To date, smallpox is the only infectious disease of humans that has been eradicated, and in 1980, the WHO officially announced its eradication. This was a worldwide effort not only involving the administration of the live smallpox vaccine but requiring the combined determination of every country to concurrently administer vaccine to all people such that the virus had no human reservoir. This was a milestone in vaccinology as this was the first, and only, human virus to be eliminated. Due to the success of the smallpox eradication campaign, the WHO and partners have tried to eradicate or eliminate other infectious diseases, most notably eradication of polio (polio global eradication initiative, http://www.polioeradication.org/) and measles (measles initiative, http://www.measlesinitiative.org/), and elimination of neonatal tetanus. In the case of neonatal tetanus, it is impossible to eradicate as it is caused by a neurotoxin produced by *Clostridium tetani*, and the bacterium survives in the environment. Nonetheless, the disease can be prevented by immunizing women of childbearing age, which provides protection to the mother, who transfers anti-tetanus antibodies to her baby. Thus, elimination would be declared if the number of neonatal tetanus cases fell to a figure below 1 case per 1000 live births per year in all parts of the world. However, these campaigns have not been successful due to the inability to immunize all people in all countries of the world because society accepts that individuals have the right to decline immunization.

In veterinary health, the livestock disease rinderpest, caused by rinderpest virus (a paramyxovirus related to measles virus), was declared eradicated in 2010 by the United Nations Food and Agriculture Organization. Rinderpest is a highly infectious viral disease that can destroy entire populations of cattle and buffalo. Although the virus does not affect humans directly, in regions that depend on cattle for meat and milk products, it has caused widespread famine and serious economic damage. Thus, a veterinary vaccine has indirect impact on human health.

Implementation

Vaccination is probably the most effective public health intervention of all time, other than safe drinking water. This is especially true in developing countries, where poverty limits those who can afford health care. Given the large quantity of research undertaken on vaccine development over a long period time (centuries), it is somewhat surprising that only a total of 31 vaccines are in use today. This is in part due to the long and complex road to the development of a vaccine. The characteristics of a vaccine in the 21st century are shown in Table 19.3. There are expectations that a vaccine will not only give long-term protective immunity from the infectious disease but it will be 100% safe, such that any side effects due to immunization are unacceptable. The vaccine will give immunity following one or few doses, and can be coadministered with other vaccines. A number of vaccines have been successfully either coadministered (i.e., two vaccines administered at different anatomical sites) or administered as what is termed "combination vaccines" (i.e., multiple vaccines as a single formulation; see Table 19.4). In addition, health providers want a vaccine that is stable for long periods of time, even in the high temperatures of tropical climates, and will be cheap to purchase, while producers want a vaccine that is cheap and easy to manufacture

---

Table 19.3 Characteristics of a Vaccine

- Protective immunity—gives long-term protective immunity
- One or few doses needed to give protective immunity
- Safety—no side effects
- Stability—retains activity for a long time at different temperatures → cold chain
- Ease of administration
- Coadministration (administration of multiple doses of vaccines by different routes or multiple anatomical sites at the same visit) or as combination vaccines (multiple vaccines given as a single formulation)
- Manufacture—ease of scale-up
- Low cost

Table 19.4 Examples of Combination Vaccines

- DTP: Diphtheria, tetanus, and pertussis
- MMRV: Measles, mumps, rubella, and varicella
- Hepatitis A&B: Hepatitis A and hepatitis B
- DTPw-HB-Hib: Diphtheria, tetanus, whole-cell pertussis, hepatitis B, and Hib
- DTPa-HB-IPV-Hib: Diphtheria, tetanus, acellular pertussis, hepatitis B, inactivated poliomyelitis, and Hib

to maximize profits. Given these expectations, at the present time the process of human vaccine development from discovery to licensure takes 15–20 years, and consequently is very expensive at $500 million to $1 billion. However, veterinary vaccine development is quicker (5–8 years) and cheaper ($50 million to $100 million), and this reflects the expectation of low cost of vaccines in veterinary markets, often in cents per dose.

Routine immunizations

As in developed countries, there are routine immunizations given to children and adults in developing countries. The WHO has recommendations for vaccines for all age groups: childhood, adolescent, and adult immunizations that vary by geographic region due to the varying prevalence of infectious diseases (for more information see http://www.who.int/immunization/policy/Immunization_routine_table1.pdf and http://www.who.int/immunization/policy/Immunization_routine_table2.pdf).

This information is frequently updated as new vaccines become available, and detailed information on all vaccines can be found at www.who.int/immunization/documents/positionpapers/. Many of the vaccines recommended by the WHO are the same as those used in developed countries, such as the USA (see www.cdc.gov/vaccines/recs/schedules/default.htm), but there are some differences. For example, the WHO recommends BCG vaccine (Bacillus Calmette–Guérin is a live attenuated vaccine against tuberculosis) for all children and the live attenuated poliomyelitis vaccine for all children, but does not recommend the live attenuated chickenpox (varicella) vaccine. However, the US FDA does not recommend BCG vaccine, utilizes the inactivated poliomyelitis vaccine, and has incorporated the varicella vaccine into the routine childhood immunization schedule. National vaccine schedules differ based on requirements of the national ministry of health. It should be emphasized that the WHO only provides recommendations as not all vaccines will be required in all regions of the world. There are a number of vaccines that are required only in certain areas of the world where the diseases are found; many of these vaccines are used for travelers who visit these areas from other parts of the world (see below). Examples include yellow fever, where the disease is found in tropical

South America and sub-Saharan Africa but not Asia, while Japanese encephalitis is found in Asia but not Africa or South America. The objective is to aid decision making to create the most advantageous immunization schedules for health care providers in each region or country to prevent vaccine-preventable diseases and maintain lifelong immunity. In this situation, health care providers include not only those who are responsible for administering the vaccine but also national decision makers, immunization managers, regulatory authorities, and ministries of health personnel. This process is important not only for public health officials, but it also helps vaccine producers to evaluate potential markets.

Vaccines for travelers

In the 21st century, air travel makes it possible to reach any destination in the world within 24 hours. The WHO estimates that at any one time more than 500,000 persons are in aircraft. Travel vaccine portfolios are an important component for most vaccine producers, and travel medicine clinics are equally important as sites to provide the appropriate vaccines for travelers. The emphasis is on appropriate vaccines, as it is important that individuals receive only vaccines for which there is demonstrable risk of the traveler being exposed to the natural disease. For example, individuals visiting Peru would want to receive yellow fever vaccine if they were visiting the jungle areas of Peru but would not need to receive the vaccine if they were visiting Lima, the capital of Peru, as this city is on the coast of Peru where the mosquito vectors that transmit the virus are not found. Similarly, intracountry travelers need to be considered for vaccination when they travel to different regions of a country (i.e., movement from an area where a disease is nonendemic to an area where the disease is endemic). Public health agencies such as the US Centers for Disease Control and Prevention (www.cdc.gov) and the European Centers for Disease Control and Prevention (http://ecdc.europa.eu/en/Pages/home.aspx), plus many other national public health agencies, have websites that provide continually updated information on recommendations of vaccines for residents and travelers to different regions of the world (www.cdc.gov/travel/content/vaccinations.aspx).

Economics of vaccine development

By the end of the 20th century, vaccine manufacturers produced routine childhood vaccines (both killed and live versions) that cost US$5–15 per dose. This translated to lower profits, compared to drug development, which when combined with problems of litigation due to vaccine-related adverse events, resulted in very few companies remaining interested in producing human vaccines. However, vaccines are complex biological entities, and, as such, there are not "generic vaccine" equivalents to "generic drugs,"; therefore, each vaccine has a long market life. The past 20 years has been marked by new advances in technology and manufacturing and enhanced investments by government and nonprofit organizations into vaccine research, resulting in a renewed interest in vaccine development and marketing.

The past 5 years has seen the global sales of vaccines increase threefold from $7 billion to over $32 billion in 2013, with the five largest multinational vaccine pharmaceutical companies (GlaxoSmithKline, Merck, Novartis, Pfizer, and Sanofi Pasteur) comprising approximately 80% of the market. The first so-called super vaccine was marketed in 2000, called "Prevnar" (Wyeth, now Pfizer), the first pneumococcal vaccine for children, which protects against seven serotypes. Prevnar rapidly became the number 2 selling product for Wyeth with over $1.5 billion in sales. This was followed in 2006 by "Gardasil" (Merck), the first HPV vaccine with over $1.5 billion in annual sales and the number 4 most profitable product for Merck after asthma, high blood pressure, and osteoporosis drugs. With these successes there is great economic interest in human vaccines. Currently it is the fastest growing "therapeutic" area in the pharmaceutical industry, with a predicted annual growth rate of 11.36% over the next 5 years (2014–2019). Since children are born continually (e.g., 4 million children born each year in the USA), there is a continual need for vaccines and so the market persists. However, as described below, the economics of vaccine development is changing. As companies tighten their belts, especially in times of economic recessions, there is a trend toward outsourcing some or all of the research and development (R&D) components. In recent years, there has been a push towards outsourcing basic discovery R&D to academic research facilities and universities.

The global veterinary vaccine market is smaller than that for humans due to lower costs of vaccines. Global sales exceeded $4 billion in 2010. There are approximately 70 veterinary vaccine producers in the world, but like human vaccines, this is dominated by a small number of companies that share more than 70% of global sales. The USA and Europe make up more than 60% of sales, with livestock vaccines constituting more than 60% of revenue. France, Germany, and the UK account for more than 40% of the veterinary vaccine sales in Europe.

Major infectious diseases in the world

Despite having very successful vaccines, there are still many infectious diseases that kill thousands of people each year (see Table 19.5). Surprisingly, a number of these are vaccine-preventable diseases. Thus there is a critical need to get vaccines to those who need them.

Given the cost to develop a vaccine, economic evaluation and economic viability are very important criteria and are based on who will pay for the vaccine and how much they are willing to pay. However, in reality, this decision-making process is more complicated as the number of people who might benefit from

Table 19.5 Major Diseases Caused by Infectious Agents in 2010

Clinical Disease	Deaths	Number Infected
Lower respiratory infections	>4 million	Not known
HIV/AIDS	>3 million	>39 million
Malaria	1 to 5 million	>500 million
Diarrhea	>2 million	>4 billion
Tuberculosis complex	>2 million	>2 billion
Measles	>500,000	>30 million
Pertussis	>200,000	20 million to 40 million
Tetanus	>200,000	>500,000
Meningitis	>180,000	>1 million
Syphilis	>150,000	>12 million

the vaccine, the population that is targeted for immunization, and the severity of the disease that will be prevented by immunization are all important points that need to be considered. Consequently, estimates of market needs are then influenced by the quantity of vaccine that is needed, the shelf life of the vaccine, and a predicted vaccine purchase price.

Until recent times, it has been considered that there are more individuals in a developing country who would benefit from a vaccine than in a developed country, but there may be fewer financial resources available to purchase the vaccine, such that market need may be perceived as insufficient to support the vaccine development. However, improvements in transportation have made it possible to travel rapidly to anywhere in the world within 24 hours, and now infectious diseases are considered a global problem rather than a problem of individual countries. The impact of financial improvements in middle-income countries provides monies for people to purchase vaccines while there are many efforts through partnerships to provide vaccines for developing countries that cannot afford them. This has opened doors for vaccine producers to have larger markets than previously thought, in particular the five large multinational vaccine pharmaceutical companies, which have formed alliances and collaborations with vaccine producers in middle-income countries. However, this is matched by the need to work with multiple national regulatory authorities.

Infrastructure

Private–public partnerships

Private–public partnerships (PPP) are government service or private business ventures that are funded and operated through a partnership of government and one or more private sector entities. Prevention of infectious diseases by immunization is advantageous due to both public health reasons and economics, and is thought to save at least 3 million lives each year. It is estimated that an additional $1 billion per year in immunizations would save 10 million more lives over the next decade. Until recently, market forces alone were insufficient to meet the health care priorities of resource-poor populations. However, the past 15 years have seen a marked change in vaccine development

for diseases found in developing countries due to large-scale involvement of entities such as the WHO, the Bill and Melinda Gates Foundation, Global Alliance for Vaccines and Immunization (GAVI), Program for Appropriate Technology in Health (PATH), World Bank, United Nations Children's Fund (UNICEF), private foundations (e.g., Rockefeller Foundation and Wellcome Trust), nongovernmental organizations, academia, governments, and developing-world vaccine manufacturers. Some of these work as product development partnerships (PDPs). These nonprofit entities work to accelerate the development, evaluation, and implementation of vaccines, drugs, diagnostic assays, and other technologies to reduce the burden of disease in developing countries. They facilitate partnerships with both public and private entities to achieve goals for a particular disease. PDPs exist for tuberculosis (e.g., Aeras, a global tuberculosis vaccine foundation), HIV, malaria, dengue, meningitis, and other diseases. Vaccine manufacturers have also been involved in these partnerships in developing countries; for example, the Novartis Vaccines Institute for Global Health is a research institute focused on translational research and development of vaccines, in particular diseases that are found in developing countries. The Merck-Wellcome Trust Hilleman laboratories also focus on diseases found in developing countries.

Global Alliance for Vaccines and Immunization (GAVI)

GAVI is a PPP of UNICEF, the Bill and Melinda Gates Foundation, WHO, and the World Bank that started in 2000 (www.gavialliance.org). The program is targeted to developing countries, and specifically only those that are the poorest. Currently, there are approximately 72 GAVI-eligible countries, which include approximately half of the world's population; however, each country is assessed for each aspect of the program and not all countries are eligible for all parts of the program.

The first phase was a 5-year plan (2000–2005) aimed at extending and improving the quality of immunization programs by two approaches: (1) supplying new and underused vaccines and (2) strengthening vaccine delivery systems. The former focused on *Haemophilus influenzae* type b (Hib), hepatitis B, and yellow fever vaccines, and the latter focused on implementation of disposable auto-disable syringes to prevent reuse of syringes and associated equipment that have the potential to cause infections. The 5-year plan provided grants for supplies of vaccines with the expectation that countries would increase their national contribution, leading to subsequent financial sustainability by a particular country.

The second phase of the program is a 10-year plan (2006–2015) and increases the range of vaccines included in the program (pneumococcus and rotavirus); however, financial sustainability is a significant problem. GAVI has an accelerated development and implementation plan (ADIP) program for pneumococcal and rotaviral vaccines that aims to shorten the period between vaccines being proven safe and effective for use and their introduction in developing countries. In addition, the "Hib" initiative has been expanded into a pentavalent vaccine program where one immunization incorporates vaccines for five diseases (Hib, diphtheria, tetanus, pertussis, and hepatitis B). A vaccine investment strategy has been developed where the WHO provided a list of 18 diseases in 2007 to be considered for investment. From this list, GAVI selected four diseases for consideration of financial support (cervical cancer [caused by HPV], Japanese encephalitis, rubella, and typhoid).

A key component of GAVI is the access to vaccines by developing countries, and this is being achieved via two financial initiatives. The first, advance market commitments (AMCs), are designed to stimulate the development and manufacture of vaccines specifically for developing countries. AMCs are typically used to guarantee a viable market for a vaccine after it is developed. This is beneficial for companies that would otherwise not consider developing or manufacturing a vaccine that ordinarily would not be profitable. The pilot AMC is for a new vaccine to target pneumococcal disease (due to *Streptococcus pneumoniae*) with the target of supporting up to 60 of the world's poorest countries to introduce pneumococcal vaccine by 2015. The second initiative is the International Finance Facility for Immunization (IFFIm) that borrows on capital markets against donor countries' pledges and raises funds through bonds. This novel financial mechanism aims to provide $4 billion in funds between 2006 and 2015.

Program for Appropriate Technology in Health

The Program for Appropriate Technology in Health (PATH) originated in the 1970s and has expanded extensively in the past 40 years and considers itself "a catalyst for global health." Active in over 70 countries, PATH focuses on a number of areas to improve public health, including advancing technologies, strengthening infrastructure, and encouraging healthy behaviors (www.path.org). One of the foci of PATH is vaccine development with projects on technologies to improve the safety, effectiveness, and efficiency of vaccine delivery in countries that are disproportionately affected by vaccine-preventable infectious diseases.

Supporting the design, development, scale-up, production, commercialization, and distribution of technologies solely through the public sector is clearly beyond available resources and not economically viable within many of the countries that need the vaccines. Thus, public–private collaborations are indispensable for investment in suitable technologies to further vaccine development in developing countries. PATH has developed and refined many approaches for identifying and advancing vaccine-related technologies, and works collaboratively in partnerships with vaccine and technology companies, public- and private-sector partners, research institutes, universities, other nongovernmental organizations, research consortia, and international agencies to further vaccine development. All of the above are keys to advancing candidate vaccines to usage in the community and improving public health. Projects have included maintaining the cold chain and issues that impact vaccine delivery and effectiveness at point of use, such as bench and field testing, technology transfer, scale-up, licensing, and market and product introduction for a number of vaccines, including *Shigella*, enterotoxigenic *Escherichia coli* (ETEC), rotavirus, Japanese encephalitis, pneumococcal disease, seasonal and pandemic influenza, and cervical cancer.

Decade of Vaccines

In 2010, the Bill and Melinda Gates Foundation launched the "Decade of Vaccines," a 10-year plan to spend $10 billion on research, development, and delivery of vaccines for the world's poorest countries to prevent, through vaccination, the deaths of at least an additional 8 million children under the age of 5 over the next 10 years. The overall goal is to achieve 90% coverage of childhood immunization. Subsequently, the Decade of Vaccines was launched in London on June 9, 2011. It has a 6-person leadership council to provide oversight, a 17-person steering committee, and four working groups: "Delivery." "Global Access," "Public and Political Support," and "Research and Development." More details and updates of the collaboration can be found at www.dovcollaboration.org.

Agence de Médecine Préventive

Agence de Médecine Préventive (AMP) (www.amp-vaccinology.org/) is a nonprofit organization dedicated to promoting preventive medicine and public health worldwide. AMP collaborates with diverse public- and private-sector partners to support countries in developing sustainable and effective immunization policies and strengthening their public health infrastructure. In terms of vaccines, the focus is on applied vaccinology, and AMP works to provide the information needed for decision making. In particular, national leaders rely on available data and analyses to determine priority health interventions, including optimal immunization policies and strategies.

World Health Organization

WHO has a number of programs that are focused on vaccines with most in the "Immunization, Vaccines and Biologicals" program (www.who.int/immunization/), whose mission is a "world in which all people at risk are protected against vaccine-preventable disease." WHO provides recommendations on policy, guidelines, and information on vaccines. These include the Initiative for Vaccine Research (IVR), Quality, Safety and Standards (QSS), Expanded Program on Immunizations (EPI), and HIV Vaccine Initiative (HVI).

Within WHO, the Strategic Advisory Group of Experts on Immunization (SAGE) was established in 1999 to be the principal advisory group for vaccines and immunization that makes the key recommendations on immunizations (including global policy, strategies, technology, research and development, vaccine delivery and relationships to other health

Table 19.6 Components of Vaccine Implementation

- Program management
- Procurement
- Vaccine quality
- Cold-chain regimen and equipment
- Vaccine handling
- Open vial policy
- Establishing recommendations for vaccine use, both universal and targeted vaccination
- Vaccine administration
- Contraindications
- Adverse events following immunization (AEFI) (also termed *serious adverse events*)
- Outbreak control
- Post-licensure assessment of safety and efficacy (population studies)
- Waste management
- Immunization coverage
- Vaccine-preventable disease surveillance
- Research
- Community outreach and education—health professionals and public
- Cost-effectiveness

Modified from www.who.int/immunization/policy/en/index.html.

interventions) and reviews and endorses all immunization-related materials prior to publication. The Weekly Epidemiological Record (www.who.int/wer) is used to publish all WHO recommendations on immunizations, in French and English, with additional translations available in Arabic, Chinese, Russian, and Spanish. Currently, the WHO provides immunization policy recommendations on most components of vaccine implementation (Table 19.6) and information about 24 vaccine-preventable diseases (Table 19.7). Details can be found at www.who.int/immunization/policy/en/index.html, and position papers are frequently updated and can be found on this website.

Global Immunization Vision and Strategy

The Global Immunization Vision and Strategy (GIVS) was established by WHO and UNICEF as a global

Table 19.7 Catalog of Available Immunization Policy Recommendations

Bacillus Calmette–Guérin (BCG)
Cholera
Diphtheria
Diphtheria, tetanus, and pertussis (DTP)
Hepatitis A
Hepatitis B
Haemophilus influenzae type b (Hib)
HIV
Influenza
Japanese encephalitis
Measles
Meningococcal disease
Measles, mumps, and rubella (MMR)
Mumps
Pertussis
Pneumococcal disease
Polio
Rabies
Rotavirus
Rubella
Tetanus
Typhoid
Varicella
Yellow fever

Modified from www.who.int/immunizations.

10-year program (2006–2015) to enhance immunizations rates (www.who.int/immunization/givs/en/index.html). The objectives are to immunize more people against more diseases, introduce newly available vaccines and technologies, manage immunization programs with respect to global relationships (i.e., implementation will depend on the specific needs of a country or region), and integrate immunizations with other health interventions. The overall goal is a two-thirds reduction in vaccine-preventable disease mortality and morbidity by 2015 compared to 2000. In its first few years, this program has significantly increased routine immunization coverage, but the challenge will be to sustain immunization coverage in future years.

United Nations prequalified vaccines

A very important issue for implementation of a vaccine is "prequalification." This refers to a service provided by the WHO to the UN for designating a vaccine from a particular producer as having suitable quality assurance (e.g., safety, efficacy, potency, thermostability) to be purchased by UN agencies. This process is very important as a particular vaccine may be manufactured by multiple producers in different countries, and a prequalification designation informs ministries of health and national regulatory authorities that a particular vaccine from a producer meets standards required for immunization. In addition, prequalified vaccines have a price negotiated between the producer and the UN. This is advantageous for both the producer (as they have a defined market) and the country (as they will know the price of the vaccine and whether or not they can afford to incorporate the vaccine in their immunization program).

As one would expect, not all vaccines manufactured by all producers are prequalified. At present, 29 of the 55 worldwide vaccine producers from 22 countries have one or more of the 37 prequalified vaccine products. Each manufacturer is prequalified for particular vaccines on a case-by-case basis. Currently, WHO has prioritized the following nine vaccines for prequalification in 2013–2014: (1) bivalent oral polio (bOPV1+3), (2) diphtheria, tetanus, pertussis, hepatitis B, *Haemophilus influenzae* type b pentavalent combination (fully liquid DTwP-Hep B-Hib), (3) diphtheria, tetanus, pertussis (DTwP), (4) inactivated polio (IPV), (5) measles, rubella, (6) pneumococcal conjugate, (7) rotavirus, (8) trivalent oral polio (tOPV), and (9) yellow fever. This list is updated annually.

Veterinary vaccines

In the international arena, two organizations play a major role for veterinary vaccines. These are the Food and Agriculture Organization (FAO) and the World Organization for Animal Health (OIE). Like the WHO, both are UN organizations.

Food and Agriculture Organization

The FAO (www.fao.org) is the lead organization of the UN devoted to defeating hunger. Its major role is to help developing countries and countries in transition modernize and improve agriculture, forestry, and fisheries practices. The emphasis of the FAO is on developing rural areas, where 70% of the world's poor and hungry people live. The FAO makes recommendations on veterinary vaccines, in particular targeted vaccination of particular animal species in geographic areas. It publishes a "vaccine manual" that provides guidelines and recommendations for methods of vaccine production and evaluation, and information on the current status of veterinary vaccine development.

World Organization for Animal Health

The World Organization for Animal Health (www.oie.int) was originally called the Office International des Epizooties and changed its name to the World Organization for Animal Health in 2003. It is the intergovernmental organization responsible for improving animal health worldwide and is recognized as a reference organization by the World Trade Organization and has 178 member countries and territories. Like the WHO, it has regional and subregional offices on every continent. It publishes the *Manual of Diagnostic Tests and Vaccines For Terrestrial Animals*, which provides information on tests and vaccines for animal diseases that are important for international trade. OIE has developed a "vaccine bank," which generates ongoing stocks of vaccine. Briefly, the supplier, which is a selected OIE-compliant vaccine production company, produces the vaccines when needed (or they remain with the supplier at its own risk) and contracts are renewed on a rolling basis under terms and conditions defined with the OIE. The goal is to enable the rapid supply of emergency stock of vaccines to infected countries in order to vaccinate animal populations at risk and to progressively achieve eradication wherever possible.

International Federation of Pharmaceutical Manufacturers and Associations

The IFPMA (http://www.ifpma.org/) is a global nonprofit nongovernmental organization representing the research-based pharmaceutical industry, including biotech and vaccine entities. Its members comprise 25 leading international companies and 45 national and regional industry associations covering developed and developing countries. The IFPMA supports a wide range of WHO technical activities, including those relating to vaccine efficacy, quality, and safety. It also provides the secretariat for the International Conference on Harmonization of Technical Requirements for Registration of Pharmaceuticals for Human Use (ICH).

Regulatory

Much of the above has focused on the vaccine development pathway. Once a vaccine gets beyond phase I clinical trials, there is a significant possibility that the vaccine producer will be seeking approval for licensure. This is a multifaceted and complex process with many variables, including whether the vaccine is to be used in the country of manufacture only or will be used internationally. Not surprisingly, each country has requirements for use of each vaccine and these are discussed below.

Vaccine safety

Significant efforts have been made in the past 20 years by regulatory authorities and manufacturers to further improve and ensure the safety of vaccines. Nonetheless, technological advances and increasing knowledge about vaccines have led to investigations focused on the safety of current vaccines, which has an ever increasingly important role on public confidence in immunization. While great efforts have been made in producing vaccines, they have little use if the target population will not have the confidence to accept the vaccine. As a consequence, it is essential that concerns regarding vaccine-related adverse events are rapidly and effectively addressed in order to maintain confidence in a vaccine, and ultimately maintain immunization coverage and reduce disease incidence. Adverse events are defined as any undesirable experience associated with the use of a medical product in a patient. In particular, serious adverse events are the major concern. These are defined by the US FDA as adverse events involving either death, life-threatening conditions, hospitalization (initial or prolonged), disability, congenital anomaly, or requiring intervention to prevent permanent impairment or damage. It was because of this that the WHO established the Global Advisory Committee on Vaccine Safety (GACVS) in 1999 to respond promptly, efficiently, and with scientific thoroughness to vaccine safety issues of potential global importance. The GACVS meets twice a year and publishes its discussions and recommendations in the WHO Weekly Epidemiological Record.

In 1999, the Brighton Collaboration (www.brightoncollaboration.org) was established at a meeting in Brighton, England, and was subsequently officially inaugurated in fall 2000. The Collaboration consists of volunteers from developed and developing countries with expertise in patient care and public health, and members of scientific, pharmaceutical, regulatory, and professional organizations who are experts in the field of immunization safety and corresponding medical specialties. The Collaboration aims to facilitate the development, evaluation, and dissemination of high-quality information about the safety of human vaccines.

National regulatory authorities

National regulatory authorities (NRAs) and national control laboratories (NCLs) play a critical role in the vaccine development process, as these entities will ultimately set the conditions for regulation, licensure, surveillance, and control of a vaccine in each country. The NRA ensures that the quality, manufacturing, storage, distribution, dispensing, efficacy, and safety of a vaccine are all appropriate for a particular vaccine product. The emphasis is often on consistency such that every lot of vaccine meets the same standards. Examples of NRAs are the US FDA, the European Medicines Agency (EMA), the China Food and Drug Administration, the Drug Controller General of India, the Egyptian Drug Authority, the Australian Thera-peutic Goods Agency, the Japanese Pharmaceutical and Medical Safety Bureau, the Korean Office for Health and Medical Care Policy, the Senegalese *Direction de la Pharmacie et du Médicament*, Biologics and Genetic Therapies Directorate Health Canada, and the Brazilian *Agencia Nacional da Vigilancia Sanitaria*.

For vaccine-manufacturing countries, the NRA has six critical functions: (1) a published set of require-ments for licensing; (2) surveillance of vaccine field performance; (3) system of lot release; (4) use of labo-ratory when needed; (5) regular inspections for good manufacturing practices (GMPs); and (6) evaluation of clinical performance. These functions are essential as not only are vaccines used in the countries where they are manufactured, but they are often exported for administration in other countries, which need to know that the NRA in the country of origin is compe-tent in its oversight.

Due to the critical role of NRAs, the WHO has estab-lished and published standards that define interna-tional expectations for a functional vaccine regulatory system. The WHO conducts audits of NRAs using international experts, particularly in vaccine-produc-ing countries, to ensure that the regulatory systems in place meet the necessary standards and that they are maintained and function in a sustainable way. Not all NRAs meet these standards.

The NCLs provide vaccine reference preparations, including antigen and antibody standards and other materials, for ensuring consistency in vaccines. These standards normally have defined biological activity expressed in international units so that vaccines man-ufactured by different producers in different countries can be compared and standardized. The NRAs and NCLs are critical, as currently 55 countries have vaccine manufacturers, and there are at least 76 NRAs. The challenge for NRAs is to keep up with the con-tinuing improvements in science and technology asso-ciated with the entire process of vaccine development. With advances in vaccine development comes an increased complexity, and this has resulted in the steady increase in requirements for each vaccine before licensure is approved. This is readily seen in the USA with the US FDA and in Europe with the EMA, but is also true of all NRAs. Due to the expanding global nature of the vaccine industry, multiple NRAs and rules present increasing challenges to the develop-ment and implementation of new vaccines. To address this growing problem, regulatory agencies and manu-facturers in the USA, Europe, and Japan established the International Conference on Harmonisation (ICH). This is complemented by the WHO, which has the Global Training Network on Vaccine Quality that was established in 1996 with the aim of improving vaccine quality practices. In addition, the WHO Expert Com-mittee on Biological Standardization consults and pro-vides consensus views on important regulatory issues and provides guidance documents for use by NRAs and industry. These are published as Technical Report Series (http://www.who.int/biologicals/technical_report _series/en/). Another important consideration is that vaccines for tropical diseases require clinical trials to be undertaken in countries where the diseases are found, while the vaccine itself may be manufactured in a different country. Thus, each NRA has a critical role in vaccine development. With this in mind, the Developing Countries Vaccine Regulators Network and Developing Countries Vaccine Manufacturers Network have been established to share the experiences of multiple countries and facilitate licensure of vaccines.

Regulation of veterinary vaccines

Animal vaccines are subject to many of the regulations of human vaccines. Each vaccine must be registered and licensed in each country that it will be used. The processes of regulation are similar with oversight of safety, effectiveness, efficacy, duration of immunity, manufacture, importation, testing, distribution, and use of veterinary vaccines. As with human products, the focus is on consistency to show that the vaccine is pure, potent, safe and effective, protects the target animal species (e.g., domestic livestock, poultry, companion animals, wildlife, and aquatic species), and helps public health and food safety by controlling domestic animal diseases and preventing the introduction and dissemination of foreign animal diseases.

Examples of national regulators are the US Department of Agriculture's Animal and Plant Health Inspection Service (APHIS), which functions similar to the US FDA (i.e., Center for Veterinary Biologics and Center for Biologics Evaluation and Resesarch, respectively), Canadian Food Inspection Agency, and the Australian Pesticides and Veterinary Medicines Authority. In Europe, the EMA regulates both human and veterinary vaccines.

Genetically manipulated organisms

As technologies rapidly evolve, so do issues regarding their regulation. Great advances have been made in recombinant DNA technology, and scientists have enormous capabilities with genetic manipulation to generate genetically modified organisms (GMOs), i.e., organisms that have been genetically modified using genetic engineering to either contain additional or deleted sequences. These organisms require careful environmental risk assessment (ERA) and must be considered on a case-by-case situation as each is unique. For example, assessment of a genetically modified virus or bacterium would be different from that of a genetically modified plant expressing a vaccine immunogen. Currently, some countries or regions have active requirements for assessment (e.g., European Union, Australia, and Canada) while others do not.

Future challenges

A combination of scientific, technologic, and economic advances in the past 30 years is leading to a very optimistic future for vaccines for tropical diseases. However, these are mostly based on candidate vaccines that are already in at least advanced stage preclinical development. Major challenges remain for a number of infectious diseases where our understanding of an immunogen that induces protective immunity is very limited or the agent has evolved mechanisms of overcoming the host immune response. Many of these diseases are found in tropical countries, and new advances are needed in discovery and basic science to generate appropriate immunogens for development as candidate vaccines.

Summary

- Vaccine development is traditionally seen as a process that takes place in developed countries; however, this is not the true situation. Infectious diseases are a global problem and not surprisingly vaccine development takes place on a global scale.

- The WHO has identified 68 diseases where vaccines can reduce the morbidity and/or mortality. There are 24 diseases for which vaccine development is a priority, either as improved vaccines or as new vaccines.

- Routine immunizations vary by country. The research and development of vaccines used in developing countries cannot be based on experiences in developed countries. Different serotypes are found for a number of bacteria, viruses, and parasites in different geographical locations such that immunogenicity and vaccine components need to be evaluated by region.

- To date, smallpox is the only infectious disease of humans that has been eradicated. Great efforts are being made to eradicate polio, measles, and tetanus.

- Public–private partnerships and product development partnerships are important to making vaccines available to developing countries.

(Continued)

- The goal of the World Health Organization is to provide vaccines for all people at risk to ensure they are protected against vaccine-preventable disease.
- National regulatory authorities set the conditions for regulation, licensure, surveillance, and control of a vaccine in each country.

Further reading

Bonhoeffer J, Kohl K, Chen R, Duclos P, Heijbel H, Heininger U, Jefferson T, and Loupi E (2004). The Brighton Collaboration-enhancing vaccine safety. Vaccine 22(15–16), 2046.

Brennan FR and Dougan G (2005). Non-clinical safety evaluation of novel vaccines and adjuvants: new products, new strategies. Vaccine 23, 3210–3222.

Duclos P, Okwo-Bele JM, and Salisbury D (2011). Establishing global policy recommendations: the role of the Strategic Advisory Group of Experts on immunization. Expert Review of Vaccines 10(2), 163–173.

Milstien JB, Kaddar M, and Kieny MP (2006). The impact of globalization on vaccine development and availability. Health Affairs (Project Hope) 25, 1061–1069.

Wolfson LJ, Gasse F, Lee-Martin SP, Lydon P, Magan A, Tibouti A, Johns B, Hutubessy R, Salama P, and Okwo-Bele JM (2008). Estimating the costs of achieving the WHO-UNICEF Global Immunization Vision and Strategy, 2006–2015. Bulletin of the World Health Organization 86(1), 27–39.

20 Political, ethical, social, and psychological aspects of vaccinology

Caroline M. Poland,[1] Robert M. Jacobson,[2] Douglas J. Opel,[3] Edgar K. Marcuse,[4] and Gregory A. Poland[2]

[1]Taylor University, Upland, IN, USA
[2]Mayo Clinic, Rochester, MN, USA
[3]Treuman Katz Center for Pediatric Bioethics, Seattle Children's Research Institute, Seattle, WA, USA
[4]Seattle Children's Hospital, Seattle, WA, USA

Introduction

The field of vaccinology is a rich intersection and interweaving of a variety of issues that together determine whether a vaccine is used at both the individual and population levels. While vaccinology is heavily dominated by the science of vaccine development, critical to the actual usefulness of a new vaccine is the willingness of governments, communities, and individuals to accept new and existing vaccines. Thus, one may consider that a logical flow occurs in vaccinology: the accumulation of a scientific base upon which to direct development of a vaccine, clinical studies to determine proper dose, route of administration, interval between doses, immunogenicity, safety, and finally, efficacy/effectiveness. From this point onward, a variety of political, ethical, social, and psychological factors determine the context within which vaccines are used. Governments must be willing to pay for the development and administration of vaccine programs, the public must be educated about the need for and safety of vaccines, individuals must be convinced of the safety and efficacy attendant to receiving vaccines for themselves and their children, and ethical, social, and legal issues arise once a new vaccine is widely administered to the populace. In turn, individuals make decisions to accept or reject vaccines based on a variety of individual social, ethical, and psychological reasons. In this chapter we explore the political, ethical, social, and psychological issues that impact individual and population acceptance or rejection of vaccines and vaccine programs.

Abbreviations

ACIP	Advisory Committee on Immunization Practices	HBM	Health belief model
		HPV	Human papillomavirus
CBER	Center for Biologics Evaluation and Research	MI	Motivational interviewing
		MMR	Measles, mumps, and rubella
CBT	Cognitive behavioral therapy	US FDA	Food and Drug Administration
CNS	Central nervous system	VFC	Vaccines for children
DTP	Diphtheria, tetanus, whole-cell pertussis	VICP	Vaccine Injury Compensation Program

Vaccinology: An Essential Guide, First Edition. Edited by Gregg N. Milligan and Alan D.T. Barrett.
© 2015 John Wiley & Sons, Ltd. Published 2015 by John Wiley & Sons, Ltd.

Politics in vaccinology

Philosophical basis for politics in vaccinology

If one defines politics as the *art and science of government*, then one might posit that vaccines and vaccination could proceed independently of politics. Theoretically, if vaccination offers substantial and worthy merit, free-market theory would hold that the supply of vaccination would rise to meet demand and therefore satisfy individual want. But since the earliest days of vaccination, governments have vigorously participated in every aspect of vaccines and vaccination, and vaccination's modern success—including the global eradication of smallpox and continental elimination of polio—is very much a *political* success. Indeed, vaccination has been acclaimed by the US Centers for Disease Control and Prevention as one of the top 10 public health achievements of the 20th century.

Successful vaccination has depended upon the synergistic benefits attributed to the vaccination of a population, rather than just an accumulation of individual benefits. Vaccination at the population level creates public health benefits that other individuals and their governments enjoy. Distinct from population-based vaccination programs are acts of mass vaccination in which a government seeks to vaccinate an entire population rapidly, such as those against smallpox that characterized the early 19th century, as well as campaigns conducted by developing countries against polio that continue today. Mass vaccination will not be the focus of this chapter; we will solely focus on population-based programs that help maintain high levels of immunity across a population.

There are a variety of bases for the benefits derived from vaccination efforts at the population level (Table 20.1). First, a significant portion—and often the group highest at risk for morbidity and mortality—of the population at risk cannot be vaccinated and instead depends upon others' immunity to reduce their risk of disease. Such are the situations for infants in regard to measles and for pregnant women in regard to rubella. In the USA, infants under 12 months are too young to reliably induce a protective immune response to the vaccine and yet are at risk for the disease. The rubella vaccine is contraindicated in pregnant women as the vaccine is a live attenuated viral vaccine yet the

Table 20.1 The Basis for Population-Based Vaccination Programs

- To protect those who cannot be vaccinated
- To protect those who do not respond well to vaccination
- To control or eliminate disease contagion
- To reduce societal expenses from disease susceptibility
- To ensure national security

basis for rubella vaccination is to prevent pregnant women from acquiring infection with the resulting complication of congenital rubella syndrome.

Definition

Herd immunity: A situation where protective immunity is achieved through attaining a high enough level of immunity in a population so as to make exposure to the organism that causes the disease extremely unlikely.

Second, a significant portion of the population at risk does not respond well to vaccines; this group benefits from the interruption in the spread of disease that helps protect them from the disease and its complications. The members of this group vary depending upon the vaccine under discussion. For example, for influenza, it is the elderly who suffer a relative hyporesponsiveness to the annual vaccine. The Japanese approach with vaccinating school children against influenza demonstrated how the vaccination of children may help to protect the elderly, as did the quasi-experimental studies with health care workers in nursing facilities who received vaccinations against influenza in order to reduce death and morbidity in their elderly patients.

Third, a significant portion of those vaccinated remain susceptible (i.e., vaccine failure) and unknowingly so. Such an individual benefits from the immunity of those in close proximity to reduce that individual's own risk of exposure. Those in close proximity include more than just family and household contacts. These exposures occur not just in the home, but also at school, in the workplace, and in public spaces.

Fourth, control of most communicable vaccine-preventable diseases benefits from the effects of herd (i.e., community) immunity in curtailing the spread of disease. In fact, through herd immunity, a disease can be eliminated or even eradicated. For example, through programmatic vaccination of populations at risk for smallpox, the disease was indeed eradicated and resulted in the elimination of the need for continued vaccination.

Measles immunization is an outstanding example of the need to maintain very high levels of vaccine coverage to achieve sufficient herd immunity to prevent outbreaks of measles in a community by interrupting person-to-person transmission of the infection when the disease is introduced. This vaccine offers personal protection with overall field-effectiveness rates of 92.5% in 12-month-old recipients and 94.1 % in two-dose recipients. However, mathematical modeling reveals that eliminating the risk of outbreaks requires rates of 95% or more in those groups with the highest rates of transmission such as high school students and young adults. Supporting these models are the measles outbreaks that still occur in schools with 95% coverage; 100% coverage with two doses must be the goal for measles given the limitations of the current vaccine. Currently, among 24- to 35-month-old children in the USA, however, only 91.5% of children have received one dose or more of measles-containing vaccine, and in some states, such as New Jersey and Montana, those rates are much lower (86.1% and 85.1%, respectively). As outbreaks in Minnesota and elsewhere in 2011 demonstrated (every US outbreak that year was traced to an introduction of measles through international travel), today measles and other vaccine-preventable diseases are just a plane ride away. In 2012, 14 individuals associated with the Super Bowl in Indianapolis developed measles after exposure to an infected person walking through Super Bowl Village.

Fifth, reduction of the disease benefits society as a whole and can reduce the burden of that disease on the government as well as the individual taxpayer by the elimination of medical and nonmedical expenses incurred, and ensuring national security. Pre-dating vaccination in the USA, General George Washington ordered his soldiers protected from smallpox through variolation in an effort to maintain the health of his troops and thereby ensure military success. In modern times, vaccine policy making often includes not only consideration of the personal protection derived from

Table 20.2 Political Issues Relevant to Mass Vaccination

- Disease surveillance
- Product regulation
- Public communication
- Product liability
- Commercial development
- Official recommendations
- Equitable access
- Vaccination mandates

vaccination, but calculations of its cost-effectiveness to society as determined by economic modeling.

Efforts to obtain and maintain high levels of vaccination at the population level have required government involvement. From investigating disease outbreaks, to assessing risk upon which to base a personal decision to vaccinate, to mandating mass vaccination to prevent personal exposure, individuals depend upon public policies and programs to pursue population-based programs of vaccination to achieve the public health benefits of vaccination. Historically, the roles for government have included disease surveillance, product regulation, public communication, product liability, commercial development, official recommendations, equitable access, and vaccination mandates (Table 20.2). In the USA, depending upon the perceived responsibilities of the governing bodies, some of these roles have been filled by the federal government, others by state and local governments, and still others shared across governing bodies. Furthermore, at the international level, the US government has collaborated with other nations in joint efforts to control disease through vaccination in developing countries. In some of these efforts, the governments have collaborated more broadly with nongovernmental organizations to fulfill roles that in other efforts.

Disease surveillance

The first role of government in population-based programs of vaccination concerns the function of modern government in the pursuit of public health and that is the role of disease surveillance across the population, which has come to be known as *epidemiologic surveillance*. (When we are referring to governments here, we are speaking of activities that occur at a variety of governmental levels. For example, in the USA, much of federally reported disease surveillance results from disease surveillance that takes place at the county and state governmental levels.) Governments first made such efforts at the time of the black plague and their roles in measuring, categorizing, and recording the population disease burden have evolved since then. At the time of the founding of the US Communicable Diseases Center (the forerunner of the modern Centers for Disease Control and Prevention) in 1946, these communicable diseases included malaria, murine or endemic typhus, smallpox, psittacosis, diphtheria, leprosy, and sylvatic or wild-rodent plague. Current efforts to catalog the incidence of vaccine-preventable diseases provide both individuals and governments the awareness needed to measure the success of existing vaccination programs as well as the need for new vaccines and vaccination programs. Epidemiologic surveillance has indeed at times served as a source of controversy (e.g., similar to the monitoring of accidental firearm injuries), perhaps because it implies a role for greater government action.

Product regulation

Governmental efforts regarding pharmaceutical and biologic safety grew out of the government's role regarding product safety, and while these roles vary from country to country, governments today play major roles in vaccine development, licensure, and production. In 1902, in response to two unrelated antitoxin- and vaccine-contamination events in Camden, NJ, and Saint Louis, MO, which took place the year before and resulted in a total of 23 deaths, the USA created a national laboratory to oversee the production of biologics such as human vaccines and disease-specific antisera. The United States Public Service Act of 1944 further required the licensure of all biologic products, including vaccines. The role of government in the regulation of safety and effectiveness cannot be overstated. The story of the Salk polio vaccine development and dissemination by a philanthropic foundation demonstrates the substantial burdens created by public demand that fell on the US federal government as well as state and local health departments for regulatory oversight of vaccine production, disease surveillance, and vaccine administration. As a result of the "Cutter Incident" in 1954 and

the failure to inactivate wild-type poliovirus in the vaccine, the US government formed the Division of Biologics Standards to oversee the production of biologics. This later became the US Food and Drug Administration's (US FDA) Center for Biologics Evaluation and Research (CBER).

Public communication

The public's awareness of the etiologies of disease, the associated acute morbidity and sequelae, and the availability, effectiveness, and safety of disease prevention are important to successful vaccination uptake. Governments routinely participate in acquiring and communicating the above data in order to achieve their public health goals. In developing countries, while surveillance for disease activity has proven important in and of itself for determining vaccine need and programmatic evaluation, the communication of the results of that surveillance has repeatedly been shown to be useful in improving the political climate to bring resources to high-risk areas, to support vaccination programs, and to achieve high rates of immunization. Of course, efforts to build and sustain surveillance systems themselves require political support for successful deployment.

In contradistinction, inappropriate communication to the public of unsubstantiated reports of harm attributed to vaccines may require political will to intervene and address public perceptions that interfere with vaccine uptake. As seen with regard to the deployment of the human papillomavirus (HPV) vaccine, as well as the development of novel avian influenza vaccines, education of those who make health care policy is critical to successful vaccine programs, such as education concerning the incidence and morbidity of the disease and the safety and efficacy of the vaccine. In addition to the political issues regarding disease surveillance and vaccine production, the rising concerns of vaccine safety that result in vaccine hesitancy and rejection, both in industrialized countries as well as developing countries, have experts calling for an increasing governmental role to inform the public about vaccines and to preserve or improve the level of public trust in immunization. The growth of vaccine hesitancy partly as a result of Internet hype and hysteria has resulted in communities at higher risk for disease outbreaks because of vaccine delay or refusal not only for measles, but other infectious diseases such as pertussis, pneumo-coccus, and varicella.

However, the reception of public communication depends on more than information transfer; public opinion is difficult to sway with just science, logic, and evidence. For instance, parents who refuse recom-mended vaccines for their children report a lower rate of trust in the government. Furthermore, education alone appears relatively ineffective, so health officials and others that advocate for vaccination must care-fully craft their messages to achieve behavior change. Part of the problem with regard to the limits of educa-tion is the epidemiologic nature of the evidence regarding vaccine safety, the inability to prove the absence of a risk, and the difficulty in communicating risks. Beyond education is the apparent undervalua-tion of the benefits of vaccines and prevention among political leaders. Observers of current trends in public communication with regard to population-based pro-grams of vaccination have expressed dismay with the apparent shift in the focus and appreciation of modern population-based programs of vaccination from the collective good (that is, the public health benefit), to (and sometimes solely for) the individual benefit. Obviously, such a shift in expressed values has impli-cations both for communication as well as for pro-grammatic success.

Injury compensation

While government regulation in the USA improved the manufacture of vaccines following the passage of the 1902 act creating the Hygienic Laboratory and the 1936 Food and Drug Act, US tort law evolved in the 20th century as a mechanism to obtain compensation from the manufacturer or from the vaccinating physi-cian for injuries resulting from vaccines. For example, following claims publicized in the media of a possible but unproven association of neurologic harm from the whole-cell pertussis vaccine, injury claims against manufacturers of the diphtheria, tetanus, whole-cell pertussis (DTP) vaccine reached a zenith of 255 cases in 1986, which resulted in all but one of the DTP manufacturers withdrawing from the US market and in an increase in the price of the vaccine from 10 cts a dose to $10 a dose over a 10-year period. The US Congress responded in 1986 with the National Childhood Vaccine Injury Act. The Act created formal programs for communicating vaccine information,

reporting vaccine reactions, and adjudicating vaccine injury. Because the adjudication moved from emo-tional appeals to juries to a more evidence-based assessment by an officer of the US Court of Claims, the number of claims of vaccine injuries tried in civil court dramatically dropped. Other industrialized countries have developed similar programs with regard to adjudication and compensation for vaccine injury.

Commercial development

The adjudication of claims for compensation for vaccine injuries required by the National Childhood Vaccine Injury Act of 1986 provided vaccine manufac-turers and providers with substantial protection from unwarranted litigation pertaining to properly manu-factured and administered vaccines, and the attendant financial risks of these lawsuits. Such approaches have significant ramifications for public trust and the viabil-ity of vaccine manufacturers. For instance, a major role for governments is the development of commerce and, specifically, support for innovation and techno-logic development; this is the basis for patent laws, for example. Yet, since the creation of the National Vaccine Injury Compensation Program (VICP) in 1986, due to factors other than product liability, the USA has suffered a number of vaccine shortages, and the costs of vaccines have increased, which resulted in calls for further government action to improve the market for vaccine manufacture and provision. Observers hold that the expense of vaccine research and development combined with the relatively small market in contrast to other pharmaceuticals has resulted in the continued departure of manufacturers from the vaccine market.

In addition to calls for general support for vaccine development, there has also been public demand for specific vaccine development such as for an AIDS vaccine. Public demand of this nature has occurred before, such as when it spurred the US and foreign governments to develop the acellular pertussis vaccine as a replacement for the much more reactogenic whole-cell pertussis vaccine. The US government has also taken major roles in developing and supporting vaccines to support the US military and to protect against bioterrorism. Furthermore, other countries have felt pressure to develop their own capabilities to ensure their citizens have access to an adequate supply to support mass vaccination in the face of worldwide demand and potential limited supply, such as with an influenza pandemic, and thereby avoid dependence on foreign vaccine manufacturers. The development and production of vaccines for developing countries requires the attention of more affluent nations as well. Writing in reference to global eradication of vaccine-preventable diseases, Obaro and Palmer posit that, "Assisting developing countries to achieve such goals should be a high priority for wealthy nations, even if only to protect their own populations and this has become a goal for nongovernmental organizations such as the World Health Organization and the Bill and Melinda Gates Foundation, among others."

Official recommendations

An additional role of the government is to promulgate recommendations and standards in health care for both individual and public health expectations for medical services, including preventive screening and interventions such as vaccination. In the USA, the federal government, through its Centers for Disease Control and Prevention, has formed the Advisory Committee on Immunization Practices (ACIP) to advise on official vaccine recommendations. Since 1995, the ACIP has issued annual editions of the routinely recommended childhood and adolescent (as well as adult) immunization schedules, harmonizing those efforts with academic societies such as the American Academy of Pediatrics, the American Academy of Family Physicians, and the American College of Physicians. These recommendations are critical for supporting clinicians' efforts to educate patients and parents regarding available vaccines as well as to guide insurance coverage and reimbursement and provide information to manufacturers on the market for their vaccine products.

Equitable access

Ten percent of US children are uninsured and another 25% live in households where incomes are below the federal poverty threshold. The US government developed the Vaccines for Children (VFC) Program in 1993 in response to a nationwide series of measles epidemics from 1989–1991 that revealed a systematic disparity in childhood immunization resulting in part from a lack of access to vaccination. Eligible children include those children who are eligible for the Medic-aid program, who have no health insurance coverage, who are American Indian or Alaska Native, or who are underinsured. The VFC program offers vaccines at no cost for eligible children through VFC-enrolled doctors or through federally qualified health centers or rural health clinics. Today more than 50% of the vaccines administered to children in the USA are purchased by the federal government. Demands for universal purchase, however, have met resistance from some manufacturers because they argue government-established purchase prices reduce revenues below what is required to sustain vaccine research and development. In particular, it is estimated that it takes 18–20 years and $500 million to $1 billion to develop a vaccine from discovery to licensure.

Vaccine mandates

For more than a century, governments have claimed a role in creating public health mandates that require vaccination. British law first mandated vaccination of all infants against smallpox in 1853. By 1898, however, the mandate was modified to permit conscientious objection. Sir William Osler himself campaigned for mandating typhoid vaccination of British soldiers in World War I but lost, and conscientious objections were allowed. In the USA the most common mandates are in the form of school and daycare requirements promulgated at the state level. These are advanced in the name of public health and most often to prevent person-to-person transmission in the schools and daycare. To be clear, these school-based rules often permit exemptions for medical, religious, and other reasons. In that sense, they can be viewed not so much as requirements for vaccination as they are requirements for notification, documentation, and informed declination. The first school rules were promulgated in 1850 by Massachusetts. By 1963, 20 states had such rules; by 1981, all 50 states had school rules.

The roles of government in vaccination at the population level are broad and long-standing. These are not purely modern concerns, but ones that have marked the history of vaccination from the days of Jenner. From surveying disease incidence to determining need, through the development, production, and distribution of vaccine, to recommendations and even mandates, those aspects that make vaccination a public health success call for political will and action.

Cognitive biases, distortions, and preferred cognitive styles in vaccine decision making

"The truth is always the strongest argument."
—*Sophocles, Phaedra*

Rationale for understanding the psychology of vaccine decision making

---

Education regarding vaccines should be a shared social responsibility including the school system, national and state departments of public health, health care providers, prenatal classes, and others.

The US Centers for Disease Control and Prevention have published that vaccines have been one of the most effective public health programs devised, with demonstrable effects on increasing the human life span. However, despite the development of an increasing number of vaccines targeted at morbid infectious diseases, and national recommendations for their routine use, the adoption of vaccines is generally slow and often controversial. Likely, this derives in part from an unfortunate current reality: the widespread questioning of vaccine safety in the popular and social media and, as a result, high levels of vaccine concern and hesitancy among parents, patients, and to some degree, providers. If parents, patients, and providers do not believe that vaccines are safe and effective, it is obvious that they will be poorly utilized. In addition, if they do not believe that they or their loved ones are at personal risk for the diseases vaccines prevent, vaccine uptake is likely to be low. The role of the provider, therefore, becomes not only one of administering a vaccine but also one of providing and reinforcing education and appropriate recommendations to the patients under their care. Notably, current economic realities are such that physicians cannot undertake this alone, nor are they reimbursed for the considerable time such education demands. For this reason, education regarding vaccines should be a shared social responsibility including the school system, national and state departments of public health, health care providers, prenatal classes, and others.

Education of parents and patients should not only include information about specific diseases but also about the vaccines intended to prevent those diseases. These latter two points are critical and form an essential crux of the issue. If educational efforts and recommendations are to be effective, then it is critical that public health workers and health care providers be knowledgeable about both the disease and the vaccine. Unfortunately, this is not always the case. In addition, while knowledge about vaccines and vaccine-preventable disease is necessary, this alone is not sufficient. Among the reasons we have failed to achieve optimal population vaccine coverage levels in the USA is the failure to understand and respond effectively to patients' and parents' concerns about vaccine safety and efficacy. This requires both an understanding of those concerns as well as insight into perceptions, beliefs, learning, and decision-making styles. Therefore, this section of the chapter is devoted to understanding the preferred cognitive styles and biases humans use in learning and making decisions about health-related matters such as vaccines.

Models in health care decision making

Several comprehensive models have been usefully applied to health behavior. One such model widely accepted in the field is the health belief model (HBM). This model is a health, behavioral, and psychological model for studying, promoting, and predicting the uptake of health services and health behaviors. The model states that individuals make health decisions based upon "perceived susceptibility to disease, perceived severity of disease, perceived benefits of preventive action, perceived barriers to preventive action, modifying facts such as demographic variables, cues to action such as advice from others, and media reporting."

Models in health care decision making

- Health belief model (HBM)
- Transtheoretical model
- Cognitive behavioral therapy
- Tailored health communication
- Social marketing
- Bronfenbrenner's ecological systems theory

Another model is the transtheoretical model, in which "behavior change is conceptualized as a process that unfolds over time and involves progression through a series of five stages: pre-contemplation, contemplation, preparation, action, and maintenance." It is perhaps obvious that not all patients will be in the action stage when they visit their health care provider. Thus, it is important for the provider to be cognizant of the stage the patient is in, such that a few key actions can help their patients move to a subsequent stage to achieve and maintain behavior change in regards to health (see Table 20.3). The value of such a framework is that "by understanding each of these stages and their importance, we can assist patients who are not even considering vaccination to accept vaccines to protect their health throughout their life-

time. Implicit in this model, and our general belief about vaccine education, is the idea that change is a time-intensive process, and this we believe identifies a key area for research in current approaches to vaccine education." Too often, health care providers rely on a quick, empiric, and untailored approach to vaccine education, which is blind to the specifics of an individual patient's needs, worries, and concerns. Rather, it should be acknowledged that parents only want to do what is best for their children, yet a parent's ability to determine what is best is compromised by an abundance of junk science as well as robust science that is difficult for the public to understand due to its complexity. Therefore, it is not surprising that perceptions of the risks of vaccine-preventable diseases and the safety and efficacy of vaccines may

Table 20.3 Stages of Change Applied to Vaccine Decision Making

Stage of Change	Definition	Application to Vaccine Decision Making
Pre-contemplation	"There is no intention to change behavior in the foreseeable future. Most patients in this stage are unaware or under-aware of their problems." (Norcross et al. 2011)	Clarify decision is theirs – don't force decision. Encourage reevaluation and exploration of information again at each visit. Provide educational material.
Contemplation	"Patients are aware that a problem exists and are seriously thinking about overcoming it but have not yet made a commitment to take action." (Norcross et al. 2011)	Discuss the pros/cons of changing the behavior, continue to point out the decision is theirs. Identify and promote new, positive outcome expectations. Continue to provide education and answer questions.
Preparation	"Individuals are intending to take action in the next month and are reporting some small behavioral changes." (Norcross et al. 2011)	Identify and assist in problem solving or overcoming obstacles, help patient identify social support, necessary support information, encourage to take initial steps. Continue education efforts.
Action	"Individuals modify their behavior, experiences, and/or environment. Action involves the most overt behavioral changes." (Norcross et al. 2011)	Focus on restructuring cues and provide support, bolster self-efficacy for dealing with concerns or obstacles (i.e., talking to others), reiterate long-term benefits.
Maintenance	"Work to prevent relapse and consolidate the gains attained during action." (Norcross et al. 2011)	Plan for follow-up support, discuss coping skills, plan for continuation, and provide positive reinforcement for decision.

Adapted From: Norcross JC, Krebs PM, and Prochaska JO (2011). Stages of Change. Journal of Clinical Psychology 67(2), 143–154.

be inaccurate, and that parents and patients act upon such perceptions.

One of the most effective theories of change is cognitive behavioral therapy (CBT). While originally implemented in mental health counseling, it has implications for health care as a whole. This theory purports that there is a strong link between an individual's thoughts, feelings, and behaviors. Essentially, thoughts provoke feelings. These feelings influence behavior. Behavior then affects feelings, and the cycle continues. Therefore, if a change in behavior is desired, the thought and feelings behind that behavior must be identified, addressed, and challenged. To change health habits, a change in attitude about that behavior must be brought to awareness and challenged before the actual behavior can be changed. In previously published work, authors Caroline M. Poland and Gregory A. Poland of this chapter provided an example of how CBT might relate to decision making about vaccines: "Perhaps an individual is exposed repeatedly through the media to the Wakefield hypothesis that measles, mumps, and rubella (MMR) vaccine causes autism. A follow-on thought might be, 'MMR vaccine causes autism and why don't the experts tell the truth about the vaccine?' This may lead to a feeling such as, 'I don't trust what I am being told and I don't want to harm my child.' This thought and feeling would then predictably lead to a behavioral decision such as 'I'm not giving my child that vaccine.'"

Another useful model is the concept of tailored health communication. A tailored health communication can be helpful in clarifying for an individual their choice of health behaviors—in this case, vaccinations. "Tailoring could enhance motivation to process health information in at least four ways: (a) match content to an individual's information needs and interests, (b) frame health information in a context that is meaningful to the person, (c) use design and production elements to capture the individual's attention, and (d) provide information in the amount, type, and through channels of delivery preferred by the individual, thus potentially reducing barriers to exposure of individuals to communication interventions." This model requires a lengthier conversation and involves intentional listening to understand the patient's worry, concerns, and positions. The complexity of a model such as this makes clear the time investment required to effect change.

Other models have also been effectively applied to methods to influence health behaviors. A particularly salient model is that of social marketing, which attempts to influence the behaviors of persons such that individual and societal welfare are improved. The latter has been used to develop a plan to increase immunization rates among infants and has been demonstrated to result in positive health behaviors in other domains of public health.

Finally, it is helpful to determine ways to not only influence the patient alone, but to address a number of systems that together influence an individual's thoughts and decision-making patterns. In this regard, Bronfenbrenner's ecological systems theory would be useful in addressing the multiple systems that influence humans. A brief description of the system levels, their definition, and possible application to vaccine decision making is provided in Table 20.4.

The influence of groups and peers

Groups and peers also play a strong role in shaping an individual's thinking and decision making. Therefore, understanding social psychology concepts can be helpful to tailoring immunization counseling to individual patient or parents' decision-making styles. The concept of "bandwagoning"—as applied to vaccines—states that individuals are more likely to accept or reject vaccination if the groups that influence the individual are supporters or opponents of vaccines or vaccine policies and recommendations. For instance, if your church leader, neighbors you respect, your health care provider, and others who you admire are vaccine advocates, you are more likely to form similar opinions.

The influence of those surrounding an individual exerts an enormous impact upon individual beliefs and behaviors. To maintain the "we feeling" that develops within groups, individuals continue to conform, fearing rejection by their peers. Furthermore, individuals tend to be most strongly persuaded or influenced by members of their own reference groups. In the context of vaccine decision making, mothers who belong to a social club formed around their children's school, for example, often develop nearly identical fears, concerns, and questions or attitudes about vaccines that they did not hold prior to membership in the "group." Studies reveal that individuals tend to conform to the group norm through

Table 20.4 The Effect of Ecological Systems on Vaccine Decision Making

System Level	Definition	Example
Microsystem	"A pattern of activities, social roles, and interpersonal relations experienced by the individual or group of individuals." (Hong et al. 2011)	An individual with vaccine safety concerns who reads anti-vaccine websites, converses with others who share similar viewpoints, and thereby experiences self-reinforcing concerns that appear to validate these concerns, and rejects vaccines.
Mesosystem	"Experiences in one microsystem or experiences involving a direct interaction may influence another microsystem." (Hong et al. 2011)	Experiences noted above, paired with media or Internet reports of vaccine harms "flow over" into the vaccine decision-making domain.
Exosystem	"Exosystem consists of connections between two or more interactions or settings" (p. 866) or "settings not directly affecting the individual but that influence the microsystem." (Hong et al. 2011)	Frequent popular media reports suggesting conflicts of interest, conspiracies, and dishonesty converge to intensify the perceived likelihood of concerns with vaccine safety.
Macrosystem	"Broader society and culture that encompasses the other systems." (Hong et al. 2011) "A 'cultural blueprint' that may influence social structures and activities in the immediate system levels." (Hong et al. 2011) Examples include race/ethnicity and policies.	An increasingly less trustful social culture is validated by the availability heuristic in regards to internet anti-vaccine sites, popular media reports, and validated by other like-minded individuals the subject comes into contact with.
Chronosystem	"Includes consistency or change over the life course." (Hong et al. 2011) Examples include historical or economic events	Vaguely understood concerns over vaccine side effects (such as Guillain–Barré syndrome [GBS] after the 1976 swine flu vaccine), paired with reports of vaccine shortages due to contaminated flu vaccines withdrawn in the recent past, and current media or internet reports of claims of harm due to current pandemic vaccine, combine to heighten fear, resulting in rejection of vaccine.

Adapted from Hong JS, Algood CL, ChiuY, and Lee SA (2011). An ecological understanding of kinship foster care in the United States. Journal of Child Family Studies 20(6), 863–872.

two primary types of influence: normative and informational. Normative influence "is based on the desire to conform to the expectations of others," while informational influence "is based on the acceptance of information from others as evidence about reality." The effects of group peer pressure can be overwhelmingly intense, and for the individual, "once having made a public commitment, they stick to it. At most, they will change their judgments in later situations.... rior commitments restrain persuasion, too.... Making a public commitment makes people hesitant to back down." A gentle inquiry into what a patient's or parent's friends believe may be illuminating and offer insight into how to address those concerns.

Cognitive biases

Humans appear to be innately wired in regard to how they make decisions and judgments when there is uncertainty. People tend to make decisions in a variety of ways; for example, individuals may use rules of thumb (heuristics) to make quick decisions or emotional decisions, or use data-driven decision-making styles. Cognitive biases, or distortions in an individual's perception of reality, play a formative role in shaping our decisions and behaviors. Failure to recognize and challenge these biases and distortions can lead to faulty decision making.

Consider examples of cognitive biases in the context of vaccines. One important heuristic in vaccine decision making is the availability heuristic, which is based in the ease of recall due to repeated broadcasting of information. The availability heuristic suggests that individuals approximate the frequency of an event based on how easily it comes to mind. For example, the individual who regularly hears anti-vaccine messages begins to assume that the ease with which messages questioning vaccine safety can be recalled is reflective of the truth—that vaccine safety is questionable and something of which to be wary. This heuristic is important today because of the importance of the Internet and mass media, both of which can have a sensationalistic quality with repeated broadcasting of what is perceived to be a good story. However, just because an event is heard frequently doesn't mean that it is actually common. The current media environment therefore creates a challenge: If patients make decisions based on what information is readily available to them, health care providers and organizations must counter such perceptions by regularly—and consistently—providing correct and accurate information. In a similar fashion, repeated stories of harms done by not receiving vaccines should also be provided on a regular and consistent basis.

Another common heuristic that commonly impacts vaccine decision making is the representativeness heuristic. This heuristic is based on the similarity of one situation to another and is frequently used in decision making. For example, an emotional story of a young child who allegedly suffered a devastating vaccine side effect may heavily influence the mother of a young child where either the child or the situation resembles her own situation or circumstances. Subconscious thoughts about the affected child (who resembles the parent's child in age and circumstance) may lead to the conclusion that great harm could

result, and hence fear and hesitancy to accept the vaccine is appropriate.

While heuristics and biases certainly play a role in processing data and making health decisions, other influencers play a role as well. For example, from a public health point of view, the central route to persuasion "occurs when interested people focus on the arguments and respond with favorable thoughts." This route works when arguments are strong, well thought out, and the individual is interested in that argument. But what happens when that individual is not interested or harbors doubt due to fear-based messages to which they have been exposed? The peripheral route to persuasion "occurs when people are influenced by incidental cues." For example, "incidental cues" such as billboards, commercials, and visual images can be used to "persuade" people to consider other alternatives to their current way of thinking. Public health should consider similar methods of educating groups and populations. Such cues also play an important role in the social marketing model, as discussed earlier.

Another common bias is that of belief perseverance, which is the idea that "individuals cling to beliefs even when the evidential basis for these beliefs is completely refuted." Once an individual develops reasons for why they believe what they believe, it is difficult for others to try to change that belief. Others have labeled this "belief-dependent realism" and belief perseverance functions such that "data" are unlikely to change an individual's belief about what they believe. As an example, once "individuals construct a causal explanation to account for the observed event, it becomes highly accessible in memory and independent of the original evidence on which it was based. If the evidence is discredited, such as after a debriefing, the explanation remains intact and available, and hence sustains the false belief."

A current example of this interplay is provided by the MMR vaccine and autism debacle, even with scores of high-quality studies, across decades and geographic settings countering claims of autism related to the administration of MMR vaccine, and acknowledgement that the originator of the claim, Dr. Andrew Wakefield, acted in such a dishonest and unethical manner in regard to his studies and data that he was stripped of his medical license. The reaction of some is instructive. J.B. Handley, cofounder of Generation

Rescue, a well-known autism support group that disputes vaccine safety, told reporters, "To our community, Andrew Wakefield is Nelson Mandela and Jesus Christ rolled up into one .... He's a symbol of how all of us feel." It is apparent that those who incorporated Dr. Wakefield's claims have great difficulty in "seeing" the data, acting upon those data, and changing their attitudes and perceptions about what the data mean.

To counteract belief perseverance and the attributional framework (defined and discussed in Table 20.5), Nestler suggested asking "the individual to explain the opposite outcome." However, in an experiment done by Nestler, he found that "participants who were asked to list many reasons favoring the opposite outcome, judged the reported outcome to be more likely and hence exhibited more belief perseverance

Table 20.5 Common Biases and Heuristics Applied to Vaccine Decision Making

Bias/Heuristic	Definition	Application to Vaccine Decision Making
Availability heuristic (ease of recall)	Individuals judge the likelihood of an event by ease of recall. (Tversky and Kahneman 1974)	Frequent dramatic media reports of MMR and autism associations result in assumption of high-risk given high ease of recall.
Representativeness heuristic	Likelihood is judged based on similarity of one issue to another. (Tversky and Kahneman 1974)	Parent is aware of concerns about DTP vaccine safety in regards to CNS side effects, and these are representative of new concerns raised about CNS side effects due to MMR vaccine, therefore judging MMR–autism link to be valid.
Belief perseverance (also known as "belief-dependent realism")	"Individuals cling to beliefs even when the evidential basis for these beliefs is completely refuted." (Nestler 2010)	Continuing belief that receipt of MMR vaccine will result in risk of autism—despite all available scientific data to the contrary
Attributional framework	"Individuals construct a causal explanation to account for the observed event, and once this causal explanation has been created, it becomes highly accessible in memory and independent of the original evidence on which it was based." (Nestler 2010)	Due to media reports, concerns of peers, Internet reports, etc., parent accepts causal explanation of autism caused by MMR vaccine. Parent, however, is unable to recall evidence upon which this belief is based. Further, fear and concern is generalized to other vaccines as being "dangerous."
Confirmation bias	"The seeking or interpreting of evidence in ways that are partial to existing beliefs, expectations, or a hypothesis in hand." (Nickerson 1998)	Accepting as evidence of cause and effect reports of a child being diagnosed with autism in near proximity to receipt of MMR vaccine.
Hindsight bias		Reports of the diagnosis of autism in near proximity to receipt of MMR vaccine is taken as cause and effect among parents who believe such a link exists.
Normative influence (also known as "bandwagoning")	"Based on the desire to conform to the expectations of others." (Kaplan and Miller 1987)	Parent makes decision to reject MMR vaccine for child based on the opinions of peer group.

Table 20.5 (*Continued*)

Bias/Heuristic	Definition	Application to Vaccine Decision Making
Informational influence	"Is based on the acceptance of information from others as evidence about reality." (Kaplan and Miller 1987)	Acceptance of claims of MMR vaccine–autism connection simply because it appears on an anti-vaccine site with an official-sounding organizational name, or from a respected celebrity.
Risk compression	Overestimating the rate of rare risks. (Fischhoff et al. 1993)	Overestimating by an order of magnitude the risk of very rare, but commonly sensationalized vaccine risks such as Guillian–Barre syndrome.
Commission/ omission bias	Actions (commissions) are riskier than inaction (omission). (Asch et al. 1994; Ritov & Baron 1990)	Parental perception that a side effect that occurs due to a vaccination (commission) is riskier than the harm done by foregoing (omission) a vaccine. (Ball et al. 1998)
Avoidance of ambiguity	Risk from a known entity is more acceptable than the equivalent risk that is considered ambiguous. (Baron 1994)	Known risk of a vaccine-preventable disease is more readily accepted compared to an ambiguous (though smaller) risk of a vaccine side effect. (Ball et al. 1998)

than subjects in a standard perseverance condition. Listing few reasons in favor of the opposite outcome, however, led to a reduction in belief persistence."

The confirmation bias is another common cognitive bias in decision making. Confirmation bias "connotes the seeking or interpreting of evidence in ways that are partial to existing beliefs, expectations, or a hypothesis in hand." Existing beliefs affect how an individual hears, absorbs, and processes information. This is similar to the "hindsight" bias wherein "upon learning the outcome to a problem, people tend to believe that they knew it all along." Hindsight bias interferes with decision making because it "provides the illusion of understanding the past and can result in a failure to learn from the past."

The implication for health care providers is that education is an iterative process and necessarily involves identifying, addressing, and challenging cognitive biases and distortions, and in moving from a heuristic or simplistic belief about vaccines, to an informed, data-driven process for decision making. To date, few tools currently exist in a form useful for providers and patients, though that is beginning to change. A further difficulty is that medical schools and residency programs offer little instruction in the psychology of decision making. We hope that physicians will seek to understand theories of judgment and decision making as related to health care decisions, and use such knowledge to positively impact their patients and communities.

Preferred cognitive styles

In a recent commentary, we introduced the concept "preferred cognitive styles" as a model in which to understand how patients (and providers) develop attitudes and opinions about vaccines. This preferred cognitive styles and decision-making model might also help organize education about vaccines (or other health decisions) for the specific patient. The concept is basic—understand the preferred method by which someone processes information and makes decisions, and mimic that process in designing your education specifically for that patient. While many physicians, because of their training, may utilize cognitive styles that are very analytic, educating a patient should first involve determining their preferred cognitive style. A patient who utilizes a cognitive style that is based more in emotion is likely not going to be swayed when presented with a fact-filled sheet giving statistics specific to that vaccine, but may be influenced by pictures and stories of children who have contracted vaccine-preventable diseases. Unfortunately, the majority of current vaccine educational efforts are characterized by a highly analytical fact-based cognitive style. A more informed strategy may be to understand decision-making style at the individual level, and use this information to design style-specific message framing and educational tools. Table 20.6 provides example styles and a brief example of how education about vaccines might be organized specific to that style.

A method potentially useful in patient education about vaccines is motivational interviewing (MI). MI "focuses on responding differentially to client speech, within a generally empathic person-centered style... a guiding principle of motivational interviewing is to have the client, rather than the counselor, voice the

Table 20.6 Preferred Cognitive Styles Applied to Vaccine Decision Making

Cognitive Style	Main Effect	Verbal Expression	Approach
Denialist	Disbelieves accepted scientific facts, despite overwhelming evidence. Prone to believe conspiracy theories	"I don't care what the data show, I don't believe the vaccine is safe."	Provide consistent messaging repeatedly over time from trustworthy sources, provide educational materials, solicit questions, avoid "hard sell" approach, use motivational interviewing approaches
Innumerate	Cannot understand or has difficulty manipulating numbers, probabilities, or risks	"One in a million risk sounds high, for sure I'll be the 1 in a million that has a side effect, I'll avoid the vaccine."	Provide nonmathematical information, analogies, or comparators using a more holistic "right brain" or emotive approach
Fear-based	Decision making based on fears	"I heard vaccines are harmful and I'm not going to get them."	Understand source of fear, provide consistent positive approach, show risks in comparison to other daily risks, demonstrate risks of not receiving vaccines, use social norming approaches
Heuristic	Often appeals to availability heuristic (what I can recall equates with how commonly it occurs)	"I remember GBS happened in 1977 after flu vaccines, that must be common, and therefore I'm not getting a flu vaccine."	Point out inconsistencies and fallacy of heuristic thinking, provide educational materials, appeal to other heuristics
Bandwagoning	Primarily influenced by what others are doing or saying	"If others are refusing the vaccine there must be something to it, I'm going to skip getting the vaccine."	Understand primary influencers, point out logical inconsistencies, use social norming and self-efficacy approaches
Analytical	Left-brain thinking, facts are paramount	"I want to see the data so I can make a decision."	Provide data requested, review analytically with patient

From Poland and Poland (2011). Reprinted with permission from Elsevier.

arguments for change." The use of MI may also be a key component in addressing behavior change. "MI is a directive (goal-oriented), client-centered counseling style for helping clients to explore and resolve ambivalence about behavior change." Chapter authors Caroline M. Poland and Gregory A. Poland state in their editorial on this subject: "The idea behind this technique is that an individual tends to respond more favorably to the accurate empathy of the health professional in dealing with resistance to a health behavior. When the patient is simply told what to do, the health care provider isn't addressing the resistance, and may actually make the patient more firm in their belief." For those who do not desire behavior change (i.e., receiving vaccinations), simply handing the patient a vaccine information fact sheet will likely do little to invoke behavior change.

Understanding and processing the patient's resistance and fears, and specifically discussing their concerns, is more likely to induce a higher likelihood of behavior change. Motivational interviewing is more time consuming than a simple, pre-written program that involves simply providing facts to the patient, but may lead to a more successful behavior change process.

Summary

The concept of understanding cognitive biases, distortions, and preferred cognitive styles at the individual level is foundational to designing effective vaccine education and message framing. The goal of effective education programs is to increase immunization coverage rates at the individual and population levels, resulting in the prevention and control of vaccine-preventable diseases. We have previously articulated suggested "next steps" in developing 21st-century vaccine education programs, which at a minimum, include the following broad tasks:

• Expand the spectrum of vaccine education. As discussed, providers need education in understanding the role of preferred cognitive styles and psychosocial theories of health-related decision making. In turn, this information informs the design and deployment of vaccine education materials and programs.
• Understand vaccine psychology and cognitive decision making. Further research and development is needed in the psychology of decision making in regard

to vaccine acceptance or rejection. Such research is critical to educational efforts. In this regard, the contribution of scientists from the social sciences and other content areas (psychology, sociology, anthropology, design, education theory, etc.) is needed.
• Learn from other health education endeavors. New regulations in the USA will require highly emotional photographs and written warnings on individual packs of cigarettes. Emotion is effective in forming memories, which are then accessed in thinking about, and acting upon, new information. Might this be useful in vaccine educational efforts? We note that anti-vaccine Internet sites routinely use highly emotionally charged words, phrases, and stories.
• Expand the platform of vaccine education. New technologies including social media, gaming, information "push" technologies, podcasts, and others have not been adequately applied to vaccine education efforts. Research funding to test the value of such technologies is needed.
• Using Bronfenbrenner's ecological systems theory, we would be wise to engage other professionals and design belief-forming "cues" to educate the public in regard to vaccines. For example, it is critical to engage counselors, social psychologists, social workers, cultural anthropologists, and others in developing and employing high-impact vaccine-education communications. Schools are critical to forming beliefs and transferring information, and they too must be part of the solution to low coverage rates.

Conclusion

We note that every single Healthy People 2010 vaccine goal for adults devised at the beginning of this decade for the USA has failed to be met. Despite the ready availability of MMR and influenza vaccines, for example, the USA is experiencing a higher number of cases of measles than in the past 16 years. A more pressing example in many ways is that even among health care workers (only 34%, the minority) received pandemic influenza vaccine in 2010, with many questioning the safety of the vaccine.

After decades of public health and provider efforts, inadequate population coverage with vaccines is evident. Cognizant of these data, new research efforts are needed to identify issues, frame questions, develop models, and test hypotheses relevant to new models of vaccine education and decision making.

Ethical issues in vaccination

Intrinsic to public health immunization programs is a tension between two goods: preserving individual freedom and protecting the public's health. While high rates of vaccination can effectively protect the health of a community, sometimes the rates required can only be achieved by limiting individual freedom of choice. The Reverend Henning Jacobson captured this tension poignantly in 1902. Faced with a requirement to be vaccinated against smallpox during an outbreak in Cambridge, MA, Jacobson stated that such a requirement was "unreasonable, arbitrary and oppressive, and, therefore, hostile to the inherent right of every freeman to care for his own body and health in such way as to him seems best, and that the execution of such a law against one who objects to vaccination, no matter for what reason, is nothing short of an assault upon his person."

Jacobson's appeal to individual freedom was ultimately considered by the US Supreme Court. Jacobson lost. In the landmark decision, the Court determined that liberty itself is not without restrictions: "liberty ... does not import an absolute right in each person to be, at all times and in all circumstances, wholly freed from restraint. There are manifold restraints to which every person is necessarily subject for the common good. Real liberty for all could not exist under the operation of a principle which recognizes the right of each individual person to use his own, whether in respect of his person or his property, regardless of the injury that may be done to others." *Jacobson v. Massachusetts* has subsequently served as the basis for US compulsory vaccination laws and, more broadly, affirmed the state's police powers to safeguard the public's health and safety.

The tension between individual liberty and public health is as controversial a topic now as it was in 1902. In fact, it continues to factor prominently in ongoing deliberations about vaccination law and policy in federal and state courts. This tension endures in part because immunization programs are constantly evolving as the science of vaccinology advances; as our ability to prevent disease with vaccines changes, so too does our concept of what constitutes a threat to public welfare. For instance, while restricting individual liberty to protect the public's health may have been justifiable in the context of smallpox, is it equally so in the context of chickenpox? Questions like this shape current discussion and are key to helping ensure necessary public health powers are exercised with appropriate restraint. Ultimately, all public health programs rely both on a broad societal consensus and on the prudent, judicious exercise of the state's extraordinary powers to protect the community's health. In this section, we will describe two current ethical controversies involving childhood immunizations—parental refusal of childhood immunizations and exemptions from required school-entry immunizations—and discuss how this tension manifests in both.

Parental refusal of childhood immunizations

A growing minority of US parents choose to not immunize their children by refusing one or more of the recommended childhood vaccines. Parental reasons for doing so are multiple and varied, but are predominantly centered on concerns about the safety of vaccines. The consequences of this parental choice, however, can be dire. Underimmunized children are at increased risk of both contracting vaccine-preventable disease and transmitting it to others. In the USA, there are more than 4000 cases of vaccine-preventable disease per year in children younger than 5 years old, resulting in an estimated 300 deaths annually. Worldwide, there are 1.4 million deaths annually in children younger than 5 years old from vaccine-preventable disease, representing 14% of total mortality globally in children younger than 5.

Imminent risk of serious harm

Parental refusal of immunizations raises a fundamental ethical issue regarding the limits of individual freedom: When is it justifiable for the state to intrude upon a parent's right to make this decision on behalf of their minor child? Like individual freedom, parental autonomy is highly valued in US society, and, as such, parents are given wide discretion in their decision making on behalf of their minor children. However, parental autonomy is not an absolute right, and the state can intervene if the parent's decision places the child's health, well-being, or life in jeopardy. The threshold for state intervention is specifically defined as those decisions that "present an imminent risk of serious harm."

It is important to recognize that the determination of the threshold at which the state is justified in limiting parental autonomy is value laden. Whether a risk is *imminent* or a harm is *serious* is fundamentally a subjective assessment. As such, where this threshold lies is dependent on societal values. As societal values change over time, so does the threshold that is considered acceptable. For example, a parent's decision to refuse surgery for duodenal atresia in a child with Down syndrome in the 1970s was respected. Today, this would constitute medical neglect and state intervention justified.

The relevant issue when a parent refuses one or more routinely recommended vaccines for their child, then, is whether their decision poses an imminent risk of serious harm to their child. Generally, in the USA, the answer is no. This is primarily because it is difficult to make the argument that a parent's refusal presents an imminent risk. Not only are the incidence rates of vaccine-preventable diseases in the USA low, but the current immunization coverage among US children for these diseases is high, both of which make the risk of contracting a vaccine-preventable disease less than imminent for an unimmunized child. Second, it is usually difficult to make the argument that the parent's decision presents a serious harm to the child. Even though serious harm is possible, if a child were to contract a vaccine-preventable disease, the likelihood of suffering serious complications from a disease is typically low in most cases.

Of course, specific characteristics of each situation are relevant and affect calculations of risk and harm. For instance, there are differing propensities for contracting and suffering complications from a disease based on factors such as a child's age and underlying health. In addition, the specific vaccines (or more accurately, antigens) that are refused matter. Each vaccine has a different efficacy and safety profile and prevents diseases with different epidemiological characteristics and individual and public health consequences. Lastly, the physical environment plays a role in the determination of risk and harm since incidence rates of vaccine-preventable disease vary based upon geography and time. Taken together, it is therefore conceivable that the parent's refusal of the diphtheria, tetanus toxoid, and acellular pertussis vaccine for a 2-month-old child with chronic lung disease amid a state-wide epidemic of pertussis might reach the threshold of imminent risk of serious harm and justify state intervention.

Vaccine-hesitant parents

Although the risk and harm to a child from his or her parents' refusal of an immunization may not warrant state intervention, we are still left to grapple with the fact that there is still some increased likelihood of risk of harm to the child and to others. That is, if the unimmunized child were to contract a vaccine-preventable disease, the child is at some risk for developing serious complications, and while infectious, presents some risk of transmitting the infection to those who are too young to be immunized, have a contraindication to being immunized, or whose immunization was ineffective. Due to this increased risk of harm to the child and community, as well as strong beliefs in the science supporting the safety and efficacy of immunization as a standard component of pediatric care, some pediatric providers consider removing parents from their practice if, after repeated counseling, parents refuse one or more childhood immunizations.

This approach is very controversial and not supported by the American Academy of Pediatrics except in the unusual circumstance that the provider/parent relationship has deteriorated to a point that compromises the quality of care for that child. There are several compelling reasons not to remove parents. First, doing so can be counterproductive. There is growing evidence that most parents who refuse vaccines are not staunchly opposed to vaccines, but simply hesitant, and this hesitancy can be modifiable. For instance, many vaccine-hesitant parents change their minds after information or assurances from their child's provider. Ending a relationship with them may lead to missed opportunities to modify their opinions about immunizations. Further, if or where parents may take their child for subsequent care is unknown. Second, trust in a child's provider is critical to parental acceptance of recommended immunizations. In fact, vaccine-hesitant parents desire a trustworthy health care provider for their child and have a high interest in receiving vaccine information from that provider. An approach to immunization communication with a parent that includes removing them if they do not comply likely undermines the trust-building process essential to parental acceptance of immunizations. Third, and perhaps most important, dismissal of parents who refuse one or more immunizations disregards the central importance of parental values in the medical decision-making process. While the nature and magnitude of a risk can be objectively stated, the perception of a risk—how it is weighted and its acceptability or unacceptability—is subjective and dependent on one's values. Parental refusal of a recommended immunization, therefore, often simply conveys a difference in values from their child's provider. For example, the remote risk of a simple febrile seizure may seem relatively trivial to a physician but be viewed by a parent as life threatening and horrific. Respectful exploration of these value differences is likely to be more productive for the provider/parent relationship and more rewarding for both parent and provider than severing their relationship.

Practically, it is also not clear whether removing a parent who refuses immunizations achieves one of its main objectives, which is to decrease the risk of infection to others. Although keeping underimmunized children out of a crowded waiting room will decrease the risk of transmission to other patients in those same waiting rooms, it does nothing to decrease this risk in other venues the child visits (e.g., daycare, school, etc.). Furthermore, there may be less drastic ways to minimize potential transmission risk without removing them from a practice, such as sequestering unimmunized kids in a separate room. Nonetheless, little research or data are available on this controversial practice.

Exemptions from required school-entry immunizations

Immunization policy in the form of school immunization laws generates unique challenges for balancing individual freedom and public health. School immunization laws, initially developed to control disease in a setting where a highly infectious agent could infect others through ordinary close contact, are an important part of the protection of the safety of the school environment and, therefore, the protection of the state's duty to educate. If enforced, school immunization laws are also very effective: They decrease disease outbreaks and increase vaccination coverage.

Making a child's entrance to public school contingent on being immunized, however, interferes with parental choice. To reduce this intrusion and perceptions of coercion, exemptions exist in many state school immunization laws to allow parents to opt their child out of the required immunizations. Currently, all

states permit parents to claim an exemption for their child for medical reasons, 48 states permit exemptions for religious reasons, and 20 states permit exemptions for personal belief or philosophical reasons. These personal belief or philosophical exemptions have currently been at the forefront of a debate regarding how best to address the tension between parental autonomy and public health, given that exemptors quantitatively increase the risks of outbreaks.

The debate over personal belief exemptions

One argument in the debate over personal belief exemptions is that they should be eliminated for those vaccines that are deemed both very safe and are associated with severe contagious diseases, such as those diseases that have high rates of childhood mortality or permanent sequelae. As such, this policy prioritizes the protection of public health over the respect for parental autonomy. However, the additional intrusion upon parental autonomy created by eliminating personal belief exemptions would only be in those circumstances where the benefit of immunization is most clearly and considerably greater than the risk. This policy is congruent with legal precedent, such as *Jacobson v. Massachusetts*, in which individuals can be forced to be immunized or quarantined in the setting of an outbreak of a deadly infectious disease. It is also decidedly more just. By compelling all parents to immunize their children with vaccines that target certain diseases that constitute the greatest threat to the individual child and to the public health, no parent is allowed to reap some of the benefits of those vaccines through herd immunity without assuming any of their risks (i.e., be a "free rider").

Another argument is that personal belief exemptions should remain, but the ease in which they can be claimed should be modified. There are also several justifications for this approach. First, evidence suggests that it is not merely the existence of personal exemptions that is associated with higher exemption rates, but also the ease in which these exemptions can be claimed. It should be no easier to claim an exemption than to get an immunization. Second, eliminating personal belief exemptions in a climate in which vaccine hesitancy is on the rise may be perceived as coercive and therefore may have the paradoxical effect of bolstering anti-vaccine sentiment. Third, the reasons parents opt out of vaccines include concerns about vaccine safety and the process with which vaccines are developed, regulated, and recommended. Therefore, rather than removing a parent's ability to opt out of immunization requirements in order to increase immunization coverage, the more acceptable alternative would be to focus efforts on these root causes of noncompliance by investing in vaccine safety research, improving the transparency of the vaccine development and recommendation process, and fostering informed public discussion of the role of immunization in protecting individual and public health. Lastly, an immunization policy that permits personal belief exemptions can also minimize unfairness.

An intersection of knowledge and values

This contemporary debate regarding personal belief exemptions is illustrative of the constant evolution in vaccine policy regarding the tension between individual freedom and public health. Vaccine recommendations and mandates evolve based on reevaluations of the risks and benefits associated with the vaccines and the diseases they prevent, as well as shifts in societal values. The smallpox immunization recommendation, for instance, was withdrawn before the disease was eradicated, but at the point when it was judged that the risk of the vaccine exceeded the risk of disease.

Vaccine policy, therefore, demonstrates the need for the integration of both knowledge and values. Current knowledge alone is not sufficient to dictate policy. The interpretation of evidence and its application to policy development requires subjective judgments by policy makers about priorities and the weighting of risks and benefits for individuals and communities.

Policy makers must foster discussion, listen, and reflect, not simply articulate the truth as they perceive it. The US Advisory Committee on Immunization Practice's recent determination to differentiate between evidence, expert opinion, and explicitly stated values encourages this process. A systematic approach to policy making is advocated both to protect against unexamined biases and to achieve the level of transparency in policy making that is required to withstand public scrutiny and garner and sustain broad public support. Only through the sort of thoughtful and informative discussion required by such a systematic approach will respect for differing values be maintained, and the appropriate balance between respecting individual freedom and protecting public health be achieved.

Summary

- Vaccinology encompasses scientific, social, ethical, political, and psychological issues in terms of vaccine discovery and vaccine use at both the individual and population levels.

- Ensuring the success of immunization programs to truly impact the health of a population will require that scientists, regulators, public health officials, and providers take care to address all of these components of vaccinology.

- Each of the components of an immunization program is imperative to building demand for vaccines and in turn drives and motivates vaccine uptake at the individual and population level.

- While vaccine discovery is critical to a good vaccine program, the vaccine will not be successful unless patients and providers believe such a vaccine will be safe and efficacious.

- More coordinated research that encompasses all elements of vaccinology is needed to develop cohesive and successful immunization programs.

Further reading

Abdelmutti N and Hoffman-Goetz L (2009). Risk messages about HPV, cervical cancer, and the HPV vaccine Gardasil: a content analysis of Canadian and U.S. national newspaper articles. Women and Health 49(5), 422–440.

ACIP. ACIP: Evidence-based recommendations–GRADE. 2012. http://www.cdc.gov/vaccines/recs/acip/GRADE/about.htm#resources. Accessed March 6, 2012.

Asch DA, Baron J, Hershey JC, et al. (1994). Omission bias and pertussis vaccination. Medical Decision Making 14, 118–123.

Ball LK, Evans G, and Bostrom A (1998). Risky business: challenges in vaccine risk communication. Pediatrics 101(3 Pt 1), 453–458.

Baron J. Thinking and Deciding, 2nd edition. New York: Cambridge University Press, 1994.

Barringer PJ, Studdert DM, Kachalia AB, and Mello MM (2008). Administrative compensation of medical injuries: a hardy perennial blooms again. Journal of Health Politics, Policy and Law 33(4), 725–760.

Bellamy R (2004). An introduction to patient education: theory and practice. Medical Teacher 26(4), 359–365.

Benin AL, Wisler-Scher DJ, Colson E, Shapiro ED, and Holmboe ES (2006). Qualitative analysis of mothers' decision-making about vaccines for infants: the importance of trust. Pediatrics 117(5), 1532–1541.

Bernstein DM, Erdfelder E, Meltzoff AN, Peria W, and Loftus GR (2011). Hindsight bias from 3 to 95 years of age. Journal of Experimental Psychology. Learning, Memory, and Cognition 37(2), 378–391.

Blume S and Zanders M (2006). Vaccine independence, local competences and globalisation: lessons from the history of pertussis vaccines. Social Science and Medicine 63(7), 1825–1835.

Brafman O and Brafman R. Sway: The Irresistible Pull of Irrational Behavior. New York: Doubleday, 2008.

Brandt AM (1978). Polio, politics, publicity, and duplicity: ethical aspects in the development of the Salk vaccine. International Journal of Health Services: Planning, Administration, Evaluation 8(2), 257–270.

Briss PA, Rodewald LE, Hinman AR, et al. (2000). Reviews of evidence regarding interventions to improve vaccination coverage in children, adolescents, and adults. The Task Force on Community Preventive Services. American Journal of Preventive Medicine 18(1 Suppl), 97–140.

Bronfenbrenner U. Ecological models of human development. In International Encyclopedia of Education, 2nd edition (eds T Husen and TN Postlethwaite), pp. 1643–1647. New York: Elsevier Science, 1994.

CDC. Vaccination coverage among children in kindergarten—United States, 2009–10 school year. 2011. Report No.: 60(21).

CDC. 2010 Table Data. 2012. http://www.cdc.gov/print.do?url=http://www.cdc.gov/vaccines/stats-surv/nis/data/tables_2010.htm. Accessed February 9, 2012.

Centers for Disease Control and Prevention (1999). Ten great public health achievements–United States, 1900–1999. MMWR. Morbidity and Mortality Weekly Report 48(12), 241–243.

Centers for Disease Control and Prevention (2010). Interim results: influenza A (H1N1) 2009 monovalent and seasonal influenza vaccination coverage among health-care personnel–United States, August 2009–January 2010. MMWR. Morbidity and Mortality Weekly Report 59(12), 357–362.

Centers for Disease Control and Prevent (2011). Notes from the field: measles outbreak–Hennepin county, Minnesota, February–March 2011. MMWR. Morbidity and Mortality Weekly Report 60(13), 421.

Center for Disease Control and Prevention (2011). Notes from the field: measles outbreak–Indiana, June-July 2011. MMWR. Morbidity and Mortality Weekly Report 60(34), 1169.

Child Abuse Prevention and Treatment Act, Reauthorization Act of 2010, 45 CFR 1340, Child Abuse Prevention and Treatment Act, Reauthorization Act of 2010, (2010).

Clements CJ, Greenough P, and Shull D (2006). How vaccine safety can become political–the example of polio in Nigeria. Current Drug Safety 1(1), 117–119.

Clements CJ and Ratzan S (2003). Misled and confused? Telling the public about MMR vaccine safety. Measles, mumps, and rubella. Journal of Medical Ethics 29(1), 22–26.

Cohen J (1993). Childhood vaccines: the R&D factor. Science 259(5101), 1528–1529.

Colgrove J (2005). "Science in a democracy": the contested status of vaccination in the Progressive Era and the 1920s. Isis 96(2), 167–191.

Colgrove J (2007). Immunity for the people: the challenge of achieving high vaccine coverage in American history. Public Health Reports 122(2), 248–257.

Copper BK (2007). Notes and comments "High and dry?" The Public Readiness and Emergency Preparedness Act and liability protection for pharmaceutical manufacturers. Journal of Health Law 40(1), 65–105.

Diekema DS (2005). Responding to parental refusals of immunization of children. Pediatrics 115(5), 1428–1431.

Dominus S. The Crash and Burn of an Autism Guru. New York Times Magazine Online. http://www.nytimes.com/2011/04/24/magazine/mag-24Autism-t.html?_r=2&pagewanted=1. Accessed March 29, 2012.

Douglas RG, Jr (1998). The Jeremiah Metzger Lecture. Vaccine prophylaxis today: its science, application and politics. Transactions of the American Clinical and Climatological Association 109, 185–196.

Feikin DR, Lezotte DC, Hamman RF, Salmon DA, Chen RT, and Hoffman RE (2000). Individual and community risks of measles and pertussis associated with personal exemptions to immunization. JAMA: The Journal of the American Medical Association 284, 3145–3150.

Fischhoff B, Bostrom A, and Quadrel MJ (1993). Risk perception and communication. Annual Review of Public Health 14, 183–203.

Flanagan-Klygis EA, Sharp L, and Frader JE (2005). Dismissing the family who refuses vaccines: a study of pediatrician attitudes. Archives of Pediatrics and Adolescent Medicine 159(10), 929–934.

Fredrickson DD, Davis TC, Arnould CL, et al. (2004). Childhood immunization refusal: provider and parent perceptions. Family Medicine 36(6), 431–439.

Gay NJ (2004). The theory of measles elimination: implications for the design of elimination strategies. The Journal of Infectious Diseases 189 Suppl 1, S27–S35.

Gerend MA and Shepherd JE (2011). Correlates of HPV knowledge in the era of HPV vaccination: a study of unvaccinated young adult women. Women and Health 51(1), 25–40.

Glanz JM, McClure DL, Magid DJ, et al. (2009). Parental refusal of pertussis vaccination is associated with an increased risk of pertussis infection in children. Pediatrics 123(6), 1446–1451.

Glanz JM, McClure DL, Magid DJ, Daley MF, France EK, and Hambidge SJ (2010). Parental refusal of varicella vaccination and the associated risk of varicella infection in children. Archives of Pediatrics and Adolescent Medicine 164(1), 66–70.

Glanz JM, McClure DL, O'Leary ST, et al. (2011). Parental decline of pneumococcal vaccination and risk of pneumococcal related disease in children. Vaccine 29(5), 994–999.

Gostin LO (2005). Jacobson v Massachusetts at 100 years: police power and civil liberties in tension. American Journal of Public Health 95(4), 576–581.

Greenberg SB (2000). Bacilli and bullets: William Osler and the antivaccination movement. Southern Medical Journal 93, 763–767.

Gust D, Brown C, Sheedy K, Hibbs B, Weaver D, and Nowak G (2005). Immunization attitudes and beliefs among parents: beyond a dichotomous perspective. American Journal of Health Behavior 29(1), 81–92.

Gust DA, Darling N, Kennedy A, and Schwartz B (2008). Parents with doubts about vaccines: which vaccines and reasons why. Pediatrics 122(4), 718–725.

Gust DA, Kennedy A, Shui I, Smith PJ, Nowak G, and Pickering LK (2005). Parent attitudes toward immunizations and healthcare providers the role of information. American Journal of Preventive Medicine 29(2), 105–112.

Haaheim LR (2007). Vaccines for an influenza pandemic: scientific and political challenges. Influenza and Other Respiratory Viruses 1(2), 55–60.

Heymann DL and Aylward RB (2006). Mass vaccination: when and why. Current Topics in Microbiology and Immunology 304, 1–16.

Hinman AR (1984). The pertussis vaccine controversy. Public Health Reports 99(3), 255–259.

Hinman AR and Randall LH (2008). Fighting for the reputation of vaccines. Pediatrics 122(1), 224–225.

Hodge JG and Gostin LO (2001). School vaccination requirements: historical, social, and legal perspectives. Kentucky Law Journal (Lexington, Ky.) 90(4), 831–890.

Hong JS, Algood CL, Chiu Y, and Lee SA (2011). An ecological understanding of kinship foster care in the United States. Journal of Child and Family Studies 20(6), 863–872.

Irons B, Morris-Glasgow V, Andrus JK, Castillo-Solorzano C, and Dobbins JG (2011). Lessons learned from integrated surveillance of measles and rubella in the Caribbean. The Journal of Infectious Diseases 204 Suppl 2, S622–S626.

Jacobson v. Massachusetts, 197 U.S. 11. 1905. US Supreme Court. Decided February 20, 1905.

Janz NK, Champion VL, and Strecher VJ. The Health Belief Model. In Health Behavior and Health Education: Theory, Research, and Practice, 3rd edition (eds K Glanz, BK Rimer and FM Lewis), pp. 45–66. San Francisco, CA: John Wiley & Sons, Inc., 2002.

Kahneman D. Thinking, Fast and Slow. New York: Farrar, Straus, Giroux, 2011.

Kaplan MF and Miller CE (1987). Group decision making and normative versus informational influence: effects of type of issue and assigned decision role. Journal of Personality and Social Psychology 53(2), 306–313.

Kennedy A, Lavail K, Nowak G, Basket M, and Landry S (2011). Confidence about vaccines in the United States: understanding parents' perceptions. Health Affairs (Project Hope) 30(6), 1151–1159.

Lantos JD, Jackson MA, and Harrison CJ (2012). Why we should eliminate personal belief exemptions to vaccine mandates. Journal of Health Politics, Policy and Law 37(1), 131–140.

Larson HJ, Cooper LZ, Eskola J, Katz SL, and Ratzan S (2011). Addressing the vaccine confidence gap. Lancet 378(9790), 526–535.

Lilienfeld DE (2008). The first pharmacoepidemiologic investigations: national drug safety policy in the United States, 1901–1902. Perspectives in Biology and Medicine 51(2), 188–198.

Linden A, Butterworth SW, and Prochaska JO (2010). Motivational interviewing-based health coaching as a chronic care intervention. Journal of Evaluation in Clinical Practice 16(1), 166–174.

Mah CL, Deber RB, Guttmann A, McGeer A, and Krahn M (2011). Another look at the human papillomavirus vaccine experience in Canada. American Journal of Public Health 101(10), 1850–1857.

Malone KM and Hinman AR. Vaccination mandates: the public health imperative and individual rights. In Law in Public Health Practice (eds RA Goodman, MA Rothstein and RE Hoffman), pp. 262–284. New York: Oxford University Press, 2003.

Miller WR and Rose GS (2010). Toward a theory of motivational interviewing. The American Psychologist 64(6), 527–537.

MMWR. History of CDC Surveillance Activities. 1990. Report No.: 39 (SS-1).

Morris A. Ind. measles outbreak, linked to Super Bowl, raises vaccination concerns. 2012. PBS NewsHour. http://www.pbs.org/newshour/rundown/2012/02/measles-outbreak-in-indiana.html. Accessed February 20, 2012.

Myers DG. Social Psychology, 8th edition. New York: Mcgraw-Hill College, 2005.

National Research Council. Calling the Shots: Immunization Finance Policies and Practices. Washington, DC: The National Academies Press, 2000.

Nestler S (2010). Belief perseverance: the role of accessible content and accessibility experiences. Social Psychology 41, 35–41.

Nickerson RS (1998). Confirmation bias: a ubiquitous phenomenon in many guises. Review of General Psychology 2, 175–220.

Norcross JC, Krebs PM, and Prochaska JO (2011). Stages of change. Journal of Clinical Psychology 67(2), 143–154.

Obaro SK and Palmer A (2003, 28). Vaccines for children: policies, politics and poverty. Vaccine 21(13–14), 1423–1431.

Offit PA (2005). Why are pharmaceutical companies gradually abandoning vaccines? Health Affairs (Project Hope) 24(3), 622–630.

Offit PA and Peter G (2003). The meningococcal vaccine–public policy and individual choices. The New England Journal of Medicine 349(24), 2353–2356.

Omer SB, Enger KS, Moulton LH, Halsey NA, Stokley S, and Salmon DA (2008). Geographic clustering of nonmedical exemptions to school immunization requirements and associations with geographic clustering of pertussis. American Journal of Epidemiology 168(12), 1389–1396.

Omer SB, Pan WK, Halsey NA, et al. (2006). Nonmedical exemptions to school immunization requirements: secular trends and association of state policies with pertussis incidence. JAMA: The Journal of the American Medical Association 296(14), 1757–1763.

Omer SB, Salmon DA, Orenstein WA, deHart MP, and Halsey N (2009). Vaccine refusal, mandatory immunization, and the risks of vaccine-preventable diseases. The New England Journal of Medicine 360(19), 1981–1988.

Opel DJ and Diekema DS (2012). Finding the proper balance between freedom and justice: why we should not eliminate personal belief exemptions to vaccine mandates. Journal of Health Politics, Policy and Law 37(1), 141–147.

Opel DJ, Diekema DS, Lee NR, and Marcuse EK (2009). Social marketing as a strategy to increase immunization rates. Archives of Pediatrics and Adolescent Medicine 163(5), 432–437.

Opel DJ, Diekema DS, and Marcuse EK (2008). A critique of criteria for evaluating vaccines for inclusion in mandatory school immunization programs. Pediatrics 122(2), e504–e510.

Orenstein WA, Douglas RG, Rodewald LE, and Hinman AR (2005). Immunizations in the United States: success, structure, and stress. Health Affairs (Project Hope) 24(3), 599–610.

Orenstein WA and Hinman AR (1999). The immunization system in the United States—the role of school immunization laws. Vaccine 17 Suppl 3, S19–S24.

Parikh RK (2008). Fighting for the reputation of vaccines: lessons from American politics. Pediatrics 121(3), 621–622.

Parker AA, Staggs W, Dayan GH, et al. (2006). Implications of a 2005 measles outbreak in Indiana for sustained elimination of measles in the United States. The New England Journal of Medicine 355(5), 447–455.

Poland CM and Poland GA (2011). Vaccine education spectrum disorder: the importance of incorporating psychological and cognitive models into vaccine education. Vaccine 29(37), 6145–6148.

Poland GA and Marcuse EK (2011). Developing vaccine policy: attributes of "just policy" and a proposed template to guide decision and policy making. Vaccine 29(44), 7577–7578.

Rimer BK and Kreuter MW (2006). Advancing tailored health communication: a persuasion and message effects perspective. Journal of Communication 56, S184–S201.

Ritov I and Baron J (1990). Reluctance to vaccinate: ommision bias and ambiguity. Journal of Behavioral Decision Making 3, 236–277.

Roush SW and Murphy TV (2007). Historical comparisons of morbidity and mortality for vaccine-preventable diseases in the United States. JAMA: The Journal of the American Medical Association 298(18), 2155–2163.

Salmon DA, Haber M, Gangarosa EJ, Phillips L, Smith NJ, and Chen RT (1999). Health consequences of religious and philosophical exemptions from immunisation laws. Individual and societal risk of measles. JAMA: The Journal of the American Medical Association 281, 47–53.

Salmon DA, Moulton LH, Omer SB, deHart MP, Stokley S, and Halsey NA (2005). Factors associated with refusal of childhood vaccines among parents of school-aged children: a case-control study. Archives of Pediatrics and Adolescent Medicine 159(5), 470–476.

Schwartz JL, Caplan AL, Faden RR, and Sugarman J (2007). Lessons from the failure of human papillomavirus vaccine state requirements. Clinical Pharmacology and Therapeutics 82(6), 760–763.

Shermer M. The Believing Brain: From Ghosts and Gods to Politics and Conspiracies–How We Construct Beliefs and Reinforce Them as Truths. New York: Times Books, 2011.

Slovic P, Fischhoff B, and Lichenstein S (1977). Behavioral decision theory. Annual Review of Psychology 28, 1–39.

Smith PJ, Chu SY, and Barker LE (2004). Children who have received no vaccines: who are they and where do they live? Pediatrics 114(1), 187–195.

Stern AM and Markel H (2005). The history of vaccines and immunization: familiar patterns, new challenges. Health Affairs (Project Hope) 24(3), 611–621.

Taylor S (2009). Political epidemiology: strengthening socio-political analysis for mass immunisation—lessons from the smallpox and polio programmes. Global Public Health 4(6), 546–560.

Tversky A and Kahneman D (1974). Judgment under uncertainty: heuristics and biases (Biases in judgments reveals some heuristics of thinking under uncertainty). Science 185, 1124–1131.

US Department of Health and Human Services. Healthy People 2010: Understanding and Improving Health and objectives for improving health. 2nd edition. 2000.

US Department of Health and Human Services, Health Resources and Services Administration, Maternal Health Bureau. Child Health USA 2008–2009. 2009.

Uzicanin A and Zimmerman L (2011). Field effectiveness of live attenuated measles-containing vaccines: a review of published literature. The Journal of Infectious Diseases 204 Suppl 1, S133–S148.

Weiss MM, Weiss PD, and Weiss JB (2007). Anthrax vaccine and public health policy. American Journal of Public Health 97(11), 1945–1951.

Winkler JL, Wittet S, Bartolini RM, et al. (2008). Determinants of human papillomavirus vaccine acceptability in Latin America and the Caribbean. Vaccine 26 Suppl 11, L73–L79.

World Health Organization. Immunization surveillance, assessment and monitoring: Vaccine-preventable diseases. 2002. http://www.who.int/immunization_monitoring/diseases/en/. Accessed February 8, 2012.

Yeung LF, Lurie P, Dayan G, et al. (2005). A limited measles outbreak in a highly vaccinated US boarding school. Pediatrics 116(6), 1287–1291.

Zhuo J, Hoekstra EJ, Zhong G, Liu W, Zheng Z, and Zhang J (2011). Innovative use of surveillance data to harness political will to accelerate measles elimination: experience from Guangxi, China. The Journal of Infectious Diseases 204 Suppl 1, S463–S470.

Zucht v. King, 260 U.S. 174. 1922. U.S. Supreme Court. Decided November 13, 1922.

Index

Note: Page entries in *italics* indicate figures; tables are noted with *t*.

MVP. *See* Meningitis Vaccine Project
MVS. *See* Master vaccine strain
Mycobacterium bovis, 2, 3, 142, 156
Mycobacterium tuberculosis, 65, 142
Mycoplasma, quality control
    testing, 201*t*
Mycoplasma tuberculosis lipoprotein
    Mtb19, 141
MyD88, defined, 76

NA. *See* Neuraminidase
NadA. *See* Neisserial adhesin A
NADPH. *See* Nicotinamide adenine
    dinucleotide phosphate
NAIP5. *See* NOD-like receptor proteins
    neuronal apoptosis inhibitory
    protein 5
NALP1 protein, 77
NALP2 protein, 77
NALP3 protein, 77, 149
Nanogels, 148–149
Nanomatrix, 148
Nanoparticles, 101–102, 150, 189
    defined, 123, 148
    with hydroxylated surfaces, 149
National Association of County and
    City Health Officials, 275
National Cancer Institute, Central
    IRB, 271
National Centre for Immunization
    Research and Surveillance
    (Australia), 291
National Childhood Vaccine Injury
    Act, 291, 339
National control laboratories, 332
National Foundation for Infantile
    Paralysis, 52
National Health and Medical Research
    Council (Australia), 266, 273
National Health System, 296
National Immunization
    Committee, 275
National immunization days, in
    Cuba, 53
National Immunization Survey, 43
National Influenza Centers, 258
National Institute of Allergy and
    Infectious Diseases, 9
National Institute for Biological
    Standards and Control, 199, 205
National Institute for General
    Medicine and Science, 314

National Institute of Allergy and
    Infectious Diseases, 11
National Institutes of Health, 9, 199,
    215–216
    Clinical Trials database, 38
National Microbiological
    Institute, 216
National regulatory authorities, 332–
    333, 334
    licensure of candidate vaccines
    and, 35, 36
National Vaccine Injury
    Compensation Program, 291
National Vaccine Program Office, 275
National Veterinary Stockpile, diseases
    covered with deployment of, 241
Native American children, invasive
    pneumococcal disease and, 21
Natural history
    of disease, 306–307
    time line, *306*
NCIRS. *See* National Centre for
    Immunization Research and
    Surveillance
NCLs. *See* National control
    laboratories
NCVIA. *See* National Childhood
    Vaccine Injury Act
NDA. *See* New Drug Application
NDS. *See* New Drug Submission
NDV. *See* Newcastle disease virus
Needle inoculation, transmission
    through the skin and, 60
Nef, 67
Neisseria heparin binding
    antigen, 174
Neisseria meningitidis, 22–23, 45, 84,
    167, 168, 283, 323
    purified polysaccharide vaccines
    against, 122
    subunit vaccines and, 71
Neisseria meningitidis type B candidate
    vaccine, development by reverse
    vaccinology, *174*
Neisseria spp., 67
Neisserial adhesin A, 174
Neonatal tetanus, 6, *6*, 156, 323, 324
Neospora caninum, 187
Netherlands, rulella in, September
    2002–2005, 16*t*
Neuraminidase, 114, *164*, 165, 170,
    205

Neuroscience, 110
Neutrophilic polymorphonuclear
    leukocytes, 63
New Drug Application, 225–227, 267
    Common Technical Document,
    225
    defined, 196, 225, 267
    electronic submissions, 225–226
    maintenance of, 227
    phase IIIa studies and, 264
    submission and review of, 226–227
New Drug Submission (Canada),
    229
New vaccine pipeline, 196
New York Board of Health strain, 2
Newborns, 156
    vaccine recommendations for, 277,
    281, 282
Newcastle disease virus, 135–136
NF-kB, defined, 76
NHBA. *See* Neisseria heparin binding
    antigen
NHMRC. *See* National Health and
    Medical Research Council
NHS. *See* National Health System
NIBSC. *See* National Institute for
    Biological Standards and Control
NIC. *See* National Immunization
    Committee
Nicotinamide adenine dinucleotide
    phosphate, 67–68
NIDs. *See* National immunization days
NIH. *See* National Institutes of Health
Niosomes, 100
Nipah virus, 240, 241
NLRs. *See* NOD-like receptors
NOD-like receptor proteins neuronal
    apoptosis inhibitory protein 5,
    105
NOD-like receptors, 149
    defined, 76
    innate immunity and, 76
Nonclinical research, defined, 206
Nonclinical safety and toxicology
    testing, 36
Nonclinical stage, vaccine
    development, 288
Nonclinical testing, 34, 37–38
Nonclinical vaccines, animal models
    immunogenicity and
    efficacy, 206–207
    safety and toxicity, 207

Printed and bound by CPI Group (UK) Ltd, Croydon, CR0 4YY

16/04/2025

14658511-0002